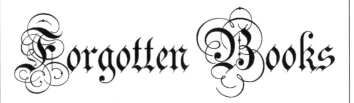

ISBN 978-1-5279-3899-1
PIBN 10931204

1 MONTH OF
FREE
READING

at

www.ForgottenBooks.com

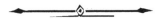

By purchasing this book you are eligible for one month membership to ForgottenBooks.com, giving you unlimited access to our entire collection of over 1,000,000 titles via our web site and mobile apps.

To claim your free month visit:
www.forgottenbooks.com/free931204

English
Français
Deutsche
Italiano
Español
Português

www.forgottenbooks.com

Mythology Photography **Fiction**
Fishing Christianity **Art** Cooking
Essays Buddhism Freemasonry
Medicine **Biology** Music **Ancient**
Egypt Evolution Carpentry Physics
Dance Geology **Mathematics** Fitness
Shakespeare **Folklore** Yoga Marketing
Confidence Immortality Biographies
Poetry **Psychology** Witchcraft
Electronics Chemistry History **Law**
Accounting **Philosophy** Anthropology
Alchemy Drama Quantum Mechanics
Atheism Sexual Health **Ancient History**
Entrepreneurship Languages Sport
Paleontology Needlework Islam
Metaphysics Investment Archaeology
Parenting Statistics Criminology
Motivational

Annals of
Otology, Rhinology and Laryngology

FOUNDED BY JAMES PLEASANT PARKER.

VOL. XVIII, 1909.

EDITORIAL STAFF.

PUBLISHED QUARTERLY,

By Jones H. Parker,
Mermod-Jaccard Building,
St. Louis, Mo.
1909.

37060
25.8.39

TABLE OF CONTENTS.

ANNALS

OF

OTOLOGY, RHINOLOGY

AND

LARYNGOLOGY.

| VOL. XVIII. | MARCH, 1909. | No. 1. |

I.

A FEW THOUGHTS CONCERNING THE PATHOLOGY OF ACUTE TONSILLITIS.

By Geo. B. Wood, M. D.,

PHILADELPHIA.

In this paper I shall deal only with acute tonsillitis, that condition which is characterized by swelling of the tonsils, soreness and congestion, and which is generally associated with the presence of purulent exudate issuing from the crypts of the tonsil. Investigations as to the bacteriology of this condition have shown that it is not a specific inflammation, in that it may be due to several varieties of pyogenic organisms. In the more severe forms the streptococcus pyogenes is generally found, while those accompanied with a large amount of exudate are generally due to the staphylococcus pyogenes aureus or albus. The pneumococcus is found in about five per cent of the cases and occasionally the bacillus coli communis. Mixed infections are more common than are infections with one variety of organism.

Goodale, of Boston, recognizes two forms of tonsillitis. The first is a diffuse inflammation of the parenchyma of the organ with increased proliferation of the lymphoid cells, and of the endothelial cells of the reticulum. This form of tonsillitis, he says, is due to the absorption of toxins formed in the crypts. The second is a suppurative process and results from the penetration of bacteria into the tonsillar parenchyma. The suppuration appears as circumscribed abscesses, starting in the follicles and eventually discharging in the direction of least resistance, namely, into the crypts. Outside of this work of Goodale's, I have not met with any scientific study of the histology of inflammatory changes peculiar to the tonsils.

My own observations have been on tonsils removed during life. In one case, I removed badly inflamed and suppurating tonsils from a boy in order to give him sufficient room to breathe, though the concomitant general edema of the pharynx necessitated a tracheotomy a few hours later. The tonsillar wound healed remarkably well, and the patient recovered very quickly after the operation, and there was not excessive hemorrhage.

To understand the pathology of acute tonsillitis, it is necessary to recall the histologic anatomy. The supporting framework of the tonsil consists of the fibrous capsule, connective tissue trabeculae and reticulum. The parenchyma of the tonsil is made up of the germinating follicles and the interfollicular tissue. The crypts of the tonsil are invaginations of the surface, lined with a specialized epithelium, the ramifications of which extend to all portions of the organ. There is very little or no subepithelial connective tissue as far as the crypts are concerned. The function of the germinating follicles is the production of lymphoid cells from what is probably the mother cell of the leukocytic group. The interfollicular tissue is the pathway through which the lymphoid cells gain access to the efferent lymphatics. The experiments of Goodale, Hendelsohn, Kayser, Pierera and Wright with dust particles, have shown that there is a definite current in the interfollicular tissue, tending toward the lymph vessels in the connective tissue trabeculae. The most peculiar feature of the tonsils is the cryptal epithelium. I myself believe that there is a direct change of the epithelial cells of the crypt into lymphoid cells.

Inflammation may be defined as the reaction of tissue to an

irritant. This irritant, in a large majority of cases, is the result of bacterial life. The first visible change in the tissue is probably the appearance of polymorphonuclear leukocytes migrating from the blood cells toward the source of irritation. In a large majority of clinically normal tonsils it is possible to find in some of the crypts numerous polymorphonuclear leukocytes associated with the desquamated epithelial cells, and these leukocytes can be seen migrating through the walls of the crypt. This must be looked upon as an early manifestation of an inflammatory reaction, and its cause is probably the numerous bacteria occupying the lumen of the crypts. This simple diapedesis of the leukocytes is frequently not accompanied by other inflammatory changes, and the condition may be simply a protective reaction, the bacteria in the crypts being destroyed by the migrated polymorphonuclear phagocytes before causing further injury.

If the toxin manufactured by the bacteria in the crypts is virulent, its first point of attack is necessarily the cryptal epithelium, and the reaction of the epithelium to this irritant is manifested by the proliferation of its cells. This is seen in the increased desquamation, the increased penetration of the cells into the tonsillar parenchyma and the presence of mitosis. It is an open question whether as long as the epithelial cells retain their vitality, bacteria which produce acute reaction can penetrate as living organisms into the tonsillar parenchyma. It seems probable that under certain circumstances they can, but in the large majority of cases they gain access to the tonsillar parenchyma only after their toxins have destroyed the epithelium. When the bacteria have gained access to the tonsillar tissue, they find permanent lodgment only in the germinating follicles. The current in the interfollicular tissue tends to carry the bacteria toward the efferent lymphatics. If they are not destroyed by the surrounding cells before they reach the efferent lymph vessels they pass on to the neighboring lymph glands and are there destroyed, producing the lymphadenitis which is associated with all severe cases of tonsillitis. The lodgment of bacteria in the germinating follicles causes the local reaction which may go on to abscess formation with rupture into the crypt.

In acute tonsillitis the cellular constituents of the tonsils change in number more than in variety. In the normal tonsil we find large numbers of lymphocytes occupying the interfollicular tissue. In the follicles there are large lymphoblasts which are dividing by mitosis and giving rise to the smaller lymphoid cells. In the epithelium we have all the stages of transitional forms from the epithelial cell to the lymphocyte. These constitute the normal essential cells, but in addition to these we find in tonsils, which are clinically normal, a few polymorphonuclear leukocytes chiefly in the neighborhood of the crypts, a few plasma cells and an occasional eosinophile. Also in the follicles one may sometimes find large cells which are probably derived from the endothelium of the connective tissue epithelium.

In an acutely inflamed tonsil we find proliferation of nearly all the cellular elements, and in addition various forms of leukocytes derived from the blood. The phagocytic cells found in acute tonsillitis are probably in greater part derived from the polymorphonuclear leukocytes. These cells are phagocytic both to cellular debris and bacteria, and are found in the tonsillar substance as well as in the crypts. In the substance of the tonsil and much more frequently in the interior of the follicles, large phagocytic cel's exist which, according to Goodale, are derived from the endothelium of the connective tissue reticulum. They are not, however, the counterpart of the endothelial phagocytes which one' sees in acute proliferative inflammation of the lymph nodes, nor are they nearly so numerous. The lymphoid cells may become enlarged developing into macrophages which are phagocytic to cellular debris, but probably not to bacteria. The eosinophiles are greatly increased in number in acute tonsillitis and are most numerous where the cryptal epithelium is being most rapidly destroyed.

SUMMARY.

From a pathologic standpoint we can recognize three types of acute tonsillitis: A proliferative form with increase in nearly all of the cellular elements of the tonsil; a lacunar form, in which the cryptal epithelium shows the most severe lesions; and a suppurative form in which abscesses develop within the germinating follicles. These different forms are generally associated together in a given case, but anyone of them may be the predominating lesion. Certainly in all cases we have a proliferation of the cellular elements, and very early in the process there is associated some diapedesis of multinuclear leucocytes through the cryptal epithelium and possibly some necrosis of the epithelial cells. If necrosis of the cells is great enough to cause a break in the epithelieum, the parenchyma of the organ is open to attack, and the bacteria gaining access to the tonsillar tissue probably find lodgment in the follicles and there cause intrafollicular abscesses.

In closing it may be well to say a word concerning the forms of tonsillitis as they can be recognized clinically. We certainly can differentiate between a simple proliferative tonsillitis in which the tonsils are swollen and reddened, and a suppurative form in which the swollen reddened tonsil shows the presence of exudate, either purulent or membranous, coming from the crypts. It is not possible clinically to differentiate between follicular abscesses discharging into the crypt and necrosis of the epithelium associated with diapedesis of large numbers of neutrophiles. It is better, therefore, to class these two types under the single heading of suppurative tonsillitis.

BIBLIOGRAPHY.

E. Bloch. Die Krankheiten der Gaumenmandeln, Handbuch der Laryngologie und Rhinologie, der Rachen II.

A. Sokolowski and R. Dmochowski. A Contribution to the Pathology of Inflammatory Processes of the Tonsils. Gaz. lek., No. 29, 30, 31, 32, 1891.

Lermoyez, Helme and Barbier. Case of Chronic Tonsillar Inflammation caused by Bacterium Coli Commune. Bul. Soc. Med. d. Hop. d. Paris, 22 and 28 June. 1894.

Mad. Sophie Weinberg. Die Pneumokokken-Angina. These de Paris, 1895.

Paul Maurel. The Infectious and Contagious Properties of Acute Tonsillar Inflammation. These d. Paris, 1895.

W. C. Pakes. The Bacillus of Friedländer in Pharyngitis and Tonsillitis. British Med. Journ., March 20, 1897.

Rosa Engleman. Membranous Tonsillitis and Pharyngitis of Influenza. Journ. Amer. Med. Ass'n, July 1, 1899.

J. L. Goodale. Acute Suppurative Processes in the Faucial Tonsils. New York Med. Journ., October 7. 1899.

J. L. Goodale. A Contribution to the Pathological Histology of Acute Tonsillitis. The Journ. of the Boston Society of Medical Sciences, January, 1899.

Wm. H. Park and A. W. Williams. A Study of Pneumococci; a comparison between the Pneumococci found in the throat secretions of healthy persons living in both city and country, and those obtained from Pneumonic Exudates and Diseased Mucous Membranes. Journ. Exper. Med., 1905, VII, 403.

Charles Norris and A. M. Pappenheimer. A Study of Pneumococci and Allied Organisms in Human Mouths and Lungs after death. Journ. of Expr. Med., 1905, VII, 450.

Jonathan Wright. The Equilibrium between Infection and Im-

munity as Illustrated in the Tonsillar Crypt.   The Med. News,
March 4, 1905.
   Suchannek.   Pathologie und Therapie der Acuten Entzündun-
gen des Rachenringes.   Bresgen's Samml. Zwanglos.   Abhandl.
VIII., 8, 1906.
   J. B. Rucker.   Study of the Nature of Microorganisms found
in Mouths and Throats of Healthy Persons.   U. of P. Med. Bull.,
Oct., 1906.
   Jonathan Wright.   The Difference in the Behavior of Dust
from that of Bacteria in the Tonsillar Crypts.   New York Med.
Journ., January 6th, 1906.
   Harry A. Barnes.   Some Points in the Applied Anatomy of the
Tonsil.   Boston Med. and Surgical Journ., Vol. clix, No. 13, pp.
402, 403, Sept. 24, 1908.
   J. L. Goodale.   The Local Treatment of Acute Inflammations
of the Throat from the Standpoint of Pathology.   Boston Med.
and Surgical Journ., Vol. clviii, No. 26, pp. 974, 977, June 25,
1908.
   H. P. Mosher.   A report of some Atypical cases of Tonsillar and
Peritonsillar Inflammations with one Unusual Complication.   Discussion.   Boston Med. and Surgical Journ., Vol. clviii, No. 23, pp.
872, 874, June 4, 1908.
   Konrad Helly.   Zur Morphologie der Exudatzellen und zur
Spezifität der Weisen Blutkörperchen.   Beitr. z. path. Anat. u.
allge. Path., XXXVII, 1904-5, p. 136-275.

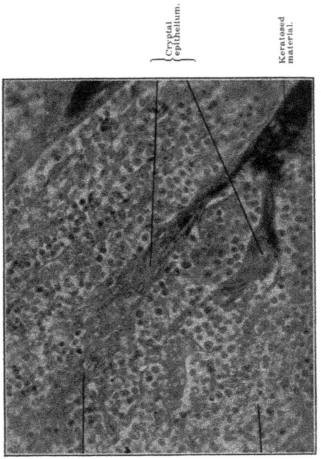

Cryptal epithelium.

Keratosed material.

Cryptal epithelium.

Interfol-licular lymphoid tissue.

Normal faucial tonsil, showing terminal portions of a crypt. Notice the keratosed material in crypt and the penetration of epithelial cells in the tonsil parenchyma.

Epithelial cells.

Crypt filled with debris, numerous polymorphonuclear leucocytes, fibrin, and broken-down epithelial cells.

Acute tonsillitis. Invasion of the cryptal epithelium.

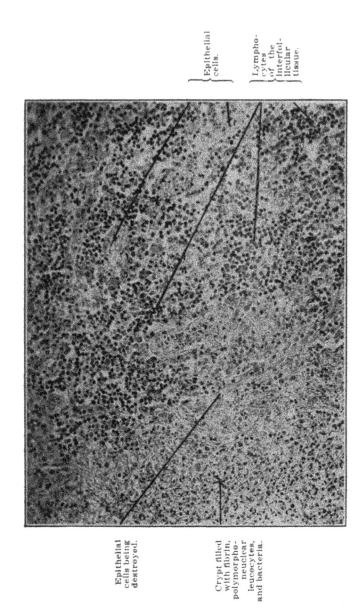

Epithelial
cells.

Lympho-
cytes
of the
interfol-
licular
tissue.

Epithelial
cells being
destroyed.

Crypt filled
with fibrin,
polymorpho-
neuclear
leucecytes,
and bacteria.

Acute tonsillitis. Extensive ramifications of the cryptal epithelium.

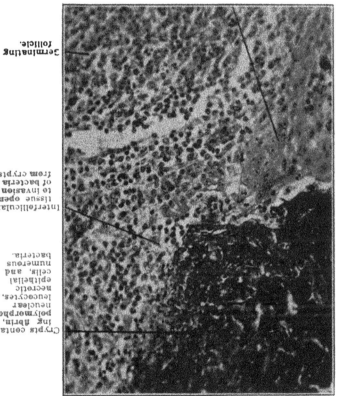

Normal healthy epithelium.

Germinating follicle.

Interfollicular tissue open to invasion of bacteria from crypts.

Crypts containing fibrin, polymorpho-neuclear leucocytes, necrotic epithelial cells, and numerous bacteria.

Acute tonsillitis. Destruction of cryptal epithelium.

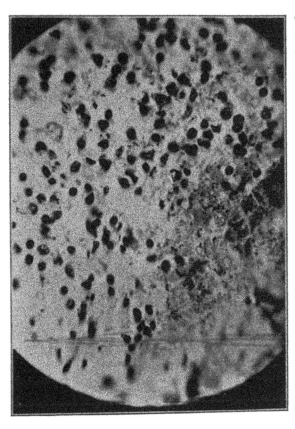

Acute tonsillitis. Numerous bacteria, mostly streptococci and staphylococci, occupying lumen of crypt.

Eosinophile cells.

Necrotic
epithelial
cells.

Living
epithelium.

Acute tonsillitis. Destruction of cryptal epithelium. Numerous
eosinophile cells.

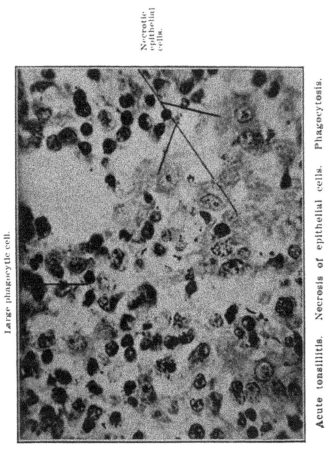

Necrotic
epithelial
cells.

Large phagocytic cell.

Acute tonsillitis.   Necrosis of epithelial cells.   Phagocytosis.

Beginning Intrafollicular abscess.

Living
epithelium.

Dehiscence
in
epithelium.

Crypt filled
with bacteria,
fibrin, polymor-
phoneuclear
and epithelial
debris.

Acute tonsillitis. Destruction of epithelium at one spot permitting
access of bacteria to tonsil parenchyma beginning
intrafollicular abscess.

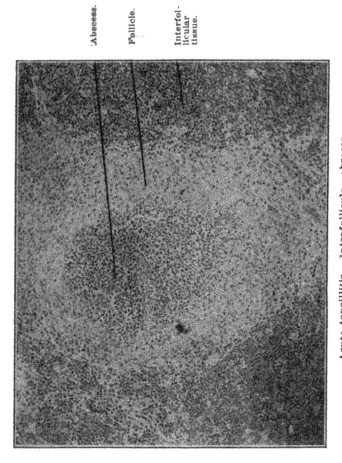

Abscess.

Follicle.

Interfollicular tissue.

Acute tonsillitis.   Intrafollicular abscess.

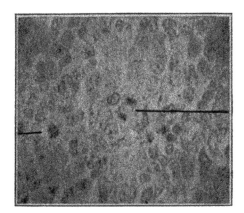

Mitosis in
wreath
stage.

Mitosis in
daughter
stage.

Cryptal epithelium, showing mitotic
division of its cells.

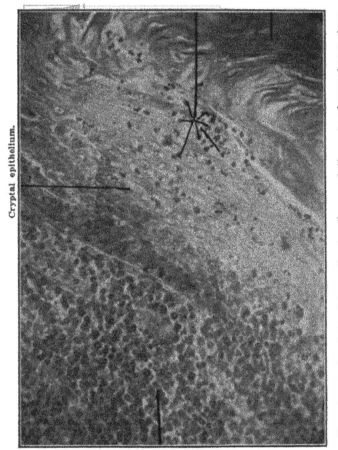

Polymor-
phoneu-
clear
leu-
cocytes.

Keratosed
mass in
lumen of
crypt.

Cryptal epithelium.

Interfol-
licular
tissue.

Hyperkeratosis of faucial tonsil, showing exudation of polymorphoneuclear
leucocytes through cryptal epithelium.

EXHIBITION OF CASES, ILLUSTRATING THE RESULTS OF THE SO-CALLED HEATH OPERATION.*

BY S. MacCuen Smith, M. D.,

Philadelphia.

The fact that the various professional periodicals, especially those devoted exclusively to diseases of the ear, nose and throat, contain so many papers repeatedly describing the various surgical procedures for the relief of aural disease, is proof positive that this branch of surgery is still an art, and has not yet assumed the dignity of a science; and yet it is only by repetition and investigation that we finally arrive at certain conclusions which embody the best that the present age has contributed. In other words, it is through the recording of our various mistakes and numerous failures that we are enabled to distinguish between the right and the wrong, and thereby to receive the stimulus of such recognition for better and more accurate work. This is true in point of diagnosis as well as in the improvement manifested in various surgical procedures for the relief of pathologic conditions involving the organ of hearing.

The evolution of operative otology from the time when the first imperfect simple mastoid operation was performed, consisting of little more than boring a hole through the cortex, up to the time when Schwartze, Stacke, and others devised the comparatively perfect radical operation, has shown great strides ·in a procedure calculated to save the lives of thousands, and in this respect is scarcely secondary to the great boon conferred upon suffering humanity when the operation for appendicitis was first devised.

In the very recent past we have heard much of what might

---

*Read before the Eastern Section of the American Laryngological, Rhinological and Otological Society, at Philadelphia, Pa.. January 9, 1909.

be expected of the so-called Heath operation, especially in its relation to the preservation of hearing. If this procedure, under whatever name it may appear, will succeed in relieving dangerous pathologic processes in the tympanic and accessory cavities, and at the same time insure not only the preservation but the actual improvement of the hearing power, the further evolution of aural surgery has certainly had a tremendous impetus.

On general principles it is difficult for one to accept as good surgical procedure that which advocates the non-disturbance of necrotic tissues, be it either diseased ossicles or carious bone that must necessarily remain in the narrow space connecting the tympanic cavity with the mastoid antrum, and yet this is precisely what is claimed for the Heath operation. In other words, we aim to perform a radical operation, which includes the complete exenteration of the cells comprising the temporal bone, with the exception of the tympanic ring and the fragment of ossicles and membrana tympani which are left undisturbed, as the extent of their necrotic involvement seems to make but little difference in the final result. In my limited experience, some of the more extensive necrotic cases have made the very best recoveries, both in the way of entire cessation of discharge and in more or less complete regeneration of the membrana tympani, while the ultimate restoration of hearing power has been carried to almost normal. On the other hand, I have to report that in some cases of shorter standing, where the necrosis seemed to be limited, I was unable to arrest the otorrhea, due, probably, to my faulty technic; nevertheless, the hearing distance was greatly increased.

In some patients, where to all appearances not even a fragment of drumhead and ossicles remained, the removal of the inflammatory debris within the mastoid antrum, tympanic cavity and aditus, preserving intact the annulus tympanicus, has certainly been the means of arresting a chronic discharge and greatly improving the hearing, without, however, causing· a regeneration of the membrana tympani. The principal contention of Heath, therefore, that the mastoid antrum is more frquently the site of a continued suppuration, rather than the cavity of the middle ear, would seem to be substantiated. Such being the case, we can readily realize how easily the narrow, unyielding aditus may become obstructed by pathologic debris, causing the antrum to fill with inflammatory products, this in turn producing a degree of pressure which may extend upward into the middle fossa, downward into the mastoid process, and backwards towards the lateral sinus.

In the past few years excision of the membrana tympani and ossicles, instead of the usual mastoid operation, has been revived and strongly urged, with a view of curing certain cases of chronic discharging ears. We have felt it our duty, in certain instances, to advise this operation, with a view of arresting the discharge. Obviously, all of us have frequently been disappointed in the results, no doubt owing to the aforementioned fact, that the principal site of the trouble, being located in the antrum, was not reached by an excision of the ossicles, and the operation did not even provide for drainage through an obstructed aditus, which omission in the end compelled us to resort to the usual radical procedure. My more recent experience, therefore, teaches me that the Heath operation, for the reasons above mentioned, will largely supplant that of the excision of the ossicles for the cure of an otorrhea.

I have performed the Heath operation in some cases of acute mastoiditis with extensive bone necrosis, where, owing to the great destruction, I should otherwise have felt obliged to perform the usual radical operation. This was especially true in cases where extensive erosion had destroyed the greater part of the bony external auditory canal, the discharge from the antrum and cells escaping through this opening.

In another class of cases I believe this operation to be of the greatest importance. We all see cases of chronic otorrhea in children involving both ears, where the hearing is practically normal. Some of these cases are persistently unyielding to any line of treatment other than operative. The simple mastoid operation does not relieve the discharge, and in performing the radical operation there is great danger of interfering with audition. If such a condition were present in only one ear in a young child, the gravity of one-sided deafness would not be so great, but suppose we should perform a radical operation on both ears of a child, for the relief of an otorrhea. There is almost a certainty that the hearing will be greatly interfered with, which condition is likely to grow worse. In this event the child, if young, will in all probability become dumb as well as deaf. Even though the aural disease may endanger the child's life, the responsibility of advising a double radical mastoid operation, in view of the possible danger to the hearing power and the consequent loss of speech that may follow, should not be lightly assumed by any surgeon. Another point in favor of this modified operation is that there is less liability of injuring the tympanic branch of the facial nerve, but the most important benefit to be derived from this surgical procedure is the eradication of the danger zone, which is located in the antrum, thus removing the source of a disease most prone to cause intracranial complications.

There are in attendance for your inspection about a dozen cases showing the results of the operation for the relief of the various forms of suppuration, and detailed histories of five of these cases follow:

CASE I. Dr. C. S. H., male, white, age 29 years. Presented himself for treatment on April 1, 1908.

History.—Eighteen years ago, he contracted a suppurative otitis media of the right ear, which has continued to date. Ten years ago, the membrana tympani and ossicles were excised with a view of relieving the otorrhea. This very materially lessened the quantity of the discharge, but it never entirely ceased. For the past year the patient has complained of increasing nausea and vertigo, both in frequency and severity, the continuation of which caused him to seek relief through operative interference.

Examination.—Right ear shows the absence of the membrana tympani and ossicles. The canal is well filled with a non-offensive, yellow, purulent discharge. The roof of the tympanic cavity has been absorbed through carious erosion, exposing the dura.

Operation.—The Heath operation was performed on April 6, 1908. The cortex looked entirely healthy, the entire process having undergone sclerotic changes, being, therefore, quite filled with new bone formation and exceedingly hard. No actual disease of the bone was noted until the antrum was reached, and at this point we found considerable granulation tissue and the exposed dura above mentioned.

The patient made an uninterrupted recovery, the discharge having ceased in six weeks from the date of operation, the membrana tympani regenerating in about the same time.

The hearing, although not in any sense acute, has improved considerably.

The chief point of interest here, however, as in some other cases, is from the fact that the discharge has entirely ceased and there is a regeneration of the membrana tympani. The patient's general health has improved considerably, he weighing more than at any time in his life.

CASE II.—H. O., male, white, age 16 years. Came to Jefferson Hospital Clinic for treatment on July 23, 1908.

History.—The patient gives a history of having suffered about nine years ago from a suppurative otitis media. It is uncertain, however, how long this continued. The present attack of otitis dates back about two weeks, the patient apparently suffering the usual amount of pain incident to such a condition.

Examination.—The canal of the left ear is filled with a yellowish discharge, offensive in character and streaked with blood. The membrana tympani is largely destroyed, very red and edematous, the inflammation involving the osseous external auditory canal, which bleeds freely on the slightest irritation from a cotton-covered probe. I have no note of the exact condition of the ossicles at this time. The boy hears the tuning fork at about three inches, aerial conduction. Ordinary conversation can be heard only in close proximity to the ear.

Treatment.—The patient was provided with an antiseptic solution for irrigation, returning to the hospital September 29, or about two months later. The examination at this time showed the discharge to be of the same character. There was not at any time during the course of his disease pain over or in the region of the mastoid process, not even on deep pressure.

A skiagraph of the mastoid was taken, and portrayed the process as well filled with pathologic debris.

Operation.—The Heath operation was advised and performed on October 16, or after three months of continuous discharge following the last attack. A separation of the soft parts showed the cortex to be rather hard, but bleeding at several points. The interior of the mastoid process was well filled with granulation tissue and extensively necrotic. There was not, however, very much free pus found. The operation consisted of the complete exenteration of the cells.

The patient states that about one month after the operation he began to notice some improvement of hearing. The membrana tympani has regenerated with the exception of a small pear-shaped opening in the posterior part. The hearing has materially improved. The boy now hears the tuning fork at about eight inches and ordinary conversation at from six to eight feet.

CASE III.—M. W., male, white, age 42 years. Patient first appeared before me on October 12, 1907.

History.—About four years ago, while swimming, he contracted an acute suppurative otitis media of the right ear. The discharge has continued to date. The patient claims that the attack occurred without pain, and that he was entirely free from suffering of any kind until about four weeks before seeking treatment, or about three years and ten or eleven months after the initial attack, at which time he began to have pain in the ear, especially over the mastoid process, which was aggravated by pressure or percussion. The patient also states that this pain was considerably increased by bending forward. The only treatment he has received up to the present time has consisted of syringing the ear with salt water.

Examination.—An examination shows the discharge to be copious, greenish-yellow in character, and very offensive. There is destruction of the lower two-thirds of the membrana tympani, Shrapnell's membrane being intact. The ossicles and landmarks are entirely obliterated on account of the swelling, and there is considerable granulation tissue in the tympanic cavity. No marked bulging of the superior and posterior wall of the external auditory canal is present. There is, however, rather marked tenderness on moderate pressure over the mastoid process, more especially pronounced at the tip.

The patient hears only when spoken to very distinctly and in a loud voice. Tuning fork is not heard by aerial conduction. Bone conduction, however, appears to be fairly good.

Operation.—The Heath operation was performed on October 25, 1907. The patient noticed a considerable improvement in hearing about two weeks after the operation. This improvement was progressive for about four months, he retaining this improvement in hearing power to the present time.

Examination.—January 2, 1908, the membrana tympani in this case has never regenerated. The discharge, however, has entirely ceased. The fragment of malleus and also that of Shrapnell's membrane remain about as they were before the operation. The hearing power, according to the patient's statement, assumes that of almost normal. Hears tuning fork at about four inches and a low voice at about five or six feet.

CASE IV.—E. S., female, white, age 11 years. Presented herself at the Jefferson Hospital Clinic for treatment on November 10, 1908 .

History.—Eight years ago, without known cause, she contracted an acute suppurative otitis media of the left ear, which has continued recurrently to date. The mother states that the discharge is usually less during the warm weather.

Examination.—Examination shows the canal well filled with thick, yellowish pus, without any particular odor. The membrana tympani is practically destroyed except Shrapnell's membrane. There is marked redness and some edema of the external auditory canal, especially the superior and posterior part adjacent to the tympanic ring. There is no pain over the mastoid, even on deep pressure. The child has great difficulty in hearing at school, it being necessary to place her near the teacher so she can properly receive instruction.

Operation.—The Heath operation was performed on November 17, 1908. The exposed cortex was found to be practically normal in appearance, but unusually hard and thick. The entire mastoid cells, however, were necrotic, which required their complete removal. The sinus was more superficial than normal and pushed far forward.

Six days after the operation the patient was discharged from the hospital and returned to the Out-Patient Department for the usual dressings.

The mother feels that the hearing has gradually improved somewhat, although she lacks the marked improvement that is shown by some of the other patients. The discharge, however, has entirely ceased and the membrana tympani has regenerated.

CASE V.—H. D., male, white, age 18 years. Came to Jefferson Hospital Clinic on October 11, 1907.

History.—Family history good. Only disease from which patient has suffered is whooping-cough, which is said not to have had any influence on the aural disease. Has suffered from a recurrent suppurative otitis media of the right ear from infancy, the trouble recurring at intervals ever since. Pain is worse during the period of cessation of discharge. The last exacerbation occurred about two years ago, causing severe suffering. The discharge continued uninterruptedly until patient came to the clinic. With each acute exacerbation the patient becomes quite ill, and before the appearance of the discharge suffers from high fever, nausea and vomiting, severe headache, and great prostration. The hearing power is very much impaired, the patient involuntarily turning the good ear toward the speaker, feeling that the right ear is more or less useless for ordinary conversation.

Examination.—Examination at this time revealed a discharge in the external auditory canal, the greater part of the membrana tympani being destroyed. The history of the case does not define the character of the secretion nor state definitely as to the presence of granulation tissue in the tympanic cavity. Deep pressure over the mastoid process elicited some tenderness.

Operation.—The Heath operation was performed on December 6, 1907. The mastoid process was found to be of the diploic variety, the accompanying osteomyelitis extending backward beyond the mastoid bone. The cells were extensively necrotic, the carious erosion exposing the sinus for almost its entire length.

The boy was entirely well about six weeks following the operation, that is, the discharge had ceased, there was a complete regeneration of the membrana tympani and the hearing power had improved almost to normal, the patient reporting that he was free from all discomfort.

Examination.—January 2, 1909. Improvement has continued uninterruptedly, and if anything there is still further betterment in hearing and the entire absence of any discharge. Hears ordinary conversation at from twelve to fifteen feet.

Notwithstanding the fact that the results seem to justify this surgical procedure in certain cases, yet it is most difficult to reconcile myself to the belief that it is sound operative technic to deliberately retain pathologic products, however minute, within the organ of hearing. However, as you will see from the cases present for your examination, the results generally are good and in some instances brilliant. Therefore, the manifest betterment of the aural condition of the patients compels us to give some recognition to this procedure, and at the same time serves to stimulate us to still further investigation.

Generally speaking, the operation should not be performed in the presence of suppurative or necrotic diseases of the labyrinth, where cholesteatomata are present within the cavities of the tympanum or antrum, or abscess formations involving the interior of the skull, especially if the infection gains entrance through the tegmen tympani.

On the other hand, we would feel inclined to advise the operation in appropriate cases, from the fact that it does not interfere with the membrana tympani and ossicles, thereby not jeopardizing the power of hearing. It would seem best, as a rule, for this reason, that the operation be performed early, before the disease has caused much destruction of the conducting apparatus. Some other points in its favor are that the danger of injury to the facial nerve is very much reduced; the shock from the surgical procedure is considerably lessened; and the recovery is notably quick, while at the same time it corrects the pathologic process within the danger zone, the antrum.

This procedure, furthermore, not only preserves the hearing present at the time of operation, but actually improves it to a noticeable degree, in the majority of cases. Then, again, it is suitable in both the acute and chronic variety of cases, and will probably supplant the operation known as ossiculectomy for the cure of an otorrhea.

III.

SOME POINTS IN ANATOMY, PATHOLOGY AND SURGICAL TREATMENT OF THE FAUCIAL TONSIL.*

By Joseph C. Beck, M. D.,

Chicago.

The purpose of this paper is to dwell on the anatomy, pathology and surgical treatment of the faucial tonsil only in so far as it is necessary in the operation of complete enucleation of this structure, based upon personal experience in a large number of cases during a period of four years. (Previons to this time I had never performed a complete enucleation.)

Almost any modern text-book on nose and throat diseases treats the subject of the tonsil in a satisfactory way, and from the point of view of a radical procedure in its removal the one of William L. Ballenger is to be highly recommended. In light of that fact it seems superfluous to add another paper on this subject, if nothing new can be presented. Beyond a slight modification in the technic of the operation, extensive macroscopic and microscopic study of tonsils removed from patients who had distinct tonsillar diseases, or diseases depending on tonsillar affections, I have nothing but corroborating statements to make. At the same time, I am sure that this subject needs to be brought before the medical profession constantly, especially the general practitioner, because too many diseased tonsils are allowed to remain in the throats of individuals, especially adults, causing not only local disturbances, but general toxemias and secondary infections. Again, when these diseased tonsils are recognized, they are often improperly managed by local applications or incomplete removal. The great but unwarranted fear of hemorrhage is what stands in the way, and yet, if the technic is understood, it is very, very rare; I have always been able to control it without difficulty.

*Read before the International Medical Congress at Mexico, January, 1909.

GROSS AND HISTOLOGIC ANATOMY.

Most of the text-books and articles written on this subject are based on the studies of tonsils removed from the cadaver or animals, and as far as the capsule is concerned, the literature is not very extensive. H. A. Barnes, of Boston,[1] has recently published an article on the study of the capsule of tonsils removed from patients suffering from tonsillar disease. Histologic sections were made and his findings are so much like mine that I will not repeat them here, but refer to my own sections. This is about the first article in the direction of the study of the capsule and of tonsils removed from patient, that has come to my notice. My own studies are based on about two hundred tonsils removed (for pathologic conditions) with capsule attached, and examined macroscopically and microscopically, in order to determine the structure of the capsule, muscle tissue, vascular distribution, partienlarly the location of entrance of the tonsillar artery, the lymphoid and connective tissue framework, also the pathologic conditions, which will be,described separately.

I have further studied the vascular supply of the tonsils by injecting the arteries on one side and the veins on the other in a very fresh cadaver by means of a lead solution. Removing both tonsils thus injected I took stereoscopic radiograms of them and demonstrated the rich supply of vessels.

Before describing the tonsils removed, I desire to call attention to some of the landmarks which are important in the operation.

The structures surrounding the tonsil and intimately connected with it are:

1. Margo supratonsillaris, which is a mucous membrane that can be made out very clearly at the uppermost portion, where the anterior and posterior pillars join one another when the tonsil is drawn from its bed towards the median line.

2. Plica tonsillaris or triangularis, which can be traced from about the lower half of the anterior pillar obliquely backwards and downwards, covering the lower one-third of the tonsil, and gradually lost in the posterior pillar, and the palatoglossal fold. This plica is not always present in this form and size. In some cases it is so markedly thickened and

---

[1]Boston Medical and Surgical Journal, September 24, 1908.

developed as to cover more than two-thirds of the tonsil, and again it may be so attenuated as to be practically wanting.

3. The anterior pillar.

4. The posterior pillar.

5. The retrotonsillar areolar tissue, fascia and muscles of the pharynx.

I consider primarily two divisions of the tonsil, namely, (a) the exposed part; (b) the hidden part. The hidden part is again subdivided into three, namely, (1) the vilar or head; (2) intrapillar or body, and (3) subplicar or tail.

These subdivisions are purely arbitrary and are used for description of the radical operation.

The exposed portion which is covered by mucous membrane is seen to be marked by small depressions, corresponding to the openings of the crypts. The number and size vary a great deal. The largest ones are found in the upper portion of the tonsil. At times they may be covered over by the margo supratonsillaris. I have seen a colored paste injected into one of these openings, escape through one or more of the other crypts, which would indicate that they communicate, a fact not very well known and not shown clearly on histologic examination.

Of the hidden part of the tonsil, the vilar or head appears to be the largest. It not infrequently happens that in a flat tonsil, after the margo supratonsillaris is incised, a large mass comes into view, if sufficient traction is made upon the tonsil. This portion is less firmly connected to the surrounding loose areolar tissue. The intrapillar or body portion of the tonsil is usually much smaller and more firmly adherent. It is within the lower half of this portion that the main artery enters the tonsil and bleeding is usually encountered at this point.

The subplicar or tail portion of the tonsil is the smallest, although I have seen it larger than either of the other parts of it, and reaching very low down below the level of the base of the tongue. This portion is very intimately connected with the surrounding structures and large veins, and some smaller arteries enter it from the anterior and posterior pillars, as well as from the palato-glossal fold. This portion has few crypts and most of them are covered by the plica. In methods other than the enucleation operation this portion of the tonsil most frequently remains in the pharynx.

The cavity created by the radical enucleation operation of the tonsil may be considered anatomically about as follows: The anterior and posterior pillars stand out very prominently, and appear thin. At the bottom of this cavity, which always looks larger than the structure removed, one can see the constrictor muscles of the pharynx and number of shreds of the severed loose areolar tissue, especially at the lower region, several points of oozing, denoting the severed blood vessels, and at times a spurter at the lower third of the cavity. I shall speak of this cavity again under post-operative treatment, and ultimate results of the operation.

MACROSCOPIC STUDY OF A RADICALLY ENUCLEATED TONSIL.

If the operation was performed *lege artis* successfully, then the entire gland is preserved and in good condition, that is, not torn to pieces by the volsellum forceps, or cut into by the knife. The hidden portion is completely enveloped by a firm fibrous capsule, which merges into the mucous membrane of the severed margo supratonsillaris, anterior and posterior pillars. and plica triangularis, which are taken along with the dissected tonsil. Attached to the outer surface of the capsule are found the severed shreds of areolar tissue and some muscle fibers. I have not been able to positively determine macroscopically the entrance of the main artery through the capsule, even by the aid of a strong magnifying lens. A blunt-pointed probe inserted into the crypts will find them in most instances right against the inner surface of the capsule. If this probe penetrates without resistance through the capsule, then one can assume that the operation was not radical; that at least part of the capsule and perhaps tonsillar tissue were left behind in the fossa.

MICROSCOPIC STUDY OF A RADICALLY ENUCLEATED TONSIL.

(Fig. 1. Natural color photographs can not be demonstrated under low power.)

Sections of many tonsils that were removed on account of tonsillar disease, most frequently of a chronic lacunar inflammation, were made both in the horizontal as well as perpendicular plane, and they show the following:

1. Mucous membrane margin of the margo supratonsillaris,

anterior and posterior pillars and plica triangularis. These are distinctly adherent.

2. Fibrous capsule of variable thickness.

3. Trabeculae of connective tissue (framework), starting at the inner surface of the capsule, and running towards the mucous membrane surface in an irregular manner.

4. Lymphoid tissue masses situated between the above-mentioned trabeculae, giving the appearance of a multilocular gland.

5. Epithelial surface with the mouths of the crypts also lined by epithelium of a stratified squamous type.

6. Crypts which appear in various forms, some single slits, some divided in two or three branches, some appearing dilated. Most of them run in an irregular course and reach near the capsule. They do not appear to communicate with one another. The epithelium lining these crypts varies considerably in thickness of its layers.

7. Arteries and veins of variable sizes are seen everywhere in the section, but particularly near the capsule they are most numerous and largest. In three tonsils serially sectioned I found the largest blood vessel (artery) at the junction of the upper two-thirds with the lower one-third of the tonsil and nearer its posterior extremity. In the majority of the tonsils sectioned I found small arterial twigs entering from the mucous membranes of the pillars and plicae, particularly at the lower portion. The largest veins are seen at the lower part of the tonsil.

8. The muscle fibers on the outside of the capsule are striped and are part of the constrictors of the pharynx. The amount of this tissue depends on how cleanly one is able to dissect the tonsil, or how firmly the attachment is to the surrounding muscles. Some muscle fibers are seen to run along in the trabeculae, but are not distinctly striated.

9. I have found in some cases lymphoid tissue outside of the capsule, not near the mucous membrane margin, and this is an interesting finding, for one could only determine how much more of this tissue remains in the fossa by deeper dissection or post-morterm. This lymphoid tissue may be compared to the parathyroid glands, and may take on the function and pathology of the tonsils after they have been removed.

The histologic pathology of these tonsils will be taken up later.

PATHOLOGY.

In this sketch I do not desire to speak very extensively of the general pathology of tonsils, except so far as I found the conditions in cases that came under my personal observation, and this not in great detail. One could easily write a very extensive treatise on the pathology of any one condition of the tonsil, which, of course, is not within the province of this paper.

TONSILS OF A CHRONIC LACUNAR INFLAMMATION.

Macroscopic Examination.—These vary a great deal in size; some are so small as to make it appear impossible that they could cause all the trouble ascribed to them. The exposed portion shows usually a number of dilated mouths of crypts, many times filled with yellowish-white, cheesy masses, the size of millet seeds. They have a very foul odor. The mouth of the crypts situated uppermost is the largest and is known sometimes as the sinus tonsillaris. It harbors the greatest quantity of this material, oftentimes hidden by the margo supratonsillaris. The anterior pillar and plica triangularis may also hide some of the openings of the crypts. These mucous membrane structures, as also the posterior pillar, are thickened in many instances, and irregularly attached to the tonsil. The capsule which has a certain degree of thickness in a majority of tonsils is more firm in cases that give a history of many attacks of acute exacerbations, peritonsillar abscesses, or where previous cauterization or tonsillotomy have been performed. In these cases there are more shreds of muscle and fibrous tissue attached to the capsule. Section through such tonsils reveals dilated crypts filled with cheesy masses, particularly in the upper portions.

Microscopic Examination.—This has already been described in the histologic examination of the tonsil. All I wish to add is that in the inflammatory tissues, round cell infiltration as well as older cells vary according to the period of the attack when the tonsil has been removed. Staining for microorganisms has proven of no value. We could very seldom find any. Examination of the cheesy masses shows a mass of dead epithelial cells, fat, mucus, leptothrix threads, and a number of cocci and bacilli (not tubercular).

Special attention paid to finding tubercular foci proved negative. In about half a dozen tonsils I found areas in which there were suspicious tubercles, but only one case showed typical giant cells.

HYPERPLASTIC TONSILS.

These occur most frequently in children, associated with adenoids and are usually large and round, with a smooth, mucous membrane surface. The mouths of the crypts are not very large. The surrounding mucous membranes of the pillars, etc., are not markedly adherent, and not much thickened. The capsule is much softer and the retrotonsillar adhesions to it are very few. Section through the tonsil shows the crypts very little dilated and the absence of the cheesy masses is conspicuous.

Microscopic Examination.—Marked increase in the lymphoid tissue, and very little organized inflammatory connective tissue, or round cell infiltration. The capsule appears thinner, as also the blood supply. Barely any muscle fibers attached to capsule, and no muscle tissue within the tonsil, as found in the adult lacunar inflamed tonsil.

HYPERKERATOSIS OF THE TONSIL.   (LEPTOTHRIX.)

This condition is usually associated with chronic hyperkeratosis of the Waldeyer's ring of lymphoid tissue, characterized by whitish masses firmly adherent to the mucous surfaces of the tonsil and within the crypts. Very little inflammation accompanies this pathologic change, nor are the tonsils much enlarged. The capsule is not thickened. Microscopic examination shows the keratitic changes of the epithelial and subepithelial structures which show the bushy appearance of the leptothrix buccalis within its meshes. In some areas the tonsil appears as in chronic lacunar tonsillitis.

TUBERCULOSIS.

This was a case of possible primary unilateral tubercular tonsil. It was twice the size of the opposite (large walnut). Firm adhesion of the surrounding mucous membrane. Otherwise had the appearance of the chronic lacunar inflamed tonsil. Macroscopically, the tubercular focus could not be distinguished.

Microscopic Examination.—Usual picture of a chronic

lacunar inflamed tonsil, but many areas of typical tubercular infection, as giant cells and epithelioid cells. Considerable round cell infiltration.

LUETIC TONSIL.

(Removed under a mistaken diagnosis.)

Both tonsils very large; otherwise appearing like chronic lacunar inflamed tonsils. Cross-section showed the abscence of dilated crypts, but a number of grayish-white areas.

Microscopical Examination.—Marked round cell infiltration, with caseous gummi in the center. The arteries appear thickened, but no distinctly obliterated vessels were found.

ACTINOMYCOSIS OF THE TONSIL.

In a case of actinomycosis of the middle ear, which I published in the ANNALS, one tonsil was enlarged, and on removal was found to be firmly adherent to the peritonsillar structures. A number of fistulous tracts could be traced towards the ostium tubae. Several greenish bodies (characteristic of this lesion) were expressed from the tonsil.

Microscopic Examination.—Acute and chronic inflammatory areas all through the tonsil. Mallory-Wright stains demonstrated the actinomyces in the tissues.

ADENOCARCINOMA.

Unilateral.—About three times as large as its opposite (two and one-quarter inches in its greatest diameter). Markedly thickened mucous membrane surrounding the tonsil and firmly adherent to it. No evidence of cheesy masses. The capsule is intimately connected with the retrotonsillar tissue, and cannot be made out as a separate structure.

Microscopic Examination. — Typical adenocarcinomatous structures; however, not penetrating beyond what I take to be the capsule, which is much thickened by the resected retrotonsillar tissue. Very large blood vessels, particularly veins, are present.

SARCOMA.

Unilateral.—About the size of a small apple; smooth, and not much evidence of inflammation. The mucous membrane is thin, stretched over the tumor. No evidence of any mouths of crypts. No evidence of a capsule. Soft friable tissue in its stead. Large vessels are seen cut across.

Microscopic Examination.—Round cell sarcoma; practically no evidence of true tonsillar structure. The mucous membrane covering the tumor not involved. Large vessels and some distinct endothelially-lined blood lakes. No evidence of a capsule.

ENDOTHELIOMA.

Unilateral.—About the size of a small apple; smooth surface. The crypts of the tonsil are distinct. Over the most prominent part of the tonsil is an area of ulceration. No evidence of a capsule, but in its stead a soft tissue mass is discernible. Large blood vessels are seen cut across in many places. Section through the tumor gives the appearance of a very fleshy mass, soft in character.

Microscopic Examination.—An endothelial growth, principally endovascular. Many blood vessels seem to be filled out with endothelial cells. Very little connective tissue or true tonsillar structures present, except the mucous membrane or exposed portions. No evidence of the capsule.

The history and final outcome of these rarer pathologic cases are of great interest, but not within the limits of this paper.

SURGICAL TREATMENT.

I consider three principal procedures in the management of the tonsils, namely, (1) tonsillotomy by guillotine; (2) partial tonsillectomy; (3) radical enucleation.

The distinct indication for the particular procedure is to be found in the history and pathologic condition present.

For the first procedure, namely, tonsillotomy by guillotine, I can see but one class of cases that should be thus operated upon, and those are the hyperplastic tonsils. Even many of those do some time or another return with trouble in the stump, perhaps several years later. I shall not spend any time on the technic, as it is too well-known to every general praetitioner. All I wish to say is that I perform it less and less all the time. A snare will do much more thorough work without any other additional operative interference.

Partial tonsillectomy, which has still its many followers,

is an operation that will be followed by excellent results and until about four years ago I performed this operation in the majority of my cases. In a goodly number of cases, particularly in children under general anesthesia, I still do this operation, providing there is not a special indication to be more radical, as, for instance, some general systemic infection or many attacks of tonsillitis. The technic in these cases is simply to separate either bluntly or sharply the adherent pillars and snare the tonsil off, or remove by scissors, punch forceps, or even tonsillotome. There is no distinct attempt made to remove the capsule; in fact, the attempt is made not to remove it, and as little of the surrounding mucous membrane of the tonsil as possible. The result from such a procedure is that there is less reaction and subsequent soreness, particularly in swallowing. There is also much less contraction secondary to the healing of the tonsillar wound There is much more bleeding in this procedure than in the radical operation.

One thing is a fact, we do not know positively that this operation will cure the patient as a radical operation will.

RADICAL ENUCLEATION OPERATION.

A confrére of mine, who is evidently not in favor of this procedure, once put the question to me like this: "Why do you wish to do such an operation? The tonsil is not a malignant growth." It is true that the majority of the diseased tonsils removed are only inflammatorily diseased; nevertheless, it is a structure which, when it is thus affected, will cause much trouble from chronic septic absorption, such as chronic endo- and myocarditis secondary to what are known as rheumatic affections; so I consider these tonsils malignant, in that sense of the word, and they should be removed radically, because when done otherwise the trouble is not cured. Who has not seen cases come back after a tonsil operation, with repeated attacks, simply because stumps were left in, when they should have been cured? I have yet to see one case where the tonsil was removed with capsule intact that returned with complaint of the original trouble.

Before describing the steps of the radical tonsil operation that I pursue, permit me to illustrate the simple necessary instruments.

In Children.—In the majority of cases I employ a general anesthetic—ether. In the past year I have used the nitrous oxid-oxygen continuous anesthetic, which works very satisfactorily. The position of the patient is in the recumbent one, and on the side, with the head close to the edge of the table.

Illumination by an electric head lamp.

Assistants: Well-trained, especially in the swabbing of blood and depressing the tongue.

In a small number of cases in very young children, from four to eight years of age, I have performed the radical tonsil operation under local anesthesia, as in adults, but on general principles I would not advise it.

STEPS OF THE OPERATION.

The steps of the operation are so similar to those employed under local infiltration anesthesia that I will just mention the exceptional points.

1. Injections of adrenalin solution 1/5000, about 20 minims each, into anterior and posterior pillars to control the bleeding during operation.

2. The use of the finger for blunt dissection, after the initial incisions are made, produces a rapid and thorough enucleation of the essential portions of the tonsil.

3. The completion of the operation in the removal of the lowest portion of the tonsil is performed with the aid of the snare.

4. Spurters are grasped with the angiotribe and free oozing is controlled by a firm sponge being pressed into the cavity and held by an artery forceps, which is used as sponge holders during the operation.

5. Prevent the child from falling asleep too soundly after operation in order to guard against its swallowing too much blood. Allow the closed mouth-gag to remain in the mouth for about half an hour, so that if there should be much bleeding one can easily reopen the mouth and stop it.

In Older Children and Adults.—The technic is as follows:

1. Seated in an upright position, with head supported by an assistant.

2. Swab the general pharyngeal surfaces with a 20 per cent cocain solution.

3. Inject by means of tonsil syringe (Fig. 1) a mixture of adrenalin, 1-1000, and cocain hydrochlorate, 2 per cent, equal parts, into the anterior and posterior pillar, supratonsillar and infratonsillar areas. These injections are made by piercing the mucous membrane with the needle, and raising a bleb, as by a Schleich injection. Each bleb holds about five minims. Four such blebs usually suffice to anesthetize the area completely. One side is injected at a time; that is, the opposite side is not injected until the first side is enucleated.

4. Depress the tongue and grasp with the volsellum forceps the upper and lower portions of the tonsil, taking a good firm bite, and locking the forceps. Remove the tongue depressor.

5. Draw the tonsil toward the uvula by means of the volsellum forceps, until it appears quite prominently behind the margo supratonsillaris and anterior pillar.

FIGURE 1.

FIGURE 2.

6. With the tonsil knife (very sharp, Fig. 2) make an inverted U-shaped incison through the mucous membrane of the margo supratonsillaris, anterior pillar and through the plica. This original incision must be performed with the greatest care not to penetrate the capsule. Carefully cut the adherent fibers close to the capsule, which appears whitish. Using the opposite end of the knife, I bluntly peel off some of the supratonsillar adhesions.

7. Release the volsellum forceps; give patient a little rest, and if there is some oozing, give patient a solution of peroxid of hydrogen to gargle.

8. Reapply the volsellum forceps, except this time the upper prong of the forceps grasps the already dissected head

of the tonsil. By drawing the tonsil now down and in, we observe some large fibers of retrotonsillar areolar tissue, and some muscle fibers. Before cutting these I apply the

9. Angiotribe (Fig. 3) to these fibers, crush them, take off the instrument, and cut the fibers close to the capsule. In this way one will observe very little bleeding.

10. The mucous membrane of the plica triangularis is now severed from the anterior pillar, and the tonsil further dissected.

11. Change hands (you should be ambidextrous). With volsellum the tonsil is now pushed back into its bed and the posterior pillar is severed from the tonsil. This procedure

FIGURE 3.

should be done with great care, because undue multilation of this structure will cause secondary contractures of a very disagreeable type.

12. The tonsil is now free on all its sides, except at the bottom, which is the most firmly adherent, and one that disturbs the patient the most when manipulating. It causes most of them to gag. The traction with the volsellum is now made upwards and inwards. Before each incision the angiotribe is put on to crush the vessels, and the direction of the knife is towards the base of the tongue, as though one were going to cut it, which, however, never occurs. Thus the operation is completed and the cavity appears as described under the head of anatomy in this paper. Should there be considerable ooz-

ing or even free bleeding, then take a sponge soaked in peroxid into angiotribe, and press into the cavity created by the dissection, and press it firmly against it. This will result in a great deal of foam, and the patient must be cautioned not to insp.re a quantity of this material, because it may cause some embarrassment in breathing. After a few moments the sponge is removed and the surface can be inspected for any distinct spurter. If such be present, then it can easily be grasped with the angiotribe and closed by crushing. No attention need be paid to the venous oozing; it always stops very soon after operation. The injection of the opposite tonsil is now performed, and the same steps are followed. The second tonsil is always more difficult to remove, because the patient is irritated by the oozing from the other tonsil cavity, and besides in many instances the patient feels the effect of the operation. Not that he suffered any particular pain, but a discomfort from the pulling by the volsellum forceps.

I usually begin with the patient's left tonsil, because it is easier of removal, gives one the practice, and the patient the confidence.

Not all cases go as smoothly as described, because several conditions may interfere. In the first place, a very irritable individual who cannot stand anything on the tongue or in the throat, as even the sensation of the cocain, will gag and sputter, making the operation very difficult. Some nervous individuals faint at almost any stage of the operative procedure from sheer fright or shock from pulling on the forceps, or other causes. It therefore becomes necessary to terminate the operation more rapidly. In such cases, usually, however, one can dissect the head of the tonsil. I make use of the snare and eventually go in after the stump subsequently, that is, a few moments later.

After-treatment.—The patient is placed on the cart and not allowed to walk; placed in bed, and not allowed to speak; to rasp the throat and spit out only when absolutely necessary, for the next half hour. A glass of peroxid of hydrogen is at hand, and he is told to use it if the throat bleeds, if patient has no special nurse. Since this is a hospital operation, the chances of hemorrhage with such a mode of treatment are very slight.

The next day or two the patient is kept on liquid diet; in fact, he does not desire to swallow very much.

Cleansing solutions of 1-1000 permanganate of potash are used, and local applications of tincture of iodin to the tonsil wound. This constitutes the after-treatment.

This large cavity created by the radical operation begins to fill in very rapidly, and on the third day it is practically filled with an organized blood clot and granulations. In about two weeks after operation one would scarcely believe that the entire tonsil had been removed, and many cases show a mass between the pillars having the appearance of a tonsil stump.

I have removed some of these tonsil stumps and found no lymphoid tissue microscopically; only inflammatory structure.

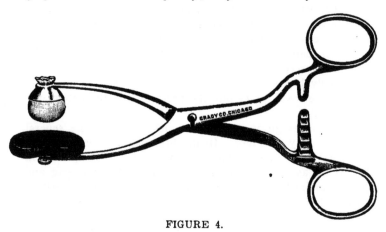

FIGURE 4.

In quite a few cases, especially where the surrounding tissues were mutilated, I have seen some had contractures and scars, although very little complaint was made of them by the patient. Such complaints as a burning sensation in the throat, easily tiring when speaking, some difficulty in swallowing, belong to the greatest minority.

Should one have such a disagreeable complication as primary or secondary hemorrhage that could not be stopped by grasping the spurter or by local applications of the various styptics and cauteries, I would recommend, instead of the use of the Mikulicz clamp, what has proven of service in a case of a colleague of mine, namely the author's tonsil hemostat, as

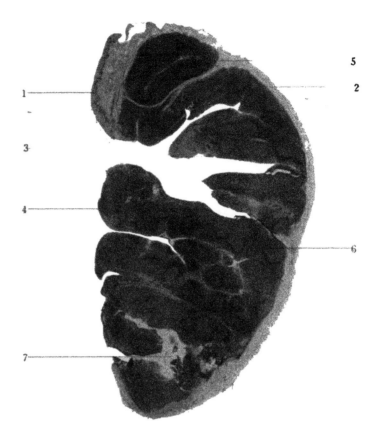

5

2

1

3

4

6

7

Colored Photograph—Lumiere's process—
of a Section of a Tonsil, radically removed
on account of Chronic Lacunar Disease

1 Margo supratonsillaris
2. Fibrous capsule of tonsil
3. Dilated tonsillar crypt
4. Epithelial surface

5. Trabeculae or septa
6. Lymphoid tissue
7. Degenerated and mechanically
lacerated crypt

shown in Fig. 4. Of course, whenever a spurter can be grasped. it had better be done, in preference to any other method.

In all my experience I have had but two severe tonsil hemorrhages after the removal of chronically inflamed tonsils, and both recovered. That does not mean that I have not had patients who bled quite a good deal.

IV

OUR EXPERIENCES WITH THE KILLIAN FRONTAL-SINUS OPERATION.*

By Dr. von Eicken,

Freiburg i. Breisgau.

Translated by Clarence Loeb, A. M., M. D.,

St. Louis.

Gentlemen: Since the Krauss-Killian paper on Killian's radical operation on the frontal sinus in 1903, an extensive literature has appeared dealing with this method. Killian himself, very thoroughly explained his method at Heidelberg in 1904, gave some modifications of the technic. and above all defined its indications. Since then, much has ben written pro and con, and this contest has not yet been settled. It is therefore in order to relate the results collected in our clinic during the last six years. The shortness of the time allowed to me forbids my going thoroughly into all the points coming into consideration, but these will be given in a larger article.

I am able to report 100 cases observed from 1902 to the end of 1907. Of these, 58 were men and 42 were women. Many of you will be astonished at this large number, but you will understand it when I analyze it a little more. Forty-two of these cases come from the private practice of my chief, and of these, only 16 are from Freiburg and its vicinity, while 27 were sent to him for operation from a considerable distance. In the cases belonging to the poorer classes—the patients of the third class—it should also be noted that 13 of them were sent to us.

A bilateral operation was necessary 20 times; of these, 7 were performed at the same time, and 13 were operated on the two sides at different times. By far the greater

---

*Read before the International Laryngo-Rhinological Congress at Vienna, 1908.

number of cases were operated by Killian himself, 23 by me, and 2 by the other assistants in the clinic.

In 20 cases, an operation had been performed by some one else, without curing the frontal sinus. Six of these had cicatricized wounds and 14 had fistulae. In these the radical operation seemed absolutely indicated. The diagnoses was based, in the other cases, on the endonasal findings and the results of lavage of the frontal sinus.

In 4 cases, the fear of intracranial complications was the indication for the operation. These were cases that had formerly suffered from accessory sinus affection and then had acute attacks with severe pain, while lavage of the frontal sinus gave foul-smelling pus. Only in one case, where there previously had been no frontal sinus involvement, where removal of the anterior end of the middle turbinate in no way influenced the terrible pain, and where even morphin gave scarcely any relief, were we compelled to make a radical operation 14 days after the beginning of the acute trouble. I would add that to-day, when we have in Bruening's headlight-bath a wonderful aid in combating pain in acute cases, even such a case could probably have been cured without operation. Where scarlet fever or trauma has caused the disease, we advise our patients against endonasal operations and at once perform the radical operation. The same is true in cases of extensive polypus formation complicated by asthma, where the endonasal treatment previously carried out by other physicians was followed always by only temporary amelioration. The urgent desire of the patient to be freed as soon as possible from the suffering he has undergone for years is a very good reason for the radical operation, if the results of radiography and transillumination make the possibility of endonasal cure of the affection very problematic. We advised the radical operation in a case where neurasthenia had followed numerous unsuccessful endonasal operations. In all other cases, more than 60, there was a chronic affection where the lack of success from endonasal operations was the reason for the radical. In a large number of these patients, numberless operations—without exaggeration—had been performed on the nose without obtaining the desired cure.

As to the technic of the operation, some improvements

have been made lately. In the first place we now make the incision through the soft part the same throughout its entire length, check the hemorrhage, and before opening frontal cavity, detach the periosteum from the lateral nasal wall and the orbit, tampon this with gauze, and only then proceed to open the sinus over the nasal portion of the supraorbital ridge, when we can count with certainty upon finding a cavity. If the relationships are not so distinct, we resect the processus frontalis of the upper maxilla, the upper portion of the lachrymal bone, a part of the lamina papyracea, the anterior ethmoidal cell, and the floor of the frontal sinus, and thus open the frontal sinus beneath the nasal portion of the supraorbital ridge, so that we eventually lay bare the mucosa which extends upward into the frontal bone, above the supraorbital ridge.

We cannot approve of the numerous, different propositions to partially or totally preserve the anterior frontal wall. The danger of overlooking a portion of the frontal sinus because of the smallness of the opening, and thus allowing diseased mucosa to remain, is much too great. This has been clearly proved by the numerous cases of fistulae coming to us from other places for treatment. If we are to attack the frontal sinus from without, the operation must be so performed that all recesses can be clearly seen. In two cases operated by me years ago, when we could not diagnosticate the extent of the sinus by means of the Roentgen picture, I saw that overlooking a recess and allowing the mucous membrane to remain, even in a circumscribed place, could cause a relapse, even after years of apparent cure. It is of great importance to thoroughly exenterate the orbital recesses, which are found so frequently, as well as the anterior ethmoid cell, which developes towards the root of the nose. When all the recesses and spaces in the frontal sinus have been sought out and their mucosa radically removed, there comes the second postulate, viz., that a broad exit from the operated cavity into the nose be made, which demands the resection of the processus frontalis maxillae superioris. The removal of this bone, which is often very thick, never causes such technical difficulties as to cause one to refrain therefrom. The hemorrhage from the nasal mucosa can always be controlled by tamponing the back of the nose from the interior of the nose. It is important in obtaining free outflow of the secretion that the nasal septum does not curve too much toward the operated side, otherwise there may be synechial formation and retarded cure. When it is possible, we should try to correct high degrees of septal deviation some time before the radical operation.

The retaining of an arch was only partially possible in several fistulae cases, on account of preceding operations, likewise in 3 cases of caries of the anterior wall and region of the ridge itself. In the great majority of cases, however, an arch could be formed, but I should state that in 3 cases with very thin bone, it collapsed either during the operation, or later on account of a trauma. We have entirely given up the formation of a mucous flap. The sizes of the sinuses were very different. Very large cavities were found 36 times, medium sized 42 times, small 28 times, and of the latter, 4 were so small that their contents could be removed without opening over the ridge. Twice, an actual frontal sinus was absent. Extensive subdivisions of the sinus were frequently found, and once the interesting observation was made that two completely separated cavities had been formed, the medial of which was diseased while the lateral was healthy. As to the contents of the cavities, a more or less swollen mucosa was found in most cases—7 times distinct polypi formation in the frontal sinus itself—furthermore, more or less secretion, sometimes mucous, sometimes muco-purulent, sometimes purely purulent, and not rarely the pus had a very foul odor. Acute inflammatory changes shown by strong hyperemia or greyish-green discoloration of the mucosa, were seen five times. In the cases with fistulae formation, we frequently saw distinct granulations in addition to the hypertropie mucosa. This was also found in 3 cases with caries, and in these cases both anterior and posterior walls were carious. The dura, covered with granulations, lay bare.

If we could not decide before the operation whether a severe disease of the ethmoid was complicated by frontal sinusitis, and consequently exploratively laid bare the latter's mucosa, we found six times no definite disease, and three times confined ourselves to making a large hole in the floor of the frontal sinus, after exenteration of the ethmoid. Yet we were forced to regret this procedure, as the frontal sinus invariably became secondarily involved, and later had to be radically operated. Apparently the removal of the floor of the frontal sinus injured the very important blood vessels, which are developed from those of the nasal mucosa, in such a way that a locus minoris resistentiae for a new infection was formed as a result of a deficient blood supply. In the other three cases, we decided to remove the normal mucosa at once, since these cavities were not very large. In the operations on one side, we sometimes accidentally perforated the septum interfrontale. If the mucosa appeared healthy, we refrained from operating on the other cavity. Twice, however, the typical operation was done on the other side also; once, because there was a foul discharge, and the other time because we wished to obtain a better drainage for a diseased sinus that extended far towards the healthy side. If the sinus opened through the septum was found diseased, we frequently removed only its anterior wall, without performing the radical operation on the other side. In these cases, we could not expect a cure, and were actually compelled later to perform the typical operation on the other side.

Unilateral, isolated frontal sinusitis was not once observed. The anterior ethmoid cells were always involved, and in the majority of cases the antrum also. Many patients came to us with tubes in their alveolae, through which for a long time they had been accustomd to wash out their antra. Several antra were bored into or radically operated by us before the frontal sinus operation, and for this we have been using for the last three years only local anesthesia.

Thirteen times, radical operation on the antra immediately preceded that on the frontal sinus. In twenty cases we were later forced to operate radically on the antrum after the frontal sinus had healed, and I would like to state here that whenever we found pus during the after-treatment of our cases, the antrum was almost invariably the source. Doubtless we have ascribed to the regular lavage of the antrum a greater curative power than it actually possesses, and it is my advice to operate on the diseased antrum either before or simultaneously with the frontal sinus, or at least to make a large opening into the lower nasal meatus.

With the above sentence we touch upon the chapter of after-treatment of operated frontal sinuses. Permit me to say something about the care of the wound itself. With the exception of 17 cases, we closed the wound primarily, yet not less than 19 cases showed greater or less disturbance in wound healing, which frequently appeared as stitch abscess, but sometimes as retention symptoms, and compelled us to reopen the wound to a greater or less extent. Three times there was an erysipelas of the wound. The secondary suturing, which usually took place two to five days after the operation, was sometimes followed by inflammatory symptoms, which caused us to reopen the wound and tampon. Upon reviewing the material, I come to the conclusion that we undoubtedly used the primary closure too frequently. This ought to be done only when drainage is very good, symptoms of acute inflammation of the mucosa are entirely wanting, and the pus has no foul odor. In all cases where we know from earlier operations that there was a tendency to disturbances in the course of the healing, it is much better to suture secondarily. Of the other, transitory inflammations which followed our operations, I would mention that angina follicularis frequently appeared; once there was a tonsillar abscess; twice, otitis media, which healed after paracentesis; once, a pneumonia of the right apex which resorbed completely.

It is very important to remove carefully and completely all strips of gauze, drains and tampons which have been introduced into the nose. If one is forgotten, the course of healing is disturbed, for which we were to blame three times. To avoid such an oversight as much as possible, we have for a long time used only one gauze drain, whose outer end was knotted. Only when this knot had been drawn out of the nose could we be sure that no gauze had become detached and left in the wound.

A hemorrhage into the orbital tissues happened to us once, but was resorbed without any bad symptoms. We had, also, two hemorrhages into frontal sinuses upon which we had operated. Both times, the clot was discharged in a short time through the nose, and the wound did not break open. A severe hemorrhage from the anterior ethmoidal vessels compelled us once to reopen the field of operation and ligate the vessels. · Rarely did diplopia follow the operation. It usually disappeared in a few days. It was complained of for longer than one month in only five cases, but it always sooner or later disappeared. One case, however, upon which I operated ten months ago, still suffers from double vision, which, however, does not disturb the patient very much. Whenever a diplopia lasts for some time, there is always a cavity whose extent upward was very slight, and which, therefore, extended so much deeper into the orbital roof and outward. The postulate, to remove all diseased mucosa, compelled us to detach the periosteum of the arcus supraorbitalis more externally than usually in order to obtain sufficient access to the lateral recesses. Wherever such a detachment can be avoided, one should not expose the patient to the danger of a long continued diplopia, even though the operation thereby becomes more difficult and tedious.

Of the other ocular disturbances, we once saw a very transitory paralysis of the levator palpebrae superioris, probably caused by pressure of the drain, and a stubborn entropium spasticum in a man who since childhood had been blind on the operated side from old iridocyclitis and amotio retinae. We were compelled in the latter cases to put a ligature through the lower lid, and thereby draw the lid downward for several days.

Anesthesias and paresthesias, caused by severing the nervus supraorbitalis, were frequently complained of by women, but these symptoms sooner or later disappeared. We were especially careful in these cases where the frontal sinus suppuration was apparently complicated before the operation by neuralgia of the supraorbital nerve. Ten times, during the radical operation, we removed the nervus supraorbitalis by slowly pulling it out. We have learned thereby to remove the whole nerve, which, as it leaves the foramen supraorbitale divides into two branches; one of these ascends perpendicularly, and the other runs outward parallel to the arcus supraorbitalis. This latter is very easily overlooked. Twice it had to be removed secondarily. The nervus supratrochlearis, a portion of the nervus frontalis, compelled us three times to make a secondary operation, on account of neuralgia.

The most frequent cause for secondary complaints was the antrum. As I have already stated, twenty times after the frontal operation, an extensive one—usually the Luc-Carlwell's—was required for the antrum. More rarely, it was necessary later to remove nasal polypi, usually in those cases where the ethmoid had been insufficiently exenterated. Only in two cases could we give no exact reason for the reappearance of polypi. In both cases, numerous operations had been made within the nose before the radical operation, resulting in atypical changes in the nasal mucosa such as synechiae and cysts. In some cases the sphenoid had to be opened secondarily.

If we would estimate the value of an operative procedure, we should know above all to what extent the life of the patient is threatened. Formerly, we did not think that Killian's frontal sinus operation, when the proper technic was observed, had any appreciable danger, and we were confirmed in this belief by a review of the 80 cases published by Krauss-Killian, which healed normally. Unfortunately, we have discovered that the otherwise beautiful method is not entirely without danger. We have seen two patients die, soon after the operation, from meningitis, and one, after suffering for a long time, with osteomyelitis of the cranial bone die of subsequent frontal and temporal lobe abscesses. It is a question whether we are to blame the operation for these three cases, and whether similar conditions can be prevented. There were no mistakes in the operative technic. Perhaps we were wrong to suture the wound primarily in the patient who later died of osteomyelitis. The inflammatory process in this case started from the lateral nasal wall and progressed in spite of repeated extensive operations. Both of the cases which died of meningitis possessed on the operated side suppurating antra, which in one case was easily accessible from the middle meatus, and in the other from the alveolar process. In the first case, the infection began at the margin of the remaining portion of the middle turbinate, apparently from the tampon impregnated with antral pus. It ascended through the lymph channels which surround the olfactory fibres, through the lamina cribosa to the bulbus olfactorius and the pia, and rapidly caused a meningitis. In the other cases the patient, in addition to the diseased antrum, had a sphenoid sinus filled with thick mucous exudate. This was not opened at the frontal sinus operation, since the posterior ethmoid cells were entirely normal. In the most posterior angle of the cavity, some drops of pus were found, and from here we could follow the path of the pus from the mucosa, along the hypophysis to the dura of the base of the brain through the intact sella turcica.

Since this last death, we have had 22 cases, which healed normally.

Ever since, we have made it a rule to operate on antral suppuration either before, or at the same time as the frontal operation. In every case, we try beforehand to diagnose the sphenoid disease, so that we will not neglect its opening and exenteration, even when the posterior ethmoid cells are healthy. Primary suturing is confined to chronic cases with mucous and mildly mucopurulent exudate, and in the other cases suture on the third or fourth day. By taking pains, this secondary suturing gives good results. Thus, we trust to have no other osteomyelitis case.

To test our results, we have made extensive re-examinations. We were able to examine 78 of our old patients, and from 14 we received complete written communications. One case, which will be well shortly, is still under treatment. We have lost track of four cases.

Before I communicate our results, I will explain what I mean when I call a patient cured. There must be no more pain, suppuration or polypi formation. Such an ideal result was obtained in 60 patients; among them are all cases with earlier fistula formation. From the written communications, we may conclude that 9 other patients were completely cured. A distinct improvement was obtained in 16 cases, and in these the frontal sinuses were likewise completely healed. There were, however, other sinuses with greater or less discharge. This came 6 times from nonoperated antrum, once from the antrum and sphenoid, once each from the ethmoid and sphenoid alone. In the other 7 cases, two required polypi removal; in one there remained a slight secretion with tendency towards formation of crusts. In two neurasthenic patients, painful sensations persisted, for which no cause could be found. One patient complained of severe pain when she had catarrh, and in the seventh case, without polypi or secretion from the nose, there reappeared asthmatic attacks, however much less severe and rarer than in the many years before the radical operation. That the patient was in general much better, is attested by the fact that she took on several pounds in weight. One case of ozena remained uncured, where by operating radically all the cavities on one side, we attempted to influence the disease. Repeated abscesses of the operated side was present once, but for this the diseased but not operated other side was responsible. When the patient came to us, she had had no new abscess for six months, consequently was not ready for another operation, which would have explained the abscess formation. Furthermore, 5 cases remained uncured, from whom we received written communications. In one man, there was malnutrition on account of repeated operations, also, perhaps, on account of treatment with Roentgen rays; he still had an open wound in the forehead. In two cases there was an ethmoid suppuration still present, and in the last there was neurasthenia and a chronic nephritis as the cause of the present trouble. There were, therefore, 3 fatal, 7 still uncured, 16 distinctly improved and 69 cured cases. I think that these are results such as no other method before Killian's has shown, especially when we remember that several very severe cases were among our material, which gave our method a very severe test.

The results obtained encourage us to continue in the way we have started. The few bad results which befell us cannot cause us to discard it. We have tried to learn from them and hope to be able to avoid them hereafter.

V.

EXPERIENCES IN THE ENDONASAL RADICAL OPERATION UPON THE SPHENOID CAVITY AND THE POSTERIOR ETHMOID LABYRINTH.

By M. Hajek, M. D.,

Vienna.

Translated By Julius Rotter, M. D.,

St. Louis.

I take advantage of the great opportunity offered by this celebrated congress, devoted to the progress of laryngology, to present the rhinologic theme in question in a few words, and to touch upon the amazing progress in the diagnosis and treatment of the diseases of the sphenoid cavity. The pessimistic aspect of earlier days and the words used to express the same, relative to the endonasal inaccessibility of the sphenoid cavity, are well known to all of us, namely, that this route would never open to satisfy our curiosity. That this is not true is evident; that furthermore the sphenoid cavity will in the course of time become most accessible to endonasal treatment is an ironically colored answer to the pessimistic prediction formerly expressed. In no other sinus is it possible by widening the endonasal opening to inspect all the walls of the cavity with detailed precision, as is the case with the sphenoid cavity. The sphenoid cavity lies in the sagittal direction and, therefore, directly in our view by rhinoscopic examination, while all the other accessory cavities depart more or less from the sagittal direction, on account of which the accurate inspection often occasions unsurmountable difficulties. In order to approach my particular theme more quickly, you will permit me to omit the individual steps in the evolution of the diagnosis of the affections of the sphenoid cavity. I may now (in this circle of professional men, thoroughly familiar with the literature) begin at once at the point, which is shown by my article published in the *Archiv. fuer Laryngologie*. I have in the above-mentioned publication called attention for the first time to the fact that the anterior wall of the sphenoid cavity is under ordinary circumstances too narrow to permit an opening large enough for good drainage. If, besides, we consider the well-known tendency of such openings towards stenosis, then it will be admitted that a sufficiently large and permanent opening can seldom be made by means of the endonasal method. On account of the anatomic relations which exist between the anterior wall of the sphenoid cavity and the posterior ethmoid labyrinth, I came to the conclusion that the anterior wall of the sphenoid cavity is accessible by the endonasal route only after the removal of the posterior ethmoid labyrinth to a large extent. Upon frontal section these relations become immediately clear. The anterior wall of the sphenoid cavity consists, as is known, of the inner narrow part, the pars nasalis, and of the outer wider part, the pars ethmoidalis. The pars nasalis is, as a rule, 2-3 mm. in diameter, so that an opening in this area can only amount to a few mm., and, therefore, is not at all sufficient for permanent drainage. If, on the other hand, the posterior ethmoid cell is removed, then the entire width of the anterior sphenoid cavity wall remains free for establishment of an artificial opening, which is not hard to do with the instruments which I have devised. Experience shows that while in the neighborhood of the pars nasalis the surrounding bony wall of the ostium sphenoidale offers very much resistance, the pars ethmoidalis of the anterior sphenoid cavity wall, as a rule, is very thin and therefore is easily removable. Only after removal of the largest part of the anterior wall of the sphenoid cavity is it possible to maintain permanently a large opening into the sphenoid cavity, and this only when the opening made can be controlled until complete cicatrization of the wound margins. It is remarkable, but as large experience shows, without a doubt, that, just after removal of the largest part of the anterior wall of the sphenoid cavity the resulting opening may in a few weeks entirely granulate over, if the edges are not thoroughly cicatrized by cauterization of the granulations. Abundant growth of granulations, resulting almost everywhere from injury of the bony wall, cause oozing of marrow from the spongy interspaces of the bone after inflammatory reaction. The cauterization of the granulating edges is done once a week, until complete cicatrization is accomplished; only then is it certain that the opening established will retain its original size. In this manner we also treat the affections of the sphenoid cavity, at the ambulatorium, where without further measures one may inspect the inner lining of

a large part of the sphenoid cavity through the large openings.
The above-mentioned cases have remained cured for years, and
only during an acute attack of catarrh is the inside of the sphenoid cavity as well as the remainder of the nasal mucous membrane affected. This secretion loosens up as the cold passes
away without any further assistance, this being proof that the
large drainage opening always guarantees the spontaneous
cure and prevents the permanency of the inflammation. I
have up to date over 18 cases of permanent cure, and with exception of two post-operative hemorrhages nothing ever happened to excite any apprehension. I have never considered the
question of removing the mucous membrane of the sphenoid
cavity, and have guarded against such action, because I am
of a different opinion in regard to that from many prominent
colleagues. I determined only in few cases to remove
the largest part of the inner lining of the sphenoid
cavity, because I have found that portions of the mucous membrane, which are greatly altered, retrograde spontaneously
after a wide opening of the sphenoid cavity. It is an undenied
fact, to which I called attention four years ago in the
publication of this radical operation in the *Archiv. fuer Laryngologie,* that a very much swollen and edematous mucous
membrane does not necessarily point to an irreparable disturbance of the same; much more this change not uncommonly
has the appearance of an acute and subacute inflammation,
which under favorable conditions returns to normal. I was
able to see very plainly, after broadening the opening of the
anterior wall of the sphenoid cavity, that such a swelling of
the mucous membrane may be of a transient nature. After
enlarging the opening of the sphenoid cavity and cleansing
the same we sometimes see circumscribed thickenings of the
mucous membrane. A few days later, however, the whole
mucous membrane of the sphenoid cavity may be changed into
a very thickened edematous cushion, which nearly fills the
entire cavity. This high grade, diffuse swelling of the inside
of the sphenoid cavity coming on in a few days is the result
of the acute, severe reaction of the cavity lining, together with
the progressing operative interference. This is proved by the
fact that in a few days the entire condition spontaneously re-
solves. We also notice after post-operative opening of the
sphenoid cavity, that a part of the altered mucous membrane
retrogrades after a few weeks, so that it is almost never neces-

sary to remove the entire inner lining of the sphenoid cavity, but it is sufficient to remove the circumscribed parts. Before curetting the inside of the sphenoid cavity we should, in view of the common occurrence of defective places in the outer upper wall of the sphenoid cavity, generally examine the same. The question now before us is to decide the indication for the external against the endonasal method of radical operation. According to my contention, the endonasal method is suitable in all cases. The only possible obstacle, a highly-situated deviation of the nasal septum, can be removed by subperichondrial resection. The external method, according to my view, is of use only in cases of combined empyema, in which some of the other diseased adjoining cavities necessitate a radical operation. In connection with such a radical operation, the operation upon the sphenoid cavity can also be done. It is possible, in connection with the Killian radical operation of the frontal sinuses, to evacuate the ethmoid and sphenoid cells, and in connection with the radical operation on the maxillary sinus the sphenoid cavity may be operated upon after the method of Jansen.

VI.

SOME INTERESTING MASTOID CASES WHICH HAVE COME UNDER MY OBSERVATION DURING THE PAST YEAR.

By Frank Allport, M. D.,

Chicago, Ill.

A recitation of cases is, of course, not always interesting to the reader, and yet I have had under my observation during the past year or so some cases that were of sufficient interest to me to make me feel that they might also be of interest to my colleagues. I have, therefore, in the following article endeavored to give the history of these cases in as brief a manner as possible, dwelling simply upon the salient and interesting features of each case.

Case i.—V. C., age 22 years, was seen July 31st, 1908. History: June 19, 1908, he was stabbed by a man with a red-hot iron. Iron pentrated head at apex of left mastoid, causing instant left-sided facial paralysis.

Remarks.—This case is merely mentioned on account of its rarity. I have never seen a similar case, nor have I read of one in aural literature. The iron, of course, injured the nerve shortly after its exit from the stylomastoid foramen. I have not seen the case since the first visit.

Case ii.—J. O., age 32 years. This man was operated by me in 1905 for an acute mastoid abscess and was dismissed in about one month. He returned in 1908 with a red swelling over the antrum, which was opened and pus evacuated. Granulations and necrosis were found in the antrum, which were scraped away as thoroughly as possible in the office, without the performance of a major operation. The cavity was cleansed and packed daily and aromatic sulphuric acid occasionally applied to the bone. The discharge was staphylococcic in character and an auto-vaccine was prepared and twice used. In about two weeks after using the vaccine he was apparently cured and sent home. I heard from him about six months later and he was well.

Remarks.—This case is reported because, I presume, in my original operation I was not as thorough as I should have been in cleansing the antrum, and because I wish to give all due credit to the auto-vaccine. It seems strange, however, that no antrum outbreak should have occurred for three years if the fault was mine in not sufficiently curetting the antrum in 1905. This brings up the possibility mentioned by some authors of the occurrence of post-operative necrosis. It seems strange also that the outbreak was confined to the antrum, to the entire exclusion of the tympanic cavity. Whether the vaccine had anything to do with the cure must, of course, be conjectured, as other treatment was used at the same time. Judging, however, from past experience and observations of other similar cases, I believe it had.

CASE III.—Miss A. I., age 35. I operated this woman in May, 1908, for an acute mastoid abscess. She left the hospital in about one month and became an office patient. The discharge from her ear ceased in a few days. The parts healed thoroughly, with the exception of a fistulous canal leading from the skin to the antrum. This canal refused to heal, indicating, I presume, as in case two, that I had not thoroughly removed all of the antrum necrosis at the operation. This fistula was treated for weeks and still stubbornly refused to heal. Finally, the drumhead broke down again and a profuse middle-ear discharge occurred. I had about made up my mind to reoperate this case and perform a radical mastoid operation, but concluded to first try auto-vaccination. The discharge proved to be staphylococcic in character and the auto-vaccine was prepared and used twice. Within three days the tympanic discharge ceased and in about two weeks the fistula entirely closed. Seven months have now elapsed since this occurred and the patient is still apparently perfectly well.

Remarks.—I mention this case because I wish to distinctly give credit to the auto-vaccine for having cured the case which had been previously treated in every possible manner without success. The cure occurred too suddenly to have been produced by anything but the vaccine.

CASE IV.—D. F., age 4. I operated this case for acute mastoid abscess in June, 1906, and the patient was discharged as cured in about six weeks. I saw him again in June, 1908, at which visit he had a red, fluctuating swelling over the antrum, which was opened and disclosed a fistulous canal leading into the antrum. Pus was evacuated, the canal and bone curetted of granulations and necrosis, as well as could be done at the office. This case was treated exactly like case two and case three, without result, for several weeks, at the end of which time a staphylococcic autovaccine was prepared and used twice with a resulting cure in about two weeks, which has continued up to the present time.

Remarks.—I have, I think, reason to believe that the vaccine cured this case. At all events, I had no success in treating it by other means. I hope these three cases will not give the reader the impression that such cases are frequent with me and that I do not thoroughly remove the necrosis from the antrum. I give them, however, just as they occurred, because it shows the possibility of such results, and also because I desire to give the autovaccine its just credit, whatever that may be.

CASE V.—Miss A. C., age 45, consulted me August 3rd, 1908. She is a neurotic. About two years ago she contracted an attack of influenza, followed by excessive pain in the right ear and mastoid. No aural discharge. Nose and accessory sinuses normal. Mastoid very painful to the touch. Her family physician, who is an exceptionally skillful practitioner, administered most if not all forms of treatment for neurasthenia, neuralgia, etc. The right drumhead was inflamed, but intact. The mastoid was exquisitely painful to the touch, and she was unable to secure any rest or quiet, except by the administration of powerful drugs. I felt that a mastoid operation was permissible, not only for the purpose of investigation, but also for the relief of pain. An ordinary mastoid operation was, therefore, performed August 4th, and she was discharged from the hospital August 31st, and allowed to go home with a healed mastoid the middle of September. No pathologic conditions were found inside of the mastoid bone, but she has never had a recurrence of pain since.

Remarks.—This case is reported on account of its peculiarity in many ways and as being one of the few cases where I considered that a mastoid operation was indicated for the relief of pain.

CASE VI.—P. M., age 6, first seen April 21st, 1908. Had very large tonsils and adenoid vegetations, which were re-

moved April 21st. This boy had been exposed to measles
before I saw him, a fact which I did not ascertain until April
23rd, when he had an afternoon temperature of 102° and
came down with an attack of measles. He was, of ·course,
isolated in the hospital. April 24th his highest temperature
was 104°. This was also his highest temperature on April
25th and 26th, which was accompanied by an almost continual
cough. April 29th he complained of pain in both ears, and
the next day both ears discharged profusely. His temperature
kept up to 104°, and May 4th his white blood count was 20,000
and his polymorphonuclear count was 83 per cent. Streptococci were found in the discharge from both ears. May 4th
his white count was 15,000 and polymorphonuclear 80 per cent.
May 6th his left ear was much better, but his right ear was
very painful. His temperature was 104°, white count 36,000,
and polymorphonuclear 91 per cent. May 7th, the right mastoid being very painful, I did an operation for acute mastoid
abscess on the right side and found considerable necrosis and
much pus. His highest temperature this day was 105°. May
8th his left mastoid process became red and painful to the
touch, and I made an acute mastoid operation on this side
with the same result as on the right. His temperature this
day was 104°. May 9th he complained of severe pain in the
front and back of his head. Highest temperature was 104°,
white count 11,500, polymorphonuclear 82 per cent. He became irrational during the night, and May. 10th showed a positive Kernig sign and negative Widal test, as the possibility of
a typhoid involvement had been brought into question by attending physicians. His highest temperature on this day was
103°. This night he was extremely restless and complained of
severe pain in the back of his head and neck, and was irrational
all night. The next day highest temperature was 104°, white
count 10,000, polymorphonuclear 84 per cent. He complained
of great tenderness along the course of the right jugular vein,
and the question of a sinus operation was seriously discussed,
but as he had already taken an anesthetic three times and was
very much exhausted, we concluded to wait for more positive
indications. A blood culture was taken and found to be negative. May 13th his condition was about the same as the previons day. May 14th, although he still complained of pain in
the head, his highest temperature was 101°, white count 9800,
and polymorphonuclear 65 per cent. His condition May 15th

remaining about the same, the idea of a sinus operation was abandoned. May 16th his highest temperature was 100°. He now began to improve steadily, and June 7th was discharged from the hospital and treated as an office patient. He went on to an uninterrupted recovery on both sides and retained perfect hearing.

Remarks.—This case teaches us several lessons, the first of which is before operating on enlarged tonsils, etc., we should endeavor to ascertain whether there is any reasonable danger of the possible occurrence of measles, scarlet fever, etc. This case also teaches the value of the blood count, especially of the polymorphonuclear percentage as an indication of the condition of the patient. I might add that this child came very near having a sinus operation performed, and while we should be on the alert to counsel such operations when necessary, I think the case teaches us that we ought not to be in too great haste in the performance of such a serious operative procedure.

CASE VII.—K. R., age 8. I made a radical mastoid operation on this case, which was followed by excessive granulations in the inner recesses of the bone. These were at various times curetted, etc., but they continued to form. I therefore applied chromic acid to the growths, which was followed the next day by a distinct facial paralysis, from which the patient fully recovered in about one month.

Remarks.—I mention this case because this accident never occurred to me before and, I am sure, never will again, and it shows how careful we ought to be in the application of strong caustics in the neighborhood of the facial nerve.

CASE VIII.—M. D., age 18. Patient, family and family physician, agree as to the non-existence of any previous ear disease in her life. May 12, 1908, she developed double tonsillitis with pain in left ear. No discharge, and drumhead congested, but otherwise normal.

May 20th meningitis developed with a chill, coma and a temperature of 106°. Slight discharge from left ear noticed for first time. I advised immediate operation, which was performed that evening at the hospital. A radical mastoid operation was made, and much pus and necrosis were found. The bony covering of the sinus was softened by necrosis and was extensively removed, and a perisinus abscess evacuated.

May 21st. The highest temperature was 105°. Patient

conscious at intervals. Normal salt solution administered by rectum. No ophthalmoscopic findings.

May 22nd. Temperature 105°. Much headache and restlessness and frequent mental aberration. Head shaved and Crede's ointment rubbed into scalp and retained by a head bandage. This was freshly applied for several days.

May 23rd and 24th. Condition about the same.

May 25th. She began to improve, made an interrupted recovery. Left the hospital June 16th, and was discharged as cured in September.

Remarks.—This case is reported as the patient was nearly dead when operated upon and because perisinus abscess was present. Besides this it raises the question of the possibility of Crede's ointment being of at least some benefit in cases of meningitis. Last, but not least, the blood count is shown and its value as a septic indicator emphasized.

Date.	Temperature.	Leucocytis.	Polymorphonuclear percentage.
May 20	105	29,500	93
21	103	25,600	90
22	104	24,600	89
24	103	16,000	90
25	102	14,000	85
26	101	11,350	81
27	99	10,350	80
28	99	10,300	79
29	98½	9,100	77
30	98½	9,100	75
31	98½	8,100	75
June 1	98½	8,100	73
3	98½	7,850	71
8	98½	7,000	69

CASE IX.—M. H., age 33, first seen February 27th, 1908. One week ago contracted influenza with tonsillitis on left side. She has had a chronic discharging ear for years, and had been treated by several competent men at various periods of her life without success. Shortly after the influenza developed she complained of intense pain in her left ear with extreme tenderness over the mastoid process. Pus was found in the left maxillary antrum, anterior ethmoidal cells and left frontal sinus. These were all opened intranasally, irrigated and drained. Her temperature was 100°. Her blood count showed white cells 20,000, polymorphonuclear 89 per cent. She was sent to the hospital and put to bed and her nasal accessory sinuses and ear irrigated and treated until March 1st when, as she showed no improvement, a radical mastoid operation was performed. The entire bone was extremely necrotic. A large area of the sigmoid sinus was uncovered and the softened bone of the tegmen antri was removed, exposing quite a large area of the dura of the middle lobe of the brain. The tympanum proper and attic were extremely necrotic. The bony covering of the facial nerve was almost completely destroyed and immediate facial paralysis followed this operation. March 2nd her temperature was 100°, white count 19,000, polymorphonuclear 98 per cent. Her condition gradually improved and by March 9th she had normal temperature and a good blood count, was able to sit up and felt quite well. Her improvement continued until March 16th, when she developed profuse vomiting, and her blood count was, white cells 9600, polymorphonuclear 70 per cent. Temperature was normal. March 21st she had a distinct chill with some vomiting and temperature of 102°. March 22nd about the same condition, with white count of 6700, polymorphonuclear 73 per cent. March 23rd she developed delirium and another chill. Temperature 103°. March 24th, temperature 101°, white count 5700, polymorphonuclear 72 per cent. March 25th, another chill with vomiting. Temperature reached 104°. A spinal puncture was made, but no pus or bacteria found. March 26th the mastoid wound was reopened and the sigmoid sinus freely opened and a large streptococcus thrombus removed, and the wound partially closed. From this time on she improved in every way. On May 2nd she was discharged from the hospital and became an office patient. In about three months the facial paralysis disappeared and her ear became entirely cured.

Remarks.—This case is reported because it was a very severe case and because it gives me an opportunity of reporting the operation upon the sinus, which was entirely successful. It is also interesting because she developed facial paralysis. which became entirely cured in the usual length of time, although it was a most complete and pronounced case. The blood count is also of interest.

CASE X.—C. E. S. (a physician), age 55, has had chronic purulent otorrhea on both sides for years. In 1898 left eye was hit and scratched by delirious patient, which accident was followed by extreme exophthalmus, this condition remaining until his death, although useful vision persisted. April 18th, 1908, he was seized with severe pain in the right ear, followed by nausea and dizziness. His temperature was 103°. April 19th he fell and became almost unconscious and powerless. April 20th the same trouble appeared in his left ear. He had frequent twitchings of the muscles of both legs and arms and his tongue was thick and heavy and he had great difficulty in articulation. Temperature continued high. April 25th he was brought to the hospital and I saw him for the first time. Both mastoids were very tender to pressure. Urinalysis at this time was negative. Blood culture was negative. The discharge from his ears showed a streptococcus infection. A spinal puncture was made, showing also streptococcus infection. Blood count showed 13,500 whites and 87 per cent polymorphonuclear. Temperature 103°. He was put to bed, kept quiet, bowels open, ears irrigated, etc. April 26th his highest temperature was 99°. An operation on the right mastoid bone was proposed and performed on the morning of April 27th. A radical operation was made and much necrosis and granulation tissue was found. The sinus and temporal lobe were freely exposed, but no abnormality perceived. April 27th highest temperature was 103°. He was very nervous, sometimes delirious, sweat profusely, had frequent twitchings of his extremities and complained of great pain in various portions of his head. April 29th highest temperature was 103°. He seemed more comfortable. His eyes were examined and no optic nerve disease was found. He was examined by Drs. Wood, Hardie and Church, and a diagnosis of meningitis was made and operation advised, which was performed next day, April 30th. An ordinary mastoid operation was made and all portions of the bone thoroughly explored. Much necrosis and granulations was found as upon the right side and the sinus and temporal lobe exposed, but no abnormality discovered. At this same operation the dressings were removed from the right side and the temporal lobe and cerebellum freely exposed and explored. One or two drops of pus exuded from beneath the covering of the cerebellum and a drainage tube was put in at this point. He sank into a comatose condition immediately after the operation and died May 1st at 2 o'clock in the morning.

The postmortem was performed May 1st by Dr. H. Gideon

Wells and the patient was found to have been suffering from acute, diffused, suppurating leptomeningitis. Some turbid fluid not distinctly purulent was found on the convex surface of the brain beneath the pia-arachnoid. The convolutions were sligthly flattened. There was no fluid in the subdural space. There were no changes in the meninges on the floor of the cerebrum. The fluid of the third ventricle was turbid. The meninges of the pons was reddened. The meninges in the region beneath the cerebellum and medulla showed a small amount of purulent material. This extended along the groove between the cerebellum and hemispheres. There was a slight purulent mass over the cerebellum. The arteries were unchanged at the base of the brain. In the right border of the cerebellum was a recent operative wound about 5 mm. deep, surrounded by hemorrhagic tissue. Purulent exudate was seen along the superior line of the cerebellum. More of it was found on the cruri cerebri. The cut surface of the cerebellum showed no abnormalities. The left chorioid plexus was reddened and slightly swollen. The vessels were slightly congested and the fluid slightly turbid. The dura over the middle cranial fossae was reddened. On the left side, the temporal bone in that region seemed to be wanting and the other bone in the vicinity was rather spongy. These changes were, of course, due to the mastoid operations. On the right side the condition was the same, with the addition of a pin-hole perforation at the roof of the operative incision, where the mastoid had been removed. An ante-mortem thrombus was seen at the right lateral and sigmoid sinuses. There was an operative defect in the temporal bone on the right side admitting the little finger. There was a corresponding hole in the dura and cerebellum. On removing the left orbital plate some tissue bulged up as if in tension. The ocular muscles seemed to be hypertrophied. After removing the muscles and fat tissue the left eyeball was found pushed forward by a dark reddish black mass apparently larger than the eyeball itself. This mass had a distinct capsule in which blood vessels could be seen. The optic nerve ran over the middle of this mass and was lifted up by it so that in crossing it from the optic foramen to the eyebulb it described approximately a third of a circle. The measurements in situ were as follows: Transverse diameter, 3 centimeters; antero-posterior diameter, 21 mm. The measurements after the mass was taken out were as follows: Transversely,

30 mm.; superior-inferior, 20 mm; antero-posterior, 25 mm. The mass was solid and had a consistency of about that of normal liver tissue. The tumor was not adherent to the surrounding tissues and was completely encapsulated throughout. Pictures of this interesting case are herewith submitted. The histologic examination of the tumor showed it to be a typical cavernous hemiangioma. The thrombus in the lateral sinus was probably of recent origin, as was shown by its structure, and was rich in leucocytes. Smears from the meninges and lateral ventricles showed streptococci in long and short chains and were very abundant.

Remarks.—I think no apology is necessary for reporting this interesting case. One interesting feature was the appearance of the man when first seen. With a double mastoiditis and an extremely bulging and protruding left eyeball, and with his symptoms, both subjective and objective, it would not have been difficult to have made a diagnosis of cavernous sinus thrombosis. This diagnosis, however, would have been quickly suspended, not only from a closer examination of the case, but from the fact that he had had this appearance for many years, beginning with the injury he received to his eye years ago, of which mention has already been made. In a case of this kind with no focal symptoms for a guide it was also hard to decide upon which ear to operate first. This decision was arrived at more through choice than judgment.

Something should perhaps be said with regard to the thrombus found in the right sinus. It is possible that this sinus should have been opened, but this matter was thoroughly discussed at the consultation and it was felt that his symptoms were meningitic rather than thrombotic in character. Besides this the histologic examination showed that the thrombus was of recent origin and it might have occurred only a few hours before death. In any event, it would not have altered the fatal issue of the case, as the postmortem examination showed diffused acute suppurative leptomeningitis. I do not believe that the infection reached the brain through the labyrinth, as a careful examination of the bone showed no pathologic avenue of approach. The orbital tumor, eyeball, etc., which were removed formed one of the most interesting pathologic orbital specimens I have ever seen, and for this reason alone the case is worthy of report.

CASE XI.—T. H., age 26. In February, 1908, I operated upon her for an acute mastoid abscess. In one month she was discharged, cured. In June, 1908, she returned with a red swelling over the antrum, which was opened, pus evacuated, granulations removed and the antrum curetted as well as could be done in the office. The canal was treated, packed, etc., and an auto-vaccine (staphylococcus) used. In about two weeks she was again dismissed as cured and has not been heard from since.

Remarks.—This is another case of apparently insufficiently operated antrum. The effect of the vaccine is conjectural, but I do not believe that such a quick healing would have occurred without it. I seem to have had a flood of such cases during the year 1908, more, I think, than in all my life before. Nevertheless, I give them as they came, because I believe that they are instructive and that we often learn more from failure than success. I think I am as thorough as most operators and yet these cases have taught me to be most careful in my treatment of the antrum, both in ebonic and acute cases. I also report these cases because they certainly have a bearing on the principle enunciated by Ballance, that in any case where a mastoid operation is determined upon, where the aural discharge has lasted for six weeks, the radical operation should be performed. I cannot say that I am prepared to accept this conclusion, and yet such results as are enumerated in cases two, three, four and eleven of this article certainly must make one think.

CASE XII.—Mrs. K. C., age 29. In January, 1907, she had a Heath operation performed upon her left ear. The result was entirely unsatisfactory. In September, 1908, she consulted me. There was redness, soreness, swelling and pain over the mastoid and the meatus was almost completely closed by an extensive stricture, through which it was almost impossible to pass even the smallest probe. I performed a radical mastoid operation and found the tympanic cavity, antrum, etc., back of the stricture extensively necrotic. This lady was dismissed as cured in January, 1909, at which time her hearing by the watch was three inches and for whispers 20 feet.

Remarks.—This case is reported on account of the performance of the Heath operation by a good operator, which proved to be entirely unsatisfactory in its result and which was afterwards cured with preservation of hearing by the orthodox radical mastoid operation.

CASE XIII.—A. B., age 12, a thoroughly healthy boy, was

taken ill with apparently a light attack of influenza February
21st, 1908. In a few days he had apparently recovered. March
10th he suffered severe pain in his head, accompanied with earache on the right side. A few days later he also had earache
on the left side. March 16th a small amount of discharge appeared in both ears. He developed some temperature each
day and about the 22nd of March began to have chills each
day. The discharge from his ears ceased, the drum membrane
healed, but he still complained of some pain in each ear, particularly the right. About March 20th he developed edema
from both frontal sinuses until about the 24th of March, when
his eyelids were completely closed. He complained of great
pain in the back of his head and through the forehead. From
the beginning of his trouble he complained that it hurt him to
open his jaws and masticate food. He was taken to the hospital March 25th, with temperature of 103°, white count
20,000, polymorphonuclear 80 per cent. His right drum membrane was incised, but no pus escaped.

I saw him first on March 27th, 1908. (He lived in another
State.) He had hardly any mastoid symptoms, no pain, tenderness or swelling of the posterior-superior wall of the meatus, no ear discharge, no redness of the drum membrane. The
redness and swelling over the frontal sinus would have led one
to suppose that if any operation was to be done it should be
made there. Consequently, an exploratory opening was made
into the right frontal sinus, but nothing found. I then opened
the right mastoid process and found some necrosis and very
little pus. This day his highest temperature was 103°. March
28th his condition was no better. Highest temperature 103°,
lowest 102°, white count 16,000, polymorphonuclear 87 per
cent. He had severe chills on this day. March 29th his
highest temperature was 102½°. lowest 99½°, white count
18,000, polymorphonuclear 84 per cent. I was requested to
see him that night, but was unable to do so and sent my part-
ner, Dr. Frank Brawley, who thoroughly examined the accessory sinuses and found nothing abnormal. He therefore
opened the left mastoid process and found considerable necrosis, pus and granulation tissue. March 31st his highest
temperature was 100°, lowest 98½°. He had several chills
and complained of great soreness near the right breast. April
1st his highest temperature was 100½°. lowest 98½°, white
count 18,000, polymorphonuclear 80 per cent. April 2nd temperature about the same, with chills. The family surgeon

opened a swelling near the right breast, but found no pus. I saw him again April 3rd, at which time he complained of severe (right) earache. On this day his highest temperature was 102°, lowest 98½°. He was having chills. At the site of the right mastoid operation I opened the right sigmoid sinus, from which blood instantly escaped and forced out a small streptococcus thrombus. April 4th his highest temperature was 98½°, lowest 97½°, pulse as low as 58, white count 8700, polymorphonuclear 81 per cent. April 5th highest temperature 98½°, lowest 97½°, pulse 60, white count 7000, polymorphonuclear 83 per cent. April 7th highest temperature 98½°, lowest 97½°, pulse as low as 60, white count 6000, polymorphonuclear 77 per cent. His urine now showed blood, albumin and casts. April 9th his white count was 8000, polymorphonuclear 75 per cent. April 14th white count 6000, polymorphonuclear 71 per cent. April 22nd white count 10,000, polymorphonuclear 66 per cent. His urine cleared up gradually. April 25th he left the hospital and in a few weeks entirely recovered.

His blood was examined at various times during his illness, from which, together with the examination of the thrombus, the infection was shown to be streptococcus in character. The swelling over the frontal sinus gradually disappeared. He had at various times throughout his illness very slight mental aberrations.

Remarks.—This case is worthy of record, because it shows what serious pathologic conditions can occur without adequate objective symptoms. The diagnosis in this case was exceedingly blind. There were practically no symptoms to cause one to suspect a mastoid or sinus involvement and yet reasoning by exclusion there seemed to be no other cause for his profound infection. Each operation was made with the feeling that very likely it was an unnecessary procedure, but with the exception of the exploratory incision into the right frontal sinus, none of the three major operations were unnecessary, as pus was found in both mastoid cells and a streptococcus thrombus in the right sigmoid sinus. Cases like this should show us that even though there is no redness, swelling or pain over the mastoid process, and while the drum membrane may look healthy, there may still be a serious infection going on inside of the bone demanding operative interference. The consistency existing between his blood count, his infection and his general condition are also worthy of record.

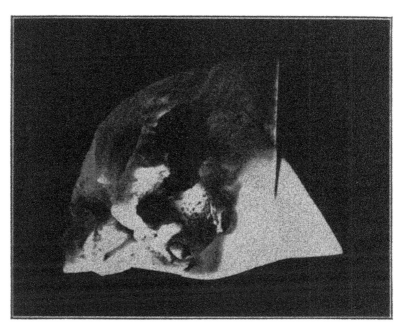

FIGURE 1.

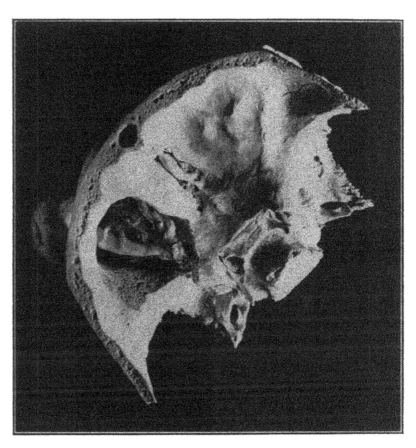

FIGURE 2.

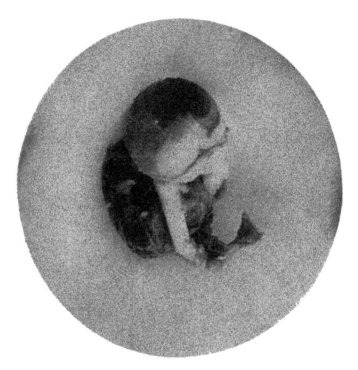

FIGURE 3.

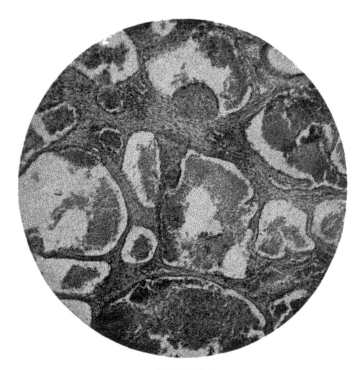

FIGURE 4.

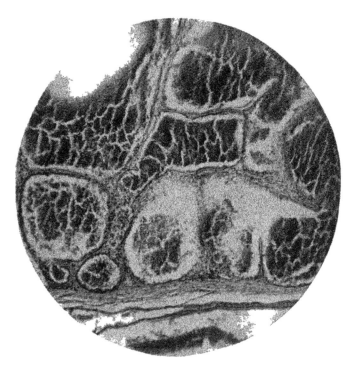

FIGURE 5.

VII

VINCENT'S ANGINA.

By Charles W. Richardson,

Washington.

I would describe Vincent's angina as a peculiar type of ulcero-membranous lesion affecting the mucous membrane of the fauces and occasionally the buccal and pharyngeal mucosa, in all probability due to the activity of a dual organism. This type of angina affects most frequently the tonsils, palatine folds and uvula. It also occurs in and about the gums, tongue and pharynx. Without going extensively into the history of this affection, it will be sufficient to state that Vincent, in 1896, gave apparently the first definition of the disease, describing the microorganism present, with histories of cases. The disease since then has been known as Vincent's angina. Vincent's right to the priority of description is questioned through a study of similar conditions by H. C. Plaut and reported by him under the title, "Studies Regarding the Bacteriological Diagnosis of Diphtheria and the Anginas." Plaut gives credit to Miller for the discovery of the microorganism made in 1883. Bernheim in 1898 published a paper evidently upon independent research in which he described thirty cases, in all of which the characteristic microorganisms were found. A number of interesting papers have oppeared in the French and German journals, describing this lesion and citing cases during the past two years. In America several excellent papers have appeared describing this interesting condition. It is my belief that the angina is not as generally known and recognized as it should be. I feel also quite firmly convinced that its occurrence is not quite so rare as many observers seem inclined to believe. The importance of disseminating knowledge with regard to the occurrence of this affection, its characteristic lesion, its diagnosis and differentiation become manifest when we recognize how readily it can be mistaken for syphilis or diphtheria. It is also interesting to note the almost universal absence of the consideration of this type of angina in all the recent text books on disease of the nose and throat.

This type of angina is apparently due to the presence of the Vincent's bacillus, a fusiform bacillus, and a spirillum. The fusiform bacillus designated by Vincent as the bacillus fusiformis is from 7 to 14 mikra in length and 1 to 2 in greatest thickness. This microorganism is readily recognized, as there is no other germ occurring in the mouth that is quite like it. It is described by some as motile, by others as non-motile.

The spirillum is a true spirochaete. This organism is stated to be motile. All culture experiments so far have been attended with uniform failures. The most striking feature of this disease is the dual association of two such dissimilar microorganisms.

Most of the authorities which I have consulted show a large preponderance in reported cases as having occurred in children. This may due to the fact that many of those who have made reports of cases are pediatricians. In my experience the disease has been entirely manifested in young adults, and almost exclusively limited to the male sex.

The angina is usually ushered in by slight general disturbance. The fever is rarely high and only endures for two or three days. There are thirst, impairment of appetite and slight headache. Locally the most annoying symptom is pain, which is very intense, and most of my patients have sought relief on account of this pain. Dysphagia is also quite pronounced. The breath is usually foul. The local appearances are quite characteristic. It is described as occurring in a diphtheroid form, which rarely extends beyond the mucosa and in an ulceromembranous form which is quite extensive in its destructive influence. The local evidence in the fauces is generally manifested in the upper angle of the tonsils and the neighboring portion of the arch and uvula. I have never seen the diphtheroid variety, all of my cases having been of the phagydenic form. It is described as being limited to one tonsil, and such has been the rule observed in my cases, except in one individual in whom both tonsils were affected, and who also had a recurrence in both tonsils a couple of months after recovering from the primary attack. The appearance of the affected area of the tonsils is more that of a sloughing ulcer than of a membranous deposit. The mucous area contiguous to the ulcer is only slightly congested and there is no infiltration of the tissue. The surface of the ulcer is slightly depressed and of a faint cream color, the edges are quite irregular and inflamed. The use of a curette will demonstrate how deep the slough has extended. L'uder the use of the curette the slough comes readily away, leaving an irregular granulating cavity, often extending to the capsule in depth and frequently involving half or more of the tonsil in extent. The slough has more the appearance, to me, of very finely broken-up bread crumbs which have been moistened. The pillars of the fauces and the uvula are occasionally involved in the destructive ulceration. The lymphatic glands in the neck and submaxillary region on the side affected are frequently enlarged and painful. The local symptoms usually persist for a period of one to two weeks. The exudate in its reaction to litmus is slightly acid.

Complications.—There is no doubt that Vincent's angina may be complicated with or complicate other conditions of a zymotic type in the mouth and fauces, such as diphtheria, scurvy, scarlatina and syphilis.

The prognosis is usually favorable as to life. There may be more or less destruction of the tonsils and adjacent tissue. In one of my cases the tonsil was completely destroyed. H. W. Bruce, of London, narrates a case terminating with death. Relapses occur and one attack does not confer immunity.

It is interesting to note that Vincent states that, in some cases of hospital gangrene and ulcerative stomatitis observed by him in Algiers, he found in great numbers a bacillus and spirillum, which, in their form, their straining reaction and in their resistance to all efforts to cultivate them, were identical with the microorganisms found in the condition which we are describing.

The Diagnosis.—The clinical evidences are so characteristic in many of the cases coming under observation that there should be no difficulty in recognizing this form of angina. Examination of smears will enable one to come to a positive diagnosis. If a properly prepared smear shows no Vincent's bacteria there can be no Vincent's angina, for the germs of this disease are present from the initial lesion and persist over the surface, indeed until after the ulcer is healed.

The treatment which I have found most efficacious is the curetting out of the slough, the use of cleansing antiseptic solutions and the daily application of a five per cent solution of nitrate of silver.

These observations are made from the study of fifteen cases which have come under my notice.

VIII.

BRONCHOSCOPY AND ESOPHAGOSCOPY — THE TECHNIC, UTILITY, AND DANGERS.*

By E. Fletcher Ingals, M. D.,

Chicago.

The history, anatomic conditions, instruments and technic
of this procedure have been so admirably presented and in such
detail by Chevalier Jackson in his excellent monograph on the
subject that I need not take your time with a exhaustive paper.

I shall therefore present only those features that appear to
me of special importance to the operator, but in doing this I
shall necessarily repeat some things that I have said before and
also some that are dwelt upon by Jackson and other authors.
I feel that much has yet to be done in the development of this
most valuable operation, especially in learning to avoid its dangers.

Before attempting bronchoscopy on the living patient, one
should make every possible effort to acquire dexterity by practice with the tubes, lights and forceps. For a beginning one
may practice with a tube, the distal end of which is held in
the closed hand. In this way he may learn something of the
difficulties and the means of overcoming them; but the view
thus abtained is much more distinct than in a congested and
swollen bronchial tube, more or less filled with secretions and
blood. The same statement applies to rubber manikins designed to represent the trachea, bronchi and esophagus, and it
appears to me that they are little if any better than the closed
hand. Practice on the cadaver is only a little more valuable
than the methods just spoken of, because the pale dry, motionless air tubes are so very different from the conditions found

*Abstract of paper read at the Southern Section of the Ameri-
can Laryngological, Rhinological and Otological Society, Richmond, Va., February, 1909.

in the living patient. A medium sized dog furnishes the best subject for practice.

Diagnosis.—The diagnosis should be as carefully made before attempting this operation as before almost any other surgical procedure. We must inquire very carefully into the history. The physical examination should be thoroughly made and every laryngologist should be an expert diagnostician of thoracic diseases. Metallic bodies, pebbles, bone and glass as well as some of the more compact organic substances cast shadows which may be more or less readily seen in a good radiograph. These can sometimes be seen with the fluoroscope. Seeds, small pieces of wood, particles of food, etc., do not cast shadows. With no history excepting that of a suddenly developed cough, a radiograph will sometimes reveal a metallic foreign body, as in a case I have seen recently where the friends had no suspicion that anything had been inhaled, yet a small nail was found in the lung.

Having established the diagnosis beyond a reasonable doubt, the next question is whether one shall perform an upper bronchoscopy, through the nasal passages, or a lower bronchoscopy through an opening in the trachea. I have come to believe that whenever marked dyspnea is present, safety to the patient demands a preliminary tracheotomy. In other cases it would generally be better first to attempt upper bronchoscopy. Where the foreign body is deeply seated in the lung and at a considerable distance from the median line, especially if upon the left side, lower bronchoscopy would nearly always be better. Experience has led me to believe that in nearly all cases, unless one succeeds in finding the foreign body within 10 or 15 minutes by upper bronchoscopy, the trachea should be opened, because lower bronchoscopy is much less difficult than the upper; for the tubes may be better illuminated, they can be more easily passed into the bronchi, and shorter and larger tubes may be employed. It would generally be safer to defer the lower bronchoscopy a few days, until all irritation has ceased.

Anatomy.—A knowledge of the anatomy and physiology of the air passages and esophagus are essential to good results in bronchoscopy and esophagoscopy. The teachings of the older anatomists were misleading, especially regarding the trachea and bronchi and the majority of physicians (even laryngologists) have not had their attention called to the errors. The demonstrations of Aeby (Der Bronchialbaum des Menschen und der Saugetiere, Leipsig, 1880), which have since been confirmed by other anatomists and are now generally accepted, show that the teachings of the older anatomists that the right bronchus runs nearly horizontally into the right lung and the left much more obliquely downward into its lung are rarely if ever correct. Prof. R. R. Bensley, of the University of Chicago, confirms Aeby's statements, and Prof. J. Gordon Wilson, formerly of the University of Chicago, now of the Northwestern University Medical School, from numerous recent dissections, has arrived at nearly the same conclusions. There is considerable variation in the direction of the bronchi in different individuals, but in a considerable proportion the right runs at a much smaller angle from the median plane downward and backward into its lung than does the left. In some cases indeed, the right bronchus is almost a direct continuation of the trachea. The left bronchus turns more nearly horizontally to the side running downward and backward. Aeby states that on an average the right bronchus makes an angle of 24.8 degrees to the mesial plane, whereas the left bronchus diverges on an average of 45.6 degrees to this plane; in children the bronchial angle is less than in adults. The left bronchus which is in the adult about 10 mm. in diameter, is usually from 1 to 2 mm. smaller than the right bronchus, but it is nearly twice the length of the latter, and not infrequently its first branch which passes upward and outward to the upper lobe, is even larger than the continuation of the main stem. This branch is usually larger than the corresponding branch of the right side, its average diameter being 9 mm. Prof. Wilson's observations show that the first branch from the right main bronchus runs downward and outward to the upper lobe of that lung, and that it averages 8.5 mm. in diameter.

It was formerly taught that the bronchi divide and subdivided dichotomously. It would generally be better to consider the bronchus of each lung as one main stem starting at the bifurcation of the trachea, running downward, more or less backward and outward toward the posterior part of the lung to a position about 8 cm. from the middle line of the body. From these main stems large branches are given off to the upper lobes, which shortly give off two or more smaller branches. Upon the right side a branch is also given off to the middle lobe. The main stems also give off branches arranged in anterior or ventral and posterior or dorsal sets. The ventral, which are also the outward of these branches, are often nearly as large as the stem from which they are given off. The branch to the upper lobe on the right side is usually given off about 1.5—2.6 m. from the beginning of the main bronchus, but that on the left is given off at about 5 cm. from its origin. The left main bronchus generally runs more nearly horizontally than the right, and it is probably from this condition that foreign bodies lodged in the branch going to the left upper lobe are often much more difficult to detect than those in the subdivisions of the right bronchus; indeed, in not a few cases, owing to the position of this branch, the congestion and swelling of the mucous membrane and the secretions and the blood in the bronchi, the operator will be unable to detect foreign bodies in this bronchus at all. The dimensions are:

Average length and size.
Adult.

	Male.	Female.	Child.	Infant.
Diameter of trachea	14-20mm.	12-16mm.	8-10mm.	6-7mm.
Length of trachea	12 cm.	10 cm.	6 cm.	4 cm.
Length of right bronchus	1.2-2 cm.	1.2-2 cm.	1.3 cm.	1 cm.
Length of left bronchus.	4.5 cm.	4.5 cm.	3 cm.	2.5 cm.
From upper teeth to trachea	15 cm.	13 cm.	10 cm.	9 cm.
From upper teeth to bifurcation of trachea.	27 cm.	23 cm.	16 cm.	13 cm.
From upper teeth to secondary bronchi going to the upper lobes of the lungs........	29-32 cm.	25-28 cm.	17-19 cm.	14-15 cm.
From upper teeth to branches going to lower lobes........	32-35 cm.	28-31 cm.	20-23 cm.	

From recent dissections on adult bodies, Prof. Wilson furnishes the following table:

Right bronchus.	Distance from bifurcation of trachea.	Diameter.
Branch to upper lobe of lung....	1.2 cm.	10 mm.
Branch to middle lobe..........	4. cm.	8.5 mm.
Main bronchial stem at this point.		8-9 mm.
First lateral branch to lower lobe.	4.3 cm.	4.5-6.5 mm.
Left bronchus.		
Branch to upper lobe of lung....	4.8 cm.	9 mm.
Main bronchial stem at this point.		8-9 mm.
First lateral branch to lower lobe.	5.6 cm.	6 mm.

These measurements, however, are only approximate and are subject to much variation. They do not allow for the dilatability of the air tubes during life, nor do they allow for the

contraction. The dilatation that can be done with safety is, I
think, very little, but unfortunately for the operator, the expiratory contraction of the bronchi, especially in the young,
and the swelling of the mucous membrane, may make the tubes
very much smaller than they would be in the cadaver. It is
especially important to know the length of the trachea and
bronchi and the probable distance from the upper teeth to the
bifurcation of the trachea and to the first and second divisions
of the bronchial stem.

Usually the bronchoscope should be from 4 to 6 cm. longer
than indicated by these measurements in order to allow for
error in the estimate and for convenience in manipulation.
Occasionally tubes much longer than just suggested will be
needed. Jackson states that to reach below the first branches
of the main bronchi tubes 45 or 50 cm. in length will sometimes
be required. I call special attention to this because I was
obliged to learn it by painful experience. Throughout the
lungs the pulmonary arteries and veins accompany the bronchi.
The bronchial arteries and veins also run along the posterior
walls of the bronchi.

Preparation.—Careful aseptic precautions should be taken for
this operation, even though perfect asepsis cannot be secured because there are so many microbes constantly in the mouth; yet,
we must protect our patients from every avoidable risk. Jackson
very properly suggests that when lower bronchoscopy is to be
done, it is advantageous to do it immediately after the trachea
has been opened, for if delayed a few days there is more chance
of carrying infection to the lower portion of the lung from a
suppurating tracheal wound.

In doing bronchoscopy, I have several times received severe
electric shocks, and I suspect that patients have also received
them. For this reason it is desirable to have a table with rubber castors and to have the floor covered with rubber sheets,
so that the operator and all the assistants will be insulated;
or everybody who is about the patient should wear rubbers and
rubber gloves.

It is desirable to have two or three sources of light, all of
which should be carefully tried out before the operation, otherwise at a critical point one may be left in darkness. All have
their advantages and defects. I think that the secretions and
blood getting into the auxiliary tube of Einhorn's or Jackson's
bronchoscopes make it more difficult to keep the lamps clean

than when they are introduced through the bronchoscope. The main objection, however, to Einhorn's and Jackson's bronchoscopes is that they necessitate using an instrument 1 or 2 mm. smaller in caliber than the Killian bronchoscope that could be employed in the same case. Usually the largest size that can be safely used is needed. I have used the Kirstein and Killian lights and Jackson's and my own small lamps, and I have at least two kinds in readiness at each operation. In one operation both of them gave out at the same time before I had finished. I have used the street currnt with reducing rheostats for all of these lamps, but I believe we should adopt Jackson's suggestion and use only a primary battery for the small internal lamps, because by this method the patient could not get a severe shock. It is also important that the conducting cords for the aspirator pump and the various lights should not come in contact with each other.

An aspirator for removing the secretions and blood or pus from the bronchi is provided with most of the sets and is important, but the hand aspirator acts slowly and not very satisfactorily as compared with a small pump driven by an electric motor. I have used with great satisfaction the pump which I think was devised by Dr. Jackson for the purpose of massage for the ear drum.

A gag is necessary. Killian's split tubular spatula or Jackson's tubular spatula, one side of which may be opened by removing a slide, or my similar open-tube spatula, are very helpful in introducing the bronchoscope, though in most of my operations I have used my introducer. I have used Killian's, Bruning's and Jackson's bronchoscopes, but on the whole I like Killian's the best. The size of the bronchoscope will depend upon the age and size of the patient, the larger the tube that can be used with safety the better. In infants, for upper bronchoscopy, the tube should not exceed 5 mm. in diameter. In older children it may be 6 or 7 mm., and in adults 9 mm. in diameter. Ordinarily, for children, bronchoscopes 7 mm., for adults 9 mm. in diameter are employed. Mandrins are usually desirable, that will just fit these tubes, with smooth ovoid ends projecting beyond the bronchoscope, and that are so made as to allow the patient to breathe through them. It is important, too, that the bronchoscope should have several openings through its wall, beginning about 4 cm. above the distal end, in order that when one bronchus is closed by the tube, the patient may respire through these openings. A number of cotton holders long enough to reach through the bronchoscope must be on hand, and they should be so made that the cotton will be fastened firmly. I have used only the cotton holders furnished with Killian's set, but those devised by Dr. Coolidge that are fastened by a ferrule which is screwed down, are better. Numerous forceps have been devised, any of which, if small enough and long enough, may be satisfactory to different operators. I like the Killian forceps best. Different forms of blades are necessary, according to what is to be accomplished. Blades that will grasp firmly any small object, are essential, others that when closed have 4 to 5 mm. between them are necessary in removing such objects as peanuts and beans, in order that they be not crushed. Cutting blades are occasionally needed and blades roughened exteriorily that may be introduced within tubular objects and then sprung out so as to hold them, are sometimes necessary. Blades that may possibly do damage by catching and tearing the soft tissues, should not be employed, if it is possible to get along without them. In two or three cases I have derived great advantage from a little instrument that I have named a pin finder, made somewhat on the principle of a corkscrew with a blunt end, the object of it being to work the pin as nearly as possible into the center of the lumen of the bronchus, so that the bronchoscope may be slipped down over it. Ingenious safety pin closers have been devised by Mosher and Jackson. Various hooks are also recommended and will sometimes be found very useful, but I wish specially to caution operators against the use of a hook bent so far that it may possibly catch into a bronchus. A hook 4 mm. across could easily be passed into a bronchus only 3 mm. in diameter, but on attempting to withdraw it, it might catch into a branch of this small bronchus, and in such case it might be impossible to disengage it without tearing the lung. Tearing the lung in this location would almost necessarily result in emphysema, which would probably prove fatal; it might be attended by serious hemorrhage, or it might be the starting point of a dangerous broncho-pneumonia or pleurisy.

A sterilized tracheotomy set should always be on hand in case it should be necessary to open the trachea. An O'Dwyer's intubation set is sometimes valuable. In a recent bronchoscopy I accomplished the same end very quickly by introducing my tubular director 5 mm. in diameter through the glottis.

I think it will be better for emergencies than either of the others. For the removal of granulation tissue and tumors, small curettes set at right angles to the stem are very useful.

Anesthetic.—Local anesthesia has been relied upon largely by Killian, von Schroetter and others, but I have preferred general anesthesia. For short examinations, cocain and suprarenaline are better where the patient is not too nervous; but in children general anesthesia appears preferable, though von Schroetter told me that he relied on local anesthesia even for these little patients. Chloroform is usually employed as a general anesthetic. Before beginning an operation, a moderately full dose of morphin and atropin, appropriate to the patient's age and size, will make it possible to get along with a smaller quantity of the anesthetic, and at least in adults I believe will render the operation safer. The use of cocain combined with some of the suprarenaline products also enables one to get along with smaller quantities of the general anesthetic. In my operations the patients have not been kept profoundly under the chloroform. Some operators consider cocain perfectly safe, but from the numerous unpleasant symptoms that I formerly saw when using it in the nose and from many recorded fatal cases of cocain poisoning, it seems necessary to employ it with considerable caution. Two fatal results following bronchoscopy in children in whom I employed cocain, and in one or both of whom moderate amounts of morphin and atropin were also used, have made me fearful about these drugs, although I have not yet been able to reach any satisfactory conclusion as to the exact cause of death in either case.

Technic.—Dr. Jackson gives very precise instruction about the arrangement of tables and the positions of the various assistants. I have found it important to have a reliable man to hold the patient's head; indeed, I feel that my first difficult bronchoscopy was successful largely because my assistant held the head in such a vise-like grip when it had been placed where I wished it, that it did not move.

Nearly all of my bronchoscopies have been done with the patient lying upon the back, the head hanging over the end of the table. Killian and von Schroetter have done nearly all of their bronchoscopies under cocain, and I judge have usually had the patient in a sitting position.

Care must be taken that the bronchoscope does not injure the patient's lips; this may be avoided by placing a folded napkin under it over the teeth, or the lip may be watched by an assistant.

Whatever method is employed in the introduction of the bronchoscope, one should be careful not to get it into the esophagus, which is much easier to enter than the larynx. If the tube should be passed into the esophagus, it must always be cleaned and again sterilized before again attempting to pass it into the trachea.

Among the difficulties that will be met in doing broncho-scopy are: rigidity of the neck, especially when only a local anesthetic is used, spastic muscular contractions, cough and excessive secretions, and respiratory difficulties due either to the foreign body or to the inflammation it has caused.

When the bronchoscope has entered the trachea, it should be passed down gently while carefully inspecting the parts until the antero-posterior septum at the bifurcation is found; then it should be inclined to the right or left, according to the lung that we wish to enter, the head and neck being turned at the same time in the opposite direction and the bronchoscope to the opposite side of the mouth so as to minimize the strain on the trachea and bronchi. In most cases there will be little dif-ficulty in finding the main bronchus, but sometimes the lower portion of the trachea is filled with secretion that must be re-moved before the parts can be seen. In young children the trachea may contract in expiration in the same way that the bronchial tubes do in adults, therefore it will not always be found easy, even to get into the main bronchi; but generally the operator, after a little experience, will not have much trouble in this respect. In passing the bronchoscope into the right lung, we expect within about 1½ cm. of the bifurcation, at its upper outer part, to find the mouth of the bronchus which supplies the upper lobe of the lung. On the left side, after the bronchoscope enters the main bronchus, it should be passed along gently for 4 or 5 cm., while the operator carefully inspects the upper outer wall for the beginning of the branch going to the left upper lobe.

There are numerous branches given off the main bronchial stems, but it must not be supposed that the operator will be able to recognize the orifices of all of them. Three to five at most are all that can usually be seen on either side.

The operator is sometimes confused by the reflections of light from the inner surface of the tube. This is best overcome by employing a small lamp carried down to the end of the bronchoscope. The secretions and pus or blood in the trachea or bronchi may prevent inspection of the parts, and sometimes it is very difficult to remove them sufficiently to make a thorough examination. Vision is not infrequently interfered with by swelling of the mucous membrane or granulation tissue, sometimes by contraction of the bronchus above the foreign body by cicatricial tissue, and it is always more or less interfered with by the normal contractions of the bronchial tube that may be exaggerated or may even be continuous in the presence of a foreign body. Foreign bodies, after remaining for a long time in the air passages, may become encysted, so that they cannot be seen at all. Gentle probing may enable the operator to discover the foreign body. I like best for this purpose the long slender tube that I generally use for aspirating the secretions.

In the case of small bodies like pins or needles, the pin finder will someties bring them into view and enable one to pass the bronchoscope over them so that they can be grasped by the forceps. Small bodies in small bronchi may very easily escape detection, especially when they are not of metallic character, so that their location can not be determined by the radiograph.

One is not justified in searching long through the bronchial tree unless he is sure that a foreign body is present. Foreign bodies lodged in the branches of the bronchi that run to the upper lobes, especially that of the left lung, have in my experience been the most difficult to detect.

Utility.—Bronchoscopy may be valuable in the diagnosis of some conditions of the upper respiratory passages when they cannot be determined by other means; thus in certain cases we may discover involution of the trachea from the pressure of a goitre, enlarged thymus, aneurism or other mediastinal tumor. I am fully convinced, however, that simply for diagnosis this method should seldom be used excepting where an accurate diagnosis cannot be made by ordinary laryngoscopy and the usual methods of physical examination.

Bronchoscopy is of greatest value for the detection and re-' moval of foreign bodies from the larynx and tracheo-bronchial tree. Most foreign bodies, after they have been located, can be best grasped with tubular forceps, the blades of which cannot damage the surrounding tissues. The forceps should be marked by a narrow strip of adhesive plaster wound around it so that the operator may know when it reaches the lower end of the tube. Having located the foreign body, one may sometimes grasp it while it is in plain sight, but commonly the forceps so obstruct the view that this is difficult. In such cases, if a forcep is used that has no sharp teeth to injure the lung, the instrument may be passed down in such a position that when the blades are opened they must pass on each side of the body; then when the mark upon the stem shows that the end of the forceps has nearly reached the body, the blades are opened and the instrument passed in about 1.5 cm. farther, when the blades may be closed with as much assurance of catching the object as though it were under direct inspection. However, where the body is of such a nature that toothed or cutting forceps must be used, it should not be touched excepting under direct inspection.

Laryngeal tumors can sometimes be removed by direct laryngoscopy more easily than by the older method, especially in children, or in other patients where a general anesthetic is necessary. Whenever operations of this kind are to be done, they should usually be preceded by tracheotomy. Laryngeal stenosis from cicatrices may sometimes be readily relieved, and tracheal tumors or granulation tissue can be removed by this method. Stenosis of the trachea or bronchi has occasionally been satisfactorily treated by the aid of the bronchoscope. Edema of the larynx may be easily reached and relieved by the tubular laryngoscope. Abscesses of the larynx that cannot be opened in the ordinary way will often be found amenable to treatment by this method. Ulcers of the trachea and the bronchial tubes have been cured by the aid of the bronchoscope that could not be reached in other ways.

It has been suggested that cavities in the lungs might be satisfactorily explored and treated through the bronchoscope. While believing that this could be done in exceptional cases, I think that the exploration would not be justifiable unless there was reason to believe that the cavity contained a foreign body.

Dangers.—Those who have had a few successful cases of bronchoscopy are apt to become very enthusiastic over its possibilities without recognizing its dangers, and therefore it has been recommended in many conditions where it is not indicated. At first sight it appears a simple thing to pass a small tube through the trachea into the bronchi, and it would seem that if the operation were done gently, no harm would result. It has been shown, however, that the operation is far from being either easy, simple or devoid of danger. The primary danger comes from the anesthetic, which if general becomes especially hazardous in the presence of dyspnea. Most operators who rely on local anesthesia speak of it as perfectly safe, but one cannot understand how they overlook the possible dangers from the absorption of cocain, when numerous fatal cases have resulted from its use in other parts of the body. It would seem that cocain applied so closely to the nerves controlling the respiration and circulation might have a serious effect; a general anesthetic when the patient is suffering from dyspnea is attended by much danger, especially, unless tracheotomy has first been performed; but in any case it is important that the anesthesia be not too profound or too long continued. Even though only small amounts of chloroform are used, I have come to believe that it is not safe to continue the operation for more than half an hour, even though not more than from 3 to 8 minutes may be available for actual inspection. It may be that even less than this should be placed as the limit.

In spite of the greatest care a certain amount of local traumatism will occur which may be the starting point of a fatal broncho-pneumonia. Should hooks or other instruments become caught in any part of the air passages, so that a little force is required to remove them, the lung is liable to be torn in such a way that the air will pass out, causing either an emphysema or a pneumothorax and pleurisy, either of which may prove fatal. Patients are known to have died soon after bronchoscopy from pneumothorax, emphysema, or pneumonia and other conditions; and if the operator is blind to the dangers it is natural to attribute these fatalities to the foreign body or to the anesthetic rather than to the operation. Pulmonary edema has apparently been the cause of death in several cases, and edema of the larynx has sometimes necessitated a sudden tracheotomy. Dangerous bronchitis has also occurred. The two deaths that I have already referred to from unexplainable causes have suggested to me also that danger may arise from electric shocks communicated to the patient through the instruments.

When we consider the relation of the blood vessels to the trachea and bronchi and the very short distance from the lumen of these tubes to the intracellular pulmonary tissues, we must realize that it would not be safe to tear or cut anything within the tracheo-bronchial tree unless we were absolutely sure that it would not open a way for air to pass out into the pleura, mediastinum, or lung tissue.

Jackson found a mortality of 9.6 per cent, but by eliminating 6 cases that he thought would probably have died without the operation, the mortality would have been 3.2 per cent. This does not appear to me a sufficiently conservative analysis of the statistics; on the contrary the chances are greatly in favor of the mortality being much larger than 9.6 per cent. Of the 6 cases that he would eliminate, no one can be certain that any of them would have died without the operation, and we may be certain that some, probably a majority of the fatal cases observed by others, have never been reported.

Notwithstanding all of the dangers, I believe that this operation is of great value in many of the conditions that I have enumerated, though it should be done with extreme care and gentleness. It is indicated in nearly all cases in the presence of foreign bodies in the air passages. Many foreign bodies can be easily removed by tracheotomy, but it would be better to try bronchoscopy first, provided there were not severe dyspnea, and in every case where the foreign body cannot be extracted by tracheotomy, bronchoscopy is surely indicated. In the other affections mentioned this operation is often indicated, but the condition of the individual patient and the experience and good judgment of the laryngologist must determine what course should be adopted.

Esophagoscopy.—Those interested in the history of this operation I will refer to Jackson's monograph. The instruments that are employed are essentially the same as those for bronchoscopy, though the tubes are larger, and many of them shorter, and occasionally they are made oval instead of round. The instruments for the removal of foreign bodies or neoplasms from the esophagus, would be the same as those employed in bronchoscopy.

Esophagoscopy is done much more satisfactorily and pleasantly when the patient is fasting than at any time within a few hours after a meal.

Cocain with one of the suprarenaline products may be used as an anesthetic in a large number of these cases, but in children and sometimes even in older subjects, it is better that a general anesthetic be employed. Either chloroform or ether can be used, as we will not have to consider the effect of the anesthetic upon the lungs in esophagoscopy as we do in bronchoscopy.

The tubes that are employed for esophagoscopy may be about 25 per cent larger than those that would be used for a similar patient in bronchoscopy. A large percentage of the diseases of the esophagus occur in the upper portion of this tube, and foreign bodies are likely to lodge just behind the cricoid cartilage or immediately below that point, so that comparatively short tubes are generally employed. The oval esophagoscope gives a larger field for inspection than the round, and according to the area exposed, it is introduced considerably more easily than the round instrument. In either case, an obturator is desirable, unless the part to be examined is near the mouth of the esophagus.

From its mouth to about the level of the upper end of the sternum the esophagus is closed, the slit indicating its lumen being directed from side to side.

As the esophagoscope is passed gently the walls of the esophagus seen across the end of the tube present a mucous membrane. only a few shades deeper in color than the laryngopharynx. When the instrument has passed a little below the upper end of the sternum the esophagus is usually found to be an open tube that contracts and expands more or less with the respiratory movements. This tube continues open down to near the cardiac orifice of the stomach. In the adult it usually appears from 8 to 10 mm. in diameter.

Esophagoscopy is of value in the diagnosis of strictures, diverticula and malignant or other growths, however the danger of rupturing the walls of the esophagus must always be borne in mind because in these conditions they sometimes tear very easily and such a tear is likely to be quickly followed by a fatal pleurisy or mediastinitis.

The operation is of special service in the diagnosis and removal of foreign bodies or tumors from the esophagus. Sometimes in this operation the edematous mucous membrane rolls down over the foreign body so as to completely hide it, even though the esophagoscope may easily pass all the way down to the stomach, therefore, wherever possible a good radiograph should be taken before the operation is attempted. It should be remembered that coins or other flat foreign bodies in the esophagus practically always have their flat surfaces antero-posteriorly. A knowledge of this fact aids the surgeon greatly in searching for them and in their removal. Failure to find a foreign body as large as a nickel in the esophagus by esophagoscopy should not convince the operator that it is not present, because the swollen mucous membrane is very likely to be crowded down over it in such a way as to hide it.

There can be no question but that this operation is by far the best for nearly all cases of foreign bodies in the esophagus, though if one is so large that it cannot be removed when discovered, it may be necessary to do esophagotomy; however, some objects of large size have been successfully cut and then removed in pieces by the aid of the esophagoscope, with much better results to the patient than would probably have attended an esophagotomy. Esophagotomy has a much larger percentage of mortality than operations through the esophagoscope and therefore whenever possible, a skillful laryngologist should be called upon to remove foreign bodies before resorting to esophagotomy. It is certain that most foreign bodies that become lodged in the esophagus can be removed with very silght danger to the patient by aid of the esophagoscope. Neoplasms that can be secured in a snare may commonly be safely removed in the same way; those that would require the use of cutting instruments must be handled with extreme care, and ordinarily they are not suitable for this operation. Strictures of the esophagus that could not be managed with ordinary bougies might sometimes be overcome with the aid of the esophagoscope and as diverticula are dependent upon strictures it is probable that some of these might be greatly benefited through this procedure that could not otherwise be satisfactorily treated.

As an illustration of the difficulties and dangers attending bronchoscopy and as a contribution toward perfecting the operation and making it safer, I wish to place on record concise histories of two recent cases.

On the 14th of November, 1908, a girl 3½ years of age was brought to the hospital with symptoms of some pulmonary trouble but no history of having inhaled a foreign body, however, a radiograph showed that there was a small nail in the air passages. A surgeon did tracheotomy and attempted to remove it. He felt the nail but was unable to extract it and finally it passed down out of reach. Before the operation the pulse was 128, temperature 98 and respiration 28; 10 hours afterward the pulse was 144, irregular and intermittent, and the temperature 104.6. The next day the pulse, temperature and respiration continued high but on the following day the pulse ranged from 128 to 160, the temperature 101 to 102.3 and respiration 60 to 72. On the succeeding day the pulse dropped to 120, the temperature to 100 and the respiration to 54. The 4th and 5th days the symptoms were better but on the 6th day (the 20th of November) it is noted that there was pneumonia of the left lung, although the temperature was not much, if any, higher. I was then asked to attempt to remove the object by bronchoscopy and at 4 p. m. on the 21st, the child was given chloroform and the operation made. A radiograph showed that the nail was at this time deep down in the left lung and the operation demonstrated that it was in the bronchus going to the upper lobe. I searched with the greatest care for about an hour examining the main stem of the left bronchus and its branches going to the lower lobe, but, probably on account of the swelling of the mucous membrane and the contraction of the bronchus, I was unable to see the opening of the bronchus going to the upper lobe and could not feel the nail. The operation was then abandoned with the intention of repeating it another day. Three hours later the pulse was 180 and weak, and the respiration over 90. At the end of 4 hours the pulse was 160, temperature 102.2 and respiration 84; 4 hours later the temperature was 103.2; the next forenoon the pulse was 160, temperature 102.6, respiration 88, but by noon, 20 hours after the operation, the pulse was 176, temperature 104.4, respiration 76. The conditions continued unfavorable and the patient died of pneumonia 48 hours after the operation.

In this case pneumonia was already present though the symptoms were not marked at the time of the operation and the bronchoscopy was done through a suppurating wound in the trachea. The patient's condition at the time of the operation and possible carrying of the pus from the wound into the lung, undoubtedly contributed to the fatal result.

How could the difficulty in seeing the bronchus going to the upper lobe of the lung have been overcome? Would it have been better to have delayed the operation until this patient had recovered, or died from the pneumonia? I await answers from others to both of these questions.

The second case—a child 17 months of age—was brought to

me on the 7th of January, 1909, with the following history:
Four weeks previously the child while in perfect health was
playing with an older brother and both of them fell upon the
floor. The patient was immediately seized with a severe
paroxysm of cough which nearly strangled it. The cough
had continued ever since and there had been several paroxysms
which the parents reported came near being fatal. An examination revealed a great many large and small mucous rales
all over the chest, but no dullness and no ·disparity in the
respiratory murmur on the two sides. A radiograph gave no
shadow of a foreign body, but the history and signs made it
practically certain that some foreign substance was in the air
passages. At 4 o'clock the same afternoon chloroform was
given and I operated with extreme care. I gave neither opiate
nor atropin, and I used a weak solution of cocain with
suprarenaline only two or three times in the larynx. The
bronchoscope was introduced easily and quickly and I made
a most careful and gentle search of the trachea and bronchial
tubes of both sides. Owing to the great quantity of secretion
the operation was much prolonged, at least 9/10ths of the time
being spent in pumping and wiping out the secretions. The
child was taking very little chloroform and I thought no
damage was being done. I designed to abandon the operation at the end of an hour, but the condition of the patient was
so favorable and my anxiety to find the foreign body so great
that I unconsciously kept up the search half an hour longer,
but nothing could be found.

At the time of the operation, temperature per rectum was
101° and at midnight it was 105.4°, pulse 122, respiration 140.
The next noon conditions remained the same and much the
same the following day, but during the afternoon of the third
day after the operation the temperature and pulse fell to normal. The fourth day the temperature went once to 103°, the
fifth to 100.8° and the sixth to 102.3°; afterward there was
steady improvement for three or four days, but subsequently
the temperature daily ranged from normal up to 2 or 3 degrees higher for four weeks. The nurse said that the child
had occasional paroxysms of dyspnea during the night for
three or four nights, but the bronchial rales greatly diminished,
although the physical signs showed a slowly resolving pneumonia of the lower lobe of the right lung. When the temperature first went up the Interne reported a broncho-pneumonia

and I ordered 1/200 gr. of strychnia and ½ drachm of liq. amm. acet. every three hours, and the chest was covered with an oiled silk and cotton jacket. This treatment was continued until the immediate danger was passed.

How could the difficulty due to excessive secretion have been avoided? Possibly by the administration of atropin in one or two full doses for a child of this size and age.

How could the unfavorable after-results have been prevented? In this case unfavorable symptoms followed the bronchoscopy promptly and the patient certainly was near death.

Since writing the foregoing, or a month after the first bronchoscopy on this patient, after consultation with several of my colleagues, I decided to operate again. The extreme dullness over the lower lobe of the right lung, with absence of breath sounds—the outline of the dullness and the negative results of three exploratory punctures—suggested obstruction of the bronchus going to that portion of the lung with collapse and eliminated the diagnosis of pleurisy. The patient's temperature had been running up to 102° or 103° F. about every third day for two or three weeks, which pointed strongly to sepsis. At 4 p. m. February 8th, when the patient was sent to the operating room, rectal temperature was 102.7° F. Morph. sulph. gr. 1/50 and atropin sulph. 1/500 gr. had been given hypodermically—chloroform narcosis—bronchi of right lung thoroughly explored down to a caliber of 3 mm. with negative results. Examination lasted 15 minutes. Patient removed to ward and temperature found to be more than a degree lower. Patient placed in croup tent, air of which was kept very warm and moist, for forty-eight hours. By midnight the temperature was normal and the next day it was only 99.2° and patient was in excellent condition. The danger in this case seems to have been avoided by the short operation and the warm, moist atmosphere.

I incline to the belief that unfavorable symptoms after bronchoscopy are largely due to the mechanical irritation of the instrument. As I have already pointed out, the bronchi and the trachea in young children expand and contract greatly with each respiration, and (as I clearly demonstrated in a child 5½ years of age from whose right lung I removed a baby's beauty pin on Jan. 13th, 1909) the bronchi are lifted and depressed fully a centimeter with each respiratory movement.

From these movements there is constant respiratory stretching and pulling of the air tube over the end of the bronchoscope, which would cause much of the mechanical irritation. This mucous membrane is not intended to bear anything like as much mechanical irritation as the conjunctiva, therefore, it seems natural that the mere presence of the bronchoscope even without pressure and stretching of the bronchi would cause a great deal of irritation.

In order to avoid the dangers it appears to me that we must make the operation as short as possible; we must not touch any part of the tracheo-bronchial tract that can be avoided, and we should use an instrument as small as will give sufficient illumination and allow of the use of suitable instruments. The Killian tubes 6-7 mm. in diameter for children over a year of age and 7-9 mm. for adults appear to me the best. Foreign bodies in the lower part of the trachea might often be removed with a bronchoscope that only passed 1 or 2 cm. below the glottis, and foreign bodies in the bronchi may frequently be removed without passing the bronchoscope more than 5 to 10 mm. into the bronchus, providing we use a forcep that will not catch the mucous membrane on the walls of the air passages, and providing also that we are careful to open the blades in such a direction that we would not catch the tissues at the point of division of the air tube. In the trachea there would be no danger if the blades opened antero-posteriorly, for then they could not grasp the septum that runs antero-posteriorly between the two main bronchi at the bifurcation, and in the main bronchi it would be safe if the blades opened along a plane running from before downward and backward at an angle of about 20 degrees to the mesian anterior-posterior plane of the thorax, for they could not catch the tissues between the main bronchus and its first branch. Again, by using such a forceps in this way the foreign body could often be safely and quickly removed from a main bronchus without taking time to remove the secretions, so as to actually see the foreign body. Before the days of bronchoscopy I several times removed foreign bodies from the main bronchi with a bent tube forceps inserted through a tracheal opening. In the case just referred to, by upper bronchoscopy, I removed the pin quickly in this way without cleaning out the secretions after having searched for it about 7½ minutes. The whole operation requiring but 8½ minutes. There were no unfavorable symptoms afterward. The difficulties of esophagoscopy are slight, as compared with bronchoscopy, but one must remember that the swollen and edematous mucous membrane may roll over and completely hide quite large foreign bodies even though the instrument may pass without obstruction to the stomach. The dangers of esophagoscopy are much less, because the mucous membrane is designed for the passage of foreign bodies and therefore will not be much irritated by the instrument.

IX

THE INDICATIONS FOR THE RADICAL MASTOID OPERATION, BASED UPON PATHOLOGIC LESIONS.*

By S. J. Kopetzky, M. D.,

New York City.

It would hardly seem to be necessary at this late day to discuss the indications for the radical mastoid operation before a body of otologists. An operation suggested upon rational, pathologic research, as early as 1873, should, by this time, have won its proper place in otology. After 36 years, it is expected that the object to be gained by this procedure, and the conditions which can properly be submitted to operation, should have been so definitely known, that they would not require of us to-day the time and thought necessary for their discussion.

However, the status of the operation is unsettled, and the reasons for this are not hard to find.

The operation gives apparently variable results even at the hands of the most experienced. Otologists, as a whole, have expected more from the procedure than scientific inquiry into its merits warrants. The indications for the employment of the radical operation have usually been based upon symptoms rather than upon an actual diagnosis of disease. Confusion naturally ensued, and the results obtained when employing the operation to cure a symptom caused us to overlook the results of the operation when computed on the basis of cures for a given disease.

A glance through the literature demonstrates that we have rather promiscuously submitted cases of otitis media purulenta chronica, with or without accompanying mas-‧toiditis, to this operation, because after a fair and reasonable

*Read before the Eastern Section of the American Rhinological, Laryngological and Otological Society, Philadelphia, January 9, 1909.

time, with the best available therapeutics at command, we were unable to stop the persistent otorrhea, or we operated radically in these cases because acute exacerbations or intracranial or labyrinthine complications were threatening.

Excepting the symptoms in the complicating lesions, the prominent determining symptom—the otorrhea—is a common factor to many varying pathologic lesions within the middle ear and adjacent structures; and as such is not to be held as an indication for the radical mastoid operation.

A tentative classification of the pathologic lesions present in the middle ear and mastoid process, gives definite data from which so to limit the indications for the radical mastoid operation that more uniform results, under similar conditions, are obtainable.

Another element tending toward the uncertainty with which the radical mastoid operation is regarded, is to be found in the fact that we do not all perform the same operation for the same given pathologic lesions. We do not all perform a complete radical mastoid operation.

The Stacke operation is the selected procedure of many; the Zaufal operation—often designated in this country, the Schwartze-Stacke operation—has the majority of adherents, and, finally, a few—Heath, Bryant and Ballenger and their followers—have recently advocated a so-called modified radical operation, in which the ossicles are retained, and the membrana tympani preserved, in the interest of the hearing faculty.

Here again, confusion is averted, if the results obtained from these varying procedures are classified and judged separately.

The Stacke operation differs really but in slight degree from the Zaufal operation. It is rather a different route toward the same end. When we add to the Stacke method, complete evisceration of the mastoid contents, the end results of both operations are the same. A true Stacke operation limiting the surgery to the uncapping of the antrum after opening and connecting this with the tympanic cavity, and only removing the adjacent bone of the mastoid process, necessarily must only be indicated by a rather localized pathologic process.

When, however, the area of disease is extensive, i. e., if it is found spread beyond the confines of the tympanic

and the antral cavities, a removal of more tissue is indicated
than the limits of the operative endeavor as laid down by
Stacke.

Since no surgeon would stop his procedure before entirely eradicating all removable areas of disease, we hold
the Stacke operation as now practiced to be a difference
in technic rather than a separate operation from that
of Zaufal (the Schwartze-Stacke), and we may consider
the indications for both these operations together.

By the radical mastoid operation is meant a procedure
which shall cleanse the tympanic cavity of all its diseased
mucous membrane, in all its accessible and removable parts;
which shall eradicate the cellular structure about the orifice
of the Eustachian tube; which shall remove the two major
ossicles and the remains of the membrana tympani; which
shall open the mastoid antrum, connecting it with the tympanic cavity by as wide a passage as possible, thereby
freeing the aditus ad antrum, eviscerating the diseased contents of these cavities, and finally removing as much of
their respective bony walls as are found diseased and are
capable of removal, and in addition removing from the
mastoid process and temporal pyramid as much of its bony
structure and its contents as is found diseased. To these
procedures there is added a plastic. Such an operation
meets the indications for radical mastoid surgery.

The operation devised by Heath, the one advocated by
Bryant, and the so-called meato-mastoid operation of Ballenger, can hardly be held to constitute a radical mastoid
operation at all. At another section of this Society, I shall
discuss these operations in detail. Suffice it here to call
attention to the fact that in the lesions of the middle ear
and its adnexa, which are chronic in nature, and where
there has existed a purulent, fetid otorrhea, coming through
a more or less pronounced perforation or defect situated
marginally in the drum, that with lesions producing these
findings, there is usually bone necrosis in the neighboring
parts—the aditus and the tympanic walls—especially the
posterior tympanic wall. No operation devised to remove
other parts, and yet preserve intact the original seat of the
lesion is, surgically speaking, logical. Neither can the preservation of more or less diseased ossicles and the remains
of a drum membrane whose final healing means the ad-

vent of considerable scar tissue give much toward the conservation of the hearing faculty. To find proof of this contention, we have only to call to mind the demonstrable loss of hearing in those cases of chronic otitis media purulenta, which we healed by local measures, where, after a lapse of time, the scar tissue became firmly contracted.

Either the entire principle under which otology has accepted ossiculectomy is an error, or what seems more likely from a study of the greater number of the cases submitted to this modified radical operation, Heath, Bryant and Ballenger, especially the two former—since Ballenger separates his indications for the meato-mastoid operation from those he lists for the radical—have thus operated upon cases which would have responded to a simple mastoidectomy, with results as brilliant regarding the hearing faculty, as these men report having obtained from the involved technic of the so-called modified radical operation. For the present, we can therefore leave out of account this operation in discussing the indications for radical mastoid surgery.

Otitis media purulenta chronica is a generic, clinical term. It implies a diseased ear with a persistent purulent discharge. Both from the standpoint of a consideration of the indications for the radical operation and for an estimation of the results of the procedure, so general a term as this can have no place in a list of conditions indicating a surgical procedure.

The actual pathologic lesions grouped under this term are: (See Chart, appended herewith.)

1. Caries of the ossicles accompanied or not by a suppurative inflammation of the mucous membrane lining the tympanic cavity and adnexa.

2. Chronic suppurative inflammation of the mucous membrane lining the tympanic and the adjacent cavities, including the Eustachian tube, especially at its orifice, without there being any disease present in the underlying bone at any point.

3. Caries of portions of the temporal pyramid (non-tubercular and non-syphilitic in nature) accompanied by a suppurative inflammation of the mucous membrane lining the middle ear cavities.

4. Necrosis of greater or lesser portions of the bony

walls of the middle ear spaces and mastoid process, with
destruction of large areas of mucous membrane lining the
tympanic and adjacent cavities, and exudative inflammation
in the remaining sections of the mucosa of the middle ear
spaces.

5.　The erosive lesions, pressure necroses in various parts
of the middle ear, caused by the ingrowth of psuedo—and
true cholesteatomata or other malignant growths; part of
the clinical picture being caused by the disintegration of
the cholesteatomatous or other new-growth masses, in
addition to the pus caused by the bone necrosis.

6.　The specific lesions of parts of the temporal bone,
especially when found to involve the middle ear spaces and
mastoid process: that is, the tubercular and syphilitic
lesions.

It is not within the scope of this paper to take up the
details of the differential diagnosis between these groups
of cases.

These six groups of cases all present ears evidencing all
or part of the following: A persistent discharge, usually
fetid, coming through a perforation in the membrana tympani, of varying size and location, and often, in addition,
presenting the presence of polyps or polypoid granulations
on the visible portions of the mucous membrane, or inflammatory excrescences sprouting through the perforation.

The radical mastoid operation is not indicated in isolated
caries of the two greater ossicles. This condition is rare,
and on the whole, the removal of the diseased ossicles and
the establishment of intratympanic drainage will suffice to
cure these cases. When ossicular caries is accompanied
by an exudative inflammation of the lining membrane of
the tympanic cavity—a product of the irritation locally by
the dead ossicles, plus insufficient drainage, or the result
of disease in the nasopharynx which has spread by contiguity through the Eustachian tube, there also the radical
mastoid operation is not immediately indicated. If after
ossiculectomy and the proper treatment of the nasopharynx,
large quantities of pus continue to emanate from the anterior wall of the tympanic cavity, or seem to come away
from the upper chambers of the tympanic cavity, from the
aditus especially, then radical mastoid surgery is indicated

to remove detritus, lay open the disease-containing cavities, and render these accessible to subsequent after-treatment.

In cases where the mucous membrane lining the tympanic cavity and its adjacent structures is the seat of a chronic exudative inflammation, and there is no lesion present in the underlying bone, the pathologic process present in the mucous membrane is the product of the spread by contiguity of an exudative process in the nasopharynx and Eustachian tube. Removal of the primary foci and the performance of ossiculectomy may stop the exudative inflammation, and thus cause a cessation of the otorrhea. When the disease is of long standing and has thoroughly blocked the Eustachian tube by inflammatory exudate, and when the continuance of the process in the middle ear, by developing plastic inflammatory adhesions about the stapes and at the niches of the labyrinthine windows, threaten a gradual but progressive loss of hearing, then it would seem better in the interest of the patient's hearing and the prevention of a superimposition of an acute exacerbation, to clean out the middle ear spaces thoroughly, especially curetting the orifice of the Eustachian tube, and removing diseased mucous membrane, thus rendering the middle ear spaces in toto accessible to further local after-treatment.

In both the above groups of cases, which in a recent monograph,* I designated as of the nondangerous type of otitis media purulenta chronica, the disease may go on indefinitely without threatening intracranial involvement. This class of cases is, however, often subject to acute exacerbations, resulting in acute mastoiditis superimposed on the chronic disease of the mucous membrane of the middle ear. A simple mastoidectomy to relieve the acute symptoms will sometimes suffice in this particular class of cases, although I prefer the radical procedure for the reasons already given.

Radical operation is often demanded in the group of cases under discussion, because of the progressive loss of hearing which these cases evidence. The radical mastoid, by removing the major part of the diseased mucous membrane, eventually causes the suppuration to stop, because the instituted after-treatment permits a logical, rational

*The Surgery of the Ear.   Rebman Company, New York.

therapeusis to be applied to the remains of the diseased tissue necessarily left in situ. The radical operation, even in its most extensive limits, is unable to effect a complete evisceration of the mucous membrane lining the middle ear spaces, and there generally remain portions of diseased tissue about the labyrinthine windows and in the more inaccessible parts of the Eustachian tube. Here then is a group of cases wherein the radical operation, although indicated as a step toward its cure, will not stop the otorrhea. The discharge from such ears only ceases when these remains of mucous membrane either become converted into epidermis, or become healed because their entire surroundings are healthy. Regarding the hearing in this group of cases, it is generally found slightly worse after the operation than before, provided the operative procedures have not been delayed too long in the course of the disease, but it is vastly better than it would be were the suppurative inflammation to be allowed to continue for years unchecked.

In necrosis of part or all of the bony tympanic walls, in caries located in the various parts of the temporal bone, mastoid process, sections of the petrosa, etc.; in pressure necrosis due to epithelial ingrowths from cholesteatoma, and in the syphilitic and the tubercular lesions of the mastoid process and petrosal pyramid, whether accompanied or not by a syphilitic or tubercular involvement of the tympanic cavity, the radical mastoid operation is indicated.

In ordinary bone necrosis, more or less localized in area, with or without sequestra formations, and in cases with cholesteatoma and tuberculosis of the mastoid process, the radical mastoid operation gives the most satisfactory results, although in cases with cholesteatoma, supervision is afterwards necessary to prevent recurrences. The predominating symptom—the otorrhea—is usually stopped as soon as the lesion is eradicated. In syphilitic lesions, I have often been unable to secure healing, because I could not secure proper epidermatization, although, generally speaking of these cases as a class, the results obtained warrant me in classing these lesions as indicating a radical mastoid operation.

When symptoms referable to intracranial involvement, or intralabyrinthine disease become evident, or when symptoms demonstrate an acute process superimposed upon any of the pathologic lesions constituting otitis media purulenta chrónica, then the complete radical mastoid operation is immediately indicated.

Summarizing, we contend:

1. That the various diseases for which the radical mastoid operation is indicated should be classified and studied according to their pathologic aspect.

2. That the cessation of otorrhea is not the only condition for which the radical mastoid operation is indicated.

3. That the radical mastoid operation does not stop the otorrhea in a certain definite group of cases, but the operation is eventually indicated in these cases, notwithstanding failure to check this one symptom. In these cases, the operation is but one step toward their final cure.

4. That in bone lesions, located both in and beyond the tympanic cavity, the radical mastoid operation is the only procedure which is indicated by the pathologic lesions present in the mastoid process, temporal pyramid or tympanic walls. That the removal of the diseased bone cures the suppurating ear, and the result in these cases is proportionate to the thoroughness with which the lesion is eradicated.

5. Finally, that the so-called modified radical operation does not meet the indications for radical mastoid surgery.

Group.	Otoscopic Picture.	Lesion.	Complicating Lesions.	Operations Indicated.
A.—Non-dangerous type.	Centrally located perforations.	Suppurative inflammation in Eustachian tube, pharynx and mucous membrane of middle ear spaces.	Acute mastoiditis.	Surgery to nasopharynx, ossitmy and mostly radical mastoid operation. Occasionally, simple mastoidectomy suffices.
B.—Dangerous type.	Perforations located at margin of membrana tympani.	Bone fixed in middle ear, and petrosal pyramid, caries, cholesteatoma, new growths, tuberculous or syphilitic in the bony structure.	Acute mastoiditis, intralabyrinthine or intracranial, and any local intratympanic lesion causing facial palsy.	Radical mastoid operation as soon as diagnosis of bone lesion is made.

Otitis Media Purulenta Chronica.

X

A SERIES OF PAPERS ON SINUS DISEASE.

First Paper.

REPORT OF A CASE OF CYST OF THE FRONTAL SINUS, COMMUNICATING WITH THE FRONTAL LOBE.*

BY CLEMENT F. THEISEN, M. D.,

ALBANY, N. Y.

The following case. because of the apparent rarity of one feature of it, was considered of sufficient interest to be reported:

Cysts of the frontal sinus, particularly mucoceles, are not so very rare, but it is fairly uncommon to find an absence of a large part of the posterior or cerebral wall of the sinus.

The patient, Miss M. B., aged thirty-four years, consulted the writer July 27, 1907. The only interesting point in her history is a severe fall, striking her head, when she was nine years old. She stated that she was unconscious for three days at that time. From that time she has been a sufferer from severe headaches, more intense on the left side. She is a worker in a textile mill.

In 1905 she had a nasal operation, the exact nature of which she could not tell me. This gave her some relief. For a number of years she had had a discharge from the left nostril. This, she believed, followed some work on the teeth on that side. About a year before consulting the writer her left maxillary antrum had been opened through the canine fossa, and for a time she thought she was a little better.

Her physician, Dr. J. B. Ledlie, of Saratoga, who referred Miss B. to me, told me that since July, 1907, her headaches had been unusually severe, particularly on the

---

*Read at the thirtieth annual meeting of the American Laryngological Association, at Montreal, May 11, 12 and 13, 1908.

left side. She also complained of a pressure and fulness over the eyes. There was slight ptosis of the left eyelid, but no orbital swelling nor displacement of the eyeball. When she turned her head quickly to the left, or bent forward suddenly, she had great vertigo, and would fall if she could not get hold of some support. Pupils reacted to light and accommodation.

On examination nothing particularly wrong could be discovered in the nose. There was a small amount of a thin, mucopurulent secretion in the left nostril, which came from the antrum. On transillumination the left antral region was slightly darker than the right, but there was good illumination of both, and the pupils were also illuminated.

The left frontal region was darker than the right. This region was also slightly more prominent.

The headaches were becoming so frequent and severe that she was anxious to have any operation that would relieve her. While there was no direct evidence of a purulent frontal sinusitis, the result of transillumination, with the headaches confined to that side, appeared to the writer sufficiently suspicious symptoms to warrant an operation. This was performed in the Saratoga Hospital in August, 1907. The usual incision through the eyebrow was made and a portion of the anterior wall of the sinus carefully removed. A fluctuating tumor, having the typical appearance of a cyst, presented in the opening. It appeared to contain considerable fluid. An incision was made through the cyst wall and a large amount of a fluid very much like thin mucus escaped. This was, unfortunately, lost, so that no examination could be made of it. The anterior wall, as well as the floor of the sinus, was found intact, but a considerable portion of the posterior wall was missing, so that the pulsation of the meningeal vessels could be seen. The cyst wall, in fact, appeared to extend through to the frontal lobe.

The sinus was large and somewhat dilated.

The anterior ethmoid cells were then investigated through a separate incision, following the method employed by Coakley. No pus and very little bone necrosis was found. At this time the patient went into a condition of collapse, and it was with great difficulty that we succeeded in reviving her. We could not get a probe through into the nose from the frontal sinus, so that, as in cases of mucocele, the ostium was probably occluded. As much of the cyst wall as possible was removed, and the frontal wound, with the exception of a small opening in the inner angle, closed. A small wick of gauze was carried into the sinus for drainage, but in about ten days the gauze was no longer inserted and the wound allowed to close. The patient made an uninterrupted recovery, and now, about ten months after the operation, is apparently perfectly well. She works twelve to fourteen hours a day and has no headaches.

I received a letter from her physician, Dr. Ledlie, a week ago, in which he stated that she was all right and able to do her work every day.

A. Logan Turner, in his interesting paper on mucocele of the accessory nasal sinuses, reports two cases in which, as in the writer's case, absorption of part of the posterior wall of the sinus had taken place.

In six out of seven cases reported by him absorption of a part or the whole floor of the sinus had taken place.

I will briefly report the two cases in which part of the posterior wall was missing.

Case 1.—C. S., a woman, aged forty-three years. During the operation it was found that a portion of the posterior, or cerebral, wall the size of a half-crown had been absorbed, so that the dura mater was seen pulsating.

Six months after the operation there was no discharge from the cavity. A drainage tube was carried into the nose at the time of the operation and worn for six weeks. It was then removed, and the patient was instructed to wash out the sinus with a curved canula.

In the second case reported by Turner, a woman aged thirty-seven years, the dura was found exposed over an area as large as a sixpence. The right eye-ball was displaced downward, outward and forward. This was so in the other case also.

In the writer's case there was no orbital swelling, a common symptom of cyst of the frontal sinus. The anterior ethmoid cells are frequently involved. Patients, as a rule, do not complain of much pain unless infection of the sinus takes place.

In Turner's cases there was displacement of the eye-ball in seven out of ten.

The displacement depends upon the size of the orbital swelling. Turner states that when the affected sinus extends backwards for a considerable distance along the roof of the orbit, and the mucous contents escape into the orbital cavity after the floor has been absorbed, the eye-ball is pushed forward and downward. A previous catarrhal condition of the nasal mucous membrane is the probable cause of such cases.

The ostium of the sinus becomes occluded, causing an accumulation of mucus in the frontal sinus and a gradual thinning and absorption of one or more of the bony walls.

Killian believes that traumatism is an important cause for the development of such cysts.   '

The writer was able to find records of only a few other cases of cysts of the frontal sinus, in which a large portion of the posterior wall of the sinus was absent, in the literature of the past ten years.

Casali has reported the case of a man, aged forty-one years, who had had a fall, striking the right side of the head, eighteen years before consulting him. There was a fluctuating swelling above the supraorbital ridge, extending down to the middle of the upper eyelid.

There was also a right exopthalmos.

A clear, sterile fluid was obtained on puncturing.

A radical operation was performed. After the anterior cyst wall was removed the pulsation of the meningeal arteries could be seen. Two hundred ccm. of clear fluid was evacuated.

Histological examination showed that this was probably not a cyst, but an enormously dilated frontal sinus. Another interesting case has been reported by Mayer.

This patient, aged fifty-three years, had been twice operated on for a cyst of the frontal sinus.

A large amount of a yellowish fluid had been evacuated, and it was found that the posterior wall of the sinus was missing.

The patient survived the first operation, but in a year there was a recurrence, and the second operation had a fatal termination. In the region of the right frontal lobe there was a deep depression produced by the cyst.

In a case reported by **Zamazal** of severe left-sided head-aches for two years there was a sudden flow of pus and blood from the nose just before the patient died. There was an abscess in the region of the frontal lobe which broke through into the frontal sinus.

BIBLIOGRAPHY.

A. Logan Turner. Mucocele of the Accessory Nasal Sinuses. Edinburgh Medical Journal, November and December, 1907.

Kelling. Wiener medicinische Wochenschrift, No. 32, 35, 1902.

Killian. Heymann's Handbuch, Bd. III, 16.

Angelo Casali. Ref. in Internat. Centralbl. für Laryngol. etc., 1908, No. 4, p. 187.

Mayer, L. Kyste du sinus frontal avec compression cerebrale. Journal Med. de Bruxelles. No. 51, 1903.

Zamazal. Ein Fall von chronischer Gehirnabscess mit Durchbruch im Antrum frontale. Wiener med. Wochenschr., No. 26, 1897.

XI

ANATOMY AND DISEASES OF THE STYLOID EPIPHYSIS.

By John J. Kyle, M. D.,

PROFESSOR OF LARYNGOLOGY, RHINOLOGY AND OTOLOGY, INDIANA
UNIVERSITY SCHOOL OF MEDICINE,

Indianapolis.

In late years, the laryngologist has found it necessary to consider many faulty embryonal developments, especially those occurring about the ear and in the roof of the mouth. Pathologic conditions resulting from normal embryonal anlage of the mouth and throat are infrequent, yet of sufficient interest to warrant a most careful study of the subject. These conditions have more often come within the field of the general surgeon and for that reason, have probably been neglected by the rhinologist and laryngologist.

The branchial arches and clefts are the essential formations necessary to the differentiation of the head and neck structures. The pharynx is the dilated end of the cephalic primitive gut tract, and within this structure about the twenty-first day, we have a bulging outward of the ectodermic surfaces, forming pharyngeal pouches or furrows on the external surface, which are designated as visceral clefts. The visceral arches are composed of mesodermic tissue and separate the clefts and furrows from each other. About the fifth week of fetal life, obliteration of the arches and clefts begins by the permanent formation of the head and neck structures. Some of the arches undergo absorption, and we have to deal in this paper with the imperfect absorption.

The visceral arches are five in number. The first has to do with the formation of the upper and lower maxillary bones, mouth cavity, malleus and incus. The second visceral arch, the one especially under discussion, becomes obliterated with the exception of a bar of cartilage, designated Reichert's cartilage.

At its uppermost portion, Reichert's cartilage becomes the stapes, and the lower portion subdivides into segments, denominated by Geoffrey Saint-Hilaire as the tympanohyal, stylohyal, and epihyal. The tympanohyal is the base of the process, articulates with the temporal bone, is immediately attached to the inner surface of the tympanic plate, and appears externally to be wedged between the tympanic plate and the petrosa, anterior to the stylomastoid foramen. The stylohyal forms the styloid process proper and the epihyal as a rule remains fibrinous and becomes the styloid ligament. The petrostyloid articulation is fibro-cartilaginous or a synarthrosis, and thus may admit of some motion.

Dr. Dieulafe (L'Echo Medical, July 20, 1901) reports such a movable styloid and refers to Cruveilheir, who says such a condition is not very rare.

Mr. Porter (Reports of the Dublin Pathological Society, February, 1873) reports three cases of abnormal styloid process, very slender and flexible, and attached to the temporal bone by cartilage, possessing no styloid muscle and ligament.

Von Thaden (Deutsche Zeitschrift für Chirurgie, 1874-5) also reports one case in which the joint was slightly movable.

From these observations, it may be concluded that a movable articulation is not uncommon, and with such a condition existing, the whole process may be deflected towards the fauces and become, under favorable conditions, a source of annoyance, as we shall show later on.

The epihyal becomes normaly the stylohyoid ligament and articulates with the ceratohyal, which becomes the lesser cornu of the hyoid bone. The epihyal instead of changing into the stylohyoid ligament, may become osseous in structure and be firmly united to the hyoid bone or the process proper may develop to such an extent that only a few fibers of the ligament remain. The process may also be firmly united to the hyoid bone by bony union. The styloid process becomes completely ossified between the twentieth and thirtieth year.

It is interesting to consider the influence of the variation in the length of the styloid process upon the voice. The length of the styloid process varies in individuals and as long as the process is directed downward and parallel with the carotid artery, probably no trouble other than disease of the bone may be expected; however, if the process is deflected inward, from its natural development or from traumatism, more or less voice affection and irritation in the throat may occur.

According to Gruber, the normal length of the styloid process is about one and one-quarter inches. The styloid process was observed to be two inches long by Hildebrandt, Meckel, Cruveilhier and Humphrey, and in the old museum at Wilna, Winslow observed one process three inches long. Gruber examined over two thousand skulls and in this number found one specimen with a styloid three inches long, eleven were nearly two inches, and the remainder were near the normal.

Interesting as the study of the styloid process may be, it is of special importance to the laryngologist because of the pathologic sequences which have their origin in, or are the sequelae of, the process. For convenience, and because heretofore no classification has appeared, as far as I know, diseases of the styloid process may be divided into the following classes:

1. Inflammation.
2. Necrosis.
3. Deflection (producing obstruction in swallowing and disturbance in speech).
4. Fracture.
5. Exostosis.

INFLAMMATION AND NECROSIS.

von Thaden reports the case of a woman thirty-five years of age, who suddenly and without any apparent cause, was attacked with pain in the right ear and tinnitus aurium, followed in a few hours by swelling in the retromaxillary region of the affected side, extending into the cheek and neck, causing almost impossibility of swallowing. On the eighth day an abcess ruptured into the oral cavity and discharged a quantity of foul smelling pus. A week later the pus reaccumulated and an incision five centimeters long, following the sternocleidomastoid muscle, was made, evacuating pus and decayed cellular tissue. Examination showed the pus cavity to extend to, and surround, the styloid process, which was roughened and covered with softened tissue. Recovery followed with the exception of a partial facial paralysis, which followed the onset of the infection.

DEFLECTION.

Because the articulation with the temporal bone may be bony or fibrinous, deflection of the styloid process may occur from natural development, or it may occur from traumatism, due to fracture or injury to the neck from a fall or blow. Deflection of the process is of more especial interest because it is a condition which is probably more often observed than inflammation or necrosis. In many cases this condition is only observed following the removal of the tonsils. Physicians report observations of a bony pointed growth in the supratonsillar region after the removal of the tonsils, and also particles of bone removed at the time of the operation or in the tonsillar structure, without associating the bony structure with the styloid process. Since conditions of this character may occur, it would probably be wise to palpate the tonsils before attempting their removal, not alone for the detection of a deflected styloid process, but for abnormal pulsations in the tonsil or pharynx.

In the differentiation of hard immovable bodies in the lateral wall of the pharynx, Wyatt Wingrave (British Medical Journal, 1900) says, "The existence of the subpharyngeal cartilage of Luschka seems to have been overlooked. This structure is by no means rare, and from the frequency of its occurrence I am inclined to think that this body was probably mistaken for a displaced styloid process. The cartilage occurs not only in the lateral wall of the oropharynx, somewhat behind and below the faucial tonsil, but also in the tonsil itself, which I have often verified by microscopic examination, attention having been drawn to it by experiencing an exceptional resistance to the guillotine. It consists of hyaline cartilage embedded in a capsule of white fibrous tissue, and is supposed to be a vestige of the third post-oral arch."

The results of a deflected styloid process from fracture, abnormal elongation, or twisting from traumatism, may be obstruction in swallowing, painful deglutition, disturbances in voice, sensation of a tumor in the tonsillar region, and the presence of a hardened, blunt-pointed object, which is detected upon compression of the tonsil or the surrounding tonsillar region. The symptoms enumerated are usually progressive in character and are confined to one side.

Rethi of Vienna (Internationale klinische Rundschau, 1888) reports two cases observed by Professor Weinlechner, with the general symptoms as enumerated. In one instance, Dr. Weinlechner made compression with his finger inserted in the mouth, sufficient to fracture the process, when all symptoms disappeared. However, after nine months the irritation in the throat returned. By making compression again, the process was fractured in two places and the symptoms disappeared entirely.

In the second case, patient age forty-six years, Professor Weinlechner reported that at the lower end of the left tonsil and near the palatoglossus muscle, a hard knob was felt, which was painful to the touch. He tried to fracture the bone, but did not succeed, all symptoms remaining.

Rethi reports his own case: a man of twenty-eight years began to have progressive irritation in the left tonsil, producing great pain and distress in deglutition and necessitating medical assistance. The styloid process was removed by splitting the tonsil, followed by relief of the symptoms.

In my own case, a physician of thirty years, a veteran of the Spanish-American war, in his personal report of the case said that on September 30, 1907, he was thrown from a wagon, striking his head and shoulders and fracturing the first and second metacarpal bones of the left hand. His neck was very stiff and painful for a couple of weeks. On December 1, 1907, he began to suffer from hoarseness in the afternoon and evening, with little or no hoarseness in the morning. This condition continued until the latter part of December, when he could hardly speak above a whisper. There was no pain present. During the months of January and February following, there was nearly complete aphonia. He took mineral baths for the condition and while engaged in this treatment, discovered that the left tonsil was enlarged, with a hard growth immediately beneath it. The tonsil and growth were cauterized and the aphonia was partially relieved until April, when it again appeared. There began now a sensation of constriction in the throat when speaking or singing. The singing voice was almost lost. The growth beneath the tonsil was now so prominent that by depressing the tongue he could readily see it. Pressure upon the growth caused pain and irritation.

On June 24th, 1908, I examined this patient. A distinct mass with small blunt point could be seen beneath the tonsil, and by palpation I could readily outline the hardened bone, external and posterior to the tonsil. X-ray photograph gave us the accompanying picture, which distinctly shows two elongated styloid processes with a large exostosis on the one, presumably the left, due, we think, to the fracture of the process, which, from the history of the case, one is justified in concluding occurred at the time of the alleged injury, producing the symptoms enumerated.

Under local anesthesia, the tip of the process was first exposed, in doing which the inferior aspect of the tonsil was loosened, and the tonsil entirely removed, leaving the process exposed. Reflecting the anterior pillar and with a narrow ringed tongue depressor, the process was encircled and the tissues lifted as far as possible from the process without injuring the surrounding structures, and with a bone forceps, the process was severed. The portion removed measured one and one-quarter inches in length. The patient made an uninterrupted though slow recovery.

FRACTURE AND EXOSTOSIS.

From the foregoing enumeration of cases, it is readily perceptible that fracture may occur from any traumatism, and if the process is deflected, serious consequences may follow. With a history of traumatism of the head and neck, followed by throat symptoms, we should always take into consideration the possibility of injury to the styloid process and its influence upon these symptoms.

Exostosis and neoplasms of the process, though infrequent, may likewise be encountered and may be mistaken for disease of the neighboring lymph glands. Surrounded as the styloid process is by tissue susceptible to infection, it is reasonable to presume that the process is more often involved that we may now suspect. Abscesses designated now as peritonsillar or quinsy, in which foul pus is evac-

uated, should be looked upon with suspicion as having
their origin in or about the styloid process.

REFERENCES.

1. L'Echo Medicale, 1901.
2. Deutsche Zeitschrift fuer Chirurgie, 1874-75.
  . Virchow's Archives, 1870.
     Dublin Journal of Medical Science, 1873.
  . Internationale klinische Rundschau. 1888.
 . British Medical Journal, 1900.
7. Embryology (Heisler).

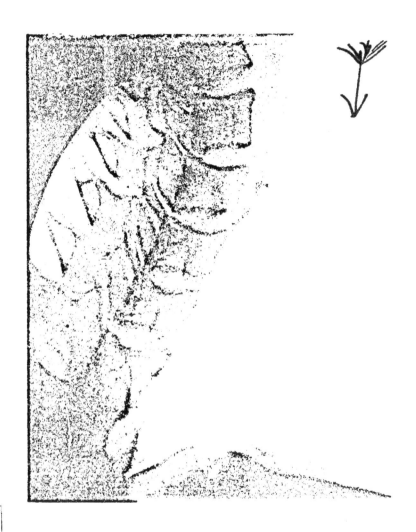

XII.

CASE OF DOUBLE MASTOIDITIS FOLLOWED BY LEFT SIGMOID SINUS AND JUGULAR VEIN THROMBOSIS. OPERATION. RECOVERY.

By John F. Barnhill, M. D.,

PROFESSOR OF OTO-LARYNGOLOGY, INDIANA UNIVERSITY SCHOOL OF MEDICINE,

INDIANAPOLIS.

Francis D——, age 16, Vincennes, Ind., was brought to the Deaconess Hospital by her family physician, Dr. Jones, February 26, 1908. A night trip had been made in order to reach the hospital early, the patient's condition being one of emergency. The history of the case was, briefly, as follows: The young lady had suffered from a severe attack of measles five weeks ago, at which time both ears discharged. In three weeks she had so far recovered from the measles that she was able to sit up a part of each day, and Dr. Jones had believed it unnecessary to continue his visits. On February 24, two days preceding the date of the patient's entering the hospital, the doctor was called on account of rigors, high temperature, double vision, fainting on attempts to rise up in bed, and especially on account of the rather profound deafness and unbearable pain in the region of both mastoid processes. The temperature was at this time 104° F., the pulse rapid and weak, there was exquisite tenderness over both mastoids and both ears were discharging very profusely. Mastoid surgery was advised and the patient was hurried to the hospital.

I saw the case at 8:00 a. m. February 26, and found conditions as above stated. The temperature remained at 104° F., the mastoid tenderness being still very acute, the discharge from the ears very profuse, the diplopia marked and the prostration very great. A double mastoid operation was advised just as soon as the patient could be properly prepared, and at 1:00 p. m. the same day both mastoids were thoroughly cleaned out and free communication was established between the mastoid wound and middle ears of each side for the purpose of securing free drainage from every infected cavity. The entire operation lasted only 50 minutes. The patient took the ether rather badly, and at the conclusion was weak and much cyanosed, on which account oxygen was administered by inhalation. The cellular structure of the left mastoid contained pus everywhere, whereas the osseous structures of the right contained but a few drops but were found much softened, and on the whole it was a question as to which was most diseased.

The temperature at 5:00 p. m. was 99.4° F., pulse 70 and general condition good. It was at that time believed that the foci of infection had been entirely removed and that rapid recovery might be reasonably expected. The temperature remained below 101 until noon February 25, when it was 102.4° F., and at 1:00 p. m. it was 104.2°. Chilly sensations were recorded as preceding the last temperature rise. Phenacetine was ordered in gr. iii doses, and, when the temperature should subside to 102°, gr. x of quinin sulphate in three doses one-half hour apart.

For the next week the temperature ranged between 99 and 104. March 2, 3 and 4 the temperature did not exceed 101.4, the general condition was good, the mastoid wounds were healing rapidly and a careful analysis of the situation indicated the convalescent stage. March 5, however, the temperature again rose to 104, and on March 7 to 105.5. Operation for the relief of sinus thrombosis was performed March 8.

Subsequent to the mastoid operation the patient complained of absolutely no pain, the mentality was at all times acute, and several times during my visit she would recite off-hand verses of poetry which she seemed to compose on the spur of the moment, and which had both sense and melody in them. At no time did any symtoms other than the septic curve of the temperature and the slight chilly sensations point to sinus thrombosis. Such a complication was, however, suspected from the first, but since the mastoid tissues of each side had been equally septic, and each had been thoroughly exenterated it seemed impossible to determine which sinus, and which side, might be causing the trouble. Malaria was considered and quinia administered in large doses without effect. The abdomen was at first distended and tender, and typhoid fever or appendicitis was thought of but at once eliminated. On the fifth day after the mastoid operation a blood examination showed

Hemoglobin 65
Red cells 3,360,000
Leukocytes 18,000

Differential count:
Polymorphoneuclear 80%
Lymphocytes 20%

No examination of the eyegrounds were at any time made. Except on the day of admission to the hospital, when diplopia was present, no complaint whatever was made of any eye difficulty.

At the time of the operation for sinus thrombosis the left side was chosen for the rather illy defined belief that this was the worse of the two. The old mastoid wound was curetted and as thoroughly cleansed as it was possible to do. The soft structures were incised to the bone backwardly from the line of old incision, and the skull was thus laid bare over a large area by the reflection of a superior and an inferior flap. With mallet and gauge the sigmoid sinus was widely exposed toward both the torcular and jugular ends. The vessel had an almost normal appearance, and felt soft and healthy to the touch. It was incised for a distance of almost two inches, the upper end being filled with a firm coagulum, while the jugular end contained creamy pus. In order to avoid carrying this septic material to parts of the vessel which contained flowing blood, all of the exposed contents of the sinus were removed before efforts at curettage of either the upper or lower ends were attempted. The clot was easily dislodged from the torcular end by means of the curette, but no fluid blood could be secured from the direction of the jugular bulb. The mastoid wound was therefore packed with gauze, the instruments and hands sterilized, and the internal jugular vein was exposed from the entrance of the thyroid vein upward. It was found thrombosed from the entrance of the facial vein upward, and hence was ligated below the facial and completely resected above as far as possible. A small cigarette drain was inserted the full length of the neck-wound, the whole extent of which was immediately sutured except the point of exit of the drain. The temperature became normal in three days, the neck-wound healed by first intention and the cavity into the mastoid and sinus was completely filled in four weeks.

There were three interesting points connected with this case: (1) It was decidedly atypical, since there was never a pronounced chill, no sweating and no pain except that due to the mastoiditis. The only prominent symptom present after the mastoid operation was the septic temperature. (2) The appearance and feel of the sigmoid and lateral sinuses were almost normal, although when extensively incised they were entirely filled with clot and pus. (3) Owing to the fact that both mastoids were about equally involved it was difficult to state with certainty on which side of the head the thrombosis existed, and this point was of course not definitely settled until the sinus was uncovered and incised.

XIII.

OBSTRUCTED NASAL RESPIRATION AND ITS RELATION TO DENTAL DEFORMITIES.*

BY JOHN HOWARD ALLEN, M. D.,

PORTLAND, MAINE.

A consideration of the influence upon the teeth of factors external to the mouth, brings to the attention the constantly widening scope of modern denistry; and while I do not feel competent, nor is this the occasion, to consider such a subject, I hope I may be pardoned if I preface this discussion of the relation of impaired nasal respiration to the dental structures with a word in regard to the relation of the practice of dentistry to that of medicine. I am not sufficiently familiar with the trend of dental thought to know whether the question of an alliance of denistry with medicine is favorably regarded or not. Very likely there are many present who are able to look forward somewhat definitely to such a coalition at a not distant time. There seems to be no more reason for giving over to an independent profession the care of the mouth and teeth than for a similar disposition of the eye or ear. If the oculist needs also to be a physician, no less does the dentist. Surely the relation borne by the oral cavity to the general organism is as intimate and as important as is that of the ear or the nose, and dentistry has as much claim to be considered a specialty in the practice of medicine as has otology or ophthalmology.

No phase of the ever-broadening field of dentistry is more eloquent of the changes which are taking place in its practice, than is the development of preventive dentistry. Preventive medicine, as it is termed, has come to be recognized as the highest and worthiest branch of medical art, and with the introduction of preventive dentistry the dental

---

*Read before the Northeastern Dental Association, at its annual meeting in Portland, Me., October 16, 1907.

profession allies itself with that which is best in medicine. Physician or dentist, our art is the art of healing, but more and more are we learning to add to this the science of prevention. He who by the magic of his skill transforms a decayed and torturing tooth into a sound and painless member, with years of usefulness before it, is deserving of much gratitude from his patients. But he who by wise forethought and intelligent care is able to forestall pain and prevent decay is far more a benefactor, and deserving of greater praise. It cannot be doubted, either, that the doctor of dental surgery or the doctor of medicine who seeks to guard the welfare of his patients by the prevention of disease and the anticipation of deformity will have a higher standing in the community, and will not only deserve but receive more at its hands, than he who contents himself merely with the repair of injuries.

It is with the desire of directing attention to a condition which is perhaps responsible for more dental malformations than any other that this paper is written. The influence of enlarged adenoids upon the dental structures is a subject which, while it has received some attention at the hands of the dental profession, has, it seems to me, been accorded but a very small part of the consideration which it deserves; and I wish to emphasize the importance of this condition to the dentist, and urge the necessity of its early recognition and treatment, in order that the dental deformities which so commonly follow it may be prevented.

Obstructed nasal breathing is in my opinion the prime factor in the production of a large percentage of dental malformations.

There are several secondary factors, among the more important of which may be mentioned—loss of occlusion resulting from the parted jaws of the mouth-breather, and the pressure upon the lateral alveolar processes resulting from the increase of tension of the buccal muscles which obtains when the lower jaw is dropped.

I shall try to show that a large percentage, perhaps the majority, of dental deformities, whether consisting of a narrowed V-shaped upper arch, a unilaterally flattened arch, rotated or displaced teeth, or an undershot or so-called prognathous lower jaw, are directly or indirectly the result of impaired nasal breathing. In order to appreciate this statement we must consider the mechanism by which these changes are brought about.

In the first place, we have to take into consideration an elemental anatomic condition, viz.: that the floor of the nose and the median portion of the palatal arch are composed of the same bony structures—the palate processes of the maxilla and the horizontal plates of the palate bone; and secondly, a well-established biologic truth—which is, that any organ which is not used does not properly develop. To the latter law the nasal cavity is no exception.

Interference with nasal breathing during the period of the body's growth necessarily inhibits the development of the nasal structures. Through impairment of function the organ fails to expand, and in a mouth-breathing child of twelve the intranasal dimensions may be but little greater than they were at the age of five or six. In a normally developing child, as the nasal structures increase in size the distance from the cribriform plate of the ethmoid to the floor of the nose gradually increases, but in a mouth-breather growth in this direction, as in all others within the nose, is restricted. As related to the other bones of the face, we find the floor of the nose and the roof of the mouth assuming a constantly higher position. The roof of the mouth is anchored, so to speak, to a dwarfed nose. The alveolar processes of the maxilla, on the contrary, are more affected in the direction than in the extent of their growth. Being somewhat outside the zone of restricted growth, they are able to develop freely in a downward direction, but their lateral expansion is interfered with by the pull of their connection with the central portion of the hard palate.

We have, then, as a result of the forces operating as described, the median portion of the palate held high up in its early premature position. The alveolar processes, less restricted in their development, lengthen and enlarge, but are drawn to a greater or less extent toward the median line, obliterating the broad dome shape of the hard palate and converting it into a narrow inverted U or V shape. Such a palatal arch is necessarily narrow; sometimes more constricted upon one side than on the other, it is asymmetric or unilaterally flattened. Having less than the normal breadth, the teeth have insufficient room for eruption, and are rotated or displaced; the incisors are pushed forward and project, and in extreme cases, where the development of the entire jaw is sufficiently interfered with, we find the lower jaw, which has gone on in unrestricted growth, projecting beyond the upper. This, it seems to me, is the simple, natural, and entirely adequate explanation of the relation between mouth-breathing and the high-arched palate, and I have entered into it at some detail, not only because there seems to have been a great deal of misunderstanding and misinterpretation of the condition, but because a proper appreciation of the principles involved is necessary to a rational understanding and intelligent treatment of such cases.

ADENOIDS IN CHILDREN.

There is no condition in childhood which operates to produce nasal obstruction and mouth-breathing to anything like the extent adenoids do. The adenoid vegetations, so called, consist in an hypertrophy of the pharyngeal or so-called Luschka's tonsil, situated in the vault of the pharynx. When normal this tissue, of course, produces no ill effects, but when enlarged it is capable of producing a series of disturbances which for variety and far-reaching consequences is equalled, perhaps, by no other condition of disease. Adenoids are found at all ages, being occasionally seen in the new-born, while remnants of them have been observed in the septuagenarian. The condition more commouly manifests itself, however, between the ages of two and fourteen, and may then be found in all degrees of enlargement, from the slight thickening which produces but very few symptoms of any kind, to the enormous growths which completely block the posterior nares, and which, untreated, are capable of wrecking the development of a child physically, mentally, and even morally.

Under ordinary circumstances adenoids if untreated will atrophy and disappear at or about maturity; but this brings no encouragement to the situation, inasmuch as the damage caused by them will then be largely beyond repair. The removal of this obstruction in the nasopharynx at maturity, by atrophy, does not avail to restore normal breathing, because the nose, not having developed, is not sufficiently roomy to supply by this channel the air needed by the mature organism, and the bony formation of the face having become fixed at maturity no further natural enlargement is possible.

A familiar figure to the rhinologist is the mouth-breathing patient of mature years, whose nasopharynx is entirely innocent of adenoids, and yet who bears the indubitable evidence of their one-time presence. The partly open mouth; the nasal cavities of almost infantile proportions; the high-arched palate with protruding or overlapping incisors; together with the adenoid expression proclaiming the dulled mentality—all are eloquent of that which has gone before.

Pathologically several types of enlargement of this tonsil are recognized. The two most common are the soft and the hard varieties. The soft variety consists of an almost formless mass spread throughout the nasopharynx. It is pultaceous in feeling, friable in consistence, and crumbles and bleeds very easily before the examining finger. The hard variety is more resistant to the touch, though it bleeds with comparative ease, and possesses the typical lobulated form which has caused the sensation imparted by it to the finger to be likened to that of a bunch of angleworms. Both varieties, instead of being confined to the central portion of the nasopharynx, are frequently found invading the fossa of Rosenmueller, in which location they press upon and produce congestion of the openings of the Eustachian tubes and are responsible for ear disturbances of various kinds. Sometimes they run so far down upon the posterior wall of the pharynx that they can be seen below the level of the soft palate, especially during the raising of the palate in gagging. In the rhinoscopic mirror they can be seen depending from the vault of the pharnyx, and to a greater or lesser extent encroaching upon the opening of the posterior nares.

The evil effects of enlarged adenoids, as has been intimated, are almost endless. I shall not try to enumerate them all, as such an attempt would probably exhaust your patience as well as my powers of description, but will content myself with calling attention to a few of the more common. When of sufficient size to be obstructive the most prominent symptom is the nasal obstruction with the attendant mouth-breathing which we have been considering, though oral deformities are not the only results of obstructed nose-breathing, nor are they the most serious. The consequences of impaired nasal respiration are numerous and far-reaching. One of the inevitable results of mouth-breathing is the admission to the throat and lungs of air that has not been properly prepared. Air passing through the nose is not only filtered but also warmed and moistened. By virtue of the large secreting surfaces of the turbinals the air is charged with moisture, and their extensive convolutions act with surprising efficacy as radiators in supplying it with heat. It has been shown that air breathed into the nose at zero temperature is raised to blood-heat by the time it reaches the posterior nares. It can be easily seen, then, that air taken directly through the mouth, without this preparation, must have a very injurious effect upon the mucous membranes with which it comes in contact. Inflammatory processes are set up in the pharynx, larynx, trachea, and bronchi, and the lung tissue is weakened and rendered more susceptible to various forms of disease, of which the "great white plague" is the most prominent. It can be readily understood, too, that this unnatural use of the mouth must result in alteration of its secretions and the production of a condition of dryness which will have a pernicious effect upon the teeth.

One of the most constant, and to the otologist and rhinologist the most important, of the phenomena attending the adenoid condition is impairment of hearing. In just what way adenoids operate to affect the organ of hearing is a disputed question and one which cannot be entered into here, but deafness of considerable degree is very frequently caused by them, while acute inflammations of the middle ear often occur, with an occasional final result in mastoiditis, chronic suppurative otitis media, brain abscess, meningitis, or sinus thrombosis. The operation for adenoids in children suffering from a considerable degree of deafness often results in a restoration of the hearing in a few days or weeks.

Neurotic and psychic disturbances of various kinds are constantly found, and range from a slight hebetude or inability to concentrate the attention, through nervousness, irritability, peevishness, and ill-temper, to mental dulness of an extreme type.

Nasal obstruction, mouth-breathing, the high-arched palate with dental deformities of all degrees; impairment of hearing, inflammation of the middle ear, and even death; the whole range of catarrhal conditions of the nose, throat, and lungs, and a broad and easy pathway laid for tuberculosis; impairment of the intellect, and mental and moral obliquities of many kinds—surely this is a mighty crop to spring from so small a seed! and yet this is but a part of the harvest.

Probably all are familiar with the extreme type of mouth-breathing which is produced by adenoids of large size. There is the open mouth with dropped jaw; the crowded teeth and dull eyes. The nostrils not being in use are collapsed and flattened. The muscles whose function it is to keep open and dilate the nostrils being atrophied, that part of the face about the nose and the upper lip has a peculiar dead and expressionless appearance. Such cases are not uncommon, and the diagnosis may be made from across the street. It is not always so easy, however. Not every child who is ill-tempered, deaf, or even a mouth-breather, has adenoids; and it may be said at the same time that many a child has adenoid obstruction and breathes with slightly parted lips, who would not ordinarily be suspected of mouth-breathing.

Fortunately for the dentist, however, he does not need to concern himself with the niceties of diagnosis in regard to this condition, and need only inquire into the matter when he is confronted with dental malformations associated with a high-arched palate. And again, fortunately, there is no single external indication of the presence of adenoids more diagnostic than the high-arched palate, of the existence and degree of which no one, of course, can better judge than the dentist. Having, then, a high-arched palate, what other signs or symptoms may we look for to justify or dispel our suspicion of adenoids? I shall speak of but five, which are the most common, and which in all ordinary cases will suffice to make a diagnosis.

SOME SIGNS SUGGESTING THE PRESENCE OF ADENOIDS.

The first is mouth-breathing. Often it is evident enough, but in other cases the child must be watched carefully to determine its presence. When there is doubt, the mother should make careful observation at night to see if the child sleeps with the mouth entirely closed. Many children breathe properly during the day who breathe through the mouth at night.

Second in importance come affections of the ears. Inquiry should be made as to the presence of deafness and the occurrence of earaches.

Third. Frequent colds, often associated with a slight cough, are very common in children with adenoid vegetations, and their occurrence even without other symptoms should arouse our suspicion.

Fourth. Is the child backward in mental development? Children having adenoids are as a rule behind their classes in school.

Fifth. Nervous symptoms. Is the child a so-called "nervous child"? Is he subject to night terrors, and does he wet the bed? There are a hundred other manifestations of an unstable nervous system, but these are the common ones.

These symptoms of course are not all found in every case, but there are usually present more than one, and sometimes all are seen together. Absolute information as to the extent and location of the growth can be obtained as a rule in but one way. Digital examination is not difficult, and with a little experience can be made so rapidly that little pain is inflicted. Nevertheless, such an examination always alarms children, and as the dentist is traditionally persona non grata to them, perhaps it would not be the part of wisdom to invest himself with any new horrors.

When it is necessary to make a digital examination, someone should grasp the child's hands; the doctor, standing behind it, should hold the head firmly in the hollow of his left arm; the palm and fingers of his left hand are placed under the chin, and the child being asked to open the mouth widely, the thumb of the left hand presses the cheek between the teeth so that the mouth cannot be closed. The index finger of the right hand is then introduced behind the soft palate and into the nasopharynx, the posterior border or the septum is felt for and the finger swept from side to side, covering the entire surface of the nasopharynx and outlining any growth which may be present. Such an examination, if adenoids be present, usually causes bleeding from the nose, and the examining finger is found to be covered with blood.

There is but one method of treatment worth considering; radical removal is quick, safe. and effectual. It should be attempted, however, only by an operator thoroughly competent in such work, as partial removal usually means recurrence and the necessity for further operations, while the danger of inflicting damage upon the mouths of the Eustachian tubes by unskilful instrumentation in the nasopharynx is considerable.

In conclusion, it should be unnecessary to say that I do not intend to assert that all high-arched palates are the result of nasal obstruction, nor that all·nasal obstruction is due to adenoids, but I think it is beyond question that a large percentage of this class of deformities is the result of adenoid obstruction, and that the dentist who fails to take it into account does his patients and himself a serious injustice. Any attempt to correct dental deformities resulting from this condition, without first removing the cause, is working against the forces of nature, and must result in only partial success, or in many cases a recurrence of the condition which may have been overcome by such tedious and painful efforts. If, on the contrary, the causative factor is recognized and removed as a preliminary step in corrective work, nature's powerful aid is enlisted in behalf of the operator, and with the establishment of nasal breathing and the normal development of the nose, the dentist may be assured that he is paddling with the current and not against it, and that—the wonderful achievements of orthodontia being established upon a rational basis—corrections once made will stay corrected.

XIV.

SOME OBSERVATIONS ON THE ACOUSTIC FUNC-
TION OF THE EAR.*

By Ernest de Wolfe Wales, B. S., M. D., (Harvard),

CLINICAL PROFESSOR OF OTOLOGY, LARYNGOLOGY AND RHIN-
OLOGY, INDIANA UNIVERSITY SCHOOL OF MEDICINE.

The most important office of the otologist is to improve
the acoustic function of the ear. It is self-evident that
where life is endangered, the life becomes more important
than the function of hearing, but this is fortunately a rare
condition. To improve the acoustic function of the ear the
otologist, to work intelligently, must make hearing tests.
We all know how many reports of cases in otology are
without scientific usefulness because of lack of adequate
hearing tests. I know of clinics where hearing tests are
never practiced and old chronic cases are treated year after
year without benefit. It helps to swell the number of old
cases treated. What would we think of an oculist who
applied glasses without testing the vision? It is just as
necessary for the otologist to find out the limits of the
hearing field. Hearing tests enable us to make a better
diagnosis, to give prognosis, and it is the most important
means by which we can say that our treatment is doing
good. It is untruthful to tell a patient that he has improved just because he thinks he has; it is not honest to
tell a patient that treament will improve his hearing because we do not know; we must experiment, and before
and after the experiment we need careful tests. If the
patient has otosclerosis which can only be diagnosed by
hearing tests, tell him so and get rid of him and later
after having spent time and money with many doctors he
will come back to you wishing he had taken your advice.
If a patient has total deafness in one ear from labyrinth

*Read before the joint meeting of the Western and Middle
Sections of the American Laryngological, Rhinological and Otological Society, at Chicago, February 23, 1909.

diseases we can establish the fact by the experiment of Voss. This experiment will save the patient many unnecessary visits. In a progressive deafness we have no way of estimating the rate of progression without hearing tests and many times the patient comes to us having had much treatment but never any hearing tests. We have all had cases where the patient had been treated for cerumen in the canal, instead of treatment for a catarrhal deafness overlooked for want of a hearing test.

Our facilities are often poor for testing the hearing, perhaps our offices are small and noisy, possibly our voices are husky and our articulation not plain, but nevertheless tests under these adverse conditions are valuable because the tests are relative and each doctor must establish his own standard. Deaf people are deaf or considered so because they do not hear what a normal hearing person hears. We do not have voices of uniform pitch or clear cut articulation.

Hearing tests with the tuning forks are very imperfect, but so is the hearing of most of us. Our patients are not all trained musicians. In testing we do not consider the temperature, the barometric pressure, air currents, external noises or the state of the patient. Our instruments are not all made by Edelmann and few of us possess the Bezold-Edelmann series of tuning forks, but for all practical purposes, the Hartmann set of forks with a fork of 80 v. s. and the Galton whistle are usually sufficient. I will not deal with the technic of the different tests in this paper. Dr. George Bönninghaus in his "Lehrbuch der Ohrenheilkunde" has written best on this subject.

Let us consider the C_1 fork of 512 v. s. It is impossible even with the aid of magnets to set the tuning fork in vibration with equal intensity, for changes in the electric current, the temperature, the barometric pressure, and in the wear of the fork itself, are constantly taking place. Ostmann inserts a separator between the arms of the fork, Gradenigo ties a lead weight by a string to one of the arms, then burns the string to get uniform intensity. A weight of 500 grams gives ten times the intensity of 50 grams. If a patient hears with his diseased ear, a sound made by 500 grams weight and a normal ear hears the same fork with a weight of 10 gr. the acuity of the deaf ear is

1/50 of the normal ear; 2/100. The low forks including 512 v. s. may be pressed together between the thumb and forefinger, slipping the fingers off at a given time. This gives a fairly uniform intensity. Hitting the forks against blocks of cork or the palm of hand loosens the clamps and the fork is soon worthless. The tone produced by the fork has the same pitch in the handle as in any part of the arms but the intensity varies; in other words the wave lengths are equal but the amplitude varies. The greatest sensation of loudness of sound is at right angles to the broad or I side or at right angles to the narrow or U side, near the prongs; these intensities are equal, but the intensity of sound grows less as the ear approaches the handle of the fork. One cannot listen to a sound of a given intensity and then distinguish a sound which has half that intensity; all one can say is that the intensity is greater or less than a given intensity. Turning the tuning fork in its vertical axis, we find four nodes where the sound is only slightly heard or not heard at all. By interference the waves neutralize with each other. The I side must begin with a crest and the U side with a hollow so the waves cancel each other.

Another interesting fact about the 512 v. s. tuning fork is that if the fork is set in vibration and the handle is carried into the external auditory canal the sound will be heard as long as that of the weighted end of the fork. Therefore I find it more satisfactory to make the air-conduction hearing tests with a combined fork and rubber tube. Take a rubber tube two or three feet long which fits snugly over the handle of the hearing fork. On the end which is placed in the patient's auditory canal I insert one of Jansen's tips. A 512 v. s. fork heard 50 seconds by the usual method will be heard about 50 seconds by the tube method with the further advantage of non-interference with the vibrating fork. There is no danger of touching the auricle or hairs of the tragus. The wavy hair falling over women's ears is very annoying at times. With the tube method there can be no variation in intensity according to the position in which the fork is held. The rubber tube is slipped over the handle about half an inch and the fingers hold the part of the handle covered by the rubber, so that the part in contact with the fingers is fairly constant.

Below is a table worked out from the ordinary imperfect tuning forks found on the market, called Hartmann's set, together with a low fork of 80 v. s. and F_4 fork. We can feel, see and hear the vibrating tuning fork. We hear it in two ways, by air and so-called bone-air conduction. We can see the vibrations without special devices only when looking at the U side of low vibrating forks.

Forks.	Tactile time. Thumb and Forefinger.	Sight.	Hearing. Bone-air Conduction.	Hearing. Air Conduction.
80 v. s.	8″	7″	3″	6″
C 256 v. s.	55″	30″	38″	90″
C_1 512 v. s.	30″	15″	25″	50″
C_2 1024 v. s.	10″	0″	20″	40″
C_3 2048 v. s.	0″	0″	8″	45″
C_4 4096 v. s.	0″	0″	0″?	35″
F_4 4720 v. s.	0″	0″	0″?	22″

It will be seen that the tactile pressure sense is of greater duration than the sense of sight and greater than bone-air conduction up to C_2. Bone-air conduction with C_2 and C_3 forks becomes confused because the sound is heard by air conduction.

Normally we hear by one method, namely by air, but pathologically we may be helped by bone-air conduction. The proof is easy from an anatomic and physical point of view. Let us first take a tuning fork and cause it to vibrate, then place it on different parts of the body. Roughly speaking the fork is heard longer, the nearer it approaches the external auditory canal. The intensity of the sound varies according to the pressure with which it is held against the body; that is, up to a certain degree, the greater the pressure the louder the sound. The fork is heard more distinctly when the handle is placed squarely on the pressed surface. Tipping the fork varies the intensity of the sound. The fork is heard loudest and longest when the base is pressed firmly and squarely on the surface of the tested part. All forks vary in duration, even those of the same pitch. The fork is heard for a certain length of time on the patella, longer time on the sternum, still longer over the lower part of the nasal bones, sometimes longer against the upper incisor teeth and longest over the condyle of the mandible, just anterior to the tragus. The mastoid fossa position without contact with the auricle is of shorter duration in most cases than the nasal vomer position. The velocity of sound is faster in the perilymph than in the air and faster in bone than in fluid but the distances in the human body are so short, and our estimation of time is so slow that this factor plays no part in our sense of hearing. It is not normal to hear by bone conduction. If we did hear by bone-air condition the sounds taken up from the ground and the floors in large buildings, carriages or trains would be unbearable. Even our own voices would destroy our hearing. Barth says, "that autophonia is a pathological condition existing where the Eustachian tube is wide open or where the external auditory canal is stopped up. By auscultation, the hearing tube conveys the increased sound to the examiner." The boiler maker suffers because he can't make use of his bone conduction. Nature has protected us by placing the auditory hair cells in endolymph, surrounded by perilymph of the scala vestibuli on one side and the scala tympani on the other; then comes the dense hard bone of the cochlea, and around the cochlea there are air cells or at least diploetic cells filled with marrow, and then more dense bone, and brain, mueles, or air cavities according to directions. I consider the large blood vessels the most important dampening factor. The carotid artery and the numerous blood sinuses all tend to carry away any encroaching sound. The sound made by the pulsation of the ⹁neighboring carotid artery is probably diffused by the surrounding plexus of small veins. Whenever the equilibrium of the ossicular chain is interfered with, bone conduction is prolonged, therefore bone-air conduction is of great importance to the otologist as a record of the pathology and also the acoustic function of the ear. Tonietti* says, that bone conduction is shortened in chronic alcoholism, general paralysis, brain syphilis, epilepsy, and traumatic neuroses.

Simulation is a very interesting subject. Those who simulate deafness, partial, total or one-sided deafness, are

*Arch. ital. di otol., etc., Vol. xviil, fasc. 6.

easily detected by repeated tuning fork tests. One can go quietly to work and the faker cannot tell what he should answer and soon becomes confused. The brush experiment of Gowseeff† is very good to detect those who simulate total deafness. After blindfolding a soldier, who claimed to be totally deaf in one ear I found he would only hear the whispered voice when I held my finger resting on his shoulder, so I substituted a hooked umbrella for my finger which I rested on his shoulder and he heard me when I was twenty-five feet away.

---

†Zelt, f. Ohren., LI. 3, p. 280, 1906.

XV.

A THEORY ON THE FUNCTION OF THE MIDDLE EAR MUSCLES, RESULTING IN A MODIFICATION OF THE THEORY OF HEARING*.

By Ernest de Wolfe Wales, B. S., M. D., (Harvard),

CLINICAL PROFESSOR OF OTOLOGY, LARYNGOLOGY AND RHINOLOGY, INDIANA UNIVERSITY SCHOOL OF MEDICINE.

The muscles of the tympanum are not fully understood. According to Dr. Robert Wiedersheim[1] on the auditory organs of mammals, "Two striated muscles are present in connection with the middle ear. The phyletically older stapedius, arises from the wall of the tympanic cavity and is inserted into the stapes, serving to keep the membrane of the fenestra vestibuli stretched. It is supplied by the facial nerve and corresponds to the dorsal portion of the deep constrictor inserted on the hyoid in fishes, from which the hinder belly of the biventor of mammals also arises. A tensor tympani, supplied by the mandibular division of the trigeminal and derived from the system of the adductor mandibulae (pars pterygoidea)†, also arises from the wall of the tympanic cavity, and is inserted on the manubrium of the malleus, serving to stretch the tympanic membrane."

v. Hensen[2] says, "The question of whether the Eustachian tube is wide open or closed is not yet wholly settled. Lucae has observed respiratory movements, and by in-

---

*Read before the joint meeting of the Western and Middle Sections of the American Laryngological, Rhinological and Otological Society, at Chicago, February 23, 1909.

†"In Man the tensor tympani is from the first connected with the tensor veli palatini muscle. In Ornithorhynchus it has a double origin, one part being continuous with the pharyngeal muscles and the other arising independently. A stapedius muscle is wanting in Ornithorhynchus and Echidna, and a tensor tympani in Manis; and in all these three animals the tympanic cavity is subdivided into an upper and lower portion by a horizontal septum of connective tissue."

spection, bulging was more frequent than retraction. Helmholz, believed the tube to be closed, and that only compressed air entered the middle ear." On the function of the muscles of the middle ear apparatus, Hensen and Bockendahl have experimented to determine the amount of movement made by the tensor tympani during its reaction to sound. The tympanic cavity was opened and a light, sensitive lever inserted in the tendon of the tensor tympani muscle. The higher the note, the greater the contraction. Bockendahl found that once the needle remained stationary under the influence of a continuous sound. It could have occurred through unfavorable insertion of the needle, or an actual long contraction (tetanic). In Hensen's experiments the needle sank back to a state of rest when a continuous tone was sounded. Pollock, confirmed these experiments. He found that the reaction disappeared completely with the destruction of both labyrinths. Hammerschlag experimented on cats and dogs and found that the action of the tensor reflex from the acoustic to the trigeminus nucleus, is by the corpus trapezoideus and not by the striae acousticae. Hensen, first observed that after hearing a very weak tone, if the ear was closed and again opened after a short time, the tone would again be heard. Hensen holds this for an accommodative phenomena. He found too, that a tone of 400 or more vibrations was clearly intensified, when at the same time a metronome was in action. When the beats were over 200 a minute the reaction stopped. That the membrana tympani was not in tension, but on the border between tension and relaxation and was made tense by the sound of the metronome could not be excluded or the other possibility, that of a pure contrast action could not be excluded. J. Mueller believes that these muscles act as sound dampners and protectors. Hensen shows that if an explosion is not known beforehand, and if the muscles served as a guardian angel, causing a contraction before the sound impulse struck the ear, it would be a false protector, for a tense membrane would be more easily torn than a relaxed membrane. Protection would only take place during relaxation, and then, even the labyrinth would be more protected. "Politzer[3] has experimentally proved that the action of the tensor is not confined to the membrana tympani alone, but also the

labyrinth, inasmuch as he observes a motion of the fluid
in the labyrinth on electrical irritation of the root of the
trigeminus. The tensor tympani therefore increases the
pressure in the labyrinth. The stapedius muscle, on the
other hand, must be regarded as the antagonist of the tensor
tympani, as the author has shown by irritation of the
facial nerve in the cranial cavity (Wiener Med. 1878); it
relaxes the tympanic membrane, and diminishes the pressure in the labyrinth." McKendrick[4] says, "From experiments conducted hitherto, we can only state that one of
the principal functions of the intratympanic muscles is to
relieve alterations in the position and tension of the ossicular chain and abnormal pressure in the labyrinth which
are brought about by the variable fluctuations in the air
pressures in the external and middle ear. They, therefore,
regulate the degree of tension of the hearing apparatus."
"When the tensor tympani contracts, the membrana tympani becomes more tense. The normal stimulus which
causes the tensor tympani to contract is the pressure of
sound waves on the membrana tympani. Although the
innervation of the membrane has not been conclusively
established there is little doubt that it is supplied with
sensory nerves by the fifth, and also by the tympanic
plexus, formed by fibres derived from the otic ganglion,
from the petrosal ganglion of the glossopharyngeal, and
from the carotid plexus. When pressure is made on the
membrana, there is irritation of these sensory nerves, followed by a reflex contraction of the tensor tympani, supplied by a motor filament from the motor division of the
fifth nerve." (See experiments of Hensen and Bockendahl[2].) "The tensor tympani also contracts during yawning. In a few cases the muscle appears to be under the
control of the will. We have no direct evidence of any
reflex excitation of the stapedius, but one would expect
it to respond in a manner analogous to the response of the
tensor tympani. Lucae first observed that the contraction
of certain muscles of the face, most easily the musculus
orbicularis oculi, can produce a simultaneous contraction
of the stapedius. This is made evident by a deep humming
sound in the ear, and also a relaxation of the tympanic
membrane as shown by the manometer. During such re-

flex contractions the perception for the lower and middle tones of the tuning forks is discontinued."

G. Bönninghaus[5] says, "The hypotheses are many as to the function of the muscles of the midle ear apparatus. It is generally thought that the muscles give a moderate tension to the sound conducting apparatus which is best suited for vibrations, and besides exercises a kind of accommodation analagous to the intrinsic muscles of the eye. Now, on the existence of this accommodation, opinions differ widely, although all acceptors take for a basis of accommodation, that the stapedius is the antagonist of the tensor; that, therefore, the foot plate of the stapes is raised out of the labyrinth (Politzer); whereas the action of the tensor pushes the foot plate in, an opinion which is very doubtful because the stapedius, as actual antagonist, is much too weak. A further criticism however on these opinions would be an unthankful task while the whole knowledge of accommodation is today the darkest point in the physiology of the ear."

These theories fail to meet the requirements of sound conduction. A number of facts are collected without any definite idea of relation. My theory is as follows: The atmospheric pressure presses on the membrana tympani constantly by way of the external auditory canal; it presses from within on the membrana tympani by way of the Eustachian tube only when the tube is opened. The tube is opened during the act of deglutition by the action of the levator and tensor palati (dilator tubae). At the same time the soft palate is forced upward, compressing the air in the nasopharynx. This compression plus the existing atmospheric pressure and the increase in volume by heat and moisture sends the air into the anatomic middle ear, that is, the Eustachian tube, the tympanic cavity, the mastoid antrum and the pneumatic cells of the mastoid. What happens when this bolus of air is forced into the middle ear? The pressure in the middle ear becomes greater than the extratympanic (atmospheric) pressure, hence the head of the malleus is separated from the head of the incus, the liquid in the manometer of Politzer rises; then the tensor tympani muscle slowly contracts, due to the stretch of its tendon, and the head of the malleus again locks with the head of the incus; the fluid in the manometer falls. During this adjustment vibratory pressures (sounds) are poorly transmitted. Meanwhile the air in the middle ear is being absorbed while the work of the tensor tympani is growing less, due to the lessened intratympanic pressure. The absorption of air in the middle ear causes a continuous variation in pressure. As the intratympanic pressure lessens, the tensor tympani muscle gradually relaxes till the intratympanic pressure equalizes the extratympanic pressure when both tensor tympani and stapedius muscles are at rest. Now the absorption of air continues, and the intratympanic pressure becomes less than the extratympanic pressure. The stapedius muscle begins its work to keep the foot plate from being pushed into the vestibular window, and again to establish the equilibrium of the ossicular chain. Soon, due to reflex action, another swallow takes place and the tensor tympani begins its work again while the stapedius muscle rests. (See diagram.) At the time of deglutition the stapedius muscle relaxes and the tensor tympani muscle contracts.

What are the advantages of this theory? They are many, for it gives us a rational physiologic action of muscles. These muscles do not act primarily to keep certain membranes tense or adapt them to certain sounds but to equalize constant pressures, and this adaptation to constant pressures brings about an ideal tension of the whole drum-ossicular apparatus causing this apparatus to be in a state of equilibrium, the best possible condition to conduct any and all sounds. What would result if the Eustachian tube remained open? If we had patent tubes, we would hear our own voices, as if we talked in a barrel, besides the tensor tympani and stapedius muscles would soon cease to act; for the tensor tympani would have to be in a state of constant contraction to overcome the slightly increased intratympanic pressure over the extratympanic pressure due to the increased volume by heat and moisture. Without contraction of the tensor there would be no tension and so no equilibrium. The muscle would become hypertrophied, and then degenerate, while the fate of the stapedius muscle would be atrophy, from no work to do. Muscles must have their periods of rest. Thus you see these muscles are accommodative to intra- and extratympanic pressures and only indirectly subserve sound or vibratory pressures. Physiology has taught us that it takes time for a muscle to contract. We know that after swallowing it takes a short time to hear plainly again, and also after a patient's ears are inflated the tensor tympani may be some minutes or hours before it is able to overcome the intratympanic pressure and keep the head of the malleus in locked apposition with the head of the incus. Sounds do not wait. It is difficult to think of muscles accommodating themselves to sounds. We hear immediately. These muscles are too slow to accommodate our middle ear apparatus to the sounds of an orchestra but rather they keep the apparatus in an ideal state of equilibrium. While the tensor tympanic muscle was adjusting itself to the base violin, the piccolo would be lost, according to the old theories. An explosion has no consideration for the intrinsic muscles; it ruptures the drum membrane or wrecks the labyrinth if we are close enough. Even the ciliary muscle of the eye does not act immediately to a strong light, we may watch it contract. The function of the intrinsic muscles is to keep the middle ear apparatus in equilibrium so that vibratory pressures may be conveyed to the perilymph. It is ready at all times to receive the simplest to the most complex combinations of sound.

Let us consider the drum membrane itself. We have a membrane supplied with radial and circular elastic fibres, which takes care of itself and because of its elasticity it adapts itself to circumstances. When the intratympanic pressure is greater than the extratympanic pressure it bulges out into the auditory canal; when these pressures are equal it flattens out due to its elasticity, and when the extratympanic (atmospheric) pressure is greater than the intratympanic pressure it is pressed inward, and yet, due to the tension of the tensor tympanic muscle, the general shape of the membrana tympani is always cone or megaphone shaped. (See diagram.) I have already shown why the fluid in the manometer of Politzer rises and falls after deglutition. I believe that if the tensor tympani muscle reacts to sound that all muscles will react to sound. I consider the metronome tuning fork experiment a contrast reaction. I consider the contraction of the stapedius muscle when the eyes are tightly closed a defensive reflex. This action takes place when we expect an explosion or

a blow of some kind. The tensor tympani does not contract to make the membrana tympani more tense, the
normal stimulus is not the pressure of the sound waves,
but the tensor tympani muscle does contract for reasons
I have set forth in my theory.

How does deglutition take place? Dr. Foster[6] on the
submaxillary gland says, "In life, then, the flow of saliva
is brought about by the advent to the gland along the
chorda tympani of efferent impulses, started chiefly by
reflex actions." "Thus stimulation of the chorda brings
about two events: a dilatation of the blood vessels of the
gland and a flow of saliva." "When the cervical sympathetic is stimulated the vascular effects are the exact contrary of those seen when the chorda is stimulated. The
sympathetic therefore acts as a vasoconstrictor nerve, and
in this sense is antagonistic to the chorda." "Thus the
secretion of the parotid gland, like that of the submaxillary,
is governed by two sets of fibres, one of cerebro-spinal
origin, running along the auriculo-temporal branch of the
fifth nerve but originating possibly in the glosso-pharyngeal, and the other of sympathetic origin coming from the
cervical sympathetic." Dr. J. P. Morat[7] on deglutition
says, "At the entrance of the digestive paths we are confronted by an act which forms the transition between those
of external and those of internal function, that is deglutition, which commences with an act of conscious sensibility
and voluntary movement and is completed by reflex movements. Once again it is the medulla oblongata which is
the locality for the organization of the system subserving
deglutition, the conducting fibres, both sensory and motor,
of this system being met with in a certain number of
bulbar nerves, namely, the trigeminal (mylohyoid muscles), the facial, the hypoglossal, and the vago-spinal,
which perform the function of motor nerves connected
with sensory elements contained in the palatine nerves (of
the superior maxillary), the superior laryngeal nerves, and
lastly, the glossopharyngeal which are less essential than
the preceding. The point of departure is the irritation of
the bolus of food occurring at the level of the isthmus on
the extremities of the palatine nerves. The laryngeal
nerves intervene to defend the entrance of the respiratory
paths. The center of association of these different nerves

is situated between two planes of which the superior passes
through the acoustic tubercle and the inferior through the
apex of the calamus; according to Markwald, a little above
and outside of the grey wing, above the respiratory centre.
Sections made above or below the limits just pointed out
permit of the persistence of swallowing (life being maintained by artificial respiration)."

In establishing a swallowing reflex induced during negative intratympanic pressure I do not concern myself with
the tensor tympani muscle or the trigeminal palatal muscle,
the tensor palati (positive intratympanic pressure), but
with the phyletically older muscle, the stapedius. Near
the end of the negative pressure phase fatigue of the
stapedius muscle takes place, while the negative pressure
of the midle ear increases the blood supply of the peri-
neurium of the chorda tympani. This stimulation increases
the flow of saliva from the submaxillary and sublingual
glands, while stimulation of the glossopharyngeal nerve by
the same dilatation of vessels around the nerves of the tympanic plexus would cause an increased flow of saliva from
the parotid gland. This flow of saliva would be followed
by the act of swallowing and the positive intratympanic
pressure would again be established. If swallowing does
not send a bolus of air into the middle ear, because of
paralysis of the vago-accessory group of muscles or of
inflammation around or in the Eustachian tube, then we
have the starting point of diseases in the middle ear.
There is probably no definite rhythm to this swallowing
reflex.

If there is anything in this theory of the action of the
intrinsic muscles of the middle ear, then the theory of
hearing must be modified. The theory of hearing has interested many groups of thinkers, the Physicist, the Anatomist and Histologist, the Physiologist, the Pathologist,
the Psychologist, the Mathematician, the Philosopher, the
Neurologist, the Psychiatrist, the Embryologist, the Biologist, and principally the Otologist, one of the youngest
of these groups but most important because he is in constant contact with diseased conditions of the ear, and has
opportunity to apply the work done by others to his
specialty.

Consideration of Sound.—What is sound? The definition

in the Century Dictionary is "1. The sensation produced through the ear or organ of hearing; in the physical sense, either the vibration of the sounding body itself or those of the air or other medium, which are caused by the sounding body and which immediately affect the ear." Sharpless and Philips[8] say, "Sound is a vibration. All sound is caused by a vibration of some body." Dr. M. Foster[6] says, "Sound is a vibration of the particles of matter, a series of movements of the particles from and to a fixed point. In air and other gases the movement of the particles lead to alternating condensation and rarefaction of the medium, the sound is propagated as waves of alternating condensation and rarefaction which since the to and fro movement of the particles is in the same direction as that in which the undulations are traveling are spoken of as longitudinal waves. Henry S. Carhart[9] says, "Sound may be defined as a vibratory movement excited in an elastic body and transmitted to the ear by means of a continuous elastic ponderable medium." The Standard Dictionary gives the following definition,—"Sound: 1. The sensation produced through the organ of hearing. 2. The physical cause of this sensation; waves of alternate condensation and rarefaction passing through an elastic body, whether solid, liquid, or gaseous, but especially through the atmosphere." Dr. Scripture[12] says, "Sounds are purely mental experiences, most of which are the results of vibratory movements reaching the ear through the air." These definitions vary considerably.

My conception of sound is, sound is vibratory pressure. It is kinetic energy. To the human ear vibrations between 30 and 40,000 v. s. are called sound. Wien[10], found that the faintest audible tone of 240 vibrations had energy amounting to 0.068 uumg. It is necessary to explain the two systems of physical equilibrium before we can register pressures of such slight energy. The first system I have already explained and is the equilibrium of the ossicular chain brought about by the intrinsic muscles of the middle ear; that system has to do with equilibrium of air pressures. The second system is the equilibrium between the perilymph and the endolymph, a system of equilibrium of fluid pressures, and lastly consideration of the intratympanic pressure on the oval and round window membranes.

I will now discuss the second system of equilibrium. The tube of the cochlea contains endolymph. Pressures may be transmitted to the endolymph in two ways: first, pressures from within the tube, and second, pressures from without. 1. The pressures from within may be .caused by increase of secretion from the secreting tubules (Schambaugh) and the stria vascularis of the spiral ligament. 2. Pressures from without are caused by pressures transmitted in two ways, (a) pressures from the perilymph; and (b) brain pressures exerted on the saccus endolymphaticus. The pressure exerted on Reisner's membrane from the endolymph must equal the pressure from the perilymph to keep this membrane in a state of equilibrium. The perilymph communicates by the aqueductus cochleae with the arachnoid space and so with the ventricles of the brain and the spinal canal. Any undue increase of fluid in the ventricles would increase the brain pressure which presses also on the saccus endolymphaticus and by the aqueductus vestibuli equalizes the pressure in the endolymph. Thus the pressure within and without the cochlear canal is equalized. If the endolymphatic pressure were greater than the perilymphatic pressure, Reisner's membrane would bulge into the scala vestibuli, and if the perilymphatic pressure were greater than the endolymphatic pressure, Reisner's membrane would bulge towards the organ of Corti.

Now, consideration of the intratympanic pressure on the perilymph. The vestibular window is nearly filled with the pressure plunger, the stapes. The stapes is not solid but disk shaped with two light, but strong crura made like the ribs of an umbrella. The intratympanic pressure presses on the foot plate of the stapes and the same intratympanic pressure presses on the cochlea window membrane. In other words, although the intratympanic pressure is constantly changing by renewal and absorption of air, this pressure never produces any change on the fluid of the perilymph. Now with the middle ear apparatus and the internal ear fluids in equilibrium we are prepared to receive the vibratory pressures from 24 to 40,-000 v. s. These vibratory pressures must be of sufficient intensity to register on the perilymph.

What is pressure? The definition given in the Century

Dictionary is as follows: "A force per unit area exerted over the surface of a body or part of a body, and toward the interior of the body. A force exerted upon a surface is necessarily equilibrated; otherwise, since the surface has no mass, it would produce infinite velocity until equilibrium ensued.

A pressure can produce no motion, because it is in a state of equilibrium; but a continuous variation of pressure in a given direction will tend to produce motion toward the place of less pressure." It is because of the fact that there is continuous variation of pressure, condensation and rarefaction, that sound travels. The biologist informs us that the lowest forms of life have feeling; a pressure sense, and this sense is skin deep, it is near the surface. Embryology teaches us that the ear is developed from the ectoderm. This organ is a highly developed pressure organ, the ear registering pressure vibrations which we call sound as the eye registers pressure vibrations called light. This process of development has been slow; time is of little account. Evolution is slow. It is interesting to note that the ear at birth is anatomically nearly as fully developed as in the adult. In the fish we find that the auditory nerve goes to a line of lateral pressure organs. It is a known fact that feeling blends with hearing. We feel vibrations up to 24 to 40 v. s. a second, then we begin to hear the vibratory pressures and even feel them above 1024 v. s. Some individuals have a keener sense of touch than others. The duration of a tuning fork held by thumb and forefinger might be a valuable test for neurologists. If we did not hear but could only feel a vibrating body we could soon differentiate low vibrations from higher ones, although we would receive no sensation of tone.

Before examining some of the anatomic facts of the organ of hearing which have to do with acoustics, let us consider a few laws of pneumostatics and hydrostatics, for we have to study the effects of vibratory pressure in air and in fluid. I have already shown* that vibratory pressure has largely been eliminated in solids by surrounding the cochlea with efficient non-conductors (cells filled with bone marrow and air cells) and currents of blood. It

---

*Paper on Some Observations of the Acoustic Function of the Ear.

is easier to think of the static condition of water than that of a gas like air. The similarity of water and air is striking. Both are made up of gases, and oxygen is common to both. We live at the bottom of a sea of atmosphere of a depth of one hundred miles or more, which varies from day to day and hour to hour as the barometer records. The birds of the air, correspond to the fishes of the sea, while we compare to the lobsters and crabs. Of late years we are attempting to fly. The falling of a book or stone causes waves of air to travel in all directions and this vibratory pressure we call sound. Vibrations where there is no pressure causes no sound, as the experiment of the clock in the vacuum proves, but a perfect vacuum is impossible to obtain, therefore there must be sound if there is the least pressure, although such sounds could not be heard by the human ear. As we go higher in the atmosphere the pressure becomes less, for example in climbing a mountain or ascending in a balloon. In these high altitudes sound is harder to make and does not travel so fast or so far. The sounds in the valley are heard in the mountain, but sounds of the same kind on the mountain are not heard in the valley. The denser the air, the further a given sound will be heard by the ear. Did you ever notice that patients with so-called catarrhal deafness due to inflammation of the Eustachian tube complain of their deafness in damp weather. They blame the dampness whereas it is the atmospheric pressure they should blame; the nearer the sea level such patients live the better for their ears, because there, the atmospheric pressure is at its maximum. In the large sense, sound or vibratory pressure does not travel equally in all directions but travels equally in all directions in a stratum which is subject to the same pressure, provided there are no air currents or interfering media other than air. A sound of equal pitch and intensity travels farther from a high pressure to a low pressure, than from a low pressure to a high pressure. As to atmospheric pressure, we must consider it practically constant, for except in diseased conditions it does not play much part in acoustics.

What is the organ of Corti? The organ of Corti is a hydrostatic dynamometer and registers vibratory pressures. For years we have been trying to make sound vibrate certain elements in the cochlea as though we had a piano or

some stringed instrument in the head which must resonate
to the sound heard. Sound waves travel like the water
waves when a stone is thrown into a pond. If one is not
in the radius of the air waves or if the air waves are not
of sufficient amplitude to register on the hydrostatic dynamometer the sound is not heard. Physics teaches us that
whatever pressure we apply to a fluid in a closed vessel, the
fluid transmits the pressure through its whole substance,
so that even the faintest audible sounds must register on
a perfectly equilibrated system such as we have described.
The auditory hairs in the basal coil register only vibratory
pressures which correspond to high tones, while the auditory hairs near the cupola register the vibratory pressures
of low tones. Each auditory hair or group of hairs is
sensitive to its own particular vibratory pressure which
when stimulated by this vibratory pressure sends an impulse to the cortex where tone perception takes place according to the education of the brain cortex for tones.

Anatomic considerations of the organ of Corti. We have
a mound with about 385,000 sensory hairs. These hairs
are within the tube of the cochlea which is in no way in
apposition with pressures of the outside world. The organ
of Corti is supported on a water bed beneath its own supporting basilar membrane. This water bed is the perilymph
of the scala tympani. Above the organ of Corti is the
delicate membrane of Reisner which is the transmitting
membrane of vibratory pressures from the perilymph to
the endolymph. I can consider the tectorial membrane
only as a protector and dampner. In the physical sense it
is a floating body immersed in a liquid. I find in my sections of the human tectorial membrane fibres arranged in
a transverse and longitudinal manner. There are many
more of the transverse fibres than of the longitudinal. We
do not know whether our fixing reagents give us a false
idea of this structure. It may be an artefact. In saying
that the scala vestibuli is above, I am speaking of the
microscopic picture, for in a closed cavity filled with fluid,
position plays no part, it does not effect the transmission
of vibratory or constant pressures. We hear standing on
our heads or lying down, as well as standing on
our feet. The rods of Corti give strength to the structure
which receives pressure from above. Let us consider that

we have an equilibrated middle and internal ear apparatus. Now if a vibratory pressure of 80 v. s. sets the stapes in vibration in the vestibular window, then this vibratory pressure travels equally in all directions in the perilymph, around the membranous semicircular canals, around the utricle and saccule and up the scala vestibuli pressing equally on Reisner's membrane from the beginning of the cochlear duct to the end, and then through the heliotrema, and down the scala tympani pressing on the cochlea window with the same force that was exerted on the vestibular window. The area of the vestibular window is about twice that of the cochlea window. Dr. A. G. Pohlman of Indiana University found the proportion was 1.7:8.5 in one and 1.72:9 in the other or practically 2:1. The shape of the cochlea, the very gradual winding staircase containing the cochlear duct 35mm. long with a height of 5mm. from base to apex, is so small, that depth of fluid does not play much part in the acoustic function. It is evident that it would take more pressure to influence the endolymph by way of the basilar membrane than by way of Reisner's membrane. It is impossible to think of the basilar membrane responding to vibratory pressures. Now with the middle ear muscles at work preserving equilibrium and a perfect equilibrium of the internal ear fluids, any vibratory pressure will press on the auditory hairs the whole length of the cochlear duct equally, but only the hairs or hair sensitive to that particular vibratory pressure will be stimulated. Music does not need to be reproduced as music in the cochlea to be perceived, because all vibratory pressure however complicated is registered by the auditory hairs. The combined vibratory pressures making the compound sound of any one moment forms a wave like that seen when the style of a gramophone carves deeply or lightly into the wax never making two similar waves. Every sound makes its impression on the ear if of sufficient intensity and within the field of hearing to be registered by the stapes in fluid. Thus the complex vibratory pressures exerted on the auditory hairs of the conductor of an orchestra are analyzed as to pitch, intensity and timbre at any one moment. Thus the autoist or engineer hears a new vibratory pressure or misses an old one as the eye analyzes the pressure of color, light and shade.

It is interesting to note that the savage thousands of
years ago in rubbing two dry sticks together stimulated all
his senses but taste, first feeling, then hearing and, with
the heat, odor stimulating the sense of smell, and lastly fire
whose light stimulated sight. Thus heat, electricity, sound
and light are all vibratory pressures or kinetic energy from
some one source.

The membrana tympani is shaped like a megaphone.
The membrana tympani acts like a screen to all vibratory
pressures which would tend to act directly on the membrane of the cochlea window. If the intensity of a sound
is great, some of the sound passes through, and if the sound
is still more intense, all other sounds less intense are
drowned out. The position of the cochlea window membrane at right angles to the foot plate of the stapes, and
the fact that it lies at the bottom of a short tube, is probably
for protective purposes. The middle ear pressure acts
equally in all directions and those intense vibratory pressures which pass through the membrana tympani act
equally in all directions but they do not dash against the
cochlea membrane directly. These vagabond vibratory
pressures are very interesting. The screen action of the
membrana tympani may be demonstrated by placing a piece
of gold beater's skin between a tuning fork and the ear. It
will be noticed that the sound grows dimmer when the membrane intervenes and increases on removal. This interference of waves is seen on the lee side of the boat. A membrane like that of the membrana tympani will so dampen
the tones of a low vibratory pressure that the intensity of
the waves passing through will be so weak that no tone is
heard. Sounds of high pitch with short waves and great
intensity will pass through less changed and are heard in
spite of the membrana tympani. In the same way a membrane will cast a shadow to light waves, but would let some
light through, depending on the intensity of the light, the
character of light, and the thickness of the membrane as
well as its color. The same is true of heat and electric
waves.

Jansen in 1899 first drew my attention to the fact that
the pathology of the membrana tympani gave no indication
of the acoustic function of the ear. We have all seen drums
of deafness and where the voice and fork tests could dis-

weighted with calcified areas when there was no complaint cover no limitation in the field of hearing. It does not matter so long as the equilibrium of the midle ear apparatus is maintained. If we look upon sound as a vibration which must cause some part of the organ of Corti to resonate, these pathologic conditions cannot be accounted for. Time does not permit of accounting for all conditions in the middle ear. A patient without any ossicles often hears better than a patient with a fixed or retarded ossicular apparatus. A patient without drum membrane, malleus or incus but with a moveable foot plate still hears because he has hydraulic balance and so vibratory pressures register with the exception of the low tones because of the drumossicular chain apparatus, which Helmholz[11] proved transformed motions of great amplitude and little force into motions of small amplitude and great force. Ankylosis of the stapes plus rigidity of the cochlea window membrane by new growth should render a person deaf to all vibratory pressures. I have seen many patients whose hearing had been made worse by irrational treatment and I know of two cases where commotio labyrinthi had been caused by great intratympanic pressures. If you inflate the middle ear with a gentle squeeze of the Politzer bag you cannot improve matters by increasing the pressure. I have known otologists to use a pressure of 40 pounds on the middle ear. Never use air tank pressures. The thickness of the membrana tympani is not an index to the membrane of the cochlea window, and besides the danger in wrecking the organ of Corti there is great danger of stretching ligaments and rupturing membranes or bands with resulting bleeding. From these ruptures new connective tissue is formed and finally contraction of the scar tissue renders the equilibrium less efficient and deafness rapidly progresses.

In conclusion, I hope I have gained a bit of truth in this interesting subject. If I have not I hope it will stimulate others to think along these lines. A rational conception of how we hear will help us in our treatment of all forms of deafness.

REFERENCES.

1. Wiedersheim. Comparative Anatomy of Vertebrates, p. 303.

2. v. Hensen. Die Fortschritte in einigen Teilen der Physi-

ologie des Gehoers. Ergebnisse der Physiologie, I Jahrgang, 2, 1902.

3. Politzer. Diseases of the Ear. Ballin and Heller, 1903.

4. McKendrick and Gray. Text-book on Physiology. Edited by E. A. Schafer, Vol. II.

5. Boenninghaus. Lehrbuch der Ohrenheilkunde, S. 67.

6. Foster, M. Text-book of Physiology.

7. Morat, J. P. Physiology of the Nervous System.

8. Sharpless and Philips. Natural Philosophy.

9. Carhart. Physics for University Students.

10. Wien. Ann. d. Phys. u. Chem., 1889, XXXVI, S. 834.

11. Helmholtz. Sensations of Tone. Trans. 4th German Ed., 1877, p. 134.

12. Dr. Scripture. Experimental Phonetics.

13. Shambaugh, George E. Zeitschrift f. Ohren., XXXVII, Heft 6, 1908.

Action of Pressure
on Membrana Tympani.

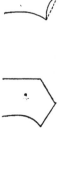

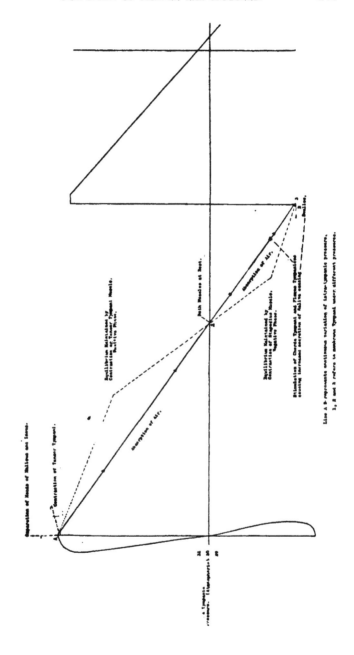

XVI

EXPERIMENTAL NYSTAGMUS AND AN APPLICATION OF ITS PRINCIPLES TO A DIAGNOSIS OF LESIONS OF THE INNER EAR AND CEREBELLUM.

By Wm. B. Chamberlin, M. D.,

Cleveland.

Nystagmus is the name applied to any oscillating movements of the eyeballs. It is a reflex and is involuntary, though cases of voluntary nystagmus have been reported. Observation has shown that all oscillating movements of the eyes are not of like character, but that all can be classed under two distinct and separate groups. The first is the undulating nystagmus. In this, both movements, the excursion from and the return to any fixed point, are equal both in extent and in velocity. The second is the rhthymical nystagmus. In this, the movements are not undulating, but follow each other with a distinct jerking motion. Closer observation reveals that in this second variety a cycle (the departure from and the return to a fixed marginal point) is composed of two distinct movements; one fairly slow and deliberate, the other quick and jerky, but both of equal extent. Successive complete cycles are equal as regards time, that is, the time of the slow plus the time of the quick component in one cycle is equal to that of any other, and the nystagmus is therefore called rhthymical. In addition, the nystagmus may be designated as horizontal, rotatory, vertical or oblique, names which will be referred to later. With the first or undulating nystagmus this paper is not concerned, but consideration will be devoted entirely to the second or rhthymical nystagmus; its experimental production, distinguishing characteristics, and observation in pathologic conditions.

TERMINOLOGY.

As before mentioned, the rhthymical nystagmus possesses certain definite characteristics. First of all, it consists of two movements, a rapid and a slow. The rapid movement or component may be in any direction, though it is usually to the right or left. The slow movement would accordingly lie in the direction opposite (the left or right). This direction of the quick component is important from a diagnostic point of view, as the nystagmus is designated as nystagmus to the right, or nystagmus to the left, according as this quick component falls to the right or to the left side. It is further designated as horizontal if the plane of the movement lies in or parallel to a second plane passing through the pupils of both eyes. It is called vertical if the plane of the nystagmus is at right angles to this plane, and oblique if the plane of the movement intersects the horizontal plane at less than a right angle or 90°. We still have a variety of frequent occurrence, the rotatory nystagmus. If we conceive of two meridians passing vertically through each pupil, nystagmus of a rolling character will be designated as rotatory nystagmus to the right, of a rotatory nystagmus to the left, according as the quick component impels the upper end of this supposed meridian to pass to the right or to the left. In addition to the above mentioned pure varieties, we may have also a variety of combinations, that most frequently observed being a combination of the rotatory with the horizontal.

Within the limits of the present paper, it would be impossible to consider the various theories of the cause of nystagmus and the paths, afferent and efferent, together with the centers through which the impulses are transmitted; but we will proceed at once to a study of experimental nystagmus and then to a study of that noticed in pathologic conditions, with some reference to the application to the pathological of the principles derived from the experimental.

NYSTAGMUS FROM TURNING.

If a subject is placed upon a revolving stool in the sitting posture and turned to the right, that is clockwise, the hands moving in a horizontal plane, the following phenomena will be observed: During the turning there will be a slow movement of the eyes to the left (in the direction opposite to the turning), and this slow movement to the left will be followed by a quick and jerking movement to the right (in the direction of the turning). If now the turning is stopped and the movements are again observed, we will find that the quick component is directed not to the right, but to the left, and that the slow component is directed to the right. In other words, we have a complete reversal of the conditions previously observed—a nystagmus to the right replaced by a nystagmus to the left. The observation of the nystagmus during the turning can only be accomplished by placing the patient upon a revolving platform sufficiently large, so that the observer can take his position on the platform at the same time. This involves not only considerable inconvenience, but also much space and fairly costly apparatus. Observation is accordingly practically limited to the nystagmus present after the turning has ceased. This is not in reality an observation of the nystagmus, but of the after-nystagmus, though results obtained from it are quite as valuable and instructive as those obtained from the nystagmus itself.

If we observe this experimental nystagmus still further we notice other characteristics. If, as before, we revolve the patient to the right, obtaining thereby, on cessation, a nystagmus to the left, we may find this nystagmus very slight if the glance of the patient is directed straight ahead. It will reach its maximum if the patient converges both eyes on the finger tip, held say twelve inches from the eye and in the extreme left position, but will disappear entirely if the glance is directed to the right, though the eyes are still in convergence. In other words, glance in the direction of the quick component increases the nystagmus; glance straight ahead, or in the direction opposite to the quick component, weakens it or causes it to disappear. In many cases the nystagmus may be very slight and may be better observed if a strong light, as from an ordinary head mirror, is thrown directly into the eyes.

Alterations in position of the head during the motion give alteration in the nsytagmus. For example, tilting the head strongly forward at an angle of 90 degrees to the axis of the body or the axis of motion gives rotatory nystagmus, while tilting the head to the right or left shoulder changes the nystagmus to vertical. Different varieties of nystagmus also give different sensations. The sensation of turning produced during the horizontal nystagmus is replaced by a sensation of falling if the nystagmus is vertical, and tilting with turning if the nystagmus is oblique.

It is a matter of common experience, that continued turning gives both during the turning as well as after its cessation, first of all, a sensation of dizziness. The objects may seem to revolve about the observer or he himself may seem to revolve as well. If the turning has been extreme, this dizziness is followed by nausea, vomiting, disturbances of equilibrium, and even loss of consciousness. These sensations are frequently varied in children by placing one ear on the top of an upright cane and running rapidly about it. This would be equivalent to placing the head on the shoulder and would give a sensation of falling, with vertical nystagmus as previously described.

NYSTAGMUS DURING MOTION.

If one sits in a railway coach and looks out of the window, for example, with the right side directed toward the engine or in the direction of motion, he himself will of course be moving from left to right; the objects on the ground will seem to be moving from right to left. If he now fixes successive objects in passing them, and keeps them within the limits of his vision as long as possible, there will be observed a slow movement of the eyes in the direction of the moving objects—from right to left. This slow movement will be followed by a quick movement in the direction of the advancing train, or from left to right. There will be, in other words, a nystagmus to the right. Similar results will follow if the observer stands upon the ground and faces a train passing to the left, fixing successive objects on the train as it passes him.

CALORIC NYSTAGMUS.

Experiments with heat or cold are best performed with large perforations in the tympanic membranes, though good results may also be obtained in experiments on those in whom the membrana tympani is still intact. For this purpose, a Hartman attic syringe is used. Attached to the syringe is a rubber tube one or two feet long and armed with a Politzer bag filled with hot or cold water. If hot water is used, it must be above the body temperature and below 110 degrees, the usual maximum point of toleration, though higher degrees may be borne by some patients. Cold water at a much greater variation from the normal is easily borne. For this reason, nystagmus can be produced by cold in many cases in which hot water produces no effect whatsoever.

With the apparatus above described, let us now inject the right ear of a- patient with hot water. This is usually performed by an assistant while the observer faces the one observed. After the injection has proceeded for some moments, the length of time varying somewhat in different individuals, if the patient's glance is directed toward the right, the side of the injected ear, a quick rolling movement of the eyes toward the right side will be observed. This quick movement toward the right will be followed by a slow movement of equal excursion to the left. We have produced experimentally a rotatory nystagmus to the right. Substitution now of cold for hot water gives the opposite nystagmus or nystagmus to the left. Similar results may be obtained by syringing the opposite ear. Hot water then in the right ear gives the same result as cold water in the left and vice versa. If now both ears are injected under like conditions with water of the same temperature, we obtain no nystagmus at all. It is interesting in this connection to note that water at say a temperature of 105 degrees, which has previously produced a well-marked nystagmus in an individual, will produce no nystagmus at all if the patient is suffering with an abnormally high temperature, for example, 103 or 104 degrees. The variation from the body temperature is too slight to produce any marked reaction.

Usually if the nystagmus is marked, dizziness, together with loss of equilibrium, is an accompaniment. This fact may explain an observation of frequent occurrence both of the general practitioner as well as the specialist. On syringing the ear of a pat'ent for the removal of impacted cerumen, especially if the injection has been long continued, the patient will not infrequently complain of dizziness and on rising he may for a few minutes be unable to cross the floor without staggering or even fall'ng. This might be a result of either the abnormal heat or cold or of the pressure as well. That nystagmus from heat or cold apart from pressure can be produced however, can easily be shown by substituting for the water, hot or cold air or ether fumes.

PRESSURE.

Nystagmus can be produced by compression or exhaustion of the air in the external canal or even by pressure on the tragus, as in cases of labyrinthine fistula. It can also be produced by direct pressure on the head of the stapes. The

· movements in many cases are exceedingly small and in others entirely wanting. There is no uniformity in the results obtained so that this method at present is of little advantage from a diagnostic view-point, except in the examination of cases of suspected openings into the semicircular canals.

GALVANIC NYSTAGMUS.

If the anode or positive pole of a galvanic battery, armed with a small electrode, is placed upon the right tragus, and the kathode or negative pole, armed with a large electrode, is held in the hand of the patient, during the passage of fifteen to twenty milliamperes of current, nystagmus can easily be produced. This will consist of a quick rolling movement of the eyes to the opposite or unstimulated side and a slow return to the right or side of stimulation. The nystagmus, however, will only be observed with glance to the extreme left (in the direction of the quick component) and not when the glance is straight ahead or to the right. It will not be pure rotatory in character, but mixed with this element will be a slight horizontal element as well.

Anode to the right ear then gives nystagmus to the left. If now the electrodes be transposed, the kathode being placed upon the ear while the anode is held in the hand, the resulting nystagmus will be reversed. The quick component will be toward the right, the slow toward the left, and the nystagmus will be observed only when the eyes are in the extreme right position. Instead of nystagmus to the left, we have now a nystagmus to the right. By comparing the results previously obtained with heat and cold, we find that the anode has the same effect as syringing the ear with cold water, the kathode the same as syringing with hot water.

Patients with galvanic nystagmus show a well-marked reaction. If placed in the Romberg position, that is, in the standing posture with eyes closed and feet together, with nystagmus to the left they fall to the right; with nystagmus to the right they fall to the left. In other words, they fall in the direction of the slow component. Turning the head about a vertical axis, to the right or left, will cause them to fall either forwards or backwards, according as the slow component falls in either of these directions.

PATHOLOGIC CASES.

We come finally to a study of pathologic cases—to an application as it were of some of the observations already made. Possibly the subject may be made clearer by an hypothesis and an illustration.

Let us take a uniform bar, for example, six feet in length, and balance it at the center. Now let us suspend from each end a weight of ten pounds. The bar will remain in balance. This balance may represent the equilibrium of the normal eyes in which no nystagmus is present; and the ten pounds the aggregate stimuli coming from both sets of semicircular canals. If the ears are normal, these stimuli will be equal, and the eyes will remain at rest. To the right arm of the bar let us now add a weight of one pound. The bar no longer remains at rest, but declines sharply to the right side. So with a labyrinthine fistula on the right side, and with it a circumscribed inflammation, we have an increase of the stimuli coming from the right vestibule and there results a nystagmus to the right. This nystagmus will be rotatory and rhythmical in character and will be increased by vision to the right or in the direction of the quick component. Let now this circumscribed inflammation become diffuse, thereby destroying completely the function of the right semicircular canals, or let them be obliterated by operative interference, and the nystagmus previously directed to the right is at once changed to a nystagmus to the left. Here, as the result of all stimuli from the right vestibule being lost, the nystagmus is extreme and manifests itself not only with vision to the left, but with vision straight ahead and to the right as well. This extreme nystagmus persists for some days. It grows gradually weaker, however; first the nystagmus with vision to the right is lost, next that with vision straight ahead, and ultimately, after a much longer interval, the nystagmus with vision to the left. We have in such cases a quantitative estimate of the nystagmus. Returning to our illustration of the balanced bar—the weight of eleven pounds on the right arm has been completely removed and the counterweight on the left arm is unopposed. The bar assumes the vertical or extreme position. As the organism gradually becomes accustomed to the loss of stimuli from the right side; as eyes, cerebellum and muscles compensate for the loss of stimuli from the right vestibule, the result is a gradual return to the normal. The nystagmus, and with it the dizziness, disappears. We can represent the condition with the bar by gradually decreasing the weight upon the left arm. When all weight has been removed, the bar again assumes the horizontal or first position.

In a condition of hyperirritation, as in a suppurative otitis with circumscribed inflammation following labyrinthine fistula, if the left ear was normal, the persistence of function of the labyrinth on the right side could easily be demonstrated. Water above body temperature would increase the nystagmus, water below body temperature would cause it to diminish in intensity or even to disappear. After destruction of the labyrinth by operation or by diffuse suppuration, neither heat nor cold would produce any effect whatever, though the ear would still react to the galvanic stimulation. We might conclude from this, that the destructive process had involved the endings of the vestibular branch of the auditory nerve, but not the nerve fibers themselves.

In these cases of irritative lesions, followed by destruction of the labyrinth, the position in bed is interesting, characteristic and also of diagnostic importance. The patient has an irritative lesion on the right side and with it a nystagmus to the right. He lies on the right side with face toward the pillow. In this position, the eyes are involuntarily turned toward the left or from the pillow—the nystagmus and with it the consequent dizziness and discomfort are decreased by so doing. If now the function of the right labyrinth is destroyed, there results a nystagmus to the left. The causes which formerly induced him to lie on the right side now impel him to reverse his position. As the nystagmus gradually disappears the patient again assumes the usual position in bed and manifests no preference for any special position.

Ear nystagmus then possesses the following characteristics:

(1) It is rhythmical in character—successive cycles being equal as regards time and extent.

(2) Each cycle consists of two distinct movements, a quick and a slow. The nystagmus is also of the rotatory type, though we may have the horizontal as well or even a combination of the two.

(3) Glance in the direction of the quick component increases the nystagmus; glance in the direction of the slow component lessens or destroys it.

If we now compare experimental nystagmus with that observed in pathologic conditions, we note the following points of similarity: hot water injections, kathode stimulation and irritative lesions all give nystagmus to the stimulated or diseased side; cold water injections, anode stimulation and destructive lesions all give nystagmus to the opposite or sound side. We may conclude then that heat and kathode stimulation, being similar in their effect to an irritative lesion, cause an increase in the stimuli from the labyrinth involved; while anode stimulation and cold, acting similarly to destructive lesions, cause a decrease of the stimuli; they exercise, as it were, a benumbing or paralyzing effect upon the labyrinth with which they come in contact.

NYSTAGMUS IN CEREBELLAR DISEASE.

As in vestibular disease, so also do we find nystagmus in lesions of the cerebellum. In these cases, the nystagmus is of extreme value in making a differential diagnosis. Nystagmus of cerebellar origin, is similar to that of peripheral origin. Its seat may be localized in doubtful cases by an exact examination of the function of the vestibular apparatus, that is, by turning, or by injecting hot or cold water. Let us now consider the nystagmus in that disease of the cerebellum most closely associated with labyrinthine suppuration—in cerebellar abscess.

Nystagmus in cerebellar abscess may be toward the sound or toward the diseased side. That toward the diseased side, however, greatly predominates. Cerebellar abscess is usually found in connection with labyrinthine suppuration, so both factors, the labyrinth and the cerebellum, would play a role in producing nystagmus. We must accordingly differentiate among the following possibilities:

(1) With nystagmus to the diseased side, we may have

    (a) A circumscribed labyrinthine suppuration, or

    (b) A cerebellar abscess.

With a circumscribed suppuration, the labyrinth would still be excitable and would react to heat and cold. We would have also the signs of a labyrinthine fistula—aspiration and compression of the air in the external auditory canal would cause movements of the eyeballs. If, however, the reaction from heat and cold was lost, we might still have reaction to pressure and to galvanic stimulation. In this case the diagnosis from the nystagmus could not be made. In such a case, with nystagmus to the diseased side and reaction to the pressure and galvanism, but not to heat and cold, the labyrinth operation would be performed immediately after the radical. After removal of the labyrinth if the nystagmus, formerly directed toward the diseased side, should then be directed to the sound side, the diagnosis of labyrinthine suppuration without involvement of the cerebellum could be made.

Cases of cerebellar abscess in the experience of the Politzer clinic do not occur in connection with circumscribed labyrinthine suppuration, but with labyrinthine suppuration of a diffuse or general character. To carry our supposition then still further, if, after operation upon the diseased labyrinth, a nystagmus was still directed to the diseased side, and did not change toward the sound side, then the nystagmus must come from some intracranial origin. For a sound vestibule, if the opposite vestibule is destroyed and the cerebellum is not involved, must always cause a nystagmus to its own side.

Our first hypothesis was with a nystagmus to the diseased side and vestibule still reacting. Our second hypothesis is

(2) With a nystagmus to the diseased side and the vestibule no longer capable of stimulation.

In this case, the nystagmus to the diseased side must be intracranial, and this intracranial stimulation must be greater than the stimulation from the opposite and intact vestibule; for, as shown before, if unopposed an intact vestibule will always cause a nystagmus to its own or to the sound side. The nystagmus to the diseased side could only point to a diagnosis of cerebellar abscess. In such a case, due attention would, of course, be given to pulse, temperature and the remaining points in the diagnosis of cerebellar involvement.

There exists now a third possible combination of nystagmus with suspected cerebellar abscess.

(3) The nystagmus is not toward the diseased, but toward the sound side and the labyrinth is not excitable.

The nystagmus here could be of either vestibular or intracranial origin and diagnosis from the nystagmus could not be made. In this case the cerebellar suppuration would have proceeded so far that all function of the cerebellum on the diseased side was lost.

If only the labyrinth is diseased, after operation the nystagmus is extreme and is directed to the sound side. As before mentioned, it decreases gradually and ultimately disappears.

If, however, a cerebellar abscess is associated with the laby-rinthine suppuration, the nystagmus after operation does not decrease in intensity, but increases instead. It is reversed and directed toward the diseased side. In this case its intracranial origin can be diagnosed with certainty.

CONCLUSIONS.

Semicircular canals and cerebellum both play a joint part in the perception of equilibrium. That other factors participate strongly is shown by the return to the normal after loss of stimuli from these organs.

Disturbances in the function of vestibule and cerebellum cause disturbances of equilibrium and also produce a nystagmus having certain definite characteristics. We might represent the condition graphically, as follows:

Right.   Left.

Normal vestibule + normal cerebellum $=$ normal vestibule + normal cerebellu
Stimulated vest. + normal cerebellum $>$ normal vestibule + normal cerebellu
Destroyed vest. + normal cerebellum $<$ normal vestibule + normal cerebellu
Destroyed vest. + stim. cerebellum $>$ normal vestibule + normal cerebellu
Destroyed vest. + dest. cerebellum $<$ normal vestibule + normal cerebellu

) Would represent the condition in a circumscribed labyrinthine suppur
he right.
) Would represent the condition in a diffuse labyrinthine suppuration on

) Would represent the condition in a destroyed vestibule with cerebellum
on the right.
) Would represent the condition in a destroyed vestibule with destroyed
m on the right.

This paper can only be offered with an apology. Many things of importance are only mentioned—others, for example, the disturbances of equilibrium and the question of nystagmus in the deaf and dumb and the signs of labyrinthine involvement in Meniere's disease are not even referred to. But it has seemed essential to me for any clear understanding of the subject to give at first as it were, a bird's-eye view of the whole rather than an exhaustive discussion of a single part—the only alternative possible in such a paper. The subject of nystagmus with reference to diseases of the ear is still in its infancy and the problems associated with it cannot help but increase both in number and importance as time goes on.

In conclusion, I wish to express my thanks to Priv. Doc.

Heinrich Neumann and Dr. Robert Barany, assistants in the clinic of Hofrath Prof. Dr. Politzer in Wien.

I wish also to mention the articles, "Der Otitische Klein-hirnabszess," by Dr. Neumann, and "Untersuchungen ueber den vom Vestibularapparat des Ohres reflektorisch ausgeloesten rhythmischen Nystagmus und seine Begleiterscheinungen," by Dr. Barany. These two articles I have used freely, and that of Dr. Neumann with reference to nystagmus in cerebellar abscess I have quoted in part. The article by Dr. Barany con-tains an exhaustive list of the literature on the subject.

XVII.

VACCINE THERAPY IN OTOLOGY AND RHINO-LARYNGOLOGY.

By Robert Levy, M. D.,

Denver.

The study of immunity to and protection against disease followed by its natural application in the development of vaccine therapy opens up a field for thought and scientific research which is practically limitless. Based upon the utilization of natural physiologic function, vaccine therapy; if considered in its purely theoretic conception, presents a vista of beautiful pictures of prophylactic and remedial results offered by no other therapeutic invention. The bacteriologic study of this subject is replete with interest, but so technical and profound that only the student trained in this department of science can grasp its numerous problems. As otologists and laryngologists we are chiefly concerned in its clinical aspects and practical application. It becomes our duty, however, to familiarize ourselves to some extent at least with the fundamental theories upon which treatment of diseases by this method is based and its rationale.

Richardson[1] states that the great mass of bacterial diseases still remains outside the antitoxin category and that speculation has been forced to seek other theories to explain immunity acquired after infection with various cocci. Trudeau[2] calls attention to the unsatisfactory state of this question by outlining the position assumed by the two theories at present in vogue, namely, that of the specific immunity to the action of the microorganism itself and that of the immunization to the chemical poison of the microorganism. In the first a stimulation of our defensive resources is attempted. In the second toxin tolerance is to be desired. In this connection it must be remembered that antitoxins are applicable only to soluble toxins, as in the cases of diphtheria and tetanus, but that for endotoxins which are insoluble, the leucocytes play

an important role and the antibodies here required represent
agglutinins, preciptitins, bacteriocidal and bacteriolytic substances and opsonins. The application of our remedy, both
as to indication for its use and its dosage, might be made
fairly accurate could it be definitely demonstrated by which
of these theories practical results had been obtained. It was
hoped that Wright's opsonic index might prove a reliable
method of measuring the degree of resistance or immunization existing in the organism during an infectious attack. Judging from the rapidly growing sentiment that the opsonic index
is of comparatively little value because of lack of standard,
we are placed in the unsatisfactory position of depending upon
clinical evidence and empiricism. A clinical study may, however, assist in clarifying the subject to a limited extent, so that
we may be enabled to calmly pursue further investigation
with neither too optimistic enthusiasm nor too pessimistic
condemnation.

The results of treatment by vaccine therapy must at this
time be considered as sub judice, especially when it is remembered that but a comparatively short time has elapsed since
this method has been advocated and because of the limited
experience of individual men. No definite conclusions can,
therefore, be presented, and when our Chairman requested me
to present a paper upon this topic, I consented reluctantly and
only with the understanding that I might be permitted to outline no positive deductions but simply the united experience of
our colleagues in my immediate vicinity. My paper, therefore,
presents an exposition or reflection of the work of men in a
limited section of our country.

To this end a carefully considered letter was addressed to
our confreres in Colorado, asking for certain definite information covering the important questions relating to vaccine
therapy in diseases of the ear, nose and throat, with more or
less complete report of cases. I was gratified and surprised at
the number and completeness of the reports, especially when
we consider that this method is used only in exceptional cases
and is rarely undertaken except where operation has failed
or has for some reason been deemed inexpedient. It has
therefore been extremely difficult to tabulate in a uniform
manner the cases so reported; nevertheless, representing
the experience of many, and uninfluenced by individual
bias, I hope the report may be of some practical value.

The total number of cases reported were 121, divided as follows:

Ear cases 48
Accessory sinus cases 15
Tuberculosis cases 58

The ear cases were divided as follows:

	Cured.	Improved.	Not Improved.	Total.
Acute Purulent Otitis Media,				
With mastoid involvement....	11	1 '	1	13
Without mastoid involvement..	8	..	3	11
Chronic Purulent Otitis Media,				
Without mastoid involvement..	13	6	5	21
Total	32	7	9	48

All of these cases received the usual conservative treatment, such as drainage and irrigation. Many of the mastoid cases were operated. In a number of cases secondary operations were performed. The most striking results were obtained in those cases in which unhealed mastoids existed, manifesting themselves in recurrences after a greater or shorter period of time.

The sinus cases were divided as follows:

	Cured.	Improved.	Not Improved.	Total.
Antrum of Highmore..........	2	3	..	5
Frontal sinus	2	1	2	5
Frontal and antrum...........	1	2	..	3
All sinuses	..	..	1	1
Antrum and ethmoid	1	..	..	1
Total	6	6	3	15

All of these cases were chronic in their nature and had received prolonged and faithful treatment by drainage and irrigation. Many of them had been operated upon as often as three times, the operation being usually conservative in character.

The tuberculous cases were divided as follows:

	Cured.	Improved.	Not Improved.	Total.
Pharyngeal tuberculosis	2	..	7	9
Laryngeal tuberculosis	3	16	30	49
Total	5	16	37	58

Many of the cases of tuberculosis reported were not considered and have not been entered in this table because of insufficient data. All the tuberculous cases received other treatment, medicinal, surgical and hygienic of the nature usually adopted in tuberculosis.

Other cases reported were as follows:

One case of tuberculosis of bronchial gland pressing upon the right recurrent laryngeal. Cured. (Cooper, Mitchell.)

One case of pharyngeal tuberculosis with suppurating cervical glands. Pharynx cured. Glands greatly improved. (Levy.)

One case of syphilitic necrosis of orbit with involvement of all sinuses. Acute sepsis. (Streptococcus.) Death. (Matthews.)

One case of acute laryngeal perichondritis. Thyrotomy, removal necrosed tissue. Pseudo-diph. bacillus. Cured. (Dennis.)

Of 63 cases exclusive of tuberculosis the reporters gave the nature of the infecting organism in 59. Of these there were cured 35, improved and not improved 24.

The infecting organisms were divided as follows:

Cases Cured.	*Improved and Not Improved.*
Pneumo., Staph. 7.	Pneumo., Staph. 3.
Staph. 8.	Staph. 8.
Strep., Staph. 3.	Strep., Staph. 3.
Pneumo. 3.	Pneumo. 2.
Strep. 3.	Strep. 2.
Pneumo-strep., Staph. 3.	Microc-Catarrh., Strep. 1.
Pneumo-strep. 5.	Pfeifer 1.
T. B., Staph. 1.	Staph., Pyocyan. 2.
Pseudo-diph. 1.	Pseudo-diph., Strep. 1.
Pseudo-diph., Microc. Catarrh. 1.	Pyog. Aureus, Coli Com. 1.

The long period over which bacterial diseases continue is explained by Wright (Matson)[3] by finding that the opsonic power hardly varies from day to day or remains uniformly low. The practical application of this is in the necessity of prolonged treatment.

Another important consideration is in the desirability of isolating the specific microorganism. Failure to accomplish this has resulted in the use of mixed vaccines and where results have not been obtained repeated re-examinations have discovered other bacteria, a vaccine of which proved more satisfactory.

One of the weakest points in bacterial therapy is the question of proper dosage, both as to amount and frequency thereof. This has been especially pointed out by Matthews.[4] One can not be guided entirely by the opsonic index because of the fact that this is subject to such variations as to make it a source of error. On the other hand, clinical evidence alone must be unsatisfactory because of *its* many sources of error and its misinterpretation. Nevertheless, careful clinical observation has been of more uniform value than laboratory reports.

In administering repeated doses one must not forget the liability to sensitization. Bergey[5] has given us some interesting experiments bearing upon this point, but draws the conclusion that the dangers are remote because the dose of bacterial vaccines is usually too small. This danger applies more to serum theapy than to vaccine therapy. The failure of response to bacterial therapy depends also upon the character of the infection. Harris[6] has shown that in nasal and throat affections the micrococcus catarrhalis produces unyielding conditions, but believes the influence of foreign particles irritating the mucous membrane prevents accurate deductions. Ohlmacher[7] shows that certain combinations of bacteriologic species are particularly obstinate in their reaction to therapeutic inoculation, and speaks especially of a combination of bacillus pyocyaneus with other pyogenic species.

Particular interest attaches to the treatment of tuberculosis in general and for us, especially in lesions of the ear, throat and nose. The local reactions which have followed tuberculin injections have been watched with much interest. Trudeau[8] has found pain and aphonia in laryngeal cases. I have seen swelling and redness of the local lesions in both pharyngeal and laryngeal tuberculosis following the use of tuberculin. Trudeau has also concluded that slight local reactions were followed by reparative changes. The ultimate result upon tuberculosis of the upper air passages and ear are necessarily modified by the coexistence of pulmonary or general tuberculosis This is especially forceful when we remember that primary lesions of the upper air passages rarely if ever occur. Nevertheless, the report of our cases shows that permanent cure of local lesions may take place under vaccine therapy, but not sufficiently often to warrant the conclusion that we have at our command a specific remedy. Tod[9] has reported improved hearing in tuberculous ears following inoculation. Cases found in the above report show occasional complete and frequent temporary cessation of discharge in tuberculous otitis. In these, tubercle bacilli were not always found but tuberculin was given with autogenetic vaccine.

Beck's[10] cases show encouraging results. Goadby[11] relates remarkable improvement from vaccine therapy in antrum cases.

Investigations in the treatment of all bacterial diseases of the upper air passages are being carried out, such as recurring colds, atrophic rhinitis, influenza and chronic nasopharyngitis, but as yet evidence is too indefinite to warrant any conclusions.

My observation and experience leads me to advise that all obstinate cases in which conservative methods, including so-called conservative operations have been adopted, should receive the benefit of vaccines This refers to all ear cases, chronic, acute, with or without mastoid involvement, and all accessory sinus cases.

In the study and preparation of this paper, I have had the assistance of the bacteriologists in my section of the country, namely, Drs. Webb of Colorado Springs, Peebles of Boulder, Mitchell and Matthews of Denver, as well as the most generous and unselfish support of the following men: Drs. Bane, Carmody, Cooper, Foster, Lockard, Strickler, Bonney, Berlin of Denver, Magruder[12] the first to report ear cases treated by vaccines, Patterson, Sollenberger, Dennis of Colorado Springs, and Spencer of Boulder. They have freely permitted me to use their cases, many of which are incorporated in this report.

BIBLIOGRAPHY.

1.   Richardson.   American Journal of the Medical Sciences, October, 1908.

2.   Trudeau.   Journal of the American Medical Association, January 23, 1909.

3.   Matson.   Medical Sentinel, July, 1908.

4.   J. Matthews.   Lancet, September 26, 1908.

5.   Bergey.   Journal of the American Medical Association, September 5, 1908.

6.   Harris.   Practitioner, May, 1908.

7.   Ohlmacher.   Journal of the American Medical Association, August 15, 1908.

8.   Trudeau.   American Journal of the Medical Sciences, August, 1906, June, 1907.

9.   Tod.   The Practitioner, May, 1908.

10.   Beck.   Laryngoscope, May, 1908.

11.   Goadby.   Journal of Laryngology, Rhinology and Otology, November, 1908.

12.   Magruder.   Laryngoscope, November, 1907.

XVIII.

OPERATION FOR MALIGNANT GROWTHS OF THE TONSIL.*

By Dr. Karl Vohsen,

Frankfort on the Main.

Translated by Wm. Baron, M. D.,

St. Louis.

Operations on malignant growths with their accompany-ing involvements of the pharynx and base of the tongue, demand a method of procedure which allows the operator a full view of the parts and permits of controlling incidental hemorrhages.

The simple enucleation of the tonsil may be considered justifiable only in those rare cases in which there is a small tumor confined entirely to the tonsil, where subsequent examination proves an intact capsule of the tumor. But even in such cases, slightly diseased, still impalpable lym-phatic glands may exist whose presence would have been revealed by an external operation.

The early stages of these tumors generally escape our diagnosis. It may be considered fortunate when the patient comes to us as soon as he notices the growth of the tonsil. He consults us, as a rule, because of pressure pains toward the ear or because of difficulty in swallowing, and then the conditions arouse suspicion that the swelling has en-croached on the anterior and posterior pillars, the tongue and adjacent lymphatics.

For the purpose of operating on these tumors, Langen-beck introduced the temporary resection of the inferior maxilla, and this method of exposing the lateral parts of the pharynx has since been the mode of procedure of all operators.

*Read before the International Congress of Rhinology and Laryn-gology, Vienna, 1908.

Kocher, in his "Operationslehre," 1907, thus describes the osteoplastic resection for exposing the upper parts of the pharynx: "After obliquely cutting through the inferior maxilla, from the back, inside and top toward the front, outside and bottom, the ascending ramus is drawn firmly upward and the horizontal ramus is drawn forward, at the anterior margin of the masseter." (p. 192.)

In conjunction with numerous modifications of the cutaneous section, assembled and illustrated by Hensell of the Czerny klinik (*Brun's Beitraege zur klin. Chirurgie*, Bd. 14, 1895), this method of resecting and drawing apart the resected parts of the inferior maxillary remains practically the same.

Only Mikulicz (*Deutsche med. Wochenschrift*, 84-86) and Kuester (ibid. 85) have resorted to another method, having recourse to a total resection instead of an osteoplastic resection of the ascending ramus. Mikulicz specifies as a marked advantage of this procedure "the complete and easy exposure, exteriorly, of the lateral wall of the pharynx and the possibility of carrying out the operation almost to its end *extra cavum pharyngis et oris."* Kuester emphasizes among other advantages of this method of operation that ankylosis of the temporomaxillary joint is avoided, which need not be apprehended at all in the Mikulicz procedure. Kuester subjoins to his description: "It is not to be denied, however, that this method has its drawbacks. The jaw is set obliquely, as both musculi pterygodei are withdrawn and those of the opposite side crowd the maxilla toward the affected side. The power of the mandibular muscles is decreased, as all of the mandibular muscles of the affected side, the masseter, the temporalis and the pterygodei, lose their points of insertion. It is true that Mikulicz has limited the detachment of these muscles by the recommendation that the section of the maxillary be made above the masseter, but even this does not remove the objections raised by Kuester. The viewpoint advanced by Kuester, that of avoiding ankylosis, seems of great moment in cases where the tumor has encroached on the fold between the superior and inferior maxillae, and in such an event, the Mikulicz method would seem to be the one to be preferred to all others.

The cutaneous section of the Mikulicz method extends

from the mastoid process of the temporal bone to the greater cornu of the hyoid bone and is serviceable in exposing and extirpating metastically affected glands along the sternocleidomastoid and the carotid sheath. In practicing osteoplastic resection it has been found, as an offset to total resection with the above described consequences, that in order to expose the field of operation to the opening of the larynx it was necessary to sever the diagastric, the stylohyoideus and the nervus hypoglossus. In a great many cases preliminary tracheotomy was performed in addition, so that temporary resection, as practiced up to the present, as well as total resection according to Mikulicz, requires a number of serious lacerations, which can only be attributed to the method of operation.

Now, I wish to demonstrate that the same final results may be accomplished with fewer lacerations. I can refer to a case in which I performed the operation to be demonstrated, on a living subject before the association of physieiaus at Frankfort-on-the-Main. It was a case of a large sarcoma of the left tonsil, encroaching on the lateral base of the tongue, with metastically affected lymphatics of the neck.

Five months ago, a man of 23, still serving his military term, felt a tickling sensation in his throat which incited vomiting. Healthy up to 7 weeks prior to examination, when he noticed an obstruction in the left side of his throat which made swallowing difficult. Appetite, sleep, stools good. No hereditary history. Parents alive. Three healthy brothers and sisters. No peculiarity of nose. Good teeth. Lungs and heart without anomalies. The left tonsil has become a superficially ulcerated swelling, the size of a small apple, rounding out the anterior part of the soft palate very considerably. It drops down over the left side of the basis linguae and obstructs the view into the larynx. The upward view is obstructed by the protuberance of the velum palati, but the still intact os tubae may yet be perceived. Slightly increased size of the pharyngeal tonsil. A large, coarse, painless, movable gland about the size of a plum lies before the upper third of the sternocleido-mastoid. No other gland palpable with the exception of one of the size of a bean in the upper part of the maxillary angle.

An examination by Prof. Albrecht of a specimen taken at a preliminary examination and of the tumor, afterward extirpated, revealed a medium-celled sarcoma, the shape of the cells indicating that it probably originated in the lymph follicles.

The cutaneous section made, according to Mikulicz, from the point of insertion of the sterno-mastoid muscle to the greater cornu of the hyoid bone. This is followed by the exposing of the superficial cervical glands adjacent to the sterno-mastoid, and all such as arouse suspicion extirpated. The skin is drawn firmly forward and up and the inferior maxilla is exposed at the anterior margin of the masseter. At the same time the facial artery is located and pushed forward. The periosteum of the inferior maxilla is cut anterior to the masseter, elevated with the raspatory on the medial side and then, avoiding injury to the medial periosteum of the inferior maxilla, the latter obliquely is sawed through, from above and behind toward the front and downward.

As a preliminary, it is proper to bore the inferior maxilla for the suturing which follows. Then the periosteum of the lower and inside of the maxilla is detached from the line of the cut to the ascending ramus, for the purpose of manipulating it as I shall now describe, which manipulation is the main feature of the new method of operation

It is now seen that the inferior maxilla, caught with a wide retractor from the back of its ascending ramus, together with uninjured fascia parotideo-masseterica in situ, can now be pushed up, out and forward far enough to accomplish the same result for which Mikulicz resorted to total resection of the lower maxilla. The mandibular joint with its very wide socket permits of very free play of the condyle. The temporalis does not in any way oppose the processus coronoideus. If, after resection, the two parts of the inferior maxillary be not drawn apart as has been generally done up to the present, but if instead, the posterior section of the inferior maxillary be pushed forward, outward and over the anterior part, a vigorous pull on a wide retractor, which catches and draws backward the sterno-mastoid, the stylo-hyoideus and the nervus hypoglossus which appears under the latter, causes a wide space between the front margin of the sterno-mastoid and the ascending ramus, so that the field is now clear for final operation.

No important blood vessel leaves the carotid artery between the internal and external maxillary arteries along this line, and if it be desirable to expose the region of the tonsils, the interna may be protected, as it is situated up higher. Only the facial vein with its anastomoses requires double ligation. We have now reached the lateral wall of the pharynx. The finger crowds the tumor, which in this case could be bluntly detached, outward from the oral cavity. As in the Mikulicz process, we have up to the present operated *extra cavum oris et pharyngis* in this case, with the exception of the section of the inferior maxilla between the second and third molars, which in this instance does not bleed very much and forms a gap very easily tamponed. Of the more important vessels and nerves, only such as were absolutely unavoidable, the inferior alveolar arteries and nerves of the lower maxillary were severed, which is not detrimental. Eight days after the operation the mucous membrane of the lower lip had regained its sensitiveness. As the preparation demonstrates, the pharynx is splendidly exposed to view. By the proper pull on the retractor the openings of the larynx and the cavum may be seen clearly, so that I consider this method adapted to any manipulation of these parts. In my case the base of the tongue was laterally diseased and had to be partially removed. The arterial supply of the tonsils did not require any ligation, which would, however, have been an easy matter, as the view was entirely unobstructed.

The breathing was not disturbed, as the slight bleeding could be entirely controlled by tamponing the exterior. An exact suture of the wound of the pharynx with catgut and the tamponing with iodoform gauze the wound of the neck (which was nearly closed) followed. The maxilla was sewed with silver wire drawn over the cheek through buttonholes and knotted. The patient was nourished for only three days through a permanent esophageal tube. On the third day he could take liquid nourishment by lying on the healthy side. Beginning with the fourth day the tampon was changed daily and gradually decreased in size. On the 11th day the patient with the external wound healed was brought before the association. The maxilla had knit, the teeth scarcely lacking normal occlusion in mastication. Later an ulceration developed in the wound of the neck, caused by necrosis of the alveolar process at the point of resection. This would not in all probability have occurred had I extracted the third molar at the time of making the resection, as I was compelled to do later. Up to the present time, seven months after the operation, there has been no recurrence.

This method of operation, the novelty of which consists in pushing the posterior section of the inferior maxilla outward, forward and over the anterior section makes possible an uninterrupted view of the pharynx, cavum and opening of the larynx. It permits the discovery and removal of metastatically diseased glands, injures no muscle, nerve or important blood-vessel and requires no preliminary tracheotomy. It seems to me that it is destined to become the generally used method in removing malignant growths of the tonsils which do not encroach on the region between the inferior and superior maxillaries. For ailments of the latter parts the Mikulicz method seems to be the preferable one, as it makes the avoidance of subsequent ankylosis possible. My method seems to be peculiarly adaptable to the removal of tumors of the cavum, at the base of the tongue and the opening of the larynx, permitting, as it does, an uninterrupted view of those parts.

XIX

RECENT OBSERVATIONS CONCERNING PHONAS-THENIA.

By Dr. Theodor S. Flatau,

Berlin.

Translated by H. Strass,

St. Louis.

The occurrence of a large number of largely serious and chronic cases of phonasthenia has given me the opportunity (since my last publication concerning this disease), to further elaborate its course, and to illustrate it by many characteristics heretofore unknown.

I will not give a description of the early symptoms of this disease, even though this be of particular importance, owing to its insidious beginnings, and the frequent misinterpretations of its connections; the period of its first or earliest development is also often very protracted. Certain forms exist, which take years to develop the earliest symptoms, until destruction and intensified phenomena make recognition easy. I will confine myself to those symptoms selected from material observed during the last few years, and which offer new and important characteristics.

First in line we must mention the pains resulting from this disease.

Connection with the phonasthenie complex of symptoms is plain because of the fact that they accompany the phonetic action, that they are intensified during its progress, and disappear gradually when it ceases. In addition to the better known phonasthenie throat and chest pains, I have frequently described in detail the phonasthenie neck pain.

As related to these pains we may consider the phonasthenic jaw or maxillary pains, easily distinguished in a number of cases, especially in those of rheseasthenia, by certain well-defined characterstics.

The given cases were all uniform in this respect, that not in one of the maxillaries was found any reason for the pains. The most minute examination of the organs, by means of our own, and also dental aid, failed to discover any reason whatsoever for the maxillary pains.

The intensity of the maxillary pain may increase enormously; beginning in the inferior maxilla, it takes its way across the chin to both sides, embraces both superior maxillaries and loses its way towards the upper part of the head, or combines with the neck pain. The patients themselves describe a laxness or tired feeling of the lip and cheek-muscles. Pressure or pain, or any objective finding, does not exist.

Hyperesthesia and paresthesia within the laryngeal mucosa are also to be considered. While laryngeal pain, particularly in its neuralgic form, is well-known, hyperesthetic conditions, and in the beginning, their resultant reactions, are generally not considered related. The result of hyperesthetic conditions are irritative symptoms which are objectively noticeable. Added to these are the cough irritations, phonasthenie clearings of the throat, the desire to gulp or swallow, and the phonasthenie swallowing.

The course of the phonasthenie cough is often peculiar, and is frequently confounded with that due to a nervous cause. The distinction lies in the fact that the phonasthenic cough, as well as the clearing of the throat, only appear during the phonasthenie action, and are caused by hyper- and paresthetic conditions. This phenomenon may easily be brought about—for instance, causing a singer, suffering from dysodia, to hold a note for some time; especially in the effort caused to hold the tone piano, the described sensation will appear, followed by a phonasthenic cough, which is dry, and only after frequent recurrence is there a slight mucous expectoration. As frequent is the phonasthenic gulping, but inducing no secretion. This phonasthenie gulping is also a little known symptom, in fact, in many cases of this kind, particularly in the earliest stages of phonasthenia, it is frequently not diagnosed as a symptom, special or local treatment being of course without beneficent results. In typically characteristic and serious cases the connection of this phenomena with the disease is easily discovered, because the motions of swallow-

ing and the described irritation appear during phonasthenic
action.

I observed a preacher who suffered from this symptom
in its most aggravated form.   After uttering a few sen-
tences of his sermon, he began to feel the irritation in his
larynx.   He was obliged to yield to the inclination to
swallow. Resuming his lecture, the phenomenon again appeared, and caused such discomfort that he was forced to
give it up.

Another case was that of a singer, whose very possibly
exaggerated practice of holding back the voice (Stanue-
bungen), was probably the foundation of his trouble.   In
all cases of this kind, close observation and functional examination strengthen the diagnosis for phonasthenia, proving the existence of objective and essentially acoustic symptoms of this disease.

We have now arrived at the objective phenomena.   To
these belong, in the train of phonasthenia, the audible and
visible swallowings, gulpings, clearings of the throat and
coughs.   As belonging to these may be considered those
expressions of fear visible on the faces of persons before
an attack of phonasthenia, the sufferers being plainly distressed.   These symptoms of fear may be so strong as
to cause palpitation of the heart, paleness and excessive
perspiration.   Added to these, in serious cases, may be a
sudden cessation of the larngeal motions, a sum of phenomena which I might call "phonasthenie collapse."   In a
number of serious cases of rhesiasthenia.   I have been
able to observe patients while they were going about their
usual occupations, and at a distance was able to notice in
what order the symptoms appeared.

First, the voice became weaker, fainter, the various irritations already mentioned multiplied, expressions of fear
appeared, paleness, and beads of perspiration were visible
on face, forehead and brow.

A number of times these attacks disappeared, helped
by drinks of water taken at regular intervals to induce artificial cessation.   In one serious case the speaker was
obliged to resort to the blackboard to make himself understood.   Laryngeal motion ceases entirely when the symptoms of laryngeal collapse are well developed and appear
simultaneously in an attack.   In many cases the impres-

sion one carries away after witnessing an attack is anything but pleasant.

Breathing, even articulation continues, while the patient seems to be struggling to regain his voice. In fact, there is a superficial resemblance to stammering. In the cases under my care the progress of the disease was so closely observed that mistake was not well possible, as the symptom appeared only at the height of the combined phonetic collapse phenomena, while gradually the objective phonasthenic symptoms decreased, to completely disappear when a cure for phonasthenia was effected.

Concerning therapeutic development, the methods of treatment described by me some years ago, and adhered to since, have proved of value. Added to these are the combined uses of electricity and vibration. In order to show the workings of this apparatus, I have brought one with me. It is a much stronger machine than the earlier ones, and fitted with removable electrodes. This stronger electrical apparatus was made necessary by the fact that in the more recent employment of electricity for treatment, particularly of the high notes, the faradic current was frequently replaced by the alternating current, with 4,400 interruptions to the second, brought about by use of the Leduc apparatus, and this, as well as the faradic application, combined with my vibrator, also each factor used separately, was applied to the collar-like contrivance here shown.

Other influences were brought to bear on those chronic cases of phonasthenia with pronounced hypokinesthenic functional derangements, and at the same time anomalies of secretion, by quicker and more thorough methods, causing improvement of the circulation and nourishment of the laryngeal musculature. As in other cases of diseased respiratory organs, operative measures have proved useful. Some time ago I called attention, in cases of atrophic rhinitis, to the favorable results obtained by the introduction of foreign bodies, bringing about a radical cure, with permanent increase of tissue and normal secretion in cases of atrophic rhinitis in its fetid form. Right here the suitable application of Bier's hyperemia has been of such service that I would like, in a few words, to speak of this method, which I have used with success to combat cases of phonasthenia.

Measured according to the size of the thyroid cartilage,

the suction cups are applied to both sides in the ordinary way and increased gradually. With gradual increase of pressure I apply suction for three-quarters of an hour. A very thorough permeation of the tissues results, followed in first place by a functional derangement lasting about three days. During this period I usually abstain from using voice gymnastics in treatment. Resuming this, an improvement is noticeable in a few days; for instance, in a case of dysodia in the form of regained upper notes, in the case of objective phenomena, a further abatement of the severe symptoms of pressure and other evils.

This is the principal form of hyperemia used in cases of phonasthenia, though I practice it in still another manner, namely, in a slight case, with mild suctional pressure, proceeding in the following manner: I produce a congestion lasting a quarter of an hour, during this period using a modified voice gymnastic treatment with progressive movements.

Laryngoscopic examination will show that during intonation, by a slight tug at the suction cups, an abduction of the cords may be brought about. It is therefore easy to see the great value of such influences during phonation, when it is a question of removing hypokinetic phonasthenic movements which have become habitual, and on the other hand to further the strength of insufficient action by mild opposing measures.

Judging by the experiences of the past few years, I consider this therapeutic factor of the greatest importance, but do not wish to take the stand that this is to be without question the sole weapon against phonasthenia, for on this subject it will always be well to take into consideration the sum total of factors of a functional therapy, not to consider but one side of it in a mechanical manner.

BOOK REVIEWS.

Chirurgie des Gehirns und Rueckenmarks.

Vol. I. Surgery of the Brain. Price unbound 12 marks.
63 Figures and 23 Colored Plates.

The first volume of Prof. Krause's "Surgery of the Brain
and Spinal Cord," which concerns itself exclusively with
the technic of surgical procedures on the brain, will be
eagerly ready by otologists whose work carries them into
this field. Nowhere is it possible, as in this comparatively
small volume of 175 pages, to find as much valuable information on a subject which is beginning to interest surgical
otologists more and more. Although the work is an expression of the author's personal experience, he has given
due credit to the investigations and teaching of Johns Hopkins and Horsley in England.

To ear specialists the chapter on the treatment of abscesses of the cerebrum and cerebellum is by far the most
interesting. The various steps of opening an abscess from
the primary osteoperiosteal flap to the proper method of
tamponing are given with great detail. The position
which he takes of never puncturing through the healthy
dura is unquestionably correct, and his flap method gives
one a more extended view of the field of operation than the
haphazard method of destroying a large portion of bone,
when the procedure is carried out from the field of the former mastoid operation.

A particularly suggestive chapter covers the disturbances
and accidents which may occur during the after-treatment.
Bone necrosis, secondary hemorrhage, the escape of the
cerebro-spinal fluid and prolapse of the brain substance are
fully considered.

The removal of tumors from the region of the auditory
nerve is an operation which but few otologists have attempted, but the detailed explanation and the magnificent
plates give one a very clear idea of the procedure. Cranio-
cerebral topography is carefully explained and illustrated, and

such important details as narcosis, asepis, etc., are not neglected.

The plates are works of art, the colors true to nature and
the text clear and convincing.   HORN.

Lehrbuch der Ohrenheilkunde.

By Dr. GEORGE BOENNINGHAUS. S. Karger, Berlin.' Price
unbound 9.80 marks. With 139 drawings in the text and
one colored plate.

In this new text-book of "Diseases of the Ear," Boenninghaus sets a standard which in the future will be difficult to surpass. The work is filled from cover to cover with
original ideas and drawings, and brings one at once abreast
of everything new in the way of physical examinations.
Even Barany's very recent work on the diagnosis of labyrinth disease is fully explained, and the newest theories regarding the functions of the internal ear are clearly and intelligently treated.

The original sketches and new diagrams are helpful and
the lecturer and teacher will be able to gather some new
points which will tend to clarify and enliven his lecture
course.

The arrangement of the text is good, the press-work per-
feet and the colored plate helpful.   HORN.

Die Komplikation der Stirnhoelenentzuendung.

PROF. P. H. GERBER (Koenigsberg). S. Karger, Berlin. Unbound 15 marks. Bound 16.60 marks. With 450 pages
text and 36 illustrations.

The magnificent monograph of Gerber's, which has just
appeared upon "The Complications of Inflammations of the
Frontal Sinus," is the most complete work of the kind in
existence and will become a classic on this subject. Although the book has been in preparation for over five years,
the work of assorting and bringing together the immense
mass of literature was delayed until the moment of its appearance. From cover to cover the scientific exactness
which always characterizes Prof. Gerber's work, gives the
reader a sense of security and puts him in touch with all the
material which can possibly bear on this subject.

A radical attack on the frontal sinus and ethmoid labyrit.th is at best no child's play, and the individual operator can draw no general conclusions from the few cases he himself has treated. Let an important complication enter the case, and one will be more than thankful if he is in a position to put his finger on the combined experience of the world's best men. It is no compliment to our profession that most of the complicated cases fall into the hands of the surgeons and ophthalmologists.

Gerber criticises, and with a great deal of truth, the loose methods of classifying the diseases of the frontal sinus. He proposes a classification, which is very similar to that of Killian, and which seems accurately to cover the ground:

1. *Antritis frontalis simplex.
   a. Blennorrhea or pyorrhea antri.
   b. Empyema antri.
2. Antritis frontalis abscendens.
3. Antritis frontalis dilitans.
   a. Empyema c. dilatatione.
   b. Mucocele, cyst.

It is impossible to give in a few words the percentage of complications to frontal sinus affections in general. The reasons are clear. It is only very recently that careful postmortem examinations of the necessary cavities of the nose have been made. The actual percentage is small, but the impression which is gained from the writings of Kuhnt and others is that cerebral complications are much more common than we have thought. In Gerber's 493 cases of disease of the frontal sinus, he found 5 per cent complications.

In Chapter II. on the pathologic changes due to disease of the bony walls of the sinus, in addition to a complete literature on the subject, he quotes 11 cases from his own experience, which illustrate all degrees of bone disturbance from a simple periostitis to caries and necrosis of all the walls of the antrum. Of the rarer complications, 5 cases of cholesteatoma, 14 cases of pneumocele and 29 cases of osteomyelitis have been collected.

The chapter on anatomy is interesting. It is shown that

---

1. a. Those cases where the discharges empty into the nose.
1. b. Those cases where the discharges have no outlet.
2. Those cases where the discharges have perforated the bony walls of the antrum and collected under the skin.
3. Explains itself.

the percentage of frontal diseases is far greater in men than in women, and much more common on the left than on the right side. An absence of the sinus is found in 5 per cent of all cases. Based on this fact and on other equally well known anatomic grounds, he lays special stress on the point "That all intranasal operative procedures, whether the sinus is present or absent, are more dangerous than the external operation." A point with which most surgeons will agree.

The full treatment allowed to the anatomy of the ductus frontalis and its many anomalies, shows what a matter of overwhelming importance it is to know the pathologic condition of this duct, for on its patency depend largely the course and complications of the disease.

The two chapters on ocular, orbital and intracranial complications occupy the second half of the book. The eye complications are lightly but thoroughly covered, as the matter has often been thoroughly treated in the writings of ophthalmologists. One becomes acquainted, however, with every change that may occur and is put on the outlook for possibilities.

Fully 150 pages are devoted to intracranial complications other than the brain abscess. Of 51 cases of leptomeningitis following inflammation of the frontal sinus, 48 patients died! Need we be on the outlook for trouble or let a case of sinus disease drift along from day to day and not demand operation?

In the chapter on etiology, syphilis is shown to be a factor of but very little consequence, contrary to what has generally been supposed, and the great importance of influenza is clearly proven. The chapter on therapeutics is headed with the sentence "One cannot burn with water or wash with fire," and he is almost completely in accord with Fridenberg (N. Y.), who considers the most radical operation the best. In accord with most of the experienced operators of today, he considers the Killian operation, with some small modifications, undoubtedly the most practical.

Space forbids a more extensive review of this great work, but to a German reading specialist it is a book which is dangerous to be without, and it is to be hoped that a translation will soon be given to English readers.   HORN.

Das Gehirn und die Nebenhoehlen der Nase.

BY PROF. H. ONODI. Buchhandler, Alfred Hoelder, Wien.
Price unbound 10 marks. With 63 life-sized plates and
13 pages of text.

"The Brain and the Accessory Cavities of the Nose" is
the fourth of Prof. Onodi's great works on the subject of
the anatomy of the nose and its accessory cavities.

As the title indicates, the present work is a series of beautiful life-sized photographic reproductions, illustrating the
anatomic relations of the brain to these cavities. The outlines of various frontal sinuses have, by means of the X-ray,
been projected directly upon the surface of the brain. One
can see at a glance what areas are covered and what enormous and important variations can occur.

In the 1200 skulls examined, an entire absence of the frontal sinus was found in 5 per cent of the cases. A comparison
with the author's results obtained by transillumination is interesting and leaves us in no doubt as to the unreliability of
this method when used alone. Here 30 per cent. showed an
apparent absence on both sides, and 10 per cent. on a single
side.

A glance at Fig. 7, showing a right-sided frontal sinus 56
millimeters high and extending over on the left hemisphere,
demonstrates at a glance how a right-sided empyema could
give rise to a left-sided brain abscess and how necessary a
correct outline of the sinus would be in case of an operation.

Only 13 pages of text precede the 63 beautiful plates;
the pictures themselves being separately described. Some
of the sagittal sections are especially fine and in fact the entire work will win for itself warm appreciation from the
anatomist, the teacher and the specialist.   HORN.

Beitraege zur Topograpisch-Chirurgischen Anatomie der Pars Mastoidea.

VON DR. H. E. KANASUGI. Alfred Hoelder, Wien. Price
unbound 8.60 marks. Postage 1 mark. Bound 9 marks.
With 40 photographic illustrations in the natural size.

This contribution to the topographic and surgical anatomy of the mastoid portion of the temporal bone is the result of a series of investigations carried out by the author
on 4000 skulls. The text covers but 25 pages, but the life-

sized photographic plates with the accompanying remarks need no further explanation. Every variation which occurs in the anatomy of this region has been covered and complete bibliography is also given.

The plates are very fine, the frozen sections especially being highly instructive. Probably no work exists where the anatomy is more thoroughly worked out.   HORN.

ANNALS

OF

OTOLOGY, RHINOLOGY

AND

LARYNGOLOGY.

| VOL. XVIII. | JUNE, 1909. | No. 2. |

XX.

THE TREATMENT OF CANCER OF THE LARYNX.*

By Prof. Ottokar Chiari,

VIENNA.

AN ADDRESS DELIVERED BEFORE THE AMERICAN LARYNGOLOGICAL,
RHINOLOGICAL AND OTOLOGICAL SOCIETY, AT
ATLANTIC CITY, JUNE, 1909.

Mr. President and Gentlemen :—

It is with great pleasure that I comply with your request to deliver an address before the American Laryngological, Rhinological and Otological Society, for this association includes among its members some of the most prominent and celebrated men in our special line of work. In spite of my many heavy duties arising from my position as official Instructor in Laryngo-Rhinology in the University of Vienna, I concluded to accept this most distinguished invitation.

*Translated by Hanau W. Loeb, M. D., St. Louis.

I have selected as the subject of my address, "The Treatment of Cancer of the Larynx," a disease which, before the invention of the laryngoscope, was only superficially known and but seldom subjected to therapeutic attention. The new method of examination resulted first in a more intimate acquaintance with the disease, made an earlier diagnosis possible, and brought out a rational therapy.

The importance of therapeutic activity against this disease depends upon the terrible fate which awaits the victims who are not treated early. Each one of you has certainly been forced to stand by, helpless, while your patient with inoperable cancer of the larynx journeyed to his distressing end. The suffering of these patients is much greater than that of others who have cancer in other parts of the body. In addition to the pain, cachexia and symptoms and fear of the spreading of the cancer to other parts of the body, there are added symptoms resulting from interference with speech, respiration, and deglutition. And while the interference with respiration may be for the moment stayed by tracheotomy, early or late in the disease, it may make its appearance again through the growth of the cancer into the trachea. Besides, deglutition may become more difficult by involvement of the esophagus and thereby make the patient's life unbearable.

It is remarkable how long, comparatively, these patients may remain in this stage without being delivered from their terrible suffering, by an inflammation of the lung or a toxic condition of the blood. They generally succumb to the ever-increasing weakness from disturbed nutrition and frequently recurring hemorrhages. On this account, any effort to cure cancer of the larynx is a real blessing to suffering humanity, and a surgeon is likewise obliged to undertake serious operations if there is merely a prospect for radical cure.

In reviewing the several methods of relief, we should discuss the prophylaxis, the causal therapy, and then the operative methods and all the means directed against the various symptoms.

Prophylaxis would be of some value if we knew the cause of carcinoma. We may, however, state with great reserve that continued irritation of the mucosa of the larynx—for instance, by excessive smoking and drinking,—and, in addition, recurring catarrh, syphilis, (especially according to Esmarch's observations), and, finally, heredity are to be considered as probable causes of cancer of the larynx. With the exception of these, the whole power of the physician avails practically nothing as to the cause.

The causal therapy should be directed against the bacterial and protozoic cause of cancer which has been extensively studied up to the present time, but without result. The investigations depend upon the effort to cure the disease by the injection of cancer serum. (Adamkiewicz and Coley.) But, up to the present time, all of these attempts have proved unsuccessful.

The use of the Roentgen rays gave much hope in the beginning; certainly these rays have a specific action upon malignant neoplasms, but, until now, it has not been possible to apply them so as to cure the disease in this way. Gradenigo, in his paper before the International Congress of Laryngo-Rhinology at Vienna in 1908, reported that a careful study of the entire literature revealed that all attempts to cure cancer of the larynx by Roentgen rays had, up to the present time, been in vain. For this reason, no time should be lost with this agent, but early surgical procedure should be undertaken wherever possible.

On the other hand, the Roentgen rays appear to be of value in inoperable cases, especially when the larynx is opened and the rays permitted to act directly on the cancer. The same observation was made by D. Bryson Delavan, in 1902, and his views presented at that time, and in 1903, before the American Laryngological Association, were concurred in by Ingals, Payson Clark, Leland, Ames, Bliss, Swain, Birkett, and Simpson. Most of the discussants emphasized the fact that in inoperable cancer the X-rays reduce or dissipate the pain and stop the growth of the neoplasms. Dr. Cott (Bryson Delavan —Meeting 1904, p. 152) was able to cure completely a cancer recurrence of the larynx by sixteen applications of the X-rays, so that there was no evidence of the growth seventeen months later. On the other hand, Lincoln reported, in 1903, a case in which the use of the X-rays resulted in necrosis and extrusion of the epiglottis and both wings of the thyroid, causing death of the patient from pulmonary inflammation.

The use of radium has given exactly similar results as shown by Gradenigo in his report made at Vienna in 1908.

Dawburn's method of influencing cancer of the larynx by ligature of the carotid is also considered by Delavan to be of value only in inoperable cases.

Clarence C. Rice reported, in 1906, a case of carcinoma of the vocal band, which was treated with subcutaneous injections of trypsin (Fairchild's) and with the internal administration of holadin. The growth was thereby reduced to one-quarter of its size, but this portion remained.

Finally, Czerny (XV meeting of the Verein deutscher Laryngologen, June 8, 1908) employed fulguration in the year 1908. He removed a carcinoma of one of the cords by thyrotomy and permitted sparks of electricity of high frequency and high tension to play upon the surface of the wound for five minutes. Czerny is inclined to ascribe to fulguration a positive influence in preventing recurrence.

From this short review it is evident that none of the methods of treatment mentioned has, up to the present time, resulted in positive cure of cancer of the larynx, and that on this account we must lose but little time in operable cases. On the other hand, these methods have value, perhaps, in preventing recurrences, or, at least, in relieving sufferings and symptoms in the inoperable cases.

The surgical methods alone remain as of demonstrated value in cancer of the larynx, as these methods alone can show undoubted cures of long duration.

The results of extirpation of cancer of the larynx are, as a rule, better than in cancer in other parts of the body. The basis of this—which I need hardly bring before this meeting of distinguished professional men—depends principally upon the fact that cancer begins generally upon the inside of the larynx, as reported by Krishaber, in 1879. The designation, intrinsic, and extrinsic cancer originated with him.

Intrinsic cancer generally affects the vocal band and in this way causes hoarseness, which induces the patient to consult a laryngologist early in the disease; more uncommonly it is located on the ventricular bands, in the ventricle, or below the glottis; in any event it has the special characteristic of not infecting the lymph nodes of the vicinity in the earlier stages and even late in the disease.

The early removal of such an intrinsic cancer results generally in radical cure. Extrinsic cancers, on the other hand, which lie about the margins of the larynx, affect the lymph nodes much earlier and give, therefore, a much graver prognosis, even if I cannot quite agree with Delavan, who said, in 1904, "Extrinsic laryngeal carcinoma is practically incurable by operations," inasmuch as some cures are reported.

A positive estimate of the value of the surgical operative methods can only be determined by reliable statistics. The value of statistics is always properly subject to doubt, as the elements of error cannot be fully eliminated. Errors are most frequently found in the statistics of the results of operative methods in general and especially in those pertaining to cancer of the larynx. As cancer of the larynx is an uncommon affection, many busy surgeons and laryngologists with large practices see few cases and operate on still fewer. This and other sources of error were brought forward by Semon in Fränkel's Archiv. in 1897, and by Delavan at the 22nd Annual Meeting of the American Laryngological Association, in 1900. I am, also, of the opinion that the general statistics are subject to error for the following reasons:

First: None of these statistics taken from the operations of the most varied operators can be complete, as many operators do not publish their cases.

Second: Many operators only publish those cases which have a favorable result, and others only those which show some unusual characteristic.

Third: It is often impossible to report the later history of the patients.

Fourth: The various operators are not alike, either in the selection of cases or in the ability to operate.

Fifth: Some cases are reported twice.

Delavan properly requires the following of each statistic component:

First: The work performed must be of the highest order of perfection.

Section: All cases must be recorded in full, not only as to result but as to the details of the operation and of the after care.

Third: Sufficient time must elapse between the operation and the final report, in successful cases, to give full credit to the method employed.

These requirements can only be obtained from personal statistics of extensive "operators of the highest standing, who appear to have reported all of their material, good and bad." Delavan did me the honor to name me with Bergmann, Kocher, Mikulicz, Butlin, Schmiegelow, Fischer and Semon. He collected the results of these operators and calculated the percentage. These results are far more trustworthy than the general statistics, even if the number of patients is not so numerous.

Finally, I have sought to classify and compare the purely personal statistics of capable operators. The general statistics, however, must not be discredited, inasmuch as they command a far larger number of cases than the other and as they give an incidental conclusion as to the progress in various periods.

The best general statistics were collected by Sendziak, of Warsaw, as he sent, in 1894, a circular to all surgeons and laryngologists in the International Centralblatt für Laryngologie, and the various surgical and laryngological journals, German, English and French, in order to study the cases operated upon, from the accounts of the operators themselves. In addition, he wrote personally to numerous operators. Three such general statistics have been published by Sendziak: one published in 1897 (Bergmann, Wiesbaden), which included all cases up to 1894, a supplementary one up to the end of 1897 (Nowiny lekarskie, 1899, Nos. 1 and 2), and, finally, in 1908, in abstract (*Monatsschrift für Ohrenheilkunde*, etc., No. 4.).

On account of the great care shown by Sendziak, these are the best statistics. He excluded all cases which were incomplete or observed too short a time. In addition, I desire to mention still another which I had made from the abstracts in Semon's Centralblatt, particularly from the beginning of 1895 to the end of 1908. All the objections previously mentioned are applicable to this which, however, will serve for comparison with Sendziak's statistics, to which it is inferior inasmuch as a direct correspondence with the individual operators was not possible on account of the lack of time.

The most important question in all of the statistics is, after what period one may consider a case of cancer of the larynx operated upon as definitely cured. According to Maydl, Scheier, Wassermann, Sendziak, and Delavan, this period should extend to three years. Semon thinks that a case remaining one year without recurrence is with highest probability, according to his experience, to be considered as cured. Still, I believe that the period should be held as three years, since even this is no absolute warrant of continued cure. Several cases have been reported in which the recurrence was much later. I wish to report several cases from my own practice.

A patient for whom Billroth, in 1889, removed the left vocal band for cancer by thyrotomy, had no recurrence until four years later and from this he died three years later.

In 1900, I extirpated a vocal band by thyrotomy in a man who, six years later, died of cancer of the esophagus without involvement of the larynx. In October, 1903, I extirpated a cancerous vocal band in a patient who was affected again with cancer of the larynx in July, 1908. A patient died seven years after a unilateral extirpation of the larynx for cancer, from a new malignant neoplasm of the neck. As to the observation of others, I mention only the case of Hahn, which died from cancer of the cervical lymph nodes eight years after partial extirpation; and a case of Novaro in which death followed six years after operation on the cervical lymphatic nodes.

These cases show that there is really no positive foundation for the statistics; still, these cases are to be considered not as recurrence, but as newly occurring cancer in predisposed individuals.

On the other hand, there are favorable cases of cancer of the larynx which exhibit a benign course without radical operation. The case of Krieg and Knaus is well known. I have reported several such cases. I wish, at this time, to speak more particularly of one (*Arch. für Laryngologie.* 1908). In February, 1888, I removed from the left vocal cord of a man who had suffered from hoarseness for two years, a soft, vascular papillary growth, which, according to the examination of Professor Paltauf, proved to be papilloma which was disposed to degenerate into cancer. The patient felt so well after the operation and had such a clear voice that he did not wish an external operation to be performed. I removed, by July, 1889, three recurrences from the same quite movable vocal band. The growth removed in July, 1889, was, according to Professor Paltauf's histologic examination, suspicious of carcinoma. The patient still refused operation. Tracheotomy was finally necessary, in October, 1892, after several additional intralaryngeal operations and total extirpation of the larynx was now advised. As the patient still persistently refused external operation, the disease continued to make further progress and he died in 1894.

In this case the carcinomatous growth was in spite of repeated intralaryngeal operations confined for two years to the vocal band and it did not interfere with the movement of the band, a good proof that intralaryngeal operations are not so dangerous as considered by many.

I must now speak of the structure of carcinoma of the larynx, as this has certainly an influence on the rapidity of its growth. The most common form of cancer of the larynx is the squamous epithelium form, originating from the framework of the glottis. Horny, squamous, epithelial carcinoma or carcinoma karatodes is less common. Cylindrical epithelial cancer and medullary cancer are much less comman, and fibrous carcinoma is the most infrequent form. The most favorable is the fibrous, which, however, is extremely uncommon. It grows very slowly and infects the nodes very late. Squamous cell carcinoma is fairly benign, particularly as it begins at the vocal bands. It affects the lymph nodes very late, while, on the contrary, the horny epithelial carcinoma and the medullary form grow very rapidly and infect the lypmh nodes very early.

The conclusions drawn therefrom for the treatment of carcinoma of the larynx were published by Navratil (*Langenbeck's Archiv.*, 1905) in Buda-Pest. According to him, the common squamous cell carcinoma may be entirely removed by thyrotomy when it is intrinsic, and when it does not interfere with the mobility of vocal band. He advises partial extirpation in simple, intrinsic squamous cell carcinoma, involving only one-half of the larynx or the epiglottis, which has caused no metastases. He advises total extirpation in the beginning stages of horny squamous cell cancer and in squamous cell cancer which has extended, if the lymph nodes are felt small and not fixed.

Total extirpation is not indicated in extensive intrinsic cancer with participation of the esophagus and in horny squamous cell cancer, except when no metastatic lymph nodes are present, and, naturally, not in the very old. ,

In general, these indications of Navratil can only be approved, but it must be remarked that Gluck achieved good results with his method of operation even when there was extensive involvement of the pharynx, tongue, trachea, and thyroid, and in large lymph node tumors. At any rate, it would be desirable if in all cases the cancer had been determined by histologic examination before he had recourse to his radical operation.

As to the question of the province of the large external

operations for cancer of the larynx, it must be conceded to the experienced surgeon. This opinion is accepted everywhere. Among the American I mention John Mackenzie and Delavan. Naturally, the physician selected must have had experience in laryngology and there can be no doubt that this operation should, in the main, be undertaken by laryngologists who have had proper training as surgeons. It is self-understood that this claim can be made for but few laryngologists.

The operations which come into consideration for radical removal of cancer of the larynx are intralaryngeal extirpation, thyrotomy, partial and total extirpation of the larynx, and, in rare cases, subhyoid, transhyoid and lateral pharyngotomy.

INTRALARYNGEAL EXTIRPATION.

It is certainly indispensable, in most of the cases, to make a positive diagnosis. It is difficult, indeed, to recognize an intrinsic cancer in the beginning by laryngoscopy alone. Many laryngologists, and especially in America, Thrasher and Simpson in 1900, and Lincoln in 1903, have given expression to this view. It is, therefore, quite natural to remove a piece of the neoplasm intralaryngeally and to have it examined microscopically by a competent pathologist. This slight operation does the patient no harm. I need only mention Semon's report in 1887 and his address delivered in 1904 before the Laryngological Section of the Academy of Medicine in New York. John Mackenzie's fear, expressed in 1900, that the patient might be subjected to autoinfection is entirely erroneous. Mackenzie's position, "The removal of the piece for microscopic examination too often means the beginning of the end," is certainly incorrect. Many operators, including myself, have never seen such a result, and the case reported in this paper also shows this. Still, I do not wish to deny that any incomplete removal of a carcinoma may increase its growth.

Upon this point, Charles H. Knight made, in 1904, an interesting report. A growth on the vocal band, held to be a singer's node, was removed with the cold wire snare and recognized to be cancer; whereupon a rapid growth of the carcinoma resulted. Therefore, as I have long claimed, the external operation should not be postponed longer than a few days, or, at most, two weeks after the removal of the piece for examination, if the carcinoma has been determined histologically. In this way the simple intralaryngeal operation can certainly do no harm.

The case already mentioned, and several others, in which, on account of the refusal of the patient to submit to external operation, I was forced to perform intralaryngeal extirpation, have taught me that a radical cure can practically not be obtained by intralaryngeal operations.

Therefore, for more than twenty years I have held the opinion that as soon as any growth in the larynx has been determined to be cancer, it must be operated upon externally, if the operation is still admissible.

Still, attempts to remove cancer of the larynx by the intralaryngeal method have not been wanting, and occasionally with good result.

Elsberg, of New York, made the first observation of this sort in 1864. Recurrence followed and it was removed three years later by thyrotomy.

The first case treated with good result was reported by Schnitzler, of Vienna, who removed, in 1867, a tumor of the vocal band by the galvano-cautery method. Histologic examination showed it to be an epithelial cancer. This patient remained cured for twenty-two years.

Indications.—Most writers consider only small circumscribed tumors upon completely movable cords as proper for intralaryngeal method. B. Fränkel, alone, includes tumors which almost cover the vocal bands. Fränkel presents the following conditions in his article ("Die intralaryngeale Behandlung des Kehlkopfkrebs," *Arch. für Laryng.*, Vol. VI, 1897) : "It must be possible to remove the entire diseased portion intralaryngeally, and one must penetrate into the healthy tissues. Even in thyrotomy, if this becomes necessary, no more should be removed than should be with the intralaryngeal method. The favorable time for external operation should never be sacrificed for an intralaryngeal operation." The patient must be under the continuous care of the physician.

B. Fränkel, Krieg, Jurasz and Bresgen report quite favorable results from this operation. B. Fränkel is especially an enthusiastic supporter. Krieg maintains, on the basis of his well-known case (*Arch. für Laryng.*, 1894), that favorable results may be obtained by this method in the uncircumscribed forms of carcinoma. It is further known that the enthusiastic advocates of this method—Fränkel, for instance—announce that recurrences are very common after intralaryngeal extirpation; as, for instance, the case of B. Fränkel where permanent cure followed only after four operations.

RESULTS OF INTRALARYNGEAL OPERATIONS.
General Statistics.

No. of patients.	Relapses.	Cures.		Not available.
		Relative.	Absolute.	
32	13 (40.7%) 4, 3, 2 years or earlier.	4 (12.5%) 2, 2, 2 and 1 years.	4 (12.5%) 22, 8, 5 and 3 years.	On account of insufficient observation, 11 cases.
		25%		
39	14 (39%)	5 (14%)	9 (25%)	11
		39%		
39	13 (33%)	18 (46%)		8 insufficient observation.
36	8 (22.2%)	8 (22.2%)	8 (22.2%)	12 (33.3%)
		44.4%		

THE NINE CASES OF B. FRAENKEL.
iblished in the Archiv. tür Laryngologie, Bd. XI, 1897.)

Among other authors than Sendziak there are only thirty cases, of which only twenty-two are of service, with twelve cures, in five of which the duration was only a half year, in three two years, and in four over three years, of which one was for twenty-two years and one for ten years.

It is clear, according to these statistics, that the intralaryngeal operation is entirely without danger. No instance of death resulted from the operation, forty-six per cent recovered, but in thirty-three per cent there was recurrence. If one observes correctly the indications of B. Fränkel, this does not render the chances of a later operation, especially thyrotomy, any worse. Still, the favorable cases are exceptional. For this reason most writers, such as Schrötter, Semon, Delavan and myself, declare the intralaryngeal operation insufficient. Nevertheless, Simpson reported a case, in 1900, a cure of four years' duration, and Ingals, in 1907, one of more than one year's standing.

TRACHEOTOMY.

Cannot be considered as a curative operation. It serves only to relieve the stenosis of the larynx caused by the cancer, or comes into play as a preliminary to the radical external operation.

THYROTOMY.

Was first undertaken in 1833 by Brauers, in Loewen, for polypi, and in 1844 by Ehrmann, in Strassburg, for carcinoma of the larynx. Ehrmann's case, however, is so imperfectly reported that it cannot be considered of worth. The honor of first properly reporting this operation for cancer of the larynx belongs to an American—Gordon Buck—who undertook it in the year 1855, before the invention of the laryngoscope. He noted, however, recurrence in five months, and the patient died in ten months.

Solis Cohen operated in 1868 and reported cure of twenty years' duration.

Paul Bruns (Die Laryngotomie zur Entfernung endolaryngealer Neubildungen, Hirschwald, Berlin, 1878), gives an extensive presentation of nineteen cases of thyrotomy performed up to that time for cancer of the larynx, with the exception of the cases of Buck and Solis Cohen. These nineteen operations were performed on fifteen cases, four being twice operated upon. In all cases, but one, there was recurrence, and this patient died twenty-two months after the operation from cancer of the kidney, the larynx being free. Two patients died shortly after the operation. Besides these, there were sixteen local recurrences. in the main a few months after the operation. Bruns says in conclusion: "That the attempt at radical extirpation of cancer by means of thyrotomy has proved itself completely unsatisfactory and worthless." We should, however, not forget that wider-spread carcinoma had been operated upon after this method and that in five the operation had to be discontinued on account of hemorrhage.

This compilation made such an impression that in the following ten years thyrotomy was performed in but few cases.

At the London International Congress, in 1881, Foulis and Czerny formulated their views that established cancer of the larynx could only be relieved by total laryngectomy and then expressed almost no contraindications thereto.

Felix Semon stated, in the discussion at that time, that he presented no theoretic objection to total extirpation as such, but that he protested against its invariable use in all cases of cancer of the larynx, as this was neither theoretically or practically established. Semon further stated that we must see to it specially that a diagnosis of cancer is made early, so that we may get along with a smaller operation, a partial extirpation, or splitting the larynx alone, and removal of the soft parts. Semon has, since that time, striven to make the early diagnosis of cancer of the larynx possible, and has materially advanced it, especially in England. Butlin, who, since 1883, was of the opinion that total extirpation should be done immediately upon the establishment of the diagnosis, now attempts more often by thyrotomy to remove the soft parts alone or small portions of cartilage also, and is convinced, finally, of the radical value of this operation in proper cases—that is, early recognized and not too extensive cases, and especially in those limited to the vocal bands.

Semon soon followed his example and the favorable results of his operation, in the lessened number of deaths from the operation and in the greater number of definite cures, are the main reasons why thyrotomy, which formerly occupied such a bad reputation, has since then been used for the radical removal of cancer of the larynx.

Indications.—This operation is, according to the consensus of opinion of most operators, only indicated when the cancer is small and circumscribed, when it involves the vocal or ventricular bands without prejudice to the motility of the vocal bands. If the arytenoid is immovable, it is an indication that the cancer has spread to the deeper portions. Even when the arytenoid is not swollen, a partial extirpation must be performed. Only Cisneros, at least up to 1905 (*Centralblatt für Laryng.*, 1905, p. 127), and Pieniazek (*Archiv. internat. de Laryng.*, etc., March and April, 1908), up to 1908, recommend thyrotomy in complete immovability of the vocal bands; and Pieniazek also in swelling of the arytenoid and large subglottic extension.

For this reason, these writers have such numerous recurrences, as we shall see later in our statistics. We must, therefore, agree with Semon that thyrotomy early enough undertaken in favorable cases is a truly ideal operation in cancer of the larynx. Even Gluck, who certainly does not shirk the most radical surgical operations, says: "Laryngofissure is not only a palliative measure in the early stages of carcinoma, but also a blissful radical and, therefore, conservative operation."

I need not speak extensively of the technic of this operation and the after-treatment, before this body of professional men. I will only mention that most operators perform tracheotomy first and then introduce a tampon-canula. Bruns (Tübingen), Moure (Bordeaux), and Pieniazek (Krakau) are content with a simple canula and permit the head to hang below. Pieniazek and his assistants have performed three hundred thyrotomies, twenty for cancer, in this way, without a death.

Butlin and Semon, who have reported very favorable results, and Moure remove the canula immediately after the operation and suture the larynx and trachea partially or completely.

The other operators, including myself, generally tampon the larynx with a Mikulicz tampon, then place an ordinary canula in and remove the tampon after three to eight days. Even Kocher, the celebrated surgeon, and most of the other operators, would not renounce this tampon, since it furnishes a positive protection against the entrance of blood, wound secretions, mucus, and saliva into the trachea during the first few days after the operation. One should not forget, in this connection, after splitting the larynx to apply cocain to the inner surface of the larynx, according to the advice of Billroth, in 1886, and the warm recommendation of Felix Semon, or, according to

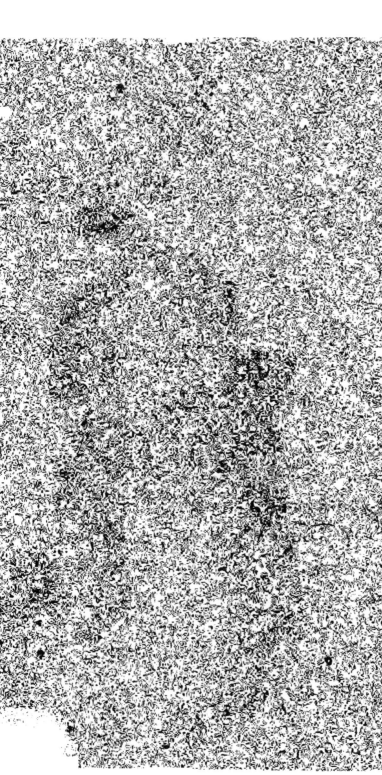

My own statistics, of forty-one completed operations, show about the average results, and, by reason of the relatively large number of cases, they give a most reliable estimate of the value of thyrotomy. The number of cures would have been much greater if there had not been thirty-nine per cent of my cases (i. e., twelve cases) without later news. These refer mainly to patients from foreign countries, the Balkan Peninsula, Russia, and to those belonging to the poorer classes whose addresses were unknown.

Very likely some of these twelve cases belong to the group of those recovered, as they had been dismissed, cured.

The bad results of Cisneros are to be explained on the basis that he included among the thyrotomies, up to 1905, every case in which the vocal band was partially or completely immovable; i. e., such cases as properly belong to unilateral laryngectomy.

The same thing pertains to Pieniazek who likewise, established too broad indications for thyrotomy.

All operators report that the voice always becomes good after the removal of one vocal band, and also after removal of the ventricular bands. One of my patients delivered scientific lectures for a year after the operation, and one in whom I had removed both vocal and ventricular bands in three thyrotomies can still, after seven years, speak quite loud and can be understood. In none of my patients was it necessary to reinsert the canula. For these reasons, thyrotomy is an operation full of blessing in suitable cases. It has very slight mortality and exhibits many lasting cures. The important factor in producing a favorable result is the early diagnosis of the cancer.

PARTIAL EXTIRPATION.

Under this head are included the atypical partial extirpation and the typical unilateral form, as well. Heine, in Prague in 1874, first introduced partial extirpation for the relief of cicatricial stenosis. The first surgeon to use it for cancer of the larynx was Maas, of Breslau, in 1876, who removed all the larynx except a piece of the cricoid and the epiglottis. Recurrence appeared in three months.

Billroth, of Vienna, who first undertook this operation in 1878, removed the whole left half of the larynx, and he gave it the name of "halbseitige extirpation." According to Sendziak, this operation was performed in 224 cases of cancer of the larynx up to the end of the year 1907.

Indications.—The most suitable cases are those in which the cancer is developed upon the vocal bands and visibly retards or prevents their mobility, without the presence of lymph node enlargement and without the pharynx being affected.

Somewhat less suitable are the extrinsic cancers which have their origin on the arytenoid or the aryepiglottic folds, and, finally, those cases in which one side of the larynx is wholly involved. If the other side becomes eventually involved, it is always possible to remove smaller or larger portions of the affected part, but the result of the operation is always more doubtful. It depends, therefore, on the opinion of the operator, whether he attaches importance to the fact that a small portion of the larynx is left in relation with the trachea, by means of which voice production is greatly facilitated.

As a usual thing, tracheotomy is generally performed five to fourteen days before the partial extirpation. This is quite necessary if severe dyspnea is present, in order that the patient may be relieved of the results of larynx stenosis. If no dyspnea is present, the tracheotomy may be performed immediately before the extirpation.

The operation is practically always performed with the aid of a tampon canula, under chloroform narcosis. Kocher, of Berne, performed, under cocain, such partial extirpations in which it was not necessary to remove so much of the cartilage.

I do not wish, at this place, to go into the details of the operation. The cricoid may be spared occasionally in partial extirpation. Under these circumstances, naturally, the operation is easier. If, on the contrary, a piece is taken away from another level of the larynx, the operation will be longer and more detailed, but the course will be the same. I have often, in such cases, removed almost the entire larynx in this way, but of late I perform total resection with previous suture of the tracheal stump, after the method of Gluck.

If the pharynx is involved, the affected portion must be cut away and removed from the healthy portion. In this particular, all suspicious lymph nodes are included.

After-Treatment.—The first tampon, which is introduced with special care, is permitted to remain as long as possible, as Koschier recommends. When the tampon no longer completely closes, in about eight days, it is replaced by another and this is changed as often as necessary. After five or six days the nourishment tube may be removed, as the patient can

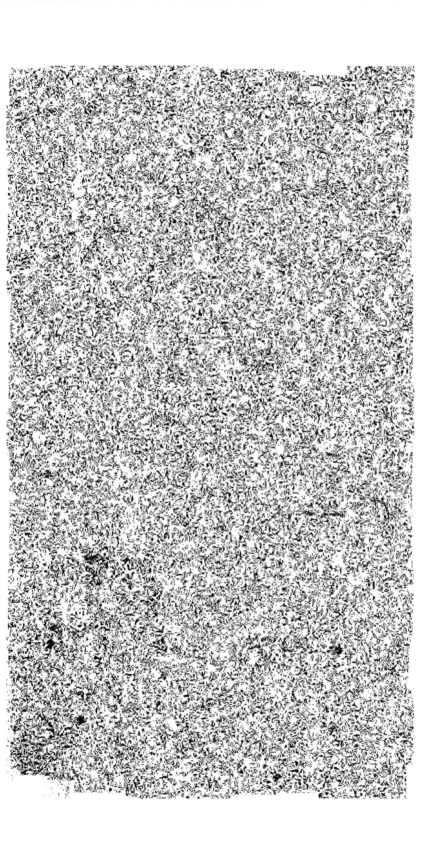

ITALIAN STATISTICS.

riter.	No. of patients.	Death following operation.	Recurrence
to 1906.............	13	2 (15.3%)	5 (38.4%)

Cure resulted in these few, very favorable cases in 46% of the cases. The large general statistics show a decided reduction in the fatal cases and recurrences, and an increase in the cures after 1888 and especially after 1895. Delavan's statistics, which were collected from the reports of seven operators (by the before mentioned and by Fischer), show the transition to the purely personal statistics.*

Of the 32 partial laryngectomies reported by me, two each were performed by my assistants, Professor Harmer, Dr. Kahler, and Dr. Marschik, at the clinic during vacation, the remaining 26 by myself. One case remained cured for six years, when I lost sight of him. Another died six years and four months after operation from carcinoma of the neck, which appeared three months before death. I have included this case under the recurrences. Two of the eight relatively cured patients have lived for two years and four months, and two years and two months, up to the present time, two lived two years and eight months and two years, and one lived eight months and then disappeared from observation. One died of pneumonia one year after operation, one died of diabetes one year after operation, and one died one year and two months after operation from a febrile disease of two days' duration, all without recurrences.

There was recurrence in fifteen cases; in four after one year, in one after six years and four months, and in ten after a few months. I removed almost the entire larynx in some of these cases.

----

*See next page.

DELAVAN'S STATISTICS.

Author	No. of patients.	Deaths following operation.	Recurrences	Cures.		Remarks.
				Relative.	Definite.	
Delavan, 1900. Results of 8 operators	56	15 (26.8%)	21 (39%)	34 (56%) { 27 (43.5%)	7 (12.5%) }	Death following inter-current disease, 14 (25%). Total, 84.

PERSONAL STATISTICS.

Author	No. of patients.	Deaths following operation.	Recurrences	Cures.		Remarks.
				Relative.	Definite.	
Billroth, 18 years (cited by Salzer)	14	5 (35.7%)	6 (42.8%)		3 (21.4%)	
Bergmann; Graf-Deutscher Laryngologen Kongress, 1897	20		8 (40%)			
Cisneros, 1908	40				6 (15%)	
Koschier, 1909	16	1 (6.25%)	10 (62.5%)		3 (18.75%)	2 (12.5%) insufficiently observed; operated in 1906, 1907, 1908.
Gluck, 1908						States that he performed hemilaryngectomy 43 times without a death since he has been making his laryngoplastic. In 13 of these cases there was a recurrence; 19 showed no recurrence.
Chiari, to end 1907	32	8 (25%)	15 (46.67%)	8 (25%) {	1 (3.1%) } (28.1%)	

The personal statistics show most varying results; the percentage of fatal cases in Koschier's cases was only 6.25, while he had 62 per cent recurrences; the results of the other operators were much more nearly uniform. An exceptional result is to be found in the report of Gluck who had no fatal issue following the 42 hemilaryngectomies which he performed according to his method. However, he does not present a statistical account of his cases.

TOTAL EXTIRPATION.

Watson, of Edinburgh, extirpated the whole larynx for syphilis, in 1866. Czerny, while assistant of Billroth, in Vienna, removed the entire larynx in dogs and showed that they were in moderately good condition afterwards. By reason for this, Billroth made the first operation in man for cancer on December 31st, 1873. The patient died, however, eight months later from a recurrence, which very likely arose from the epiglottis which was not removed. Since this time, the operation has been frequently performed. Sendziak was able to report 188 such operations up to 1894, and more than 416 up to the end of 1907.

Indications.—The opinion of specialists has been changed to the effect that total larynx extirpation, or laryngectomy as it is also called, is only necessary when both sides of the larynx are affected. In general, we can say that very many operators consider those cases only as operable where there are not many lymph nodes affected and these completely movable. Besides, not a great portion of the pharynx must be affected with cancer, and but few of the rings of the trachea or the thyroid gland. Many operators believe that those cases of intrinsic cancer which grow through the thyroid cartilage and extend outwardly can hardly give any hope of radical cure. Most operators operate, with a tampon canula, several weeks after a preliminary tracheotomy. Only a few apply a single canula and endeavor by the position of the patient, with head hanging down, to prevent the entrance of blood into the trachea.

Bardenheuer, in 1890, made the proposition that the mucosa of the posterior wall of the larynx,—that is, the anterior wall of the esophagus,—be sutured to the mucosa of the pharynx in the neighborhood of the hyoid, thus completely closing off the oral cavity from the wound remaining after the removal of the larynx. Bardenheuer also advised that the patient should lie in bed in such a way that the head would be much lower than the tracheal opening so that the discharges from the mouth could not flow into the trachea. Butlin and Semon place the patient horizontally on the side (in the unilateral extirpation on the operated side). The after-treatment is the same as in partial extirpation. I have lately heard of the excellent results of Dr. Chevalier Jackson, who had, I believe, no deaths and numerous cures.

The completed operation leaves, as a rule, a connection between the wound opening and the trachea, so that the patient, even if he wears the canula, can blow air through the window of the canula into the pharynx and oral cavity. In order to give the patient vocal speech, a tube may be introduced, in three or four weeks, from the canula to the lower end of the pharynx and a reed may be placed in this tube. This instrument is known under the name of artificial larynx. This artificial larynx, however, generally gives the patient such discomfort and annoyance that he remains content with whisper voice. This whisper voice, as a rule, becomes fairly satisfactory by exercises and the artificial larynx is discarded.

That it is possible to have a fairly loud voice after complete closure of the pharynx and oral cavity from the trachea was already known to Czermak, and was later often confirmed by Gluck.

GLUCK'S OPERATION METHOD.

In order to obviate the danger of aspiration pneumonia and an infection of the neighborhood of the wound through blood, discharge or food, Gluck recommended a procedure at the Surgical Congress in Berlin in 1881, with the report of several favorable cases, by which the trachea is cut off from the larynx one to two weeks before the operation, drawn forward and sutured as carefully as possible with its borders in the skin wound. This prophylactic suturing of the tracheal stump forms an absolute protection against the development of aspiration pneumonia. More recently, he releases the entire larynx and upper part of the trachea from their attachments and then severs the larynx from the trachea and sutures the tracheal stump.

He uses the old method only where there is serious

dyspnea. Gluck reported in 1908 that he had a cure in 128 of his own cases of total laryngectomy. None of his cases of typical laryngectomy in many years has succumbed to the operation. Out of about 300 operations on the upper respiratory and deglutition apparatus in which it was necessary to make very extensive extirpation of lymph nodes, ligatures of the large cervical vessels and extensive resection of portions of the tongue, pharynx and esophagus, the mortality reached only 13 per cent. Already in 1904 he could present a series of eleven such serious cases without fatal issue from the operation. It is unfortunate that up to the present time there are no definite personal statistics of Gluck's operations for cancer of the larynx. However, it appears from the data just mentioned that his results are better than those of any other operator. For this reason I use as often as possible his method of suturing the trachea in advance and shutting off the pharynx from the trachea and the adjacent tissues; so far I am satisfied with this method.

Of my nine cases,* eight were performed by me and one by my assistant, Dr. Kahler, in the clinic. In eight of the cases the tracheotomy was performed several weeks in advance. In my last case, it was necessary on account of severe dyspnea to open the trachea immediately before the extirpation.

Gluck's method was used in all the cases, for the trachea was sutured into the skin wound and the pharynx completely shut off below from the respiratory tract.

In general it must be said that the personal statistics are in part incomplete and in part the cases are too few to permit any definite conclusions to be drawn from them. The general statistics, which show very favorable results only remain to determine the value of complete laryngectomy. So far as mortality is concerned, the results since 1895 are better than in partial laryngectomy and are next to thyrotomy; it surpasses all other methods in regard to recurrence; as to cure, it ranks just next to partial laryngectomy and about half that of thyrotomy. Gluck's results, as already mentioned, are the best. It is true that he has had a mortality in all of his complete laryngectomies of 13 per cent, while my general statistics from 1895 to 1908 show only 12 per cent, but he had many seriously complicated

*See page 29.

GENERAL STATISTICS OF RESULTS OF TOTAL EXTIRPATION.

Author	No. of patients.	Deaths following operation.	Returns.	Cures.		Remarks.
				Relative.	Definite.	
Sendziak, 1873-1894 incl.	188	84 (44.7%)	61 (31.45%)	13 (6.9%)	11 (5.85%) 12.75%	24 cases insufficiently observed. Total, 193.
Sendziak, to 1897 incl...	267	94 (35.2%)	81 (30.3%)	24 (9%)	12 (4.4%) 13.4%	32 cases insufficiently observed. Total, 243.
Sendziak, 1873 - 1907 (416); 1888 to end 1907 (269)	269	58 (21.6%)	46 (17%)	58 (21.6%)		107 cases insufficiently observed.
Perez, 1906 (Italian operators)	73 for carcinoma laryngis.	22 (30.13%)	29 (39.8%)	5	5 10 (13.7%)	Deaths from intercurrent diseases, 6 (8.2%); insufficiently observed, 6 (8.2%).
Chiari, 1895 to end 1908	242 (including 24 complicated cases.)	29 (12%)	21 (8.7%)	24 (9.9%)	38 (15.7%) 25.6%	130 cases insufficiently observed (53.7%).

From these General Statistics it will be seen that the results are distinctly better since 1888, especially since 1895. Especially noteworthy is the decrease of deaths following the operation to 12 percent and that of returns to 8.7 per cent.

DELAVAN'S STATISTICS (1900) OF SIX OPERATORS.

(Bergmann, Kocher, Mikulicz, Fischer, Chiari, Schmiegelow.)

Author	No. of patients.	Deaths following operation.	Recurrences	Cures. Relative.	Cures. Definite.	Insufficient observation.
Delavan	34	9 (26.5%)	12 (35.3%)	11 (32.3%)	2 (6%)	Death from intercurrent diseases 16 (47%).

AUTHOR'S STATISTICS.

Author	No. of patients.	Deaths following operation.	Recurrences	Cures. Relative.	Cures. Definite.	Insufficient observation.
Billroth, 18 years (according to Salzer)	5	4	1			
Bergmann, 1883-1896	28				4 (14.3%)	
Cisneros, 1908	15					
Koschier (personal communication)	3	In uncomplicated cases practically none.			2 (66.6%)	Insufficiently observed, 1 case.
Gluck, 1908	128			25	35% { 20	
Chiari (to 1909 incl.)	9	3 (33.3%)	4 (44.4%)			Two observed only a few months (22.2%).

cases with involvement of the tongue, esophagus, thyroid gland and ligature of the large vessels. In the uncomplicated cases he had no mortality, so the superiority of his method is demonstrated. Cisneros had in one year 7 complete laryngectomies with suture of the trachea in advance, death following in only one case (*Boletin de laringologia,* Dec., 1907). v. Hacker (Graz) and Motella (Madrid) also operate accordling to Gluck's method. Patients upon whom Gluck's method of total laryngectomy has been performed learn almost always easily understood pharyngeal speech which is often loud in character. This result is attained more quickly by instruction from a specialist in speech defects.

Deglutition is difficult in those cases only in which a large part of the pharynx or esophagus has been removed. In such cases Gluck uses rubber prosthetic appliances which carry the food through the mouth. I saw such patients in London in 1905, and in Vienna in 1908, in which Gluck had removed, at the same time, the larynx, some tracheal rings and a portion of the tongue and esophagus. They wore a prosthetic appliance, were well nourished, spoke with a loud voice in spite of a large cervical fistula. They declared that they were satisfied with their lot. It is certain that this extensive resection of the larynx, pharynx, esophagus and tongue is justifiable from an ethical and social standpoint. Therefore, we must be thankful to Gluck for his tireless and oft misunderstood efforts. In spite of this it must be the endeavor of the laryngologist to recognize cancer of the larynx so early that it may be radically cured by thyrotomy, as this operation results in the most cures and but slight mortality even if there are more recurrences than in complete laryngectomy. Those operated upon breathe, speak and swallow in the natural way; but these results are attained only if Semon's advice is followed, namely, to perform thyrotomy only if the intrinsic cancer but slightly diminishes the motility of the cords. Early diagnosis, however, is only possible after intralaryngeal removal of a portion of the growth for diagnostic purposes—an operation which is not difficult.

I must therefore declare that the opinion of John Mackenzie, against the extirpation of a portion of the growth for microscopic diagnosis and against thyrotomy as a radical operation,* as unfounded in view of the experience of many distinguished laryngologists as well as my own.

Only with insufficiency of thyrotomy is partial or complete laryngectomy advisable.

UNCOMMON OPERATIVE PROCEDURES.

Subhyoid pharyngotomy (Richet), or subhyoid laryngectomy (Malgaigne), is proper for those cancers which involve only the entrance of the larynx; they are generally located on the epiglottis alone, more uncommonly on the arytenoid or aryepiglottic fold.

The following gives the results.

GENERAL STATISTICS.

riter.	No. of patient				
k up to the end 4	8	5 (62.5%)	1 (12.5%)	1 (12.5%)	1 (12.5%

Cisneros reported in 1908 two cases without special details. The operation gave very unpleasant immediate results. •Semon (*Fraenkel's Archiv.,* Vol. VI, p. 412) operated a single time, the patient dying in four days. I did it once in 1897, in connection with a lateral pharyngotomy for a cancer of the right arytenoid and of the recessus piriformis. The patient recovered, but had a recurrence in the lymph nodes at the end of that year.

Rene Lacour* collected 40 cases operated on for various conditions, with a mortality of 10 (25 per cent). It is seldom done for carcinoma of the larynx. Cisneros, epithelial carcinoma of the epiglottis, recovery (*Centralblatt für Laryngol.,* 1900); Lutz, epithelioma of the larynx, recovery (*Philadelphia Med. journal,* February 24, 1900); Lambert Lack, epithelioma of the larynx, recovery for over two years (*Centralblatt f. Laryng.,* 1906, p. 36); Brockaert (*Centralblatt fuer Laryng.,* 1905, p. 352). Subhyoid pharyngotomy with temporary resection of the hyoid bone for tumor of the ary-

---

*These de Paris, 1897. Central. f. Laryng., 1898, p. 315.

tenoid and pharynx, death in three weeks. Also, since 1895, six operations with two deaths, one recurrence and three recoveries.

TRANSHYOID PHARYNGOTOMY was introduced by Vallas, 1896. It comprehends the median splitting of the hyoid bone and membrana hyoidea, permitting the edges of the wound to be held apart by strong retractors. It is claimed that in this way the passage to the larynx is good. Cisneros stated in his report at the International Congress of Laryngo-Rhinology at Vienna that he had performed the operation eight times but did not mention his results.

MEDIAN PHARYNGOTOMY by Mouret (*Bulletins et Memoires de la Societe Franc. de Laryn. et de Rhin.*, 1908, p. 405), is a combination of transhyoid pharyngotomy and thyrotomy. It has not been used for cancer up to the present time.

LATERAL PHARYNGOTOMY has been used according to various methods, those of Langenbeck, Bergmann, Küster, Mikulicz and Cheever, and is suitable especially for carcinoma of the pharynx and tongue and less so for cancer of the larynx. I once saw Gussenbauer remove a cancer of the left arytenoid after this method; the patient however died of diabetes ten days afterwards. Lambert Lack (Proceedings of the London Laryngological Association, March 17, 1905; *Centralblatt fuer Laryng.*, 1906), removed a carcinoma of the right arytenoid and pharynx, after this method. Recovery for one year.

I repeat, in conclusion, that in such a terrible disease as cancer of the larynx, serious undertakings are permitted but the patient should be fully informed of his disease with the greatest indulgence. The results of the individual operation can be only properly determined if all extensive operators report all their cases with the utmost detail as was already suggested by your distinguished colleague, Bryson Delavan in 1900.

XXI.

A STUDY OF THE ANATOMIC RELATIONS OF THE OPTIC NERVE TO THE ACCESSORY CAVITIES OF THE NOSE.*

By HANAU W. LOEB, A. M., M. D.,

ST. LOUIS.

(FROM THE ANATOMICAL DEPARTMENT OF ST. LOUIS UNIVERSITY.)

Although a great deal has been written during the past ten or fifteen years upon the anatomy of the accessory cavities of the nose, comparatively little has been done in the direction of establishing the relation which they bear to the optic nerve. True, the exhaustive work of Onodi[20] has been of great value in this respect, but there is still much to be done.

CLINICAL REVIEW.

There has been considerable clinical evidence of this relation, as may be easily discovered by a casual view of the literature. In this abstract of cases I have purposely excluded the large number of orbital abscesses which have been reported, confining it to those in which changes in the nerve itself were noted, without symptoms of an associated infection of the periorbita.

Berger and Tyrman[2] state that 26 cases of blindness had been reported, due to disease of the sphenoid, six from caries and twenty from tumors.

Welge, according to Berger and Tyrman,[2] reports the case of a man who as a result of suppuration in the accessory cavities of the nose became blind in both eyes.

Caldwell[5] reports a case of suppuration of the sphenoid sinus and marked hyperemia of the disk with necrosing and

---

*Read before the New York Academy of Medicine, November 25, 1908.

cystic ethmoiditis, causing atrophy of the right and then the left optic nerve and blindness.

Kuhnt[9] cites a case of amaurotic amblyopia following an acute coryza.

Courtaix[6] collects several cases of ocular disease from literature which seem to be due to suppuration of the maxillary sinus: B. Travers.[43] A case of beginning amaurosis, checked by extraction of a tooth. Galezowski.[9] Amaurosis, cured after thirteen months by extraction of a tooth. Pasquier.[33] Five days after extraction of a tooth, sudden complete right-sided amaurosis developed with foul discharge from the nose. Ten days later sight returned. Joh. Hjort[16] reports a case of frontal empyema causing exophthalmus and papillitis with distinct diminution of vision.

Winckler[45] reports a case of retrobulbar neuritis cured by removal of a hypertrophied inferior turbinate.

Hansell[15] reports a case of acute loss of vision, due to disease of the ethmoid and sphenoid cavities.

Holmes[17] gives the notes of a case of empyema of the left sphenoid sinus which had been unrecognized until patient completely lost sight in the left eye. Vision became normal after opening the sphenoid sinus.

Bull[4] calls attention to symptoms from involvement of the optic nerve by tumors of the sphenoid.

De Lapersonne[20] reported at the Congress at Utrecht several cases of unilateral optic neuritis with greyish projecting papilla, with voluminous and tortuous vessels hidden by edema behind the papilla, without retinal hemorrhages. They were accompanied by well-marked amblyopia, scotoma and reduction of the visual field. In spite of treatment, they resulted in complete blindness of the affected side through papillary atrophy. Careful rhinoscopic examination revealed sphenoid sinusitis or posterior purulent rhinopharyngitis. In the discussion which followed, these observations were confirmed by Knapp, Meyer, Kuhnt and Gutmann; Meyer claiming that the attack could be arrested by treatment of the sinus disease.

Halstead[14] observed sudden blindness in the left eye in a case of empyema of the right maxillary, ethmoid and sphenoid cavities. After operation the patient recovered vision. He thought that the contralateral involvement depended upon the rupture of the sphenoid septum, but in the light of later studies of the relation of the sphenoid cavity to the optic nerve, a better explanation is found in the fact that a sphenoid sinus may be in relation with both optic nerves. (See figures 1, 7, 9, 10, 13, 14, 15, 16, 22, 24, 25, 28, 29, 30.)

Mendel[25] reported several cases in point:

(a) A patient with left exophthalmus for two years with gradual loss of sight, whole lower and part of temporal portion of the left field of vision lost; disk outlines indistinct and pale; pus found in left antrum. Operation resulted in some improvement in vision.

(b) Sudden loss of sight in left eye with large absolute central scotoma and suppuration of anterior and middle ethmoid cavities. Operation was followed by immediate improvement, eventually with almost complete recovery of sight.

(c) In (four of seven) cases of unilateral optic neuritis, the accessory cavities were involved in (four) cases, one being of the maxillary. An old amaurosis was not cured by operation, nor was a case of bilateral atrophy.

Nordquist[27] reports a case of optic neuritis, due to maxillary empyema.

Broeckaert[3] reports the case of a woman suffering from chronic suppuration of the ethmoid and frontal with detachment of the retina and numerous opacities of the vitreous. The opacities disappeared, the detachment persisted and vision became sharp in the intact portion of the retina after the suppuration was relieved.

De Lapersonne,[21] in a most detailed paper, discusses the various aspects of the subject. He calls attention to the reports of Reinhardt, Braun, Neiden and Panas, who had noted blindness, unilateral or bilateral, following infectious optic neuritis, but in these the lesions were very extensive. He maintains that sphenoid sinusitis may be complicated by optic neuritis, papillitis with more or less encroachment on the retina, and prepapillary edema, accompanied by considerable diminution of central or peripheric vision; and that while amelioration is possible by treatment, the prognosis is none the less serious.

Risley[39] describes a case of hemicrania and partial loss of sight, which were relieved by treatment of a gummi of the maxillary sinus; another case of general neuritis with blindness in maxillary empyema; and another in which a secondary neuritis from sphenoid and ethmoid empyema resulted in blindness of the right side.

Gronbak[13] had a patient, aet. fifty-one years, who was referred to him by an ophthalmologist with the statement that there was disease of the left optic nerve and several motor branches of the ocular muscles, complete amaurosis on this side, nothing on ophthalmoscopic examination, papilla normal, distinct exophthalmus. Upon removal of the nasal polypi and a large carious portion of the left middle turbinate, he found for the first time thick, foul-smelling pus coming from the ethmoid cells. The carious portions of the ethmoid were removed and the opening of the sphenoid sinus enlarged. The exophthalmus disappeared, the muscular paralysis vanished, but the amaurosis continued unchanged.

Polyak[36] reports a case of bilateral optic atrophy of three years' standing, resulting from a suppurating bone cyst of the left middle turbinate, which filled the left nostril and closed the openings of the posterior ethmoid and sphenoid, causing retention of secretions and eventually empyema of these sinuses. As there was no other way for it to grow, Polyak thought that it forced the posterior portion of the septum to the extreme right, causing retention of secretion and empyema on this side. Although the process started on the left side, the right optic became first affected. It is, however, no less rational to assume that the left sphenoid was in relation with both optic nerves, as in the case of the sphenoids shown in the figures to which reference has already been made in discussing Halstead's case; or that the last posterior ethmoid cell was in relation with both optic nerves, as in Onodi's case.

Onodi[21] addressed letters to various ophthalmologists, with the view of ascertaining the clinical proofs of the influence of disease of the posterior nasal accessory cavities upon the optic nerve. In reply, Schmidt-Rimpler stated that disease of the optic nerve is the result of an affection of the adipose tissue and that there is no real proof that empyema of the sphenoid can, of itself, cause an affection of the optic nerve. Sattler did not consider that unilateral optic neuritis and atrophy were characteristic of diseases of the ethmoid and sphenoid cavities, as they might arise from inflammation, hemorrhage, or tumors at the cerebral end of the optic nerve. Blindness in both eyes with simultaneous empyema of these cavities might indicate a causal connection if no other cause is present. Axenfeld maintained that diseases of the optic nerve are much rarer than is expected in diseases of the sphenoid. He had seen one case of empyema of the sphenoid with retinal neuritis and two tumors, causing unilateral disturbance of vision. Onodi concludes that, in general, bilateral disturbances of sight are intracranial in orgin, but may be due to disease of either the sphenoid or ethmoid.

Fish[8] presents four cases bearing on the subject:

(a) Woman, aet. 37 years, right eye normal, left eye punetate keratitis, vitreal opacities, retinitis, hyperemia of the disk, general edematous condition of the fundus. Resection of the middle turbinate and syringing out the sinus resulted in improving the sight, but the trouble returned whenever the nasal discharge was obstructed.

(b) Opacities of the vitreous, hyperemia of the disk, edema of the fundus, frontal sinusitis. Great improvement followed syringing the sinus.

(c) Attack of grip in 1898, with inflammation and pain in the eye and forehead. At present time there is retinochoroiditis, central and peripheral, disk pale, absolute central scotoma with contraction of the field of vision. Frontal sinusitis and polypi of nose present.

(d) Pain and inflammation for about a week; hyperemia of disk, keratitis, pain in ball and frontal bone, hyperemia middle and inferior turbinate, sinusitis frontalis. Syringing resulted in no improvement at first, but as soon as discharge appeared in the nostril the eye rapidly improved.

Moritz[26] showed that optic neuritis, with sudden loss of vision, may result from compression of the optic nerve at the foramen, or from perineuritis, and that a threatened affection of the optic nerve is shown by hyperemia of the disk.

Pollatschek[35] reports a case of bilateral papillitis, cured by resection of the middle turbinate, curetting of the posterior ethmoid cells and opening the sphenoid sinuses.

Galezowski[10] presented a case in which there was a maxillary sinusitis of dental origin, giving the appearance of an orbital phlegmon. The papilla was edematous, with tortuous veins and hyperemic arteries. Visual acuity was one-fourth, the field of vision being normal. Luc's operation was done; three weeks later all ocular symptoms had disappeared and the vision was normal.

Alexander[1] reports a case of a man, forty-one years of age, who suffered from bilateral optic neuritis, due to empyema of the posterior ethmoid cells and the sphenoid sinus.

Paunz[34] reports a case of papillitis with considerable diminution of vision, due to posterior ethmoid diseases; greatly improved after operation.

Glegg and Hay[11] had a patient in whom there was limitation of the field of vision and reduction of vision to six-twelfths and six-eighteenths, with other ocular symptoms, all being entirely cured by removing the middle turbinate and opening the posterior ethmoid cells.

Green[12] claims that the optic nerve is especially prone to become implicated in sphenoiditis and posterior ethmoiditis, though the involvement is usually slight. If severe and prolonged, retrobular neuritis may develop.

Knapp[18] reports a number of cases of orbital abscess and the two following cases without orbital abscess:

(a) Neuro-retinitis following influenza, recovering without treatment.

(b) Retrobulbar neuritis, congestion of the right disk, later central scotoma, deflection of septum, and turbinate hypertrophy; not much improved at first, but later complete recovery.

In the discussion which followed, Kipp stated that he had never seen optic neuritis in connection with sinus disease, except where the infection extended to the orbital tissue; but Randall had seen numerous cases.

Schmiegelow[40] reports two cases of latent empyema of the sphenoid and posterior ethmoid cells, resulting in retrobulbar neuritis:

(a) A boy suddenly taken with pain, malaise, vomiting and later diminished vision in the left eye. The papillary tissues were obscured, borders indistinct, slight swelling, veins dark, tortuous and slightly thickened, macula normal. Vision was greatly improved by resection of the posterior end of the middle turbinate, and opening of the sphenoid sinus.

(b) Young woman, aet. eighteen years, two and a half years before was taken with severe headaches on the left side with reduction of vision on the right side. Headaches improved under treatment. Later, headaches appeared on the right side. Papilla white and atrophic without showing optic neuritis, vision decreased considerably. Very decided improvement followed the resection of the posterior portion of the middle turbinate and the anterior wall of the sphenoid.

Delneuville[7] was able to relieve a patient with reduction of vision to one-half on the left side while the fingers could hardly be counted by the right eye, one meter away, with fundus and medium normal, central scotoma, retrobulbar neuritis, by cleansing and treatment of a sphenoid sinusitis which was present.

Onodi[30] found that relief followed resection of the middle turbinate, removal of polypi and irrigation of maxillary sinus in a man nineteen years of age, who was attacked suddenly with headache, exophthalmus, double vision, and lessened vision.

Packard[32] reports a number of cases:

(a) Margin of left optic nerve hazy, hyperemia of disk, left ethmoiditis and sphenoiditis; improvement of the eye under nasal treatment.

(b) Left optic neuritis, hypertrophy of the left middle turbinate, no pus, bulla ethmoidalis swollen, improvement following treatment.

(c) Right optic neuritis, hypertrophy of the right middle turbinate, improvement following treatment.

(d) Intense hyperemia and edema of both disks, cystic middle turbinates.

(e) Swelling and tortuosity of retinal vessels, acute frontal sinusitis, hypertrophied and cystic middle turbinates.

(f) Retinal vessels overfull, ethmoiditis.

Thompson[42] reports a case in which there were pain for three weeks, paralysis of the third nerve, choked disk, right eye similarly affected but less extensive. After removal of septal spur and treatment of ethmoid and sphenoid condition, vision returned to almost normal. \

Posey[37][38] makes the very pertinent remark that there were cases of retrobulbar inflammation of the optic nerve observed in earlier years, following grip and in association with catching cold or rheumatism, which, in place of simple and effective treatment directed towards the sinus, received active and often depressing and harmful general medication. As a cousequence, blindness was not the infrequent result, whereas, with proper appreciation of the circumstances attending the origin of the neuritis, complete recovery might have been the question of but a few days. Posey maintains that the nerve may be affected from the sinuses by contiguity of tissues from all stages of edema to retrobulbar neuritis.

Sluder[41] reports a case in which there was pain in the right eye for three days, with sudden blindness in both eyes. The right upper lid was edematous. Immediate improvement in vision followed operation.

Risley[39] reports an additional case of optic neuritis, with impaired central vision and contracted fields, recovering after drainage of the frontal and ethmoid sinuses, although the symptoms had lasted three years.

Alfred Wiener[44] reports two cases. (a) Absolute blindness followed an attack of rhinopharyngitis. The middle turbinate bone was resected and the posterior ethmoid cells curetted, first on the right side and then on the left, with evidence of disease at each operation. Vision returned in one eye, but not in the other. Wiener regards the condition as an acute retrobulbar neuritis, occurring in the canalicular portion of the optic nerve, brought about through a posterior ethmoiditis on both sides, probably of syphilitic origin. (b) Complete blindness in a child of nine, following an acute coryza and severe frontal headache. Vision returned in about two weeks after mild local treatment of the nose.

METHOD OF ANATOMIC STUDY.

With this array of clinical facts, a study of the anatomic relations of the optic nerve is certainly justified.

Departing somewhat from the practice of Onodi, Zuckerkandl, Hajek, and others, who used their material without special reference to uniformity, I have made these studies on fifteen heads which have been sectioned horizontally. They were first injected through the carotid with a fifty percent formalin solution, then immersed for from three to five months in a three percent solution of hydrochloric acid, in order to decalcify them; then sectioned and reconstructed after the plan designated in my previous papers.[22] [23] [24] I have taken the sections containing the optic nerve and have dissected out the optic nerve and cut away portions of the walls of the accessory cavities so as to bring into view the most important relations. In some instances the mucosa has been left intact and in others the bony walls alone are shown.

The reconstructions, I consider of great importance, for it is only in this way that it is possible to define accurately, in a series of heads, the diameters of the sinuses, their positions with respect to the optic nerve throughout its course, their variations in graphic form and, at the same time, to preserve the specimens for identification and study. Besides this, it is easy at any time to verify the findings and, if it is desired, to study additional problems in this connection. An illustration of each head is presented, accompanied by the necessary reconstructions, so that the details of this work may be used by other investigators who may be interested in this field of research.

MATERIAL FOR STUDY.

The heads, used as material for study, were all obtained from the Anatomical Department of St. Louis University, but there has been, in no instance, a possibility of ascertaining the ante mortem history of the individuals, and, in some cases, the age and sex were unknown, as the heads had been removed from the body before they came into my possession.

DESCRIPTION OF HEADS.

The heads are given numbers in the order in which they were reconstructed. Thus far I have reconstructed twenty heads, the last fifteen of which (from VI to XX, inclusive) have been used in this study. In future papers, where reference is made to these heads, the numbers will be given. In papers already published, only the first four heads reconstructed have been utilized—designated A, B, C, D, respectively. These are hereafter to be numbered I, II, III and IV, respectively.

HEAD VI. (Figures 1 and 16.)

Sphenoid Sinus.—Left, small, not in relation with optic chiasm which lies behind it. Right, large, extending more than a centimeter posterior to the optic chiasm.

Ethmoid Labyrinth.—Left, two posterior ethmoid cells in relation with optic nerve at their postero-external angles near the roof. Right, posterior ethmoid consists of but one large cell which comes into relation with the optic nerve at the postero-external angle of the cell, its roof slightly overlapping the nerve.

Frontal Sinus.—Left, covers about one-third of the bulbus at its supero-internal portion and extends a somewhat greater distance internal to the globe. Right, smaller than the left, extends over one-sixth of the roof of the globe, its main portion somewhat larger, lying internal.

Optic chiasm lies on the roof of the right sphenoid.

Optic Nerve.—Left, passes along roof of the right sphenoid and the external wall of the left sphenoid, external to the postero-external angle of the posterior ethmoid cell. Right, passes over the external wall of the right sphenoid and external to the postero-external angle of the right posterior ethmoid.

HEAD VII. (Figures 2 and 17.)

Sphenoid Sinus—Left, very large, extends to the occipito-sphenoidal articulation posterior to the carotid; optic nerve passes over anterior fourth of the roof. Right, very large, extends to the occipitosphenoidal articulation posterior to the carotid ; optic nerve passes over anterior fourth of the roof.

Ethmoid Labyrinth.—Left, anterior portion narrow, posterior portion wide, extending somewhat external to the optic nerve, but below it. Last posterior ethmoid in relation with the optic at the postero-external angle. Right, anterior portion narrow, posterior portion wide; last posterior ethmoid in relation with the optic at postero-external angle.

Frontal Sinus.—Left, though quite large, lies almost entirely internal to the globe, overlapping it but slightly. Right, similar in shape and relation to the left, but somewhat smaller.

Optic chiasm extends about an equal distance over the roof of the two sphenoids.

Optic Nerve.—Left, passes over the roof of the left sphenoid then downward to the postero-external angle of the posterior ethmoid. Right, passes over the roof of the left sphenoid and downward to the postero-external angle of the posterior ethmoid.

HEAD VIII. (Figures 3 and 18.)

Sphenoid Sinus.—Both fairly uniform, the right reaching a somewhat higher level than the left.

Ethmoid Labyrinth.—Left, posterior portion much wider than the anterior portion, but the only direct relation is at the postero-external angle of the last cell near its roof. Right, anterior ethmoid cells extend posteriorly beyond the posterior ethmoidal cells, but not in close relation with the optic nerve. The right posterior ethmoid, last cell, in relation with the optic only at its postero-external angle, near the roof.

Frontal Sinus.—Left, very small and not in relation with the globe, being more than a centimeter internal to it, but reaching about the same level as the bulbus. Right, much larger than left, extending more than three centimeters above the globe and overlapping it but slightly.

Optic chiasm lies over posterior portion of the roof of right and left sphenoid, three-fourths being over the right and one-fourth over the left.

Optic Nerve.—Left, passes externally over roof of the sphenoid to the postero-external angle of the last posterior ethmoid cell. Right optic passes externally over the posterior portion of the roof of the sphenoid sinus and over the postero-external angle of the last posterior ethmoid.

HEAD IX. (Figures 4 and 19.)

Sphenoid Sinus.—Both fairly uniform, right reaching a slightly higher level. Considerable intervening bone between the roof of the sinuses and the optic chiasm which lies above and behind.

Ethmoid Labyrinth.—Left, anterior portion broad; last posterior ethmoid cell not in close relation with the optic which lies 3 mm. from its postero-external angle. Right, anterior portion broad, last posterior ethmoid cell not in close relation with the optic which lies 3 mm. from its postero-external angle. A second cell presents an angle 4 mm. from the nerve.

Frontal Sinus.—Left, very large, extending a considerable distance anterior to the globe, but overlapping it but slightly. It extends internally beyond the median line. Right frontal much smaller than the left and not in relation with the globe, except at the supero-external portion.

Optic chiasm lies 5 mm. above left sphenoid, 2 mm. above right and behind both of them; no evidence of sulcus opticus on roof of either sphenoid sinus.

Optic Nerve.—Left, passes along lateral and upper wall of left sphenoid and the postero-external angle of the left posterior ethmoid. Right, passes along roof of right sphenoid externally and the postero-external angle of the last posterior ethmoid cell.

HEAD X. (Figures 5 and 20.)

Sphenoid Sinus.—Left, small. Right, larger, extends above the optic nerve, which runs along the external wall.

Ethmoid Labyrinth.—Left, broader posterior than anterior. Last posterior ethmoid in relation at postero-external angle with the optic nerve. Right, two posterior ethmoid cells in relation with optic nerve at their postero-external angle.

Frontal Sinus.—Left, overlaps the inner portion of the globe but slightly. Right, considerably smaller, lies 3 mm. from the globe at its nearest point.

Optic chiasm in relation almost entirely with the right sphenoid.

Optic Nerve.—Left, passes along the left sphenoid laterally and superiorly, and along the postero-external angle of the last posterior ethmoid. Right, passes along the lateral wall of the sphenoid sinus just below its roof and along the postero-external angle of the last two posterior ethmoid cells.

HEAD XI. (Figures 6 and 21.)

Sphenoid Sinus.—Both sinuses large and fairly uniform.

Ethmoid Labyrinth.—Both unusually small. Last posterior ethmoid cell on each side 3 mm. from the corresponding optic nerve, the nearest point being the postero-external angle of the cell.

Frontal Sinus.—Left, small, lies considerably internal to the globe. Right, much larger, somewhat more distant from the globe, extends beyond the median line on the left.

Optic chiasm passes over the roof of left and right sphenoid, the left being about two-thirds of the entire distance.

Optic Nerve.—Left, passes over the roof of the left sphenoid and 3 mm. away from postero-external angle of the last posterior ethmoid cell. Right, passes over the roof of right sphenoid and 3 mm. from postero-external angle of the last posterior ethmoid cell.

HEAD XII. (Figures 7 and 22.)

Sphenoid Sinus.—Left, exceedingly large, in relation with optic chiasm and both optic nerves. Right, very small, 6 mm. below the optic nerve.

Ethmoid Labyrinth.—Left, anterior portion much longer than the posterior; last posterior ethmoid cell shows the usual relation at its postero-external angle with the optic. Right, anterior ethmoid has the same antero-posterior diameter as the labyrinth, in that its posterior wall extends as far back as the posterior ethmoid cells. The last anterior ethmoid cell is here in relation with the optic nerve at the postero-external angle of the cell, having replaced the posterior ethmoid, which is quite small.

Frontal Sinus.—Left, very large, overlapping the inner wall of the bulbus very slightly. Right, very small, some distance removed from the inner wall of the bulbus.

Optic chiasm lies on the posterior third of the roof of the left sphenoid.

Optic Nerve.—Left, passes from the roof of the left sphenoid to the postero-external angle of the last posterior ethmoid cell. Right, passes over the left sphenoid and to the postero-external angle of the last anterior ethmoid cell.

HEAD XIII. (Figures 8 and 23.)

Sphenoid Sinus.—Left, exceedingly large, extending almost as far back as the fifth nerve on both sides, far behind the posterior wall of the right sphenoid (13 mm.). Left optic nerve runs across the superior wall, though the sinus roof extends to a much higher level. Right, much smaller than left, in relation with the optic nerve, which runs along its external and superior wall, though not at its highest level.

Ethmoid Labyrinth.—Left, anterior ethmoid constitutes anterior and large part of the outer portion; last posterior ethmoid cells, two in relation with the optic nerve at the postero-external angle. Right, last posterior ethmoid in but slight relation with the optic at postero-external angle.

Frontal Sinus.—Left, not in relation with the bulbus, most of the cavity being anterior to it. Right, similarly disposed, but somewhat larger.

Optic Chiasm.—Right two-thirds lies on the posterior wall of the right sphenoid, and left third on the superior wall of the left sphenoid.

Optic Nerve.—Left, runs along the superior wall of the left sphenoid below its highest level and just posterior to the postero-external angle of the last two posterior ethmoid cells. Right, runs along the supero-external wall of the right sphenoid and the postero-external angle of the last posterior ethmoid cell.

HEAD XIV. (Figures 9 and 24.)

Sphenoid Sinus.—Left, small, 4 mm. below the optic nerve.
Right, very large, in relation with both optic nerves and
chiasm.

Ethmoid Labyrinth.—Left, anterior cells very wide, extending almost as far externally as the frontal; posterior ethmoid
composed of one cell only, which is in relation with the optic
nerve at the postero-external angle. Right, anterior ethmoid
cells similar to those on the left; last posterior ethmoid cell
in relation with optic nerve at postero-external angle.

Frontal Sinus.—Left, very large, extending over the inner
wall of the orbit and beyond the median line. Right, relation
almost identical, but somewhat larger.

Optic chiasm lies posterior to right sphenoid.

Optic Nerve.—Left, runs along the postero-external wall
of the right sphenoid and along the postero-external angle of
the posterior ethmoid. Right, runs along the posterior wall
of the right sphenoid and along the postero-external angle of
the posterior ethmoid cell.

HEAD XV. (Figures 10 and 25.)

Sphenoid Sinus.—Left, in relation with both optic nerves
at its postero-lateral wall. Right, insignificant in size, 8 mm.
below the optic nerve, appearing as a mere indentation communicating with the nasal cavity by an opening of the usual
size.

Ethmoid Labyrinth.—Left, small, last posterior ethmoid in
relation with the optic nerve at the postero-external angle just
below the roof. Right, very similar to the left.

Frontal Sinus.—Left, very small, not in relation with orbit.
Right, smaller, but similar in relation.

Optic chiasm lies behind the left sphenoid about the level of
the roof.

Optic Nerve.—Left, runs along the postero-external wall of
the left sphenoid and along the postero-external angle of the
posterior ethmoid. Right, runs along the postero-external
wall of the left sphenoid and along the postero-external angle
of the posterior ethmoid.

HEAD XVI. (Figures 11 and 26.)

Sphenoid Sinus.—Left, small, 8 mm. below optic nerve,

being replaced by an ethmoid cell which is interposed. Right, in relation with the optic nerve at its roof and external wall.

Ethmoid Labyrinth.—Left, large; last posterior ethmoid in relation with optic on the external wall of the cell. Right, large, but relation with the optic nerve is only at the postero-external angle of the last posterior ethmoid cell.

Frontal Sinus.—Left, close to the inner wall of the globe, but does not overlap. Right, but slightly larger and overlaps several millimeters.

Optic chiasm lies entirely behind sphenoid sinuses, in no relation with them.

Optic Nerve.—Left, passes along the external wall of the last posterior ethmoid cell, not in relation with either sphenoid. Right, passes along the external wall of the right sphenoid and postero-external angle of the last right posterior ethmoid.

HEAD XVII. (Figures 12 and 27.)

Sphenoid Sinus.—Each sphenoid in about equal relation superiorly with the corresponding nerve and chiasm.

Ethmoid Labyrinth.—Each in relation with corresponding optic nerve at postero-external angle of the last posterior ethmoid.

Frontal Sinus.—Left, large, in relation externally and anteriorly with globe. Right, similar in shape, but smaller and at a greater distance from the globe.

Optic chiasm in relation with both sphenoids.

Optic Nerve.—Left, passes over the roof of the left sphenoid and to the postero-external angle of the posterior ethmoid, slightly below the roof of this cell. Right, passes over the roof of the sphenoid and to the postero-external angle of the posterior ethmoid slightly below the roof of the cell.

HEAD XVIII. (Figures 13 and 28.)

Sphenoid Sinus.—Both small, left in relation with optic chiasm and both optic nerves. Right, 7 mm. below optic nerve, being replaced by posterior ethmoid cell which has been interposed.

Ethmoid Labyrinth.—Left, large, usual relation with optic. Right, large, optic nerve passes along external wall of last posterior ethmoid cell.

Frontal Sinus.—Left, large, overlaps inner wall of globe. Right, relation similar to the left.

Optic chiasm in relation with left sphenoid only.

Optic Nerve.—Left, passes above left sphenoid and postero-external angle of the last posterior ethmoid cell. Right, passes over external margin of the roof of the left sphenoid and then downward and outward over the roof of the last posterior ethmoid cell and along its external wall.

HEAD XIX. (Figures 14 and 29.)

Sphenoid Sinus.—Left, small, somewhat replaced by the right. Right, extends over to the left side, coming into relation with the left optic nerve at the supero-posterior wall of the sinus.

Ethmoid Labyrinth.—Both small, usual relation to the postero-external angle of the last posterior ethmoid, the left being nearer to the nerve than the right.

Frontal Sinus.—Left, overlaps antero-inferior portion of globe. Right, has about the same relation.

Optic chiasm lies on the postero-superior wall of the right sphenoid.

Optic Nerve.—Left, one-third of the sinus portion lies over the right sphenoid, one-half over the left sphenoid and one-sixth over the postero-external wall of the left posterior ethmoid. Right, runs along and above the right sphenoid, but the anterior half of the portion in relation with this sinus lies laterally. The nerve comes in relation with the last posterior ethmoid cell only at the postero-external portion of the cell.

HEAD XX. (Figures 15 and 30.)

Sphenoid Sinus.—Left, very peculiar in shape, consisting of two portions, an upper third and lower two-thirds, united at a constricted point at the level of its nasal orifice. Only the upper portion is in relation with the optic nerves. Right, not in relation with the optic nerve, being 5 mm. below it at its nearest point, which is at the apex of a projection 4 mm. above the main cavity of the sphenoid.

Ethmoid Labyrinth.—Usual relation.

Frontal Sinus.—Left, very large, extending behind the posterior wall of the anterior ethmoid, barely overlapping the inner wall of the globe. Right, extends almost as far posteriorly, but not so far as the anterior ethmoid cells, overlapping the globe a somewhat greater distance than on the left side.

Optic chiasm lies posterior to left sphenoid sinus.

Optic Nerve.—Left, runs along external wall of the left sphenoid and on the postero-external angle of the last posterior ethmoid cell. Right, runs along the external wall of the left sphenoid and the postero-external angle of the last posterior ethmoid cell, right. side being a trifle higher than this ethmoid cell.

DESCRIPTION OF THE SINUSES.

The maxillary sinuses of the fifteen heads are not described in detail, as it was deemed inexpedient to burden the report with it, and as the maxillary sinus does not enter into the subject to the same degree as the other sinuses. However, in each case it has been reconstructed in the lateral projections which have been made, and the diameters and other important particulars are given. ·

In order to avoid repetition, the measurements are all given in millimeters. The reconstructions are all exact within a possible error of 1 mm.

SPHENOID SINUS.

There is a tremendous variation in the dimensions of the thirty sphenoid sinuses, as shown in the following table:

DIAMETERS OF THE SPHENOID SINUSES.

HEAD.	Antero-posterior.		Supero-inferior.		Lateral.	
	R.	L.	R.	L.	R.	L.
VI.	35	15	30	24	31	12
VII.	42	36	22	34	34	25
VIII.	25	20	27	25	16	12
IX.	21	14	23	17	17	13
X.	17	14	22	20	17	11
XI.	31	27 ·	26	26	14	19
XII.	9	39	8	26	7	24
XIII.	16	33	36	36	14	27
XIV.	24	10	38	18	35	10
XV.	2	23	4	27	2	21
XVI.	20	9	21	10	14	8
XVII.	24	14	24	19	17	17
XVIII.	9	19	10	19	9	24
XIX.	32	20	28	17	27	12
XX.	29	30	21	27	28	34

The antero-posterior diameter varies from 2 in Head XV to 42 in Head VII, left; the supero-inferior from 4 in Head

XV, right, to 38 in Head XIV, right; lateral from 2 in Head XV, right, to 35 in Head XIII, right.

The sphenoid sinus of Head XV (figure 25) is by far the smallest, with diameters 2, 4 and 2, the next smallest being Head XII (figure 22), right, with diameters 9, 8 and 7. That of Head VII (figure 17), right side, is the largest with diameters 42, 22 and 34, while that of Head VI (figure 16), right, is next largest, with diameters 35, 30 and 31.

The average diameters of the thirty sinuses are as follows: Antero-posterior 21.5, supero-inferior 22.8, lateral 18.4. Excluding five extremes, smallest and largest, the range of the remaining twenty, which may be considered as common, is as follows: antero-posterior 14 to 32, supero-inferior 17 to 27, lateral 11 to 27.

A glance at the reconstruction of the sphenoid sinuses (figures 16 to 30) shows the great variety of size and shape. The right sphenoid of Head XV is but little larger than its opening into the nasal cavity, which is in its accustomed position. It is replaced almost entirely by the left sphenoid, which is shown in relation with the optic chiasm, and both nerves (figure 25). Both sphenoids of Head VII are exceedingly large (figure 17) and extend far behind the optic chiasm, sharing this feature with Head VI, right (figure 16), Head XII, right (figure 22), Head XIII, left (figure 23), Head XVII, right (figure 27), and Head XIX, right (figure 29).

There is likewise great disparity in the size of the two sphenoid sinuses in Heads VI (figure 16), XII (figure 22), XIV (figure 24), XV (figure 25), and XIX (figure 29). One sphenoid only is in relation with both optic nerves in Heads XII (figures 7 and 22) left, XIV (figures 9 and 24) right, XV (figures 10 and 25) left, XVIII (figures 13 and 28) left, XX (figures 15 and 30) left. .

Each sphenoid sinus is in relation with the corresponding optic nerve, and one is in relation with the other optic nerve in addition in the following instances: Heads VI (figures 1 and 16) and XIX (figures 14 and 29).

In Head XVI neither sphenoid is in relation with the left optic nerve (figures 11 and 26). A large posterior ethmoid cell (figure 11) replaces a small left sphenoid.

The relation is fairly uniform in the following: Heads VII (figures 2 and 17), VIII (figures 3 and 18), IX (figures

4 and 19), X (figures 5 and 20), XI (figures 6 and 21), XIII (figures 8 and 23) and XVII (figures 12 and 27).

The orifice of the sphenoid sinus, while invariably opening into the nose above the superior turbinate, varies considerably in its position. The following table shows the distance between the inferior margin of the opening and the lowest level of the floor and the highest level of the roof, respectively:

DISTANCE BETWEEN THE INFERIOR MARGIN OF THE NASAL
OPENING OF THE SPHENOID SINUS AND THE FLOOR
AND ROOF OF THE SINUS.

Heads.	Right		Left	
	Floor	Roof	Floor	Roof
VI.	17	13	13	11
VII.	7	15	20	14
VIII.	13	14	11	16
IX.	10	13	4	13
X.	13	9	8	12
XI.	12	14	11	15
XII.	4	4	14	12
XIII.	15	21	17	19
XIV.	16	22	8	10
XV.	2	2	14	13
XVI.	7	14	3	7
XVII.	12	12	7	12
XVIII.	6	4	5	14
XIX.	21	7	9	8
XX.	19	2	17	10

These figures certainly show a wide variation, and yet it may be said that the orifice, as a rule, is midway between the roof and the floor. This is true for twenty out of thirty sinuses.

In XVIII, XIX, XX right and VII, XVIII and XIX left, the orifice is in the upper third; in XI right and IX, XI and XVII left it is in the lower third; in the other thirty instances it is in the middle third.

It is relatively highest in Head XX, right, where its distance from the roof is one-tenth of that between the roof and the floor. It is relatively lowest in IX, left, where it opens in the lower quarter of the anterior wall.

The more specific relations of the optic nerve and chiasm will be discussed under those heads.

ETHMOID LABYRINTH

Until Onodi pointed out that the last posterior cell was at times in close relation with the optic nerve, it was generally supposed that this relation was confined to the sphenoid exclusively, but since that time his investigations have been confirmed that the last posterior ethmoid cell may replace the sphenoid in both position and relation.

The study here presented is for the purpose of establishing how extensive this relation is and, to this end, the entire ethmoid labyrinth is reconstructed superiorly and shown in figures 16 to 30. The anterior cells occupy the space within the dotted lines, the posterior cells within the unbroken lines, while the solid black spaces represent that portion of the last ethmoid cavity in relation with the optic nerve, or perhaps it would be more explicit to say that it is a superior reconstruction of that position of the last posterior ethmoid cavity which lies at the level of the optic cells. The space outside of this, inclosed in the unbroken lines, represents that additional portion of the posterior ethmoidal cavities not in relation with the optic nerve.

The dimensions of the ethmoid labyrinth are as follows:

DIAMETERS OF THE ETHMOID LABYRINTH.

HEAD		Labyrinth			Anterior Ethmoid			Posterior Ethmoid		
		Antero-posterior.	Supero-inferior.	Lateral.	Antero-posterior.	Supero-inferior.	Lateral.	Antero-posterior.	Supero-inferior.	Lateral.
VI,	Right	37	23	18	23	22	8	28	23	28
	Left	36	20	13	22	15	9	20	17	12
VII,	Right	43	34	26	22	31	8	26	34	27
	Left	47	35	20	27	12	9	30	36	20
VIII,	Right	32	26	19	32	20	16	22	17	11
	Left	47	32	26	24	25	11	22	32	26
IX,	Right	34	39	20	21	33	18	23	26	12
	Left	30	36	20	20	32	19	21	28	23
X,	Right	35	28	14	19	25	11	20	17	13
	Left	35	28	15	21	26	15	22	19	14
XI,	Right	24	33	15	10	26	11	20	18	13
	Left	23	29	16	14	27	11	17	15	16
XII,	Right	40	20	12	40	17	12	15	6	8
	Left	34	17	12	30	17	9	13	10	11
XIII,	Right	35	31	12	14	18	9	26	23	12
	Left	35	35	18	26	35	14	25	31	18
XIV,	Right	45	59	26	26	57	26	27	30	17
	Left	46	57	28	30	50	29	32	31	12
XV,	Right	33	26	9	9	7	24	24	20	9
	Left	37	26	11	17	8	26	20	22	11
XVI,	Right	32	40	15	20	35	14	22	26	12
	Left	35	31	22	19	28	18	28	23	16
XVII,	Right	27	19	12	9	19	7	18	17	11
	Left	22	18	10	12	16	10	16	17	10
XVIII,	Right	54	33	16	22	18	14	14	28	15
	Left	38	25	15	30	34	12	33	23	15
XIX,	Right	24	25	11	16	25	13	17	18	11
	Left	25	28	11	15	28	11	17	20	9
XX,	Right	35	40	15	28	38	11	27	35	14
	Left	32	42	13	15	29	12	25	38	13

These figures show the following:

Ethmoid Labyrinth.—Range, antero-posterior diameter 22 to 54, supero-inferior 17 to 59, lateral 9 to 28. Usual, leaving out five highest and lowest, antero-posterior 27 to 43, supero-inferior 23 to 36, lateral 12 to 20. Average, antero-posterior 35, supero-anterior 31.6, lateral 16.3.

The largest is that of Head XIV, left, 46, 57, 28, and the smallest, Head XVII, left, 22, 18, 10.

Anterior Ethmoid.—Range, antero-posterior 9 to 40, su-pero-inferior 7 to 57, lateral 7 to 29. Usual, leaving out five highest and lowest, antero-posterior 14 to 27, supero-inferior 17 to 34, lateral 9 to 18. Average, antero-posterior 21, supero-inferior 25.6, lateral 14.

The largest is that of Head XIV, left, 30, 50, 29, and the smallest that of head XVII, right, 9, 19, 7.

Posterior Ethmoid.—Range, antero-posterior 13 to 33, su-pero-inferior 6 to 38, lateral 8 to 28. Usual, leaving out five highest and lowest, antero-posterior 17 to 26, supero-inferior 17 to 31, lateral 11 to 18. Average, antero-posterior 22.3, supero-inferior 23.3, lateral 14.7.

The largest is that of Head VII, left, 30, 36, 20, and the smallest that of Head XII, right, 15, 6, 8.

The anterior ethmoid cells, while constituting in part the inner wall of the orbit, are not in close relation with the optic, as may be readily ascertained by examination of figures 16 to 30. However, there is a fairly close relation in Heads VIII, XII and XIV.

Onodi mentions a case where the anterior ethmoid came into close relation with the optic nerve. Head XII (figures 7 and 22) exhibits a cell of this character.

The posterior ethmoid, on the contrary, has almost always a very close relation. It may replace the sphenoid and the nerve thereby comes into relation with the external wall, as shown in Head XVI (figures 11 and 26) and XVIII (figures 13 and 28). Under other circumstances the relation is a very slight one, being confined to the postero-external angle at the roof. That there is this slight relation may be easily ascertained by examining the reconstructions. figures 16 to 30. In practically all, the optic nerve may be seen close to this postero-external angle.

FRONTAL SINUS.

While there is a great diversity of shapes to be found in the different frontal sinuses, there is rather more uniformity of shape and size in the two frontals of the same head. The dimensions are as follows:

DIAMETERS OF THE FRONTAL SINUS.

HEAD.	Antero-posterior.		Supero-inferior.		Lateral.	
	R.	L.	R.	L.	R.	L.
VI.	15	18	24	30	20	32
VII.	32	33	28	26	22	26
VIII.	22	16	51	28	25	11
IX.	17	21	27	36	21	37
X.	17	17	40	37	27	22
XI.	22	16	38	38	22	15
XII.	16	22	34	45	10	27
XIII.	17	13	25	22	21	18
XIV.	26	21	45	37	42	37
XV.	9	12	14	24	7	11
XVI.	12	13	35	30	26	21
XVII.	26	30	35	43	17	23
XVIII.	28	21	39	41	25	30
XIX.	12	17	30	31	28	20
XX.	26	31	46	45	32	24

The variations in the size of the frontal may be summed up as follows:

Range, antero-posterior 9 to 33, supero-inferior 14 to 51, lateral 7 to 42. Usual, leaving out five highest and lowest; antero-posterior 15 to 26, supero-inferior 26 to 40, lateral 17 to 30. Average, antero-posterior 21, supero-inferior 34, lateral 23.

The largest is that of Head XIV, right, 26, 45, 42, and the smallest that of Head XV, right, 9, 14, 7.

That the frontal in these heads has not any close relation with the optic nerve, but with the bulbus opticus, is made manifest in figures 16 to 30. Thus the frontal is shown to be more than 3 mm. from the bulbus in Heads VIII, left (figure 18), XI, both sides (figure 21), XII, right (figure 22), XIII, both sides (figure 23), XV, both sides (figure 25), XVII, right (figure 27). The overlapping is considerable in Heads VI, both sides (figure 16), IX, left (figure 19), XIV, both sides (figure 24); in only one instance, Head XV, both sides (figure 25), does the frontal fail to reach a higher level than the bulbus.

MAXILLARY SINUS.

Although the upper wall of the maxillary sinus constitutes a portion of the floor of the orbit, the optic nerve is quite far from the sinus.

The following are the measurements of the diameters of the thirty sinuses, the distance from the optic nerve at the

nearest points, and the distance between the lowest margin
of the nasal opening of the sinus, and the floor of the sinus:

DIAMETERS OF THE MAXILLARY SINUS, DISTANCE FROM OPTIC
NERVE AT THE NEAREST POINT AND DISTANCE BETWEEN
THE LOWEST MARGIN OF NASAL OPENING OF THE
SINUS AND FLOOR OF THE SINUS.

HEAD.	Antero-posterior.		Supero-inferior.		Lateral.		Nearest point to optic nerve.		Distance of opening from floor of cavity.	
	R	L	R	L	R	L	R	L	R	L
VI.	39	40	42	32	30	25	10	11	36	28
VII.	40	42	41	47	28	29	13	17	32	39
VIII.	32	30	28	29	19	18	16	25	24	25
IX.	17	20	17	21	8	11	18	15	15	14
X.	39	37	37	40	33	30	7	7	36	38
XI.	40	40	37	39	31	29	10	11	33	34
XII.	34	29	28	28	28	25	12	10	21	23
XIII.	37	40	45	43	29	32	10	7	32	32
XIV.	37	42	38	40	25	25	22	17	23	21
XV.	40	33	38	34	24	26	15	16	33	30
XVI.	25	26	23	26	15	17	16	14	18	24
XVII.	35	37	31	33	32	23	13	17	22	25
XVIII.	35	26	38	26	26	19	7	7	33	21
XIX.	36	42	45	42	27	32	8	12	40	38
XX.	36	35	39	36	25	21	21	21	36	28

The variations are as follows:

Range, antero-posterior diameter 17 to 42, supero-inferior
17 to 47, lateral 8 to 33, nearest point to optic nerve 7 to 25,
orifice to floor 14 to 40. Usual, leaving off highest and lowest
five; antero-posterior 29 to 40, supero-inferior 28 to 42, lateral
19 to 30, nearest point to optic nerve 8 to 17, orifice to floor
21 to 36. Average, antero-posterior 38, supero-inferior 38,
lateral 23.8, nearest point to optic nerve 13.5, orifice to floor 29.

The largest is in Head VII, left, 42, 47, 29, the smallest in
Head IX, right, 17, 17, 8. It will be noted that leaving out a
few of the extremes, the maxillary sinuses are more uniform
than any of the sinuses.

The optic nerve comes within 7 mm. of the maxillary sinuses
in Head X, both sides; XIII, left; and XVIII, both sides.
The greatest distance is found in Head VIII.

OPTIC CHIASM.

The optic chiasm in these· heads is in the main in relation with one or more sphenoid sinuses. It is directly upon the roof in Heads VI, both sides (figures 1 and 16); VII (figure 17); XII, both sides (figure 22); XIII, left (figure 23); XV, both sides (figure 25); XVII, right (figure 27); XVIII, both sides (figure 28); XIX, both sides (figure 29).

It lies considerably above the roof in Heads VII, right (figure 17); VIII, left (figure 18); XVI, left (figure 26).

It lies posterior to the sphenoid sinus in Heads VIII, both sides (figure 18); IX, both sides (figure 19); X, both sides (figure 20); XI, both sides (figure 21); XIII, right; XIV, both sides; XVI, both sides (figure 26); XVII, left (figure 27); XX, both sides (figure 30).

It is thus seen that in more than half of the instances the chiasm lies posterior to the sphenoidal cavity. Special attention is called to Heads VI, VII, XII, XIII, XVII, XIX, where a considerable portion of the sphenoidal cavity lies beyond the anterior margin of the optic chiasm.

No other cells among these specimens come into relation with the optic chiasm.

OPTIC NERVE.

The optic nerve may described as passing externally from the chiasm along the roof, or lateral wall of the sphenoid sinus in slight relation, usually, with the last posterior ethmoid cell. and from thence to the bulbus opticus through the periorbita.

It may be divided into a sinus portion and a free portion. Under the former term, I include that part of the nerve in immediate relation with the accessory cavities of the nose, or (arbitrarily) within 3 millimeters of the sinus wall.

The following measurements show the length of the nerve in the different heads:

LENGTH OF OPTIC NERVE.

HEAD.	Right.	Left.	Free Portion.		Sinus Portion.	
			R.	L.	R.	L.
VI.	44	44	21	22	23	22
VII.	54	55	22	24	32	31
VIII.	40	40	21	20	19	20
IX.	45	45	18	20	27	25
X.	37	34	18	15	19	19
XI.	54	55	26	26	28	29
XII.	45	44	22	23	23	21
XIII.	39	40	15	12	24	28
XIV.	43	40	15	14	28	26
XV.	54	47	28	27	26	20
XVI.	43	44	19	18	24	26
XVII.	40	40	19	23	21	17
XVIII.	48	45	23	20	25	25
XIX.	39	37	15	14	24	23
XX.	44	44	21	23	23	21

The following variations are obtained:

Optic nerve: range, 34 to 55; usual, leaving off highest and lowest five, 40 to 48; average, 44.

Free portion: range, 12 to 28; usual, leaving off highest and lowest five, 15 to 23; average, 20.

Sinus portion: range, 17 to 32; usual, leaving off highest and lowest five, 21 to 28; average, 24.

It is therefore clear that, at least in these heads, the sinus portion of the optic nerve is a trifle greater than the free portion.

There does not appear to be any correspondence between the length of the optic nerve and the extent of accessory cavities. Where the sphenoid is very large, the optic nerve has its origin in the chiasm on the roof of the sphenoid, some distance anterior to the posterior wall of the sinus, as, for instance, in Heads VI, right (figure 16); VII, both sides (figure 17); XII, both sides (figure 22); XIII, both sides (figure 23); XX, both sides (figure 30).

Where the cells are small, the optic nerve leaves the chiasm generally behind the sinus, as seen in Heads VIII (figure 18); IX, both sides (figure 19); X, both sides (figure 20); XVI, both sides (figure 26).. Head XVIII (figure 28), is somewhat at variance with this rule, but, under any circumstances, it does not appear possible to assign to the extent of the sinus an explanation of the varying size of the optic nerve.

The reconstructions (figures 16 to 30) show that there is no constancy in the relation of the sphenoid to the optic nerve.

This has already been considered in discussing the sphenoid sinus; but the relation which the sphenoid opening bears to the optic nerve is still to be considered. It is seen to vary greatly in the distance between them.

The following table of measurements shows this difference:

DISTANCE LOWER SURFACE OF OPTIC NERVE AND NASAL OPENING OF SPHENOID.

Head.	Right.	Left.
VI	9	6
VII	6	6
VIII	2	6
IX	6	7
X	3	2
XI	9	12
XII	9	3
XIII	5	0
XIV	14	14
XV	8	5
XVI	12	11
XVII	5	5
XVIII	1 above	2 above
XIX	1 above	1
XX	8	12

Range, 2 above to 14; usual, leaving off highest and lowest five, 2 below to 11; average, 6.

In two instances, Heads XVIII, both sides (figure 28), and XIX, right (figure 29), the orifice is above the lower surface of the optic, and in XIII, left, it reaches the same level. In eight instances out of the thirty, the optic nerve lies within 3 mm. of the level of the orifice of the sinus.

It has already been pointed out that the usual rule is that the optic nerve comes into relation with the postero-external angle of the last posterior ethmoid cell at its roof, and from this point it passes in an external direction through the periorbita to the bulbus. The space between the nerve and the ethmoid labyrinth increases in almost direct proportion as the nerve approaches the bulbus, and its junction with the bulbus is generally the position of greatest distance from between the nerve and the ethmoid labyrinth.

In only one case, Head XII (figures 7 and 22), does the anterior ethmoidal cell come in close relation with the optic nerve, replacing a posterior ethmoid cell which lies below it. The relation which the nerve bears to the last posterior ethmoid, when that cell replaces the sphenoid, is very characteristic, for, in every instance in which this replacement had taken place in the heads examined, the nerve is found to run along the external wall of the cavity. This increases the ethmoid portion very considerably, changing it from a course along an angle, apparently made for that purpose, to a wall which it follows in an almost surprising manner.

The frontal is relatively quite distant from the optic nerve, the nearest point being, as a rule, to the inner side of the orbit, and here is much further away than the corresponding anterior ethmoid cells, which ordinarily lie anterior to it at the level of the optic nerve. In some instances, however, the frontal reaches a point far back along the anterior ethmoid cells; for example: Heads VII, X, XI, XII, left; XV, XVII, XVIII, XX (figures 17, 20, 21, 22, 25, 27, 28 and 30). In all the cases the sinus is much closer to the optic nerve than where the sinus remains anterior.

In all the specimens the periorbital fat makes a close relation with the maxillary sinus impossible, although, in some instances, the distance is less than 10 mm.

SUMMARY.

To summarize, the following has been observed in the study of these fifteen heads, with respect to the relation of the optic nerve to the accessory cavities of the nose:

1. The sphenoid sinuses vary as follows: Antero-posterior diameter, 2 to 42 mm.; supero-inferior, 4 to 36 mm.; lateral, 2 to 35 mm.; averaging, respectively, 21.5, 22.8, 18.4.

2. The opening of the sphenoid into the nose, in the great majority of cases, is about midway between the floor and the roof of the sinus. In some instances it is much closer to the roof.

3. The diameter of the ethmoid labyrinth and its component parts, the anterior and posterior ethmoid cells, vary as follows: Labyrinth, antero-posterior 22 to 54 mm., supero-inferior 17 to 59 mm., lateral 9 to 28 mm.; anterior ethmoid cells, antero-posterior 9 to 40 mm., supero-inferior 7 to 57 mm., lateral 7 to 29 mm.; posterior ethmoid cells, antero-posterior 13 to 32 mm., supero-inferior 6 to 38 mm., lateral 8 to 28 mm.

4. The diameters of the frontal sinus vary as follows:

Antero-posterior 9 to 33 mm., supero-inferior 14 to 51 mm., lateral 7 to 42 mm.

5. The diameters of the maxillary sinuses vary as follows: Antero-posterior 17 to 42 mm., supero-inferior 17 to 47 mm., lateral 7 to 33 mm.

6. The optic chiasm is usually in relation with one or both sphenoid sinuses; in no instance, in these heads, with the ethmoid. In more than half of the heads it lies posterior to the sphenoid cavity.

7. The optic nerve may be divided into sinus portion and a free portion, of which the former is usually the larger, as shown by the variations, as follows·

Optic nerve 34 to 55 mm., sinus portion 17 to 32 mm., free portion 12 to 28 mm. As far as could be ascertained, there is nothing in the extent and shape of the sinuses to account for the variation in the length of the nerves.

8. In five instances (one-third) one sphenoid is in relation with both optic nerves, the other sphenoid not participating; in two, the other sphenoid participates in the relation, and in one there is no relation between either sphenoid and one of the optic nerves.

9. There is a considerable variation in the distance between the optic nerve and the level of the lower margin of the nasal opening of the sphenoid from 2 mm. above to 14 mm. below. In four instances the opening is at the level of or above the optic nerve.

10. As a rule, the last posterior ethmoid cell (sometimes there are two) has a very slight relation with the optic nerve, at the postero-external angle just at the roof and from this point the nerve passes externally to the bulbus, gradually increasing the distance which separates it from the labyrinth. In one instance an anterior ethmoid replaces the posterior ethmoid cell and assumes the usual relation of the last posterior ethmoid cell. When the last posterior ethmoid cell replaces the sphenoid, the optic nerve runs along the external wall of the ethmoid.

11. The frontal is not in close relation with the optic nerve, except when it extends posteriorly in the region of the ethmoid cells. It is commonly in relation with the bulbus, but sometimes it is far removed from it.

12. The roof of the maxillary sinus, forming the inferior

wall of the orbit, is below the bulbus and does not reach a distance nearer than 7 mm. from the optic nerve.

CLINICAL DEDUCTIONS.

In view of the cases of optic nerve involvement, due to sinus disease, as abstracted, and of the anatomic study described in this paper, the following clinical deductions are justified:

1. Optic nerve involvement without periorbital abscess, although heretofore thought to be an infrequent sequella, is common enough to merit consideration in sinus affections.

2. There have probably been many unreported cases.

3. In all likelihood many minor symptoms resulting from transitory involvement have been overlooked.

4. Whether the infection be lymphogenous or hematogenous, or by contact, the smaller the distance from the infecting focus, the greater will be the chance of the involvement of the nerve.

5. It, therefore, is uncommon for frontal or maxillary sinusitis to be accompanied by optic nerve disease without periorbital involvement. However, from their relation to the bulbus, disease by extension through it is not to be overlooked.

6. Sphenoid sinusitis would naturally be called to account as the prolific cause of the infection, but the sphenoid is less commonly affected than the other sinuses, and, except in closed empyema, the pus is evacuated in a large measure through its nasal opening. Stagnant and decomposing pus is more or less common on the floor, in sphenoid empyema, in that part farthest removed from the optic nerve; but this factor becomes more potent where the orifice is at the level or above the optic nerve, as shown in the four heads, and the likelihood of trouble is greatly increased by the immediate propinquity of the stagnant and decomposing pus, which, in these cases, is separated from the nerve only by a thin lamina of bone and the nerve sheath.

The seven heads out of fifteen, shown and described in this paper, in which one sphenoid is in relation with both optic nerves, afford sufficient explanation for contralateral optic neuritis when caused by sinus disease.

7. The anterior ethmoid cells, which are so commonly affected with suppurative inflammation, are so far from the nerve that they are not likely to influence the optic nerve, ex-

cept through the effect on the periorbita adjoining. However, where an anterior ethmoid cell is extensive enough to come into relation with the nerve by replacing a posterior ethmoid cell, as in Head XII, trouble is more likely to occur.

8. The posterior ethmoid cells, also frequently affected, have very little influence on the optic nerve on account of the meagerness of their relation, viz., the postero-external angle at the roof of the cell, as I have pointed out in this paper. When the cell replaces the sphenoid and the optic nerve passes along the external wall, then the posterior ethmoid becomes the most potent factor of all, for the nerve is closer to the mass of pus and for a greater distance than under any other circumstances, even though the nasal opening may be in the dependent portion of one part of the cell.

9. It, therefore, becomes necessary to study more carefully the cases in which the sphenoid orifice is near the optic nerve and in which the sphenoid is replaced by a surmounting ethmoid cell.

HANAU W. LOEB.

REFERENCES.

1. Fr. Alexander. Verh. d. Deutschen Otol. Gesel., 1905, p. 191.

2. Berger and Tyrman. Die Krankheiten der Keilbeinhöhle und des Siebbeinlabyrinthes und ihre Beziehungen zu Erkrankungen des Sehorganes, 1886, p. 18.

3. Brockkaert. La Belgique Med., No. 2, 1901.

4. C. S. Bull. Some Points in the Symptomatology, Pathology and Treatment of Diseases of the Sinuses Adjacent and Secondary to the Orbit. N. Y. Med. Record, 1899, Vol. 56, p. 73.

5. G. W. Caldwell. Diseases of the Pneumatic Sinuses of the Nose and their Relation to Certain Affections of the Eye. N. Y. Med. Record, 1893, Vol. 43, p. 425.

6. Courtaix. Recherches cliniques sur les relations pathologiques entre l'oeil et les dents, 1891.

7. Delneuville. La Presse Oto-Rhino-Laryn. Belge, 1906, No. 1.

8. H. M. Fish. Some Cases of Uveitis due to Accessory Sinus Disease. Am. Journal of Ophthal., 1904, Vol. 21, p. 353.

9. Galezowski. Arch. génér. de Med. XXIII.

10. Galezowski. Sinusite Maxillaire, Exophthalmie et Nevrite optique. Guerison. Societe d'Ophthalmologie de Paris, Feb. 7. 1905. Archives de Laryng. d'Otologie et de Rhin., 1905, Vol. 19, p. 638.

11. W. Glegg and P. J. Hay. Lancet, Sept. 30, 1905.

12. J. Green, Jr. Ocular Signs and Complications of Accessory Sinus Disease. Ophthalmic Record, 1906, Vol. 15, p. 269.

13. A. C. Gronbak. Verhandlung des danischen oto-laryngolischen Vereins, March, 1904. Quoted by Schmiegelow, l. c.

14. T. H. Halstead. Empyema of the Right Maxillary Ethmoidal and Sphenoidal Sinuses with Sudden Blindness of the Left Eye. Operation; Recovery of Sight. Trans. of the American L. R. & O. Society, 1901, p. 61.

15. H. Hansell. A Case of Acute Loss of Vision from Disease of the Ethmoid and Sphenoid Cavities. Med. and Surg. Reporter, 1896, Vol. 75, p. 101.

16. Joh. Hjort. Mitteilungen vom Reichshospital in Christiana.

17. C. R. Holmes. The Sphenoidal Cavity and its Relation to the Eye. Archives of Ophthalmology, 1896, No. 4.

18. H. Knapp. The Inflammatory Diseases of the Nose and its

Accessory Sinuses in Relation with the Eye. Trans. Amer. Otol. Soc., 1906, Vol. 9, Part 2, p. 345.

19. Kuhnt. Ueber dié entzündlichen Erkrankungen der Stirnhöhlen und ihre Folgezustände, 1895.

20. de Lapersonne. Des Nevrites Optique liées aux sinusites sphenoidales et aux maladies de l'arriere cavite des tosses nasales. Arch. d'optal., 1899, p. 514.

21. de Lapersonne. Les Complication Oculo-Orbitaires des sinusites. Annales des maladies de l'or., etc., Sept., 1902.

22. H. W. Loeb. A Study of the Anatomy of the Accessory Cavities of the Nose by Topographic Projections. Annals of Otology, Rhinology and Laryngology, Dec., 1906.

23. H. W. Loeb. The Anatomy of the Middle Turbinate. Journal of the American Medical Association, 1907.

24. H. W. Loeb. Anatomie des Sinus Accessoires du Nez, Basée sur la Reconstruction de deux Têtes. Revue hebdom. de Laryng. d'Otologie et de Rhin., 1907.

25. Mendel. Ueber Nasale, Augen inbesondere Sehnerven-Leiden. Centralbl. f. Augenheil., 1901, p. 33.

26. S. Moritz. The Causes, Symptoms and Complications of the Diseases of the Nasal Accessory Sinuses in their Relation to General Diseases, Ophthalmology, and Neurology. British Med. Journal, 1905, Vol. 1, p. 174.

27. Nordquist. Gotheborg Lakaresallskaps Forhandlingar. May 22, 1901. Central. f. Laryn., 1903, p. 71.

28. Onodi. Orr Gege fulgyogyaszat, No. 2 Centralblatt für Laryng., 1906, p. 45.

29. Onodi. The Optic Nerve and the Accessory Cavities of the Nose. Annals of Otology, Rhinology and Larynology, March, 1908.

30. A. Onodi. Das Verhaltniss der Hinteresten Siebbeinzellen zu den Nervi Optici. Arch. f. Laryn., Vol. 15, p. 259.

31. A. Onodi. Disturbances of Vision and Blindness Caused by Troubles in the Posterior Nasal Accessory Cavities. Journal of Laryng., Vol. 19, p. 622.

32. F. R. Packard. Ophthalmological Manifestations of Latent Diseases of the Nose and its Accessory Sinuses; Report of Illustrative Cases. Transactions of the American Laryng. Association, 1907, p. 217.

33. Pasquier. Lancette francaise, 1839.

34. M. Paunz. Orvosi Hetilap, 1905, 17. Centralb. f. Laryng., 1906, p. 48.

35. E. Pollatschek. Orvosi Hetilap, 1905, 17. Centralb. f. Laryng., 1906, p. 173.

36. L. Polyak. Fall von latenter multipler Nebenhöleneiterung, Knochenblasenbildung, Exophthalmus und Atrophie beider Sehnerven. Arch f. Laryng., 1904, Vol. 15, p. 340.

37. W. Campbell Posey. The Accessory Sinuses of the Nose from an Ophthalmological Standpoint. N. Y. Med. Jour., Mch. 2, 1907.

38. W. Campbell Posey. The Ophthalmological Phase of Diseases of the Accessory Sinuses of the Nose. New York Med. Record, Vol. 72, p. 255.

39. S. D. Risley. Pennsylvania Med. Journal, 1904.

40. E. Schmiegelow. Beitrag zur Beleuchtung der Beziehungen zwischen Nasen und Augen Krankheiten. Arch. für. Laryng.

41. G. Sluder. Blindness due to Postethmoidal. Empyema Acute; Report of a Case. Laryngoscope, Vol. 17, 9, 883.

42. J. A. Thompson. Suppuration in the Ethmoid and Sphenoid Sinuses with Paralysis of the Third Nerve; Case Reports. Laryngoscope, 1907, p. 708.

43. B. Travers. A Synopsis of Diseases of the Eye, 1821.

44. Alfred Wiener. American Journal of Surgery, Oct., 1908.

45. Winckler. Naturforscherversammlung zu Lubeck, 1895.

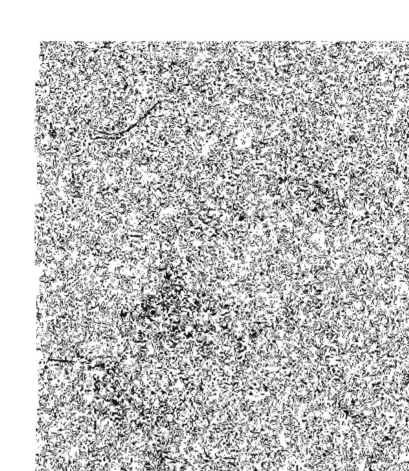

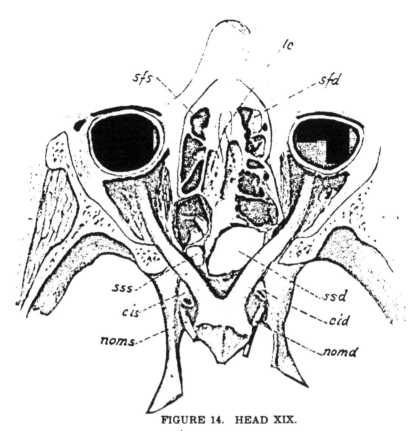

FIGURE 14. HEAD XIX.

Left sphenoid (sss) very small, in relation with left optic, but not with ri
sphenoid (ssd) in relation with both optic nerves and chiasm. Posterior eth
(ceps, cepd) in relation with optic nerves at postero-external angle; l. c.,
plate; sfs, sfd, frontal sinus; cis, cid, internal carotid; noms, nomd, oculomot

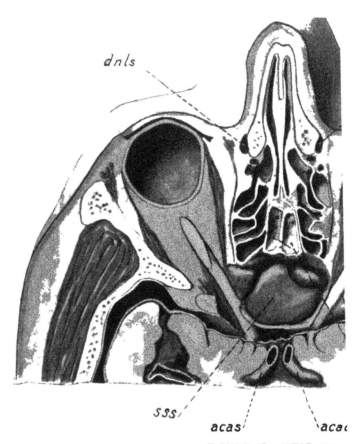

dnls

sss

acas

acac

FIGURE 15.   HEAD XX.

Left sphenoid (sss), with mucosa of root intact, in re
and chiasm; posterior ethmoid cells on either side of an
in relation with optic nerve at postero-external angle, near
cerebral arteries; dnls, dnld, nasolacrymal duct; lc, cribrif

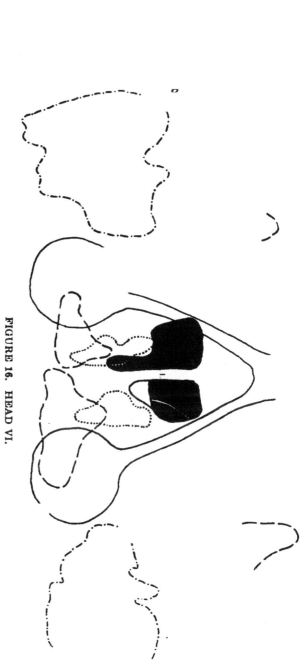

FIGURE 16. HEAD VI.

Right sphenoid in relation with left optic as well as right optic. Left sphenoid much smaller than right. Last posterio sides in relation with optic nerve at postero-external angle. Two such cells on the left side.

In this and the succeeding illustrations, the lateral reconstructions (at each side) show the frontal in parted lines, the lines, the maxillary in parted lines with a dot between each division; the superior reconstructions (in the middle) show the lines, the anterior ethmoid in dotted lines, the posterior ethmoid in solid lines, that part of the ethmoid in relation with the made black. The optic nerves, globe and chiasm are obvious. All drawings are natural size.

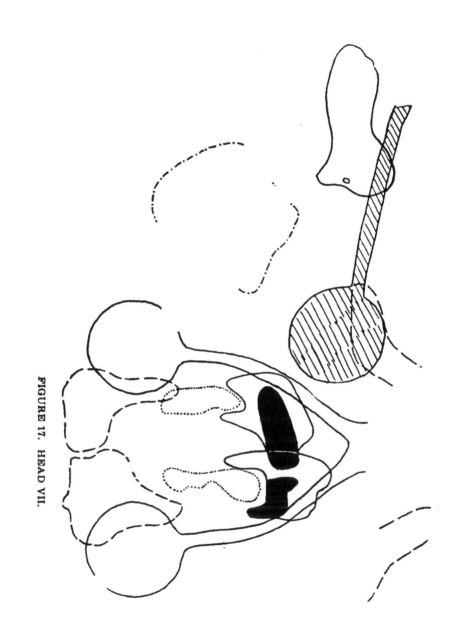

FIGURE 17. HEAD VII.

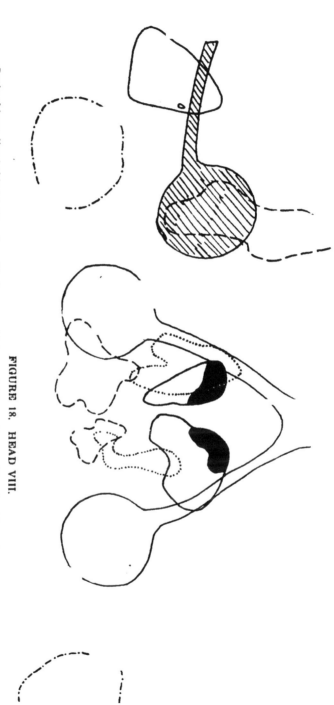

FIGURE 18. HEAD VIII.

Optic chiasm lies behind both sphenoid sinuses, which are fairly uniform. Right frontal very extensive, much larger than left. Last posterior ethmoid cells show the usual relation to the optic, at pos Right anterior ethmoid extends behind the posterior but not at the level of the optic.

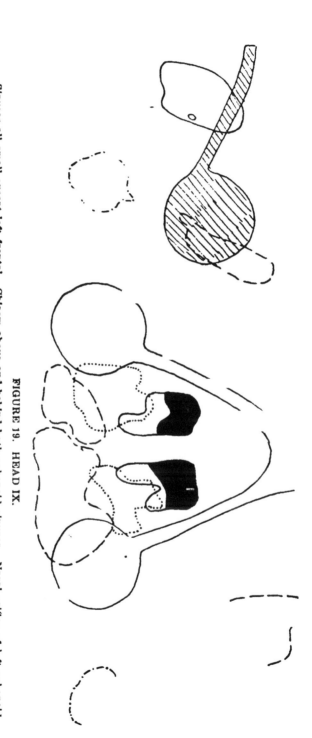

FIGURE 19. HEAD IX.

Sinuses all small except left frontal. Chiasm above and behind both sphenoid sinuses. Nasal orifice of left sphenoid sinus. Last posterior ethmoid cells in relation with optic nerve at postero-external angle of the cell.

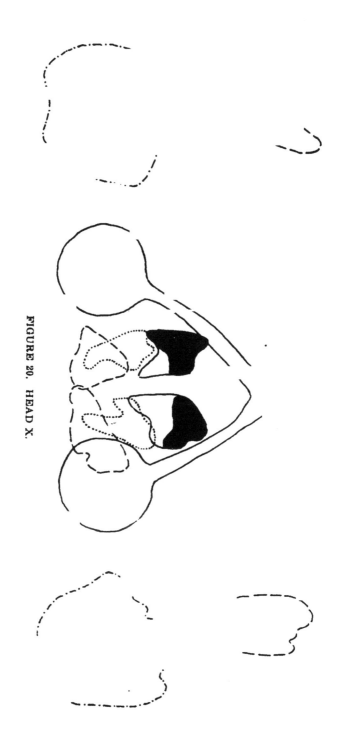

FIGURE 20. HEAD X.

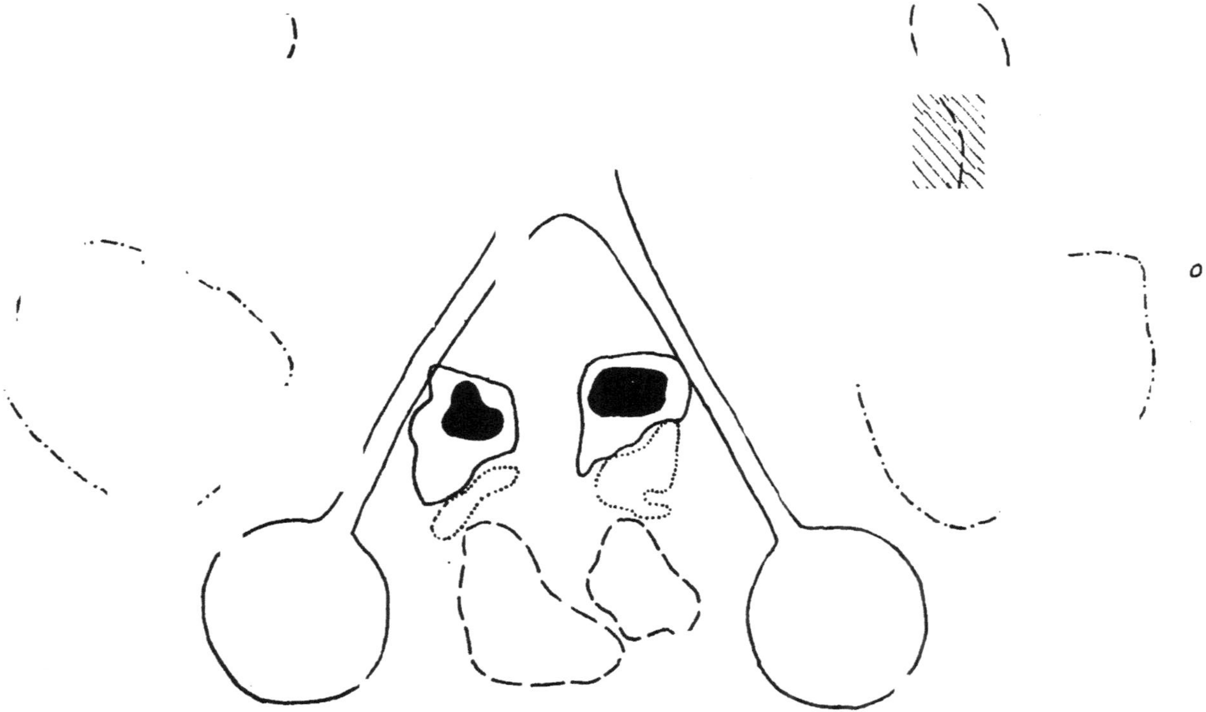

FIGURE 21. HEAD XI.

th sphenoid sinuses large, chiasm above their roofs and behind the greater portion. Last posterior ethmoid cells in relation with

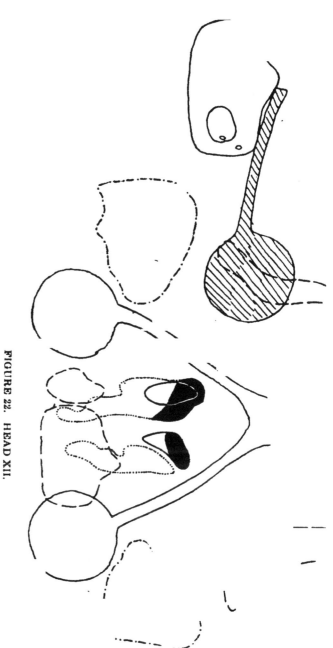

FIGURE 22. HEAD XII.

Right sphenoid very small, not in relation with optic nerve or chiasm. Left sphenoid in relation with both optic nerves. Na
this sinus near both optic nerves. Optic chiasm lies wholly on roof of left sphenoid. Last left posterior ethmoid in relation
postero-external angle. Right anterior ethmoid cell replaces small posterior ethmoid and is in relation with the optic at its postero-e

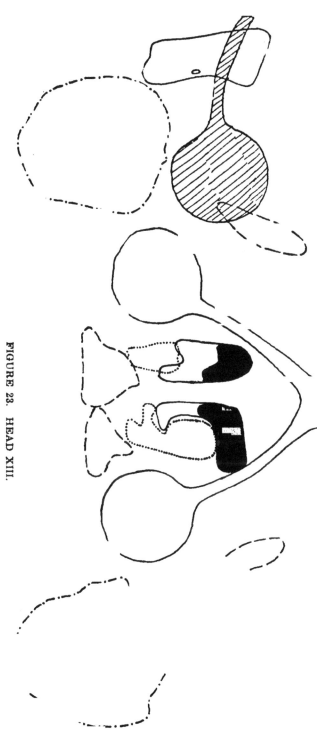

FIGURE 23. HEAD XIII.

Left sphenoid very large, right as large in a supero-inferior direction but smaller antero-posteriorly. Chiasm lies on roof of lef[t] and behind the posterior wall of the right sphenoid. Orifice of the left sphenoid just below the optic, distance slightly greater on the r[ight] posterior ethmoid cells in relation with optic at postero-external angle. Both frontals very small.

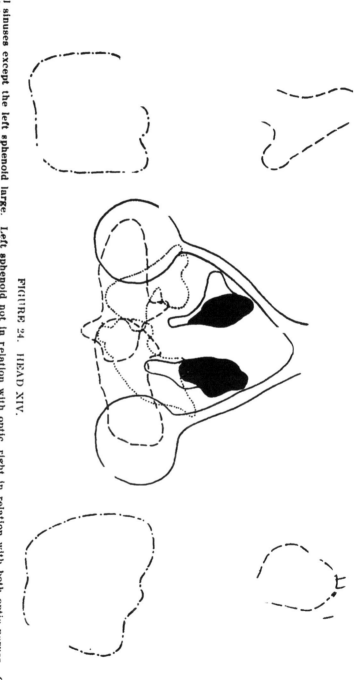

FIGURE 24. HEAD XIV.

All sinuses except the left sphenoid large. Left sphenoid not in relation with optic, right in relation with both optic nerves. Chias
ind right sphenoid. Last posterior ethmoid cells in relation with optic nerves at postero-external angle.

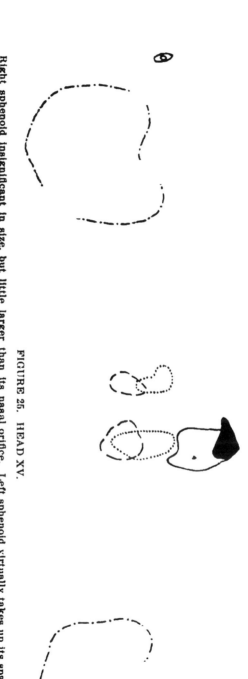

FIGURE 25. HEAD XV.

Right sphenoid insignificant in size, but little larger than its nasal orifice. Left sphenoid virtually takes up its space, com[...] with both optic nerves superiorly and with the chiasm posteriorly. Posterior ethmoid cells in relation with optic nerves at l[...] angle. Frontal and anterior ethmoid cells very small.

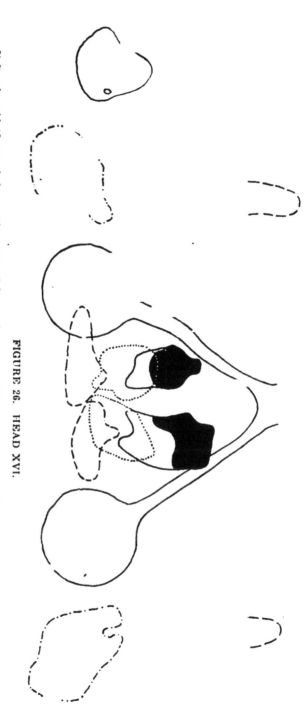

FIGURE 26. HEAD XVI.

Left sphenoid 10 mm. below optic nerve, right much nearer. Chiasm lies behind the posterior wall of right sphenoid and above
f the left. Left posterior ethmoid, having replaced left sphenoid, has a more extensive relation than usual with the optic nerve, viz.,
xternal wall. Right posterior ethmoid has usual relation at postero-external angle.

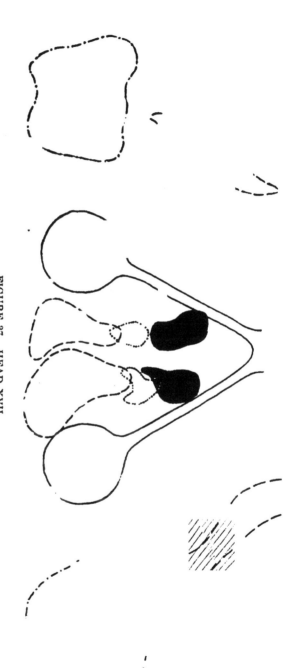

FIGURE 27. HEAD XVII.

Sinuses unusually uniform. Chiasm above and behind the sphenoid sinuses. Nasal orifice of right sphenoid nearer the optic nerve of left. Usual angular relation of posterior ethmoid cell to optic nerve on both sides.

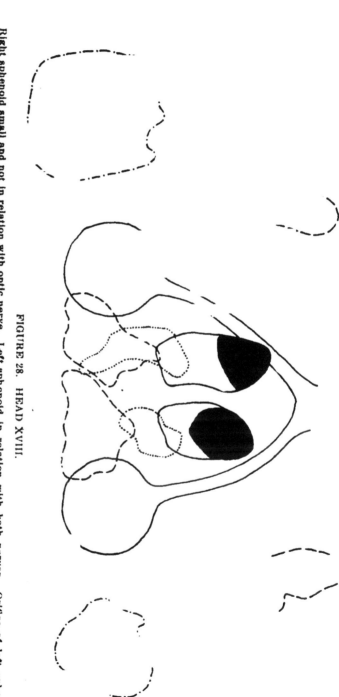

FIGURE 28. HEAD XVIII.

Right sphenoid small and not in relation with optic nerve. Left sphenoid in relation with both nerves. Orifice of left spheno lower level of both optic nerves. Chiasm above the roof of right sphenoid near the posterior wall. Right posterior ethmoid cell sphenoid and optic nerve runs along the external wall of the cell. The left posterior ethmoid has the usual relation of the optic postero-external angle.

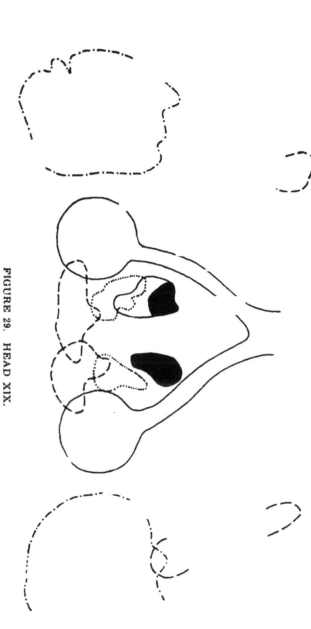

FIGURE 29. HEAD XIX.

Right sphenoid large, in relation with both optic nerves. Left sphenoid much smaller, in relation with the left optic only. O lies on roof of right sphenoid which extends a considerable distance posteriorly. Orifices of both sphenoids lie practically at the 1 optic nerve. Both posterior ethmoid cells in relation with the optic at their postero-external angle.

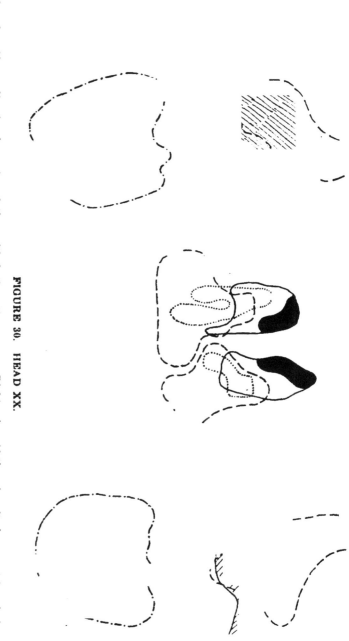

FIGURE 30.   HEAD XX.

Left sphenoid peculiar in shape, in relation with both optic nerves. Right sphenoid though quite large not in relation with either isam lies behind the left sphenoid. Both posterior ethmoid cells in relation with optic at postero-external angle.

XXII.

DISEASES OF THE EYE AND ORBIT SECONDARY TO PATHOLOGIC CHANGES IN THE NOSE AND ACCESSORY SINUSES.*

By Christian R. Holmes, M. D.,

Cincinnati.

Of late years the attention of many of the best minds among the rhinologists of Europe and America has been turned to the relationship that exists between the diseases of the nose and its accessory cavities and the resulting secondary affections of the orbit and the eye. The volume of literature upon the subject is large and is constantly growing and the industry of observers everywhere is an index and an evidence that the new pathology offered at once a key to a numerically important and a clinically obscure class of cases that previously were of doubtful prognosis as to function and even as to life itself.

The scientific study of these problems began with the discovery of the locally anesthetic properties of cocain by Dr. Carl Koller. Previous to that date we find a long list of reported cases of osteomata. benign or malignant soft growths and inflammations involving the sinuses and the eyes and adnexae. but they were only dealt with surgically when they had assumed such proportions that they had become unbearable to the patient or a source of reproach to the surgeon. Many of us have seen—and it does not seem so long ago—that an exophthalmos. accompanied by pain, tenderness and fever would be treated by the expectant method by very competent men, or, if the abscess pointed in the region of the upper or lower lid, that a bistoury would be cautiously plunged into it. evacuating the pus from the orbit while no attempt would be made to attack the primary focus of the disease, the operator not realizing that this lay in one of the accessory sinuses.

*Read before the Eastern Section of the A. L. R. and O. Society at Philadelphia, January 9, 1909.

Since the introduction of cocain, however, we have acquired a number of other aids in arriving at a complete and satisfactory diagnosis. They are adrenalin, transillumination, radiography, and a large number of clinical descriptions and pathologic reports of the macroscopic and microscopic conditions of the parts and tissues, and the non-pathogenic and pathogenic flora found therein.

By the indispensable aid of these means, we are now enabled to write down a definite pathology and symptomatology and—what is of great importance—we are able to proceed from effect back to cause and in this way to procure a radical cure in cases where our elders had to be content with more or less of palliation.

Thus we find that a number of so-called neuralgias are reflex or referred pains, due to intranasal pressure upon terminal nerve filaments in the course of acute or subacute coryza, in the paroxysms of hay fever, etc.

Epiphora often results from temporary occlusion of the lower end of the lachrymal duct—and the indications are, therefore, for attention to the nasal mucosa or other structures. Probing or slitting of the ducts under such conditions is certainly never justifiable and should be resorted to only in chronic cases of long standing where repeated inflammatory processes have left behind them areas of fibrous stricture.

The phlyctenular keratitis so often associated with nasal inflammation in children responds much more readily to constitutional treatment associated with treatment of the nose than to treatment of the eye alone—in fact, the latter method is most frequently quite ineffective. I reported cases of this character some fifteen years ago and since then have frequently omitted all direct treatment of the eyes in my management of such cases. In all cases of conjunctivitis and keratitis, whatever the age of the patient, I make it a routine practice to treat the nose if inflamed and I am convinced that this joint treatment very materially hastens the cure in almost all, if not in all cases.

In this connection I would briefly refer to three typical cases from private practice:

Mrs. S., aged 65 years, had for two years suffered from repeated, severe attacks of phlyctenular conjunctivitis and keratitis, which never appeared to be influenced by the usual forms of treatment. Recovery from one of these attacks was always prolonged and tedious. The slightest exposure would cause a return of the trouble and in the left eye useful vision was lost, because of maculae resulting from repeated corneal ulcerations. I had frequently examined the nose, but with the exception of a congestion and thickening of the membrane in general and over the middle turbinals in particular, there was nothing abnormal—transillumination was negative—the middle turbinates were, however, "wedged" in the rather narrow nares. During a violent recurrent attack, especially involving the good eye, I determined to remove the middle turbinates. The result was almost magical, and a permanent cure resulted without any other treatment. Repeated examinations after the operation failed to detect pus. Evidently the symptoms were caused by pressure resulting from a chronic hypertrophic interstitial inflammation of the mucous membrane, of the type we sometimes encounter in the middle ear.

CASE II.—Mr. W., aged 50. In 1896 this patient became totally blind in his left eye, after suffering from the most excruciating pains in the temple, occiput and back of the orbit for months at irregular intervals. There was no history of nasal catarrh and repeated examination failed to detect any. Having exhausted medicinal means of relief, I determined to open the left sphenoid cavity, and found it filled with pus (closed empyema). There was complete relief from pain and vision slowly returned to almost normal—a small central scotoma remaining as a result of too prolonged pressure upon the nerve; the delicate macular fibers having succumbed before the operation. For ten years after this operation the patient was entirely-free from eye symptoms and head pains. Then began a burning sensation with mild catarrhal conjunctivitis of both eyes and asthenopic symptoms, which for a while he attributed to the fumes from paints and varnishes with which he worked. A vacation gave only temporary relief. He was compelled to spend his evenings sitting with his eyes closed in the darkest part of the room. Treatment of the lids and re-examination of his muscles and refraction failed to improve the trouble. After a year's treatment with others, he returned to me unimproved. With an increased knowledge of the intimate relation between the nose and eyes, I finally came to the conclusion that the cause was due to pressure within the nose. The left sphenoid cavity, formerly infected, could be inspected through the opening made ten years before—and was found normal, but the middle turbinate bodies were "wedged." I operated upon both sides, with almost immediate relief. With the post-operative swelling there was a slight return of the eye symptoms, for about a week, but after the parts had healed the cure was complete and permanent.

CASE III.—Miss M., aged 32, one of my nurses, had for years been a great sufferer from head and eye pains, which became more frequent and severe. She felt incapacitated for work and contemplated giving up nursing and returning to her home in the country. Her nose had been examined repeatedly, but revealed no unusual amount of secretion and I did not think there were sufficient pathologic changes in the rather large middle turbinates to justify their removal. Only as a last resort did I consent. The relief was complete and permanent, with a marked increase in bodily weight and general well-being.

Inflammations of the orbit and of the deeper structures of the eye, involving the iris or all of the uveal tract, and optic nerve, are often secondary to inflammations of the nasal sinuses. On this relationship much has been written of late, both in this country and Europe; but here, as in other departments of medicine, we must guard against riding a hobby too hard, as I fear some of us may do in claiming too much etiologically for the nose and sinuses and overlooking many other important causative factors in other parts of the body, a mental obliquity that specialism is prone to lead us into unless we are on our guard.

The pathologic position of nasal polypi is now fixed as being a secondary manifestation of chronic purulent inflammation of one or more sinuses, and their recurrence after removal is sufficient evidence of the persistence of the empyema.

That their removal is not entirely free from danger, I have myself observed—especially when the galvanocautery or a caustic is used to destroy the base after the growth has been snared. This cauterization, in the light of our present knowledge, I hold to be most unsurgical, as it produces a more or less extensive sloughing surface affording refuge and pabulum to innumerable bacteria. A direct attack upon the sinus that is the seat of the inflammation is the only logical procedure.

Among the untoward effects of nasal cauterizations I have seen neuroretinitis, retinal hemorrhages and optic nerve atrophy—this latter result, as we now know, being due to a thrombosis following local infection.

There is one important subject that has not received the attention that it deserves—and I mention it here to bring it up for discussion: I refer to the nasal and orbital manifestation of syphilis.

The favorite seat of the orbital syphiloma occurring in the course of nasal syphilis appears to be the superior orbital margin—and the first objective symptom is the appearance of a sharply circumscribed, hard, inelastic tumor, the overlying skin in the beginning not reddened. Later redness and fluctuation, going on to sloughing and evacuation of the characteristic tenaceous secretion—with rough, necrotic bone in the bottom of the abscess. The pain prior to the evacuation is very severe, but intermittent, as in most syphilitic periostitis. Antispecific treatment generally causes rapid and total resorption. The swelling of the orbital margin may cause displacement of the globe and interfere with its mobility. There may be involvement of the ocular muscles and if the inflammation extends to the apex of the orbit serious involvement of the optic nerve may occur with secondary atrophy. The displacement of the globe in these cases is not due to the presence of pus, but to a hyperplastic process taking place in the orbital periosteum and orbital fascia. Recognized in good time in a very large proportion of cases all of the swelling, even if extensive, may subside under energetic appropriate treatment without serious or permanent damage to important structures.

It is, of course, of great importance to differentiate between these gummata and malignant or non-malignant tumors. Failure to make correct dignosis would possibly—even probably—lead to enucleation of an eye that ought to be and might be saved. The character and the amount of the pain is a valuable but not an infallible guide. The non-malignant tumors may cause great displacement of the globe with little or no pain—while in the gummata we practically always have the characteristic night pains of syphilis. No careful surgeon, however, would in a doubtful case appeal to operative measures without having applied the therapeutic test. The gummata may not spring from the orbital margin, but have their origin in the middle cerebral fossa, involving the Gasserian ganglion with resulting trophic lesions—such as corneal ulcers, anesthesias, etc. Or the syphilitic growth may begin in the nose and extend to one of the sinuses and the orbit.

Double and symmetrical syphilitic orbital tumors are also encountered, and have been reported by Goldzieher and others. Schotts reported a fatal case in a child five years of age, where a gumma involved the nose, orbit and cranial fossa. Walter reported a fatal case in a child three and one-half years of age, the growth involving both orbits and intervening parts.

In both of these cases the diagnosis had been made of sarcoma, based upon microscopic findings of fragments of the turmors removed. Macroscopic and microscopic examinations after death proved them to be gummata.

Goldzieher's case was a girl, 16 years of age, with absolutely negative history. Tumors were removed from both orbits at different times—the microscopic examination resulting in a diagnosis of fibrosarcoma. The disease was not arrested by the operation—resulting in death. The postmortem revealed the process as having its origin in the bony walls of the orbit and adjoining sinuses.

Miliary gummata in liver, spleen and kidneys—postmortem and microscopic examination made by Prosector Minich (another had examined the tumors intra vitam) showed that it was a case of syphilitic gummata. To what extent these cases involved the sinuses is not shown by the reports. They were in the hands of ophthalmologists, who in all probability did not consider the accessory sinuses very seriously, as at that time the interrelation between the nose, the sinuses and the orbit had not been very generally recognized. Even the postmortem reports fail to mention the sinuses and I question if they were opened. There was no history of acquired syphilis in any of these cases of unrecognized congenital syphilis. In one of my own cases the microscopic findings were also incorrectly reported (and by a supposedly competent microscopist) and in view of the doubtful clinical picture and of the uncertainty of the laboratory reports I believe that the strongest possible weight should be given to the effects of antispecific treatment and that it should be pushed vigorously for a sufficient length of time to allow of its failure to definitely negative the diagnosis of syphilis.

Of the sinuses the antrum of Highmore was the first to claim the surgeon's' attention, being easy of access through the alveolus. Carious teeth no doubt pointed out the way. The literature upon diseases of this sinus is very extensive. In preparing a "bibliography of diseases of the accessory sinuses" from 1748 to date I have collected over 1500 references (and no doubt many have escaped me) to publications made before 1890. The vast majority of these referred to the antrum of Highmore.

While a number of cases of empyema of the antrum in infants with involvement of the lower lid and orbit have been reported, I doubt very much if most of them were not cases of osteomyelitis or necrosis with the formation of a pocket of pus, as in the young infant the antrum of Highmore is a mere slit instead of a cavity. I wish that some specially qualified American confrere would take up the study of the minute anatomy of the lining membranes of the sinuses in health and disease—paying especial attention to the lymphatics and blood supply, along the lines laid down by Dr. J. Marc André, as published in his excellent monograph "Lymphatiques du Nez," 1905.

The lining membrane of the antrum of Highmore being thicker and richer in glands and lymphatics and blood vessels than any of the other sinuses, gives it a high degree of resistance to unfavorable influences. This probably explains why this cavity can for years remain a receptacle for the pus flowing into it from the frontal sinus—as sometimes occurs—without the lining membrane of the antrum becoming diseased, as is proven by the fact that when the pus ceases to flow from the frontal sinus, after a successful operation, and the antrum is washed, the latter has repeatedly been known to remain normal without further treatment—a possibility we should bear in mind before resorting to the radical operation on this cavity. The extra thickness of the lining membrane also explains why we encounter in the antrum greater edema of its mucous membrane than in any of the other sinuses—this swelling is principally located in the loose connective tissue layer under the layer of ciliated epithelium. When the antrum is small this layer may swell to such proportions as to fill the cavity, producing intense neuralgia by pressure; the pain radiating to the orbit and eye. In chronic cases the lining of the antrum may undergo fibroid changes forming septa and bands that almost occlude the cavity.

The relation between sinus disease and secondary involvement of the orbit and eye have recently been set forth in a masterly manner by Birch-Hirschfeld. So far as I have been instructed by my limited experience, my views and results coincide with his, and hence I have taken the liberty of translating his conclusions:

1. Sinus inflammation plays a much more important part in orbital inflammation than has been recognized up to date.

2. In nearly all cases we have to deal with an acute or chronic sinus empyema.

3. The extension of the inflammation to the orbit depends upon the local periostitis of the orbital wall, there being certain points of predilection. The infection usually follows the course of the perforating vessels.

4. The orbital inflammation may be a (1) periostitis, (2) orbital abscess, (3) diffuse orbital inflammatory infiltration.

5. The orbital periosteum often offers sufficient resistance to the inflammatory process to prevent its extension to the orbital contents and the abscess remaining subperiosteal may extend forwards, or backwards, into the orbit, causing an inflammation of the optic nerve; or if forward, evacuate itself spontaneously at the orbital margin.

6. In other cases the inflammation extends early to the orbital contents through a thrombophlebitis. These cases are more difficult to diagnose.

7. In addition to the circumscribed areas on the orbital walls tender to pressure, the direction of the dislocation of the globe is of diagnostic value.

8. Contraction of the visual field is rare.

9. Of great importance as an aid in the diagnosis of inflammation of one of the posterior sinuses (posterior ethmoid or sphenoid cavity) is the discovery of a central scotoma.

10. In 409 cases of orbital inflammation following sinus disease, 66 eyes became blind (16 per cent), blindness following most frequently empyema of the antrum of Highmore (27 per cent).

11. The ophthalmoscope *frequently* revealed hyperemia of the disc—optic neuritis—atrophy of the optic nerve *less frequently*. Thrombophlebitis of the retinal veins—retinal hemorrhage and detachment.

12. There were present ulcus corneae 18 times—panophthalmitis in 8 and glaucoma in 2 cases.

13. The mortality is highest in cases of empyema of the sphenoid (28 per cent of all fatal cases); in the frontal sinus empyema (16.3 per cent of the fatal cases).

14. Postmortem examination demonstrated:

Meningitis, 34 times.

Brain abscess, 15 times.

Sinus thrombosis, 6 times.

15. The author holds that the simple incision as made into the orbit by the ophthalmologists is inadequate and recommends free exposure of the orbital (bony) margin, with careful separation of the periosteum from the bone by means of a blunt periosteotome (using every care to protect the orbital contents). In this manner we obtain free drainage.

(To this I should add—to promptly establish thorough drainage from the affected sinuses, either by the intranasal or external operation. In cases where the orbital symptoms are not seriously threatening the functions of the eye, prompt drainage of the sinus will obviate the necessity of any operation upon the orbit, as I have several times demonstrated in my own cases.)

16. The examination and treatment of the nasal cavities and accessory cavities demand such training and experience as the ophthalmologist seldom possesses, and the writer feels that the diagnosis and treatment of sinusitis should be left to the rhinologist.

17. The importance of the ophthalmologist in these affections lies in the fact that he is often the first to establish the diagnosis, because these patients as a rule first seek relief from their eye symptoms, and in doubtful cases by a careful analysis of the ocular and orbital symptoms, he helps to arrive at a correct conclusion.

18. That from the working in unison of the ophthalmologist and rhinologist we may expect the development of the greatest amount of scientific knowledge and practical results.

In conclusion I wish to touch upon two points in relation to the diagnosis and operative management of suspected and also undoubted frontal sinus infection.

1. When the obscure clinical symptoms and somewhat negative findings of our diagnostic aids, such as the trans-

illuminator, have left us in doubt as to the condition of the sinus (and such a situation naturally precludes the presence of any very active inflammatory process) *we should not hesitate to make an external exploratory opening.* Since 1895 I have often resorted to this when in doubt—making a short incision just below the supraorbital margin above the inner canthus and exposing only enough bone to permit the removal of a disk 5 mm. in diameter by means of a hollow electric drill. If the sinus is healthy—then the wound is closed by catgut suture and hermetically sealed with gauze and collodion dressing. This latter left intact for two weeks. In another two weeks it is difficult to find the scar. I have never seen such a case fail to heal by first intention.

2. On account of its great importance, I wish to again call attention to the fact that we should not make minor intranasal operations within a period of several days before an extensive external operation in cases where we have to deal with a streptococcus infection, because of the liability to the erysipelatons infection of the skin wound. The minor intranasal operation is liable to excite the streptococci present to a high degree of virulence. While in this condition of exalted virulence infection of the external skin wound is more than likely and an erysipelatous inflammation starting in this neighborhood is extremely dangerous to the eye, if not, indeed, to life itself.

When during an acute frontal sinus inflammation it become absolutely necessary to give vent to pent-up pus, establish drainage through a small opening in the floor of the sinus, doing as little damage as possible to the skin and subcutaneous structures and postpone the radical operation upon and cure of the cause until the acuteness of the inflammation and the virulence of the streptococci have subsided.

XXIII.

ORBITAL COMPLICATIONS OF DISEASE OF THE FRONTAL SINUS.*

BY HOWARD F. HANSELL, M. D.,

PHILADELPHIA.

The subject chosen by Dr. Holmes for his essay and the discussion proposed by the president, Dr. Packard, are most opportune. Readers of recent ophthalmic literature must be impressed with the number and value of papers and clinical contributions dealing with the interrelationship of diseases of the accessory sinuses and diseases of the eye and orbit. The close anatomic connection existing between these cavities of the skull, separated only by perforated and attenuated bone from each other, and from the greatest of them all, is a sufficient reason for the frequency in association in disease, as of function in health. Moreover and independent of any precise and definite path, the coordination of function so easily unbalanced by imperfect control or failure of individual response, renders still more intimate and interdependent the combined physiologic action of the cavities and their contents. We have known since the early days of specialism that some ocular diseases, such as chronic conjunctivitis, corneal ulcer, dacryocystitis, may have their origin in pathologic conditions of the mucous membrane of the nose. Recently, owing to the valuable contributions of Zeigler, Posey, Germann, Axenfeld, Eversbusch, Gerber and Birch-Hirschfeld, we have awakened to the supreme importance of the etiologic connection in other and more dangerous ocular diseases. The investigations have been carried on by experts in both specialties and by pathologists, and as a result of their cleverness and industry we have at our disposal cumulative evidence of the greatest practical importance. I am sure that many of us may remember our treatment of patients. which, owing to our partial knowledge, was of

---

*Read before the Eastern Section American Oto-Laryngological Society, January 9, 1909.

little service. Had we fully appreciated the significance of symptoms and thought more deeply into the etiology and listened with greater patience to the story of the history, our opinions might have been more valuable. Early ignorance and neglect are all the more culpable in view of the quotation on the title page of Gerber's monograph, Komplicationen der Stirnhöhlenentzündungen, 1908, taken from Med. u. Chir. Bemerk. 2 B., published in 1813. "Die Stirnhöhlen sind zuweilen der Sitz gefärhlichen und schwer zu entdeckenden Krankheiten."

A conception of the frequency of orbital and ocular complications in accessory sinus disease may be learned from the statements of Birch-Hirschfeld (2nd ed. Graefe-Saemisch), "nearly all inflammations of the orbit are caused by empyema of the neighboring cavities," and of Mackay (Trans. Oph. Sect. Brit. Med. Asso., 1908), "evidence goes to prove not only that a large proportion, perhaps the majority of cases, of idiopathic orbital cellulitis and orbital abscess have their origin in diseases of the nasal accessory sinuses, but also that a considerable number of maladies affecting the textures of the eyeball and its appendages in a more solitary manner may at times be traced to the same source as direct or as reflex disturbances." The former writer says (*Klin. Monatsb. f. Augenh.,* January, 1908) that out of 684 cases of orbital inflammation, 409 (59%) were due to accessory sinus inflammation, and he suggests that the number would probably have been still higher if the nose and accessory sinuses had always been examined. In 129 (30%) the frontal sinus had been the starting point; in 89 (22%) the maxillary sinus, and in 25 (6%) the sphenoidal sinus. Gerber collected 177 cases of frontal sinus disease and 56% of them showed ocular or orbital symptoms. Accepting these figures as correct, the importance of the frequent coöperation of the laryngologist and ophthalmologist is demonstrated. Without expert examination of the frontal sinus the diagnosis in many cases must be doubtful. Only operation or postmortem will show the character and source of the disease. For example: A boy was admitted to the Jefferson Hospital (Trans. Sect. Ophthal. College of Physicians, Phila, 1908) who had received on the superior rim of the orbit an injury from a frozen snowball. On the day following the accident the lids were edematous, completely covering the ball, the conjunctiva was chemotic and protruded between the lids, the eye was proptosed and immovable, the cornea rotated down and out, the media clear, the retina and nerve edematous. Operation showed fracture of the roof of the orbit and commencing purulent meningitis. The patient became delirious and died in three days. In this case it was clear we had to do with acute orbital cellulitis, but the complications and the structures affected could not have been positively foretold. The frontal sinus was not sufficiently developed to figure as a prominent factor in the diagnosis, and yet the presence of purulent inflammation following so speed'ly after the injury would suggest accessibility of germ-laden air.

Affections of the frontal sinus involve the orbit in one of three ways: by displacement of the structures, by infection, by functional disturbances.

1. Mechanical displacement or insult. Protrusion downward of the floor of the sinus by a collection of foreign matter in it will cause displacement of the orbital contents according to the degree and site of the swelling. The symptoms closely resemble those of an orbital tumor interposed between the eyeball and orbital roof. A man of 40 presented himself at the Eye Dispensary of the Jefferson Hospital in July, 1908, complaining of pain in the right orbit, diplopia, partial loss of vision and dislocation of the right eyeball downward and outward. He gave a history of two injuries to the right side of the forehead. The first occurred sixteen years ago by striking the top of a doorway while running. He was thrown down backward, but was not rendered unconscious. He had moderate pain for two weeks and lost one day's work. The second happened five years ago. As he was crossing a railroad track he tripped and struck the forehead and root of the nose against a rail. The wound was quite severe, requiring several stitches, of which he still bears the marks. A swelling could be felt between the ball and the superior margin of the orbit. Believing the growth was sarcoma, because of its slow growth, the pain, its rounded anterior extremity and its resemblance to other cases seen in the clinic which had proven to be tumors, the man was treated by application of x-rays. After two months' trial the only change consisted in the partial cessation of pain. Recently the pain returned with its former violence and the rays were ineffective. An ex-

ploratory incision was made and after carefully dissecting the
tissues down to the supposed tumor, the enclosing sac of a
large collection of pus was opened. After thorough evacuation
of the pus a round perforation, 1 cm. in diameter, was found
leading into the frontal sinus. In several places on the roof
of the orbit as far back as the apex the bone was roughened
. as though denuded of periosteum. A rubber drainage tube
was inserted and the wound sutured around it. In two days
the tube was removed. The symptoms were relieved and grad-
nally the eye returned to its nomal position and regained its
power of rotation. The patient complains of slight pain in
the mornings, but is well the remainder of the day. A small
electric light applied between the eye and the roof of the orbit
gives much less reflex through the right than through the
left half of the frontal sinus. Dr. D. Braden Kyle, who frequently examined the man, believes that the sinus is free from
foreign contents and explains the dull reflex from the presence
of inflammatory exudate of the old periostitis. The large and
bright reflex of the left side indicates that the process was entirely limited to the right side and at no time invaded the left.
The optic nerve and retina were not edematous, nor was the
retinal circulation disturbed. The lowered vision was the ·
result of several factors ; pressure by the displaced orbital contents on the nerve between the ball and the optic foramen, the
use of the periphery of the retina in the act of seeing, the
foveal region having been displaced upward, hyperopia of 6 D.
and amblyopia. The last examination was made January 6,
1909. Vision was only slightly improved by glass, the media
were clear and the fundus healthy. It seems probable that the
mucous membrane and periosteum of the frontal sinus will
resume their normal condition and the perforation and the
periostitis recover without further treatment. Had the exploratory incision not been made until after the pus sac ruptured, the ocular and orbital symptoms would have been more
serious, to which would have been added the lively danger of
extension backward of the infection to the meninges through
the posterior orbital openings.

2. Infection. The pus invades the orbit directly through
the perforated bone or is carried to the orbital tissues by the
vessels. The causes of indirect infection are caries of the
orbital roof, thrombophlebitis of the orbit, thrombosis of the

cavernous sinus, infection of the brain structures and transmission of the germ along the optic nerve sheath to the ball and to the muscles, lids and lacrimal apparatus.

3. Functional, in which there are no anatomical findings. Involvement of the eye and orbit is shown by accommodative and muscular asthenopia, limitation of fields, diminution of central vision and central scotoma. Under this head are included some of those obstinate cases of asthenopia which glasses will not cure. No lesion of the eye exists. The error of refraction may be small or great, spherical or astigmatic, perfectly corrected under mydriasis and the glasses intelligently worn. It may be that no symptoms point to the existence of sinus disease and attention is not called to the sinus as a possible source of the trouble, yet the oculist's duty is not fulfilled unless he eliminates the frontal sinus from the etiology.

The diseases of the orbit commonly associated with or dependent upon primary frontal sinus disease are, according to Germann (*Mitth. a. d. St. Petersburger Augenh.*, Ht. 5, 1908) :

1. Phlegmon : Benign orbital cellulitis, non-purulent, arising from the lymphatics. Malignant—purulent caries and necrosis.

2. Cysts, consisting principally of orbital mucocele.

3. Optic neuritis leading to optic atrophy; irritation of the 1st and 2nd divisions of the 5th nerve.

4. Panophthalmitis.

The symptoms of orbital complications vary according to the nature and character of the primary affection. In 70 cases of periostitis Germann found changes in the orbit in 27, edema and infiltration of the lids in 38, of the ball in 25, uveitis, keratitis and other affections of the eye, including choked disk in 16, and lacrimal fistule in one. The usual *signs,* those common to most cases of orbital involvement, are edema, infiltration or emphysema of the lids, particularly the upper, the folds of which are smoothed away, mechanical ptosis; inflammation, chemosis and ectropion of the conjunctiva and probably tenonitis; dislocation forward and outward of the ball with partial or complete immobility; uveitis, optic neuritis; panophthalmitis. Corneal affections early in the disease are rare, owing to the protection of this membrane by the overhanging lid. The lacrimal gland and sac may become involved and, indeed, may furnish the principal signs of frontal sinus dis-

ease—leading to error in diagnosis. The signs are modified
by the progress of the disease, keeping step with its various
phases.

The principal *subjective symptoms* are headache, neuralgia
of the 5th, diplopia, vertigo, vomiting, insomnia, mental depression, and sometimes chills and fever, sensitiveness over the
frontal sinus or the inner angle of the orbit, deterioration or loss
of vision. The headache is frontal, persistent, intense and aggravated by body movements and by percussion of the skull,
by light, no se or attempts to use the eyes. The diplopia is
present only when the lid is raised, hence it is seldom annoying and cannot be regarded as the cause of the vertigo or
disturbance of the stomach. For the same reason loss of
vision is not a conspicuous symptom. The defective vision
is due to opacities of the media or pressure upon the nerve
in the orbit or in the optic canal. Birch-Hirschfeld pointed
out that astigmatism of the cornea may be produced by pressure on the ball. Schoen says the headache is characteristic
and is accompanied by cramp of the accommodation and of the
internal recti. Hajek, however, says the localization of the
pain is not typical. Radiography and transillumination are
extremely useful in determining the diagnosis and may be
employed with advantage during the course of the disease.
Naturally their sphere of usefulness is limited to the cavities
other than the orbit, excepting in cases of bony or other hard
orbital growths. Birch-Hirschfeld calls attention to two forms
of sinusitis without external signs of inflammation in the orbit
or neighboring tissues, but

(a) With ophthalmoscopic signs of optic neuritis, neuro-
retinitis, retinal phlebitis or hemorrhages, and

(b) Without ophthalmoscopic signs, but with disturbance
of vision, such as central scotoma, limitation of fields, muscular
paralysis or trophic disturbance from interference with the
function of the 5th pair of nerves. Finally, the history may
throw some light on the diagnosis, for example, traumatism,
or a record of recurring colds, rhinitis after infectious diseases, as measles, scarlet fever, or influenza, or changes
secondary to syphilis or tuberculosis of the bones or brain
tumor.

The function if not the integrity of the eye and its appendages are seriously compromised by disease secondary to sinu-

sitis. Early and radical treatment may be effective in checking the disease and saving the ocular structures. Frequently,
however, the prognosis is unfavorable, because of optic atrophy, muscular paralysis and permanent dislocation of the
ball. Attempts to drain the orbit with free incisions are almost
valueless. Opening the frontal sinus by trephining or the
operation proposed by Arnold Knapp (*Jour. Amer. Med. Asso.,*
July, 1908), is to be recommended. The latter permits of the
examination and treatment of the frontal sinus and causes
comparatively little disturbance of the eye or its muscles.

XXIV

SOME OCULAR SYMPTOMS OF DISEASES OF THE NASAL SINUSES.*

By Wm. Campbell Posey, M. D.,

Philadelphia.

During the past four years, under some such title as this, I have contributed a number of papers upon the subject under discussion this afternoon, and while I have nothing new to add to the observations of others or to the various points in the symptomatology to which I have made reference elsewhere, I am glad of this opportunity to speak of several phases of the subject which may perhaps bear further elaboration.

And first as to the symptoms of eye-strain which may be evoked by a sinusitis. In this assemblage, mention need not be made of the orbital and periorbital pain which the various forms of inflammation of the sinuses may evoke, but I would call attention very briefly to the dull ocular pain, to the photophobia and the conjunctival symptoms after any use of the eyes, which glasses fail to relieve and which disappear after rhinologic treatment. In this class of cases the oculist finds difficulty in determining the proper axis of the cylinder, in correcting the astigmatism, and observes various vagaries in the behavior of the ciliary muscle. If referred to a rhinologist, there will be found, as summarized for me by Dr. Packard, following the observation of a large number of cases studied in common with him, a "septal spur or deflection upon which the swollen turbinate impinges, or congestion of the sinuses, with possibly an accumulation of nonpurulent secretion within them, due to the occlusion of their orifices by swelling of the turbinate tissues." I take it that such intranasal conditions are often not striking and may be readily overlooked, but unless they are properly cared for, the ocular symptoms will persist

---

*Read before the Eastern Section of the American Laryngological, Rhinological and Otological Society, January 9, 1909.

despite every local application which can be made to the conjunctiva or any combination of lenses that may be ordered.

It is in this class of cases that the ophthalmologist often masks the real source of the asthenopia by drying up the nasal and sinus mucous membrane by the atropin which he employs to put the ciliary muscle at rest, the disappearance of the symptoms being due quite as much to the subsidence of the nasal as the ocular congestion.

Another conclusion of Dr. Packard's is that "there is a very large class of cases which present not only asthenopia but other ophthalmologic symptoms as well which are undoubtedly attributable to old sinus trouble, but in which at the time they are seen by the rhinologist no pus is to be found in any of the sinuses, although the history points to sinus origin of the patient's catarrhal trouble. These are cases which give a history of grippe with intense head pains, followed by a profuse purulent discharge from the nose, leaving later more or less so-called catarrhal trouble in reality originating from the sinuses."

This seems to be a most important observation, and is in line with a statement of Axenfeld, that in cases of orbital cellulitis, in which the nasal examination is negative, the original sinusitis which occasioned the orbital condition may have healed by evacuation into the nose, while the orbital condition is progressive, on account of the absence of drainage. Indeed, Axenfeld was able to actually demonstrate by exploratory trephining that the original sinusitis may be healed at the time the orbital condition is under treatment.

In this condition of active and passive hyperemia of the orbital tissues, the function of the extraocular muscles, as well as that of the intraocular, may be interfered with and double vision may result, or if diplopia be not complained of it can be obtained by careful search in the extreme periphery of the field of activity of the individual eye muscles. I have already recorded a number of such cases, and a transient imbalance of the ocular muscles is often suggestive to me of some trouble within the sinuses. More constant and serious affections of the muscles of the eye may result from a more active state of inflammation within the sinuses, and actual palsy may occur either as a consequence of the juxtaposition of some of the eye muscles with the walls of the orbit, such as the internal and superior rectus, or by an involvement of the nerves which supply them as they pass along the wall of the sphenoidal sinus.

A second point of interest is whether inflammations of the uveal tract, such as iritis and kerato-iritis, may be evoked by inflammations within the sinuses. Zeim, Fromaget, Fish and others affirm that they have observed such an association and follow treatment of the sinuses. Fage contends that ozena follow treatment of the sinuses. Fage contends that ozaena bacilli can reach the eye from the nose and there set up an iritis. Such a transference of bacteria or toxines from the nose or nasal cavities has never been proved in a single instance, and as Axenfeld says, "The occurrence of bulbar inflammations in these nasal affections can quite as well be explained by a localizing and predisposing reflex circulatory disturbance, due to the neighboring affection, while the true exciting cause of the iritis, scleritis, etc., is perhaps something quite apart from the nose,"

Although Dr. de Schweinitz has referred at length to inflammation of the optic nerve from sinusitis, I should like to again call attention to the retrobulbar edema of the nerve which sometimes occurs in acute involvement of the sphenoidal and ethmoidal cells. I have observed quite a large group of these cases after sea bathing in conjunction with Drs. Packard, Freeman, Stout and others, the patients in nearly all instances first consulting me for their ocular condition, being ignorant of any nasal affection. Examination of the affected eye, for as a rule but one eye was involved, reveals some haze of vision, but a much more marked diminution in the light sense, relative scotoma at or near fixation, pain on pressing the eyeball back into the orbit, and at one or more points in the rotation of the eye through various meridians, choking of the lymph sheaths of the central vessels of the retina, with perhaps some blurring of the edges of the nerve, and not infrequently a partially dilated pupil. The recognition of this set of symptoms and the reference of the patient to a rhinologist, is usually attended by the prompt subsidence of the ocular symptoms, whereas the failure to appreciate the proper source, condemns the patient to a long course of treatment with salicylates and may terminate in more or less serious ocular and nasal sequellae.

As a fourth point, it may not be amiss to refer briefly to the frequency with which orbital inflammation is dependent upon diseases of the sinuses. Birch-Hirschfeld has compiled some interesting figures in this connection and as his paper was published comparatively recently and in an ophthalmological journal, and thus may have escaped the attention of rhinologists, their recital may not prove tedious.

Of 684 cases of orbital inflammation Birch-Hirschfeld found that at least 409 (59.8 per cent) depended upon one of the sinuses, and he believes that the percentage would have been still higher if examination of the sinuses had been made in all cases. Of these 409 cases, 129 (29.8 per cent) showed involvement of the frontal sinus, 89 (21.8 per cent) of the maxillary antrum, 83 (20.5 per cent) of the ethmoid cells, and 25 (6.1 per cent) of the sphenoidal sinus. In 60 cases (14.7 per cent) several cavities were affected, most frequently (25 times) the frontal and ethmoidal, then the ethmoidal and antrum (12 times), and finally the ethmoidal and sphenoidal (10 times). In almost all cases the condition was chronic or acute purulent sinusitis, so-called sinus empyema, which had followed rhinitis, influenza, pneumonia, scarlet fever and diphtheria, or after traumatism.

Birch-Hirschfeld found that blindness, which occurred in 66 out of his 409 cases (16 per cent) may be produced by empyema of the frontal, ethmoidal and antral sinuses. The optic nerve may be involved by the pus burrowing its way to the apex of the orbit, or the blindness may be evoked by thrombophlebitis of the optic veins. This was especially the case in antral empyema. Fifty-two out of the 409 cases (12.7 per cent) were fatal. Of this number 28 per cent presented sphenoidal, 16.3 per cent frontal, 14.6 per cent maxillary and 6 per cent ethmoidal sinusitis. He found that the mean death rate is not so great as in orbital inflammation without sinus affection, which was 17 per cent in 275 cases, since treatment of the disease exerts a beneficial influence upon the orbital inflammation, thrombophlebitis also occurring less often than in so-called true orbital inflammation. The postmortem examination revealed meningitis in 34 instances, frontal abscess in 15, and sinus thrombosis in 6. Four patients died of pneumonia, two of sepsis.

In conclusion, let me once more urge the desirability, nay,

the necessity, of intelligent co-operation between rhinologists and ophthalmologists in the treatment of the class of cases under discussion. He who does not combine both specialties in his practice will in many instances not place at the patient's disposal all that science has achieved in the way of diagnosis and treatment of affections of the accessory sinuses, unless he avails himself of the services of a rhinologist, if he be an ophthalmologist, or of an ophthalmologist, if he be a rhinologist. Both should work hand in hand and the skill of both will often be taxed to bring obscure cases to a successful issue.

XXV

EXTRALARYNGEAL CAUSES OF LARYNGEAL SYMPTOMS.*

By Frank Smithies, M. D.,

Ann Arbor.

Modern specialism in medicine tends to segregation. The spirit of the times is an eager one. The search for new facts, the testing of new theories and the acquirement of new methods confines each of us to the particular rut along which some previous training has given impetus. This holds for all branches of the profession, whether one is doing the day's work with tuning-fork and tracheotomy tube or using percussion-hammer and stethoscope. He would, indeed, be an odd and a marvellous man who has not found, occasionally, that the limit of his own skill and wisdom lay beyond the boundaries of his particular clan, be he oto-laryngologist or internist. To many of us this limbus is reached all to soon, and we are continually impressed with the interdependence of the various branches of our art, and the disadvantages of a too rigid or a too premature specialism. The text implied in these observations furnishes the raison d'etre of this paper. It is not my purpose to wander into new fields, but to tread the much travelled paths of both laryngologist and internist. laying emphasis, so to speak, upon the sign-boards that mark the crossing of our ways. And, if, like Kipling's "Kim", I misconstrue these signs, then the faults of rendition must find excuse in the sincerity of the intention.

I believe that I but express the convictions of the large majority of internists, when I say that cases all too frequently come to our examining rooms which would compel us to submit but hesitating diagnoses and prognoses,

---

*Read, by invitation, at the Joint Meeting of the Western and Middle Sections of the American Laryngological, Rhinological and Otological Society, Chicago, February 22-23, 1909.

and certainly to administer inefficient treatment were we not able to secure certain positive facts from the laryngologic expert. And, perhaps, I shall not be considered too bold, when I state that many laryngologists have experienced the satisfaction of having, for example, such anomaly as an obscure paralysis of a vocal cord cleared up by a careful physical examination of the zone below the clavicles. If these premises are warranted, then, perhaps, it would not seem necessary to emphasize an openness of mind and hearty co-operation in both examination and treatment, when the welfare of our patients is uppermost.

The peculiar anatomic situation of the larynx permits of a bewildering multiplicity of disturbances in the functions of the surrounding structures and also gives opportunity for abnormalities in adjacent or related parts to make themselves manifest in the larynx. These manifestations may result in gross anatomic changes in the organ itself or give rise to functional disturbances in the dual work which the larynx has to perform, namely, phonation and respiration. It is to be assumed that when the laryngeal process is a primary one its recognition has been possible. It is to the class of pathologic changes apart from the larynx, but with distinct symptoms pointing to abnormal conditions within the organ that we would invite attention. To confine the subject within the limits of this paper, it will be necessary to take up the consideration of these conditions somewhat systematically. It will be recognized that the field is a broad one, and hence, if the consideration resembles Homer's famous "Catalogue of Ships", I crave your indulgence.

In the main, this class of laryngeal impairments may be due to malfunction or faulty construction of the nervous system—central or peripheral—of the circulatory system and the blood carried, of the respiratory system, apart from the larynx, of the digestive tract—adjacent and remote— of the genito-urinary system, of the supporting and contiguent parts of the larynx, as muscles, glands (thyroid, parathyroids, thymus, lymphatics), vessels, and of congenital imperfections. The evidences of faulty functionating on the part of the larynx are mainly those resulting from actual loss of function on the part of related structures or from pressure upon the larynx itself or adjacent parts.

But little attention need be given here to that class of
disturbances occurring in the so-called diatheses, e. g.
rheumatism, gout, rachitis, etc.

Fortunately for both patient and medical attendant, improper working of the intricate mechanism of the larynx,
in either of its special fields—phonation or respiration—
makes itself known very early and leads to examination,
generally local. These manifestations are commonly
dysphonia—hoarseness, whispered voice, etc.—aphonia, disturbances in respiration, cough, pain, dysphagia, hemorrhage, the presence of sputum, or external evidences of
faulty movement or construction of the larynx as a whole.
Laryngoscopy, even when the cause is not primary in the
larynx, may reveal pallor, hyperemia or abnormal pigmenta-
tion with swellings, variations in the position or movements
of the integral parts of the organ, with or without the
presence of atypical secretion.

Among the most important, and often the most puzzling
disturbances in the functionating of the larynx are those
resulting from some impairment in the nervous system.
This impairment may be central, peripheral or entirely
functional. The common central lesions are those associated with the brain and its ganglia. They are responsible
for a multitude of laryngeal symptoms. When the brain
is directly involved—as in hemorrhage, embolism, thrombosis, abscess, gummi, new growth, encephalomalacia, anemia, tophus or external pressure—there may result paralysis
of one or both cords, with or without paralysis of the extrinsic muscles, spasmodic contractures of these muscle
groups, local anesthesia or occasionally hyperesthesia. The
parts involved are frequently characteristic for the local
area of the brain diseased. Clinically, the manifestations
may take the form of cough, difficulty in respiration, aphasia, dysphonia, alterations in voice, quality and manner of
enunciation, local or general nutritional disturbances, or
alterations in the normal secretion of the laryngeal mucosa.

When the spinal cord and its nerves are involved, the results are frequently not dissimilar to those following cerebral impairment. The causative factor may be infection,
hemorrhage, tumors, scleroses, atrophy or pressure,—as
from vertebrae following injury or disease. The laryngeal
symptoms are not so marked as a rule as in those cases

where the brain is involved. There may be cough, frequently paroxysmal, hoarseness, scanning speech, yawning respirations, disturbances in sensation and tickling or burning of the mucous membrane. Interference with the proper function of the sympathetic nerves may bring about variations in the co-ordination of the individual parts of the larynx with dysphonia, cough and sometimes respiratory distress.

When the laryngeal disability results from a so-called pure neurosis, complete loss of voice, whispering, interrupted speech, inability to pronounce certain words and phrases, or to produce high tones may follow. Frequently the condition is entirely negative from the laryngeal standpoint, or the changes in the larynx may be extremely slight, sometimes just enough to focus the attention of the patient upon that organ. Generally, there is a history of mental strain or shock. Often only the most careful neurologic examination and from standpoints other than the throat is required before the true cause of the disturbance can be ascertained. It is needless to emphasize the importance of this with respect to the immediate or future prognosis of the case. During the past five years, three cases of hysterical aphonia have come under my observation. In all the cases, some intrinsic laryngeal condition could have been suspected. It was only after careful examination from every standpoint that the conditions were proven to be pure neuroses, and proper treatment instituted.

Among other neuroses I might mention those alterations in voice, frequently hoarseness and sometimes cough, associated with the normal physiologic sexual cycle of the female. These are most common at menstruation, pregnancy and the menopause. I have at present under my care three females who have annoying cough during one or more days of the menstrual period. Two of these patients were victims of marked phthisophobia, until assured that there was absolutely no condition in either larynx or lungs that could be considered causative. In one, the tuberculin test had to be resorted to before the patient and her family were satisfied. It is certainly within the experience of all of you that pregnant women occasionally complain of laryngeal tenderness and sometimes of actual pain. A few of them are bothered with troublesome cough. These symptoms are most frequently found in neurotic and anemic primiparae.

Neuroses in the male are not so common as in the female. However, they may be present. So called "habit-coughs" and "throat clearing" may occur. These may be associated with functional neuroses of the abdominal viscera, in either male or female. The most common of these is gastric hyperacidity, with more or less marked spasm of the cardiac or pyloric rings. The cough is frequently associated with gastric distress and burning sensations in the stomach, esophagus or throat. It is most common to have the patient exhibit the cough after indiscretions of diet and at the height of digestion, hence between meals and at night. The character of the cough varies. It is usually high pitched, harsh and not accompanied by sputum. There is frequently a burning sensation in the region of the larynx. The cough is often accompanied by acid eructations, and if paroxysmal, may be followed by acid vomitus. It is generally relieved by washing the stomach or by doses of olive oil or by one of the alkaline preparations. In cases of continuous hypersecretion—Weil's Disease—the cough may be almost constant, having little relation to meals, and may then result in secondary changes in the mucosa of the larynx. It is not impossible for these to be taken as the primary causative disturbance in hasty examination, and this is particularly the case when an anemnesis has been neglected or but poorly made. Other reflex neuroses, as laryngismus stridulus, angioneurotic edema, urticaria and the like, may result from gastro-intestinal irritation, particularly in rachitic and syphilitic children and in neurotic women.

Before passing to a consideration of the effects of pressure of thoracic viscera upon parts related to the larynx, it would perhaps be well to mention the effects of pressure in the neck itself. These may be from retropharyngeal abscess, injuries to the spine, enlarged cervical glands, enlarged thyroid, persistent thymus, abnormally large or cystic parathyroids, aneurysms, esophageal new growths, foreign bodies and branchial cysts. The enlargement of the cervical glands may result from an acute infection, and may, as in certain cases of diphtheria, bring about symptoms on the part of the larynx from pressure upon related parts, simulating tracheal or intralaryngeal exudation. Other causes of enlargement of the cervical glands may be tuberculosis, syphilis, Hodgkin's Disease, leukemia, sarcoma, carcinoma or cysts. Here again the effects of pressure result from direct involvement of the larynx or related parts. Pain and cough are common clinical manifestations. The cough may be paroxysmal or almost constant, leading the patient to consult the laryngologist very early. Sometimes the effects of intralaryngeal irritation are so marked that the affair may be taken for a primary, local one, and local treatment instituted, often without avail. The cough may be complicated with frothy or bloody sputum, and may be particularly severe at night when the patient is recumbent. This latter occurred in my experience in two cases of Hodgkin's Disease, one spleno-myelogenous leukemia, with terminal glandular enlargement, and one case of sarcoma, with severe anemia.

Severe cough from enlargement of the thyroid or the thymus is common. It is usually associated with external evidences of the gland enlargement in the case of the thyroid. Not infrequently, however, the thyroid may be but slightly enlarged internally and yet the evidences of pressure from internal enlargement of the whole or a part of the gland are not wanting. This is particularly the case in incipient, atypical Graves' Disease. The cough, with slight sputum, the associated weakness, loss of weight, and sometimes fever, may, on superficial study, readily lead to the diagnosis of incipient pulmonary tuberculosis or a similar process in the larynx. Sputum examinations, tuberculin tests and laryngoscopic examination are however negative. The signs of Graves' Disease should be most carefully searched for. The tremor, tachycardia and the eye phenomena may become more manifest and so clear up the picture, after diagnostic administration of thyroid extract. Appropriate treatment with thyroidectin, serum or by surgical means may result in the disappearance of the laryngeal pain and cough. Simple parenchymatous or cystic enlargement of the thyroid may also produce cough, dyspnea and pain. Thyroid extract, puncture of cysts or surgical intervention may be necessary before the effects of pressure or irritation of nerves disappear. Cysts of the salivary glands occasionally occur. They may reach great size and early cause pressure symptoms. New growths, foreign body, or diverticulum in the esophagus may be responsible for chronic cough, pain on swallowing or dyspnea. Examination with esophageal bougie or esophagoscope should be performed when slight alterations are found in the larynx. Branchial cysts are rare. I have seen two within the last three years. In both, cough, dyspnea and laryngeal pain were present.

Laryngeal symptoms from alterations in the thoracic viscera are not uncommon. The heart and great vessels, the structures of the mediastinum and the lungs themselves may be involved. The manifestations are generally the effects of pressure. The pressure may be upon the larynx itself, by extension of the aneurysm, upon the related nerves, upon the parts adjacent to the larynx or upon related ganglia.

When the heart and the great vessels are involved, the most frequent cause is aneurysm. The aneurysm may be of the heart itself, the great vascular trunks, particularly the arch, or, secondarily, the great vessels ascending into the neck. Occasionally—as happened in a young man under my care about two years ago—the formation of a heart thrombus may result in such enlargement of the right auricle with coincident embarrassment of the circulation, that the effects of aneurysm are closely simulated. The symptoms on the part of the larynx vary with the location of the aneurysmal sac. Early "brassy" cough with or without sputum leads commonly to laryngoscopic examination. This may reveal nothing beyond slight redness of the mucosa, tumefaction or extremely slight and apparently insignificant alterations in the movements of related parts. Later the cough becomes violent and frequently paroxysmal. It may be associated with bloody sputum. Even then expert laryngeal examination may reveal nothing very positive. It is at this stage that there is danger of ascribing the local hyperemia or swelling to something primary in the larynx. Superficial examination of the neck or thorax may discover nothing apparently causative. The proper diagnosis may not be returned until later when there is either external thoracic tumor, or when a most careful scrutiny of the thorax with the patient stripped, reveals the presence of such definite physical signs as atypical cardiac dullness, atypical pulsations or the presence of extracardiac bruits. The subsequent examination with fluoroscope, blood pressure machine and sphygmograph confirm the physical findings. From a somewhat varied experience, I may be pardoned if I cite the following cases to show that this thorough examination of the thoracic viscera is not infrequently neglected:

CASE 1. Mr. B. entered the University Hospital September, 1906, on account of dyspnea, cough, sharp, lancinating pains in the left back and neck, aggravated by lying down and more troublesome at night; pain in the left arm, anorexia, vague feelings of discomfort in the precordia, dizzy spells when the dyspnea was most marked. The trouble was apparently of a year's standing. The patient denied lues. There was no history of rheumatism or other infectious disease, nor of injury to the thorax. He had been treated for throat trouble and had had gargles and various cough mixtures administered for the greater part of the year previous to entering the hospital. He was finally sent to the hospital by a physician who told him that he had heart trouble. When he was stripped for examination, it could be readily seen that there was a distinctly pulsating, slightly elevated area in the thorax, over the left upper, anterior region, centering in the second intercostal space, parasternal line, extending inwards to the mid-sternal region, outwards to just below the mid-clavicular line, upwards to the clavicle and below into the third intercostal space. The prominence was nearly a centimeter higher than the corresponding region of the thorax of the opposite side. The pulsation was heaving, synchronous with the apex beat. There was no prominence to be seen in the back. There was no tracheal tug. The entire tumor area was tender. Over the tumor was a marked systolic pulsation, on palpation, followed by a diastolic shock of moderate intensity. The pulsations conveyed the impression of being slightly expansile. The radial pulses were unequal, the right being considerably fuller than the left. Percussion revealed a large, atypical area of dullness, corresponding to the position of the left end of the transverse and the upper portion of the descending portion of the aortic arch. This was confirmed by radiogram. Auscultation disclosed the presence of a systolic bruit at the apex of the heart, and over the arch of the aorta, at the site of the enlargement. The diastolic shock was moderately intense. Auscultation at the back of the thorax revealed similar but less pronounced signs. The lungs and larynx were negative. There was no Drummond's sign. The blood pressure, on the right, at the radial, with the Erlanger apparatus, 12 cm. cuff, was as follows: Systolic 139 mm. Hg., Diastolic, 103 mm. Hg.; of the left radial, Systolic 118, Diastolic 86 mm. Hg. Diagnosis: Aneurysm of the left portion of the arch of the aorta, with probably diffuse dilatation of the entire arch; cardiac hypertrophy.

CASE II. Mr. H. entered the Medical Clinic of the University Hospital, Oct. '07, on account of dry, persistent, hacking cough, dyspnea, especially when lying down, pain in the right neck and in the right side of the thorax at the level of the lower ribs, and radiating to the back, along the ribs, colicky pains after eating, loss of weight—40 lbs. since the preceding February—and weakness. The history was negative, with the exception of moderate use of alcohol and tobacco, and three attacks of gonorrhea. The patient had retired from business three years previous to coming to the hospital, on account of cough and dyspnea. Six months before entering he had had more severe attacks of coughing brought on as he suspected from exertion and getting cold. The pain in the neck and thorax had become more pronounced during the last three months. This patient had also been treated for throat trouble, intercostal neuralgia, and more lately for enlargement of the heart. The examination, with the patient stripped, revealed moderate cyanosis over face, mucous surfaces, neck and upper part of the thorax. The superficial veins over the upper part of the thorax and neck were engorged, the jugulars were prominent; the laryngoscopic examination by Prof. Canfield showed slight infiltration of both cords, especially near the vocal processes, giving the appearance of a moderate degree of internal paresis. There was slight tracheal tug when the patient sat up. Physical examination of the thorax disclosed enlargement of the heart in all directions, with fairly good compensation. At the base of the heart and to the right largely was an extensive area of dullness extending beyond the mid-scapular line, and occupying the upper sternal region; no expansile pulsation could be made out. There was faint suggestion of diastolic shock. Auscultation was as follows: Sounds muffled throughout; first sound at apex impure with suggestion of soft systolic ' bruit not transmitted to axilla; second sound faintly heard at apex; heart sounds become more distinct up the left edge of the sternum; they are very weak over the base of the heart, the aortic second being barely audible; the second sound over the upper portion of the sternum and in the second left interspace is accentuated. and impure, with a suggestion of roughening; there is no arrhythmia. The blood pressure was, systolic, 150 mm. Hg. (Erlanger.) Fluoroscopic examination revealed the presence of a large pulsating mass in the median line. occupying the upper two-thirds of the sternal space. The radiogram showed that the mass extended farther to the right than to the left. Diagnosis: Aneurysm—diffuse—of the aortic arch; cardiac hypertrophy.

It will be seen from the brief resume of these cases that cough and pain with more or less dyspnea, early directed attention to the larynx. In the first case, there was no laryngeal alteration that could have been called causative; in the second there was distinct alteration in the mucous and the vocal cord movements. Both the patients reviewed died within a year after entering the hospital. Early and careful examination of the thorax would have doubtless led to the discovery of abnormal conditions, and the lives of the patients may have been prolonged. The futile attempts to relieve cough and dyspnea by the laryngeal route are apparent.

Dyspnea, frequently referred to the larynx is not uncommon in aneurysm. It may or may not be associated with cough, cyanosis and alterations in the character of the voice. The dyspnea may be inspiratory or expiratory. The inspirations may be short, high-pitched and sometimes crowing; the expirations may be long drawn-out, wheezy or grunting. Alterations in the quality of the voice and in phonation are common. At times the patient may not be able to speak above a whisper. Hoarseness, inability to pronounce certain letters of the alphabet, disturbances in laughing or singing may be prominent. Disturbances in swallowing are occasionally present. There may be regurgitation of food after the swallowing act. Abnormal movements on the part of the larynx are not so common as the literature would lead one to suppose. So-called "tracheal tug" may or may not be present. When it is present, it is certainly significant of alterations in either the heart or the great vessels. In aneurysms as we have seen, direct examination of the larynx may reveal marked hyperemia, edema, swelling and alterations in the mobility of the parts. The symtoms are generally out of proportion to the positive laryngeal findings.

Extension of an aneurysm beyond the boundaries of the thorax should not be forgotten, as for example, the effects of pressure upon the larynx of multiple, aneurysmal dilatations of the carotid artery. In these cases, the effects of direct pressure are generally pronounced, and the conditions readily differentiated. Occasionally, however, one hears of an aneurysmal sac being aspirated for diagnostic purposes, under the impression that the case is one of cyst. Rupture of an aneurysmal sac into the larynx with acute and fatal hemorrhage sometimes occurs.

Disease of the tissues of the mediastinum may closely simulate affections of the heart and vascular trunks insofar as their effects on the larynx are concerned. These affections may be primary or secondary. The pathologic process may be carcinoma, sarcoma. lymphoma or cysts. When primary the process may have its origin in thymus remnants, lymph glands or connective tissue. When secondary, any or all of these structures may be involved.

The symptomatology, from the laryngeal viewpoint is well illustrated by the following cases:

CASE I. Mr. L. H. entered the University Hospital in January, 1907, on account of difficulty in breathing. palpitation of the heart, chronic cyanosis, frontal and occipital headaches, dropsy and general weakness. The patient said that he was in good health up to ten years ago, when he suffered several attacks of "asthma", at which times his "wind would be suddenly shut off by a pressure just above the top of the breast-bone." Occasionally, he became unconscious. When he recovered consciousness he would have palpitation for some time afterwards; blueness of the face, hands and neck became noticeable. He said that he had improved at times under medication. In 1906, the dyspnea, cyanosis, feeling of thoracic constriction and sensations of smothering became more marked. Cough developed, with hoarseness, sometimes whispered voice. The dyspnea, cough and change in the voice were paroxysmal and generally worse at night, when the patient lay down. More recently, the cyanosis has become more marked and edema of the ankles had appeared. Examination disclosed displacement of the heart inward towards the sternum. A large area of atypical thoracic dullness in the region of the mediastinum, which radiograms proved to be due to infiltration of the mediastinal tissues and the adjacent lungs, could be made out. The larynx was negative, at several examinations. There was no tracheal tug; the liver was slightly enlarged. The blood revealed marked erythremia, the red cells numbering at times more than 9,000,000 per cubic millimeter: the urine contained varying amounts of albumin and casts. Other features of the case which should be emphasized are the paroxysmal nature of the symptoms; periods of comparative freedom from cough, dyspnea or cyanosis; then again the changes would be particularly marked with whispered voice, sometimes actual aphonia, barking cough, without sputum, extreme grades of inspiratory dyspnea with prolonged, sibilant expiration. And with all these symptoms pointing to laryngeal change, expert laryngoscopic examination revealed no alterations in the larynx.

CASE II. Mr. J. W., boilermaker, entered the Medical Clinic at the University Hospital on account of sense of constriction across the upper thorax; occasional "choking sensations" in the throat; shortness of breath with gasping, crowing inspiration; insomnia; morning nausea without vomiting; weakness and headaches. The history was negative with respect to syphilis, acute infections, foreign body or excessive use of tobacco. About a year previous to entering the hospital, the patient noted gastric distress, insomnia and a sense of pressure beneath the upper sternal region. He began to "get winded" with little exertion and his face became cyanosed. His voice became husky. Dyspnea developed with "whooping" when he drew a breath. There was frequent cough without sputum. Examination revealed a slight cardiac hypertrophy, the presence of an infiltrating mass in the mediastinum, as shown by physical examination and radiograms; and of mucous gastritis. The larynx was abnormal in so far as both cords abducted to the cadaveric position and were slightly retracted; they were moderately injected; on phonation the right cord was negative; the left showed imperfect approximation to the vocal processes posteriorly. Blood and urine were negative. In this case also, the paroxysmal nature of the cough, the dyspnea, the high-pitched crowing inspirations, the hoarseness and the feeling of upper thoracic constriction should be emphasized.

When the lung is involved, as in tuberculosis, syphilis, tumor, acute infections, bronchiectasis or by foreign bodies in one of the air passages, cough, pressure symptoms, dyspnea and pain may be referred to the larynx. It is certainly not an uncommon experience to have had cases of incipient pulmonary tuberculosis receiving local treatment for the larynx in the belief that this process was primary, long after the physical signs and the clinical symptoms are indicative of considerable involvement of pulmonary tissue. While the early anemia of the laryngeal mucosa gives significant information, with respect to the diagnosis and prognosis of a case, yet one cannot feel justified in relying upon even careful laryngoscopy to segregate our doubtful cases. Frequent thoracic examinations, before and after the use of an approved tuberculin preparation, subcutaneously administered, should be coupled with local examination of the larynx. It is unnecessary to urge that in all cases of pulmonary hemorrhage, the larynx should be carefully examined. In incipient cases of pulmonary tuberculosis, this is especially important.

In syphilis and new growths of the lungs every effort should be made to locate the primary process. This can only be done by careful anemneses, physical examination and the use of such tests as the Wassermann reaction and the hemolysis reaction for cancer. This especially applies to those cases where the laryngeal alterations are slight and where the question of operation or medical treatment is a vital one for both surgeon and patient. Positive findings in the thorax frequently modify the prognosis decidedly.

In tuberculous patients, the development of a spontaneous pneumothorax may bring about dyspnea, cough, cyanosis and alterations in the voice, which in the event of discovery of a small focus of infiltration in the larynx may result in local measures entirely to the exclusion of general treatment, indicated by the results of thoracic examination.

Foreign bodies present in the trachea or the bronchi may readily give rise to laryngeal symptoms—as cough, dyspnea, pain, cyanosis and alterations in the voice—which may lead to prolonged search in the larynx for the offending agent, to the exclusion of examination with tracheascope or bronchoscope. Radiograms furnish invaluable aids to the search for foreign bodies in the air passages, and particularly when laryngeal examination directly has proven negative.

Alterations in the composition of the blood itself may be responsible for serious and frequently puzzling laryngeal symptoms. They are frequently acute and death supervenes before diagnosis has been made or treatment has been instituted. The laryngoscopic examination usually reveals general or local edema, pallor, with swelling of the cords or narrowing of the rima. The common causes of these conditions are those associated with faulty circulation, as in incompensated heart disease or uremia—those associated with changes in the cellular elements and plasma of the blood, e. g., severe secondary anemia, pernicious anemia, lymphatism, hemophilia and myxedema; and lastly, the changes following the use of such medicinal agents as nitroglycerin, pilocarpin, adrenalin, orthoform and the like.

Changes in uncompensated hearts are not frequently missed; if the onset of the edema is acute, in either heart or kidney disease. Unless the thorax is gone over or the urine examined, one may readily miss the full significance of the extralaryngeal state.

Laryngeal distress may be pronounced and acute in the various forms of anemia. This is particularly the case in pernicious anemia, leucemia and lymphatism. Cough with dyspnea, especially on exertion, is sometimes pronounced. Frothy or bloody sputum may be present. Negligence in general examination or in examination of the blood, the making of both counts of fresh blood and the differential estimation of the leucocytes from stained smears, may lead to errors in treatment and to disappointments in prognosis.

The following cases of pernicious anemia were associated with marked laryngeal manifestations:

CASE I. Mrs. L. H., aged 30, entered the University Hospital January 1, 1907, on account of anemia, cough, dyspnea, dull pain in upper thorax, and swelling of ankles and eye-lids. The patient had had a cough for eight years and had taken "all sorts" of treatment for it, but to no purpose. At the time of entry, the blood examination was as follows: Reds, 2,227,000; whites, 4,550, and Hg. 37% with the Miescher apparatus. The differential count showed a slight increase in the relative number of lymphocytes. Macrocytes and microcytes were numerous. Poikilocytosis was marked. Normablasts and megaloblasts were present. The patient remained in the hospital for about a month, showing some improvement at times. At the end of that period, there was sudden decrease in the red cell count, increase in the cough with abundant blood-stained sputum, acute dyspnea and death from glottidian edema.

CASE II. Mrs. McK., aged 21, entered the University Hospital on January 16, 1907, on account of constant cough with blood-stained sputum, nausea, vomiting and numbness of the extremities. She was evidently well so far as she can tell, until three months before coming to the hospital. Then she began to feel weak, to vomit and to cough. Her voice became weak and hoarse; sometimes she could scarcely speak; the glands in her neck began to swell and a physician diagnosed tuberculosis. When she entered the Medical Clinic she was very weak. The larynx showed moderate edema; the blood examination was as follows: Reds, 600,000; whites, 5,600; Hg. 18% (Miescher). There were many poikilocytes and megaloblasts present. The patient lived about two months and died from terminal laryngeal edema, which came on within six hours. The day of her death the blood examination was. reds, 410,000; whites, 12,000; Hg. 12% (Miescher).

CASE III. Mr. W. D., aged 46, entered the University Hospital October 13, 1903, on account of cough, dyspnea and weakness. The symptoms had been present for about nine months and were becoming worse. He had taken several varieties of cough mixture and more recently had been compelled to resort to morphine. The blood examination at the time of entry was: Reds 1,200,000, whites 2,312, Hg. 30% (Tallquist scale.) The differential count showed a great excess of lymphocytes. The reds showed moderate poikilocytosis, a large number of oval forms and there was considerable difference in the size of the individual reds. The laryngeal, examination, with the exception of anemia of the mucosa was negative. The patient remained a few days for treatment. His cough became somewhat better and he left suddenly. He returned, however, the following month, with more marked cough, shortness of breath and weakness. His laryngeal examination revealed considerable edema of the cords and glottis. The blood examination at this time was: Reds, 720,000; whites, 1,900, and Hg. 15% (Miescher). Poikilocytosis was marked; there were many microcytes and macrocytes, and an enormous number of normablasts and megaloblasts. The patient improved for a few days after entering the hospital, but then gradually grew weaker. Cough, dyspnea and laryngeal edema became more pronounced and the patient barely reached home before his death.

Finally, the effects of medicinal remedies with respect to the larynx should not be forgotten. In instances where pilocarpin is being administered for middle ear scleroses, sharp watch must be kept of the patient lest suddenly developing laryngeal and glottidian edema follow with fatal termination of the case. The excessive use of nitroglycerin may be accompanied by similar effects. Locally, the use of cocain or adrenalin, either frequently in small amounts, or in large amount at one sitting, may be followed by marked and obstinate edema. The same might be said of such a remedy as orthoform, used in painful local conditions of the larynx or where used upon related parts, as in the esophagus, pharynx or nose. Very marked, annoying and painful edema may follow which may even be fatal.

XXVI

THE CLINICAL DIAGNOSIS OF TUBERCULOSIS OF THE TONSILS.

By Lee M. Hurd, M. D.,

New York.

WITH SOME REMARKS UPON THE MICROSCOPIC DIAGNOSIS.

By Jonathan Wright, M. D.,

New York.

The physiologic relation existing between the faucial tonsil and the lymphatic gland situated at the angle of the jaw, anterior to the sternocleidomastoid muscle, has been established.[1][2][3] When these cervical glands are enlarged there is always evidence of disease in the corresponding tonsil. This glandular enlargement is due to septic absorption or to the absorption of the tubercle bacillus. Personally, I believe that all these cases of glandular enlargement start from septic absorption, after the tonsillar resistance has become weakened by disease, so that it may easily allow the tubercle bacillus to gain a foothold and soon invade the cervical lymphatics. I also believe that at times this takes place without leaving much evidence of their passage through the diseased tonsil. This has not yet been established as a fact, but the following analogous facts tend to lead me to believe it may be true.

Wood's experiment of once rubbing tubercle bacilli upon a pig's tonsil, later finding tubercular lesions in its lymph gland, but none in the tonsil.[4] The experiments of Calmette and Guerin on goats[7]—that tubercle bacilli can pass through the intestinal walls without leaving lesions, and even through the mesenteric lymph glands, making themselves first known in the pulmonary apex. The clinical diagnosis of primary tuberculosis of the tonsil was made in these selected cases on the condition of the lymph gland that drains the tonsil, as well as the condition of the tonsil itself.

The faucial tonsils may be divided into two classes clinically. First, those that are enlarged, somewhat pedunculated, with most of the tonsil hanging free into the fauces. Such large tonsils are the ones that are usually removed. They are also the tonsils that cause the least systemic harm. True, they interfere with free breathing to a certain extent, but the children that have this class of tonsils are more inclined to be healthy and robust. It seems that the freer the tonsil, the more it resists the invasion of harmful microorganisms; also it is exceptional to find associated with them much enlargement of the lymphatic glands.

The second class consists of those tonsils which are more or less buried beneath the tonsillar pillars, and which are prone to chronic inflammation rather than to acute inflammation, although they may have acute exacerbations of the chronic condition. This class causes more systemic effect. These tonsils, when diseased, will regularly give enlargement of the glands in the deep cervical chain. The children are not robust, but are more inclined to be anemic and languid, and it is in these patients that we find the proper soil for the invasion of the tonsil, primarily, then the cervical gland, with tuberculosis.

On casual examination, these submerged tonsils appear small and insignificant, because the greater portion is in the space between the pillars and crowds upward, sometimes half an inch, above the highest visible portion of the tonsil. It is in this buried portion that the tubercular evidences are usually found, closely bordering upon the tonsillar capsule. Dr. Wright examined sixty tonsils for tuberculosis, in the days when it was considered necessary to remove only the protruding portion. He did not find it in a single case.[5][6] This seems to prove two things: first, that the protruding tonsil is rarely attacked by tuberculosis; second, that if attacked the lesion is nearly always found just beneath the capsule, at the bottom of the tonsillar crypts.

The tonsil in which we find evidences of tuberculosis is usually pale, the crypts contain cheesy detritus, the edge of the anterior pillar may have a passive hyperemia, and the associated lymphatic gland is usually much enlarged and hard. From this early stage it may progress until any number of glands are involved. The question has been put to me—If the tuberculosis has reached the cervical lymphatics,* why remove the tonsil? There are two very good reasons. First, such a tonsil is allowing microorganisms to take the same route as the tubercle bacillus did, and I believe that this makes it still harder for the lymphatics to overcome the tuberculosis, which it has a fair chance of doing with the tonsil out. This is easily shown by the fact that after removal of the tonsil the lymph glands begin to subside, and if only enlarged from septic absorption will entirely disappear; and in tubercular adenitis there will be a rapid diminution in the size of the glands to a certain point, which I believe was the increased load placed upon the glands from draining a generally diseased tonsil. Also, when the tubercular cervical glands are removed, the tonsil remaining is liable to reinfect the remaining glands, as in case No. 2. The most frequent site for enlargement of the cervical glands is at the angle of the jaw, and in recognizing the tonsil as the portal of infection, its prompt removal will abort many cases and perhaps other more remote tubercular lesions.

I would here like to digress long enough to state that the tonsil must be removed in toto in order to get out the tuberculous portion, and also that the stump of a partially removed tonsil is quite as liable to tubercular infection as if originally submerged. This is probably due to the fibrous cicatrix closing up most of the crypts.

All the tonsils reported in this article were of the submerged variety. From my observations, I would say that the inflammatory enlargement—both septic and tubercular —of the lymph glands that drain the tonsil, are nearly always associated with the submerged tonsil. The tonsil removed from cases of slight glandular enlargement usually showed microscopic evidences of chronic inflammation, but in one of this class the tonsil was typically tubercular. The tonsils from cases in which clinically the glands were considered tubercular or bordering on that condition, had the diagnosis of tubercular tonsil confirmed by the microscope in nine (9) out of the twelve (12) cases.

---

*An enlarged lymphatic gland is not necessarily tuberculous.

CASES IN WHICH THE TONSILS WERE CLINICALLY CONSIDERED TUBERCULAR.

No.	Age.	Sex.	Class of Tonsil.	Condition of Cervical Glands.	Microscopic Findings.	75 per cent
1	25	M	Submerged, large.	A but 3 large glands, hard, of several ths duration.	Tuberculous.	+
2	19	F	Submerged, large stumps.	Has had 11 ns for tubercular glands.	Tuberculous.	+
3	22	F	Submerged.	Tubercular ass at angle of jaw. Opened when sil was red.	Tuberculous.	+
4	27	F	Submerged, fibrous, small.	Enlarged glands angle of jaw 2½ years. Acute periadenitis.	Tuberculosis not confirmed though suspicious.	−
5	12	F	Submerged.	Enlarged glands angle of jaw.	Tuberculosis not confirmed though suspicious.	⌡
6	4	F	Submerged.	Enlarged glands angle of jaw.	ul ous.	+
7	8	F	Submerged, small much cheesy matter	1 enlarged hard gland.	Tubercul ous.	+
8	8	F	Submerged, small.	Broken down gland, incised 3 months ago. Now several glands matted together.	Tubercul us.	+
9	3	F	Submerged, medium size.	Slightly enlarged glands.	Tuberculous.	+
10	8	M	Submerged stumps.	Slightly enlarged glands.	Tuberculous.	+
11	7	M	Submerged.	Small chain of glands.	Not tuberculous.	−
12	25	F	Submerged, small.	Large gland, two operations.	Tuberculous.	+

Note large proportion of females, 75 per cent.

CASES WHERE THE TONSILS WERE CLINICALLY CONSIDERED CHRONICALLY INFLAMED BUT NOT TUBERCULOUS

No.	Age.	Sex.	Condition of Tonsil.	Condition of Neck.	Microscopical Findings.	
1	23	F	Submerged.	Slightly enlarged and soft.	Nothing noteworthy.	—
2	12	M	Submerged.	Slightly enlarged and soft.	Nothing ... day.	—
3	8	M	Submerged.	Slightly enlarged and soft.	Chronic Inflammation.	—
4	6	M	Submerged.	Slightly enlarged and soft.	Chronic in ... mation.	—
5	6	M	Submerged.	Slightly enlarged and soft.	Chronic in ... mation.	—
6	7	M	Submerged.	Slightly enlarged and soft.	Some areas of necrosis.	—
7	14	F	Submerged.	Slightly enlarged and soft.	Mitotic-looking bodies in crypts. ...ic inflammation.	—
8	6	M	Submerged.	Slightly enlarged and soft.	...le metamorphosis.	—
9	6	M	Submerged.	Slightly enlarged and soft.		—
10	13	M	Submerged, large.	Slightly enlarged and soft.	Typical t ... cle.	+
11	5	F	...rged.	Slightly enlarged and soft.	Chronic in ... mation.	—
12	8	F	Submerged stumps.	Slightly enlarged and soft.	Chronic in ... mation.	—
13	6	M	Submerged.	Slightly enlarged and soft.	Simple hypertrophy.	—

I am unable to state the percentage of tubercular tonsils
to the total number removed during the same period. All
the cases have been selected with the tubercular and chronic
inflammatory changes of the tonsil in view, and outside·of
the throat and neck showed no other signs of tuberculosis.

No. 1. J. H. Male, aet. 25. June 29, 1908. Many carious
teeth. Large submerged tonsils, with hard enlarged glands
at angle of jaw. Clinically considered tubercular. No other
evidences of tuberculosis.

Microscopic examination, by Dr. Jonathan Wright.—This
tonsil is a good illustration of the grounds I have for calling
areas in tonsillar sections "suspicious" of tubercle. In one
of the three sections there are granular areas where the
proliferation of the round cells are becoming granular and
taking the stain badly; nearby are some old fibrous areas.
Another section shows this more marked, with the addition
of epitheloid cells and the contiguity of the fibrous areas.
Still a third section shows all this plus two imperfect giant
cells in these areas. I should, therefore, say that this appearance is strongly indicative but not yet, to me, entirely
conclusive of the existence of typical tubercle. In this case,
from the clinical history and the objective examination,
there is little doubt that the glands in the neck are
tuberculous. Later, 10 more slides were examined. In
many of them there was the well-marked identical area of
tubercle-granulum, of epitheloid cells, and in one of these
supplemental 10 slides there was in this area a fairly well
marked giant cell. Diagnosis: Tubercle of the tonsil.

I avail myself of the report of this case to furnish me with
an opportunity of making the remarks upon the microscopic
diagnosis of tubercle which have so often formed the substance of our informal conversations in the course of the
work with which you have been engaged. As you know,
some criticism has been expressed at my unwillingness in
many cases definitely to declare there were no evidences
of tuberculous processes in a given tonsil submitted to me
for examination. It is, of course, a familiar rule in making a
negative report on a specimen of sputum to remain on the
conservative side by saying that no tubercle bacilli are
found. The limitations of this negative opinion are well
understood, but when I have reported that no conclusive
evidences of tubercle have been found by me in tonsillar

structure, the position assumed has not been understood. It is the purpose of these remarks to explain the grounds of this undesirable but, to me, unavoidable uncertainty expressed in the form of speech I have sometimes adopted and which it is often so awkward to use in communication to friends of the patient the·result of the microscopic examination. This, by the way, to uninformed minds seems to be a sort of mystic shrine from which to expect the oracular infallibility not inherent in scientific terms.

Now, in my mind there is often a very large addition of doubt in the negative expression of opinion as to the existence of tubercle in the tonsil, which is not attached to the diagnosis of bacilli in the sputum. With me, this arises from the conviction that the cytolytic emanation of the tuberele bacillus which causes the crumbling of protoplasm may not in lymphoid structure give rise to any of the other structural changes thought to be necessary to the satisfactory identification of tubercle by the microscope. These necrotic areas are not infrequently present in the tonsil, and the most diligent search fails to reveal that they are accompanied by other areas in which are present giant and epitheloid cells. Now, in well recognized tubercle, as in this case, the majority of the necrotic areas do not contain these added characteristics. When areas exist side by side, one containing giant cells and epitheloid cells and connective tissue indications. and the others without them, we do not hesitate to ascribe all to the cytolytic activities of the bacillus. I do no hesitate to believe that such areas of simple protoplasm necrosis may be the sole evidence of the tuberculons nature of the lesion, but I hasten to add that they cannot be considered as processes exclusive of other origins. This, I believe is the kernel of doubt that lies at the bottom of the differences of opinion as to the frequency of the occurrence of latent tuberculosis of the tonsil.

I am convinced that if every tonsil removed in our hospital were examined microscopically (I suppose the number would mount into the thousands every year). and if the accepted evidence of the existence of tuberculosis rested only on the presence of the typical tubercle described by the text-books, the proportion of 5 per cent or 10 per cent would be found to be a gross exaggeration. On the other hand, were we to accept every area of circumscribed granular necrosis as tubercle caused by the action of the bacillus, without a doubt the proportion would be placed at a higher figure.

While we are upon this aspect of the subject, I might also remark that the word "latent" tuberculosis of the tonsil is misleading, as it is most frequently used. I suppose the term "latent tuberculosis of the tonsils", when originally used, meant a local tuberculosis without systemic clinical manifestation of tuberculosis there or elsewhere. This strict interpretation of the word "latent" involves the shrinkage in the number of cases observed under the microscope as the index of the acuteness of diagnostic acumen on the part of the clinical observer rises. These cases which we have been observing, many of them, now present to your trained eyes clinical evidences of tuberculosis which a few years ago the microscope would only have revealed as "latent." What becomes of our definition, therefore? We expect tuberculous people to have tubercle of the tonsils, but you suspect or tentatively diagnosticate a case as probably having tuberculous foci in the tonsils because you have followed the reports we have sent you and are able to appreciate shades of clinical phenomena which a few years ago you could not do. This is a fundamental weakness of all statistics, but nowhere so glaringly evident as in discussions on tuberculosis. The importance of the statistical argument pales before the mature entertainment of such considerations.

Here, confusion in figures as to the frequency of "latent" tuberculosis depends upon the definition to be applied to a number of ill-defined terms by observers of different degrees of diagnostic acumen. What is patent to you is latent to some one else. What is "tubercle' to me is not the only thing that is "tubercle" to some one else. All these fundamental differences of opinion and capacity are unexpressed in the discussion of the statistics. I think it would be well to give them what prominence we can.

To return from this quite excusable digression to the subject of the "tubercle granulum". As I have said, I know that not all the crumbling areas I see in the tonsil are tuberculous. Some I believe to be due to autolysis, with the transformation of protoplasm into fat or the substitution of fat for the destroyed protoplasm, a process taking place in the retrograde metamorphosis of the tonsil, and an entirely physiological adjustment of the organism.* Some possibly may be due to syphilis. though I am inclined to think this very rare. When occurring, the lesion is usually superficial.

The difference between these effects of cytolytic ferments,—that of the bacteriolysin of tubercle and the autolysin,—is commonly ascribed to the efforts the organism makes in the former case to remedy the damage, i. e., the production of epitheloid and connective tissue cells in and around the necrotic areas, but I know no reason why the organism should always thus respond. It may be that the tubercle bacillus in passing through from the surface to the deeper lymphatics of the neck has left this imperfect trace behind it, because of its temporary lodgment. The tonsil, no doubt, is the entry port of a great deal of infection, and if all the virulence of the germs were expended there we should have tonsillar lesions far in excess in frequeney to all other lesions of the organs of the body.

Near these spots of granular protoplasm, representing the regression of the tonsil, we have always more or less low grade fibrous tissue, such again as we have around old healed tubercle at the apex of the lungs. Thus you see why it is that I am undoubtedly often in a state of doubt as to how I am to interpret these spots of granular necrosis.

I am reminded by some recent literature upon the formation of the tubercle that in view of your intention to publish the communication I made you in regard to the problem of the microscopic diagnosis of tonsillar tubercle I should briefly refer to the conception at which I have arrived of the usual sequence of events. Virchow and Arnold, and many of the earlier writers, looked upon the formation of the giant cell and the appearance of the epithelial cells as the initial tissue-change in answer to the insult of the tubercle bacillus.

---

*In order to avoid repetition of what you may elsewhere find in print, I refer you to the details of the facts upon which this belief was founded originally, remarking that subsequent observation has only confirmed them.

The Fat Contents of the Tonsils. N. Y. Med. Jour., Dec. 15, 1906.

Cysts in Lymphoid Tissue: an Exceptional Manifestation of Tonsillar Regression. The Laryngoscope, Sept., 1905.

This they supposed to be due to the confluence of the fixed tissue-cell into a giant cell and the alteration of others into the epitheloid cells. This is subsequently followed by the accretion of leucocytes from the blood vessels with resulting coagulation necrosis. Many others,—Koch, Cohnheim, Metchnikoff, Yersen, among them,—believe that the nucleated blood cells are the mother cells of tubercle, and from them are formed the giant cells and the epitheloid cells.

So far as the tonsil is concerned, I am inclined to think the leucocytes from the neighboring lymph spaces and capillaries first form a cluster around the point of irritation,—be it bacillus or foreign body, or tissue altered by the influence of either. Epitheloid cells are soon formed, whether from the leucocytes or the fixed tissue-cells I am unable to say, but I am inclined to think they arise from the large and small lymphocytes. By this time, and often before the appearance of giant cells, a certain amount of coagulation necrosis has taken place. The giant cells, when I have been able to detect their genesis, have been arising from the endothelial cells of the capillaries, in accord with the observations of many histologists. By the confluence of these we have a multinuclear cell with feeble cytoplasmic contents. It seems very probable to me that the sequence of events in the formation of tubercle in general is not always the same. The morphological appearances of tubercle differ considerably, and it is quite probable that the giant cells of tubercle differ considerably, and it is quite probable that the giant cell of tubercle is due, like the giant cell of bone, to the confluence of other cells than those of the capillaries, and this may even be the case in the tonsil; but, for certain reasons I do not believe that the giant cell is usually the first step in the process in the tonsil,—rather the last, or next to the last,—fibrosis being more properly a process of repair. It is not necessary to say anything of the fission of nuclei in giant cells as the sole cause of their existence. While nuclei may divide in them, I suppose, I have never detected it, and I am not disposed to think of them as arising in this way.

No. 2. G. McM. Single; age 19. For the past three and a half years has had enlarged cervical glands. Two and a half years ago had first operation on glands. Subsequently has had ten more operations, making eleven in all. Three years ago had first operation on adenoids, again in four months. Two years ago had still another tonsil and adenoid operation. I found this girl on the side-walk talking to patient No. 3, and on observing large numbers of scars on her neck, induced her to come into hospital and have her throat examined. I found large submerged tonsillar stumps, flush with the pillars; no adenoids; two distant cervical glands enlarging since last operation, some two months previously. I induced her to have her tonsils out. She rather thought it was hopeless, as this made the fourth attempt, but on being informed of their relation to the neck condition she consented, and I enucleated them last April. Dr. Wright found typical tubercle in the tonsillar tissue. Her health has improved so that she has gone back to work, which she has not done in two years. The two glands that were showing a tendency to grow,—one in parotid, other above clavicle,—have receded somewhat. These two glands cannot be directly connected with the tonsillar drainage. but the removal of the primary tonsillar foci seems to have been very beneficial to the girl's general condition.

No. 3. E. McM. Female, age 22; servant. Perfectly healthy except for broken down gland at angle of jaw. Submerged tonsil that looks suspicious of tubercular involvement. Admitted to hospital; neck abscess opened; also tonsil enucleated. Neck promptly healed, and tonsil showed following condition:

Lymphoid material with much subjacent fibrous connective tissue. There are typical Langerhans' giant cells and tubercle granulum deep down in the lymphoid tissue.

No. 4. M. N., Irish, aet. 27. June 3, 1908. For past two years has had glands at angle of jaw much enlarged and gradually increasing in size. In last two months mass acutely enlarged to double former size. Tonsils very small (no history of tonsillitis), entirely submerged. The corresponding tonsil enucleated, and submitted to Dr. Wright, who reported "chronic inflammation," but he remarked that if he saw the same masses of fibrous tissue in a section of the lung he would call it healed tubercle, but was not prepared to so state regarding the tonsil. Seven days after the removal of the tonsil the acute swelling subsided, leaving the old tubercular glands their former size. These tubercular glands did not diminish in size, and about four months after removal of tonsil they showed evidence of breaking down, and a month later were a fluctuating mass. They were now entirely removed. One had become fluid, and the rest,—about six in all,—had cheesy centres. Dr. Wright said: "I presume this is a tuberculous gland, but we have been unable to find typical tubercle in the sections examined." I feel tolerably certain that the tonsil was the port of entry, for the glands first affected drain the tonsil and there is no evidence of secondary drainage into these glands.

Considering the length of time,—over two years,—between development of the adenitis and examination of the tonsil, it seems to me logical to believe that the tonsillar lesion had healed. The patient had the most pronounced enlargement of the glands, with the longest duration, of any of the cases reported, considerably over two years, she says it might be three, since she first noticed their size, and they had probably then been enlarging for some time.

No. 7. L. O'R., aet. 8. Aug. 15, 1908. Very small submerged tonsils. Glands moderately enlarged, with tonsillar gland about size of hickory nut. Microscopic report: "Typical tubercle, giant cells, etc." In the six months since operation all the glands have subsided, except the tonsillar, which is hard and about half former size.

February 18, 1909, the tonsillar lymphatic gland removed; about 1½ inches in diameter. Its tuberculous condition confirmed by Dr. Wright.

No. 8. M. V., aet. 8. June, 1908. Three months before operation, tonsillar gland and others in relation broke down and drained. Small submerged tonsils. Dr. Wright found typical tubercle in corresponding tonsil; now, after period of seven months, glands have entirely subsided.

No. 9. M. D., aet. 3. May 12, 1905. Submerged tonsils, enlarged glands. Tonsils enucleated. Report: "Sections through tonsils show undoubted evidences of tubercular process. While there are no typical anatomic tubercles, still the presence of masses of epitheloid cells arranged in groups with central coagulation necrosis and proliferating coagulation tissue fibres, the patchy appearance, nuclear fragmentation, makes the diagnosis fairly positive. In addition to this, the presence of tubercle bacilli can be demonstrated, arranged in clumps."

This child's health has greatly improved; the glands have receded, until now, after a period of over three years, they are hardly palpable.

No. 10. L. K., aet. 8. January 4, 1908. Had tonsils removed,—that is, down to the pillars,—two years ago. This boy has recurrent O. M. S. A., some adenoid; large tonsillar stumps remain that are submerged and partially covered with cicatricial tissue. The tonsillar neck glands are enlarged from size of hazel nut down. Tonsils enucleated. Dr. Wright reports as follows: "These tonsils have many fibrous bands of large diameter traversing the lymphoid tissue; near them the lymphoid tissue is undergoing coagulation necrosis with much hyperplasia of the epithelial or large plasma (epitheloid) cells. There are no giant cells, and the degenerated areas are so scattered that I am inclined to regard this rather as evidence of a retrograde metamorphosis than of old tubercular lesions. Supplementary report: "Sections stained for tubercle bacilli show them apparently in the areas of degeneration. I cannot avoid therefore regarding this as a tuberculous lesion." In the year since tonsillar removal the boy's health has greatly improved, and the glands have subsided. .

No. 12. Mrs. L., aet. 30, American. Has had tuberculous cervical glands for two and a half years. Has had two operations with recurrence. Now there is a large mass beneath the sternocleidomastoid muscle. The tonsils are very small and submerged; the crypts filled with detritus.

While this tonsil does not present the crumbling connective tissue areas which I have been accustomed to look upon as suspicious, it shows a number of places where the endothelium of the small capillaries have swollen, obliterating their lumina, and with the bodies of the cells for the most part obliterated, a number of giant cells thus formed is apparent; they do not, however, show the crumbling protoplasm and the nuclei at one pole of the giant cell body with an obliteration of the limiting cell membrane of the other pole, characteristic of the giant cell of tuberculosis.

Another feature of the tonsil is the metamorphosis of the lower line of the surface epithelium. This is being encroached upon by the connective tissue and the round cells from below, and in many cases it is difficult to reconcile the appearances with any other view than that along this line some of the epithelium is taking on the form and function of connective tissue. I have never been sure that I can detect the microphages (large mononuclear lymphocytes) destroying the epithelium at this line, though it is possible that this process may occur in the way some writers have described. There are many places,—indeed most of the places,—where this view is entirely inadequate to account for appearances.

In this chronic process of inflammation and mutation, the mononuclear lymphocytes are plainly to be seen forming the thick fibrous connective tissue bands of the fibrous tonsil. The swollen endothelium spoken of above as forming a common cell body,—or at least the appearance of it in transverse section (an atypical giant cell as noted) may be seen in many places not to have thus fused its cell bodies; but a bunch of separate cells entirely indistinguishable, at least as to shape (and, with this eosin-hemotoxylon stain, as to tinctorial reaction also) from the mononuclear lymphocytes, has formed. We thus have this later connective tissue form of cell, as commonly described, acting as an apparent transition form between not only connective tissue cells subserving different functions, but between surface epithelium and connective tissue. Further, if we imagine a mononuclear leucocyte stripped of its cell body we can at once note the transitional forms between its nucleus and the naked nuclei of the small round lymphoid cells. This has its significance coupled with the fact, now commonly admitted, that the lymph nodes in the tonsil and lymph glands are so-called germ centres arising from a mononuclear lymphocyte as a parent cell, as more fully described for the bone marrow. These lymph nodes we know as physiologic structures; but occurring in hypertrophied tonsils, we recognize a normal process of proliferation in embryonic life carried over into adult life in a pathologic process under the stimulation of inflammation, as I have instanced,—again in a pathological process,—as occurring in the genesis of the bony cysts of the middle turbinate. Now, all this prolongation or reassumption of the mutability of embryonic life in adolescence under the stimulus of irritation (itself the answer to some irritation of environment) has a bearing upon the heretical opinion I hold of the transformation of epithelium into connective tissue,—a refusal longer to accept in pathological processes the inviolability of the blastoderm layers.

I am very much indebted to the laboratory for the work it has done in these cases. It is out of the question to ask them to convert a suspicious tonsil into sections and examine every section. What has been done, however, is to take the most likely portion of the tonsil and make three or four sections. If these look suspicious, but are not positively tubercular, a few more sections are made; but in this series it has not been difficult to find tubercular evidences in most of the tonsils in the first few sections.

I wish to express my gratitude to Dr. Wright for the interest and work he has given the subject. Without his help, this article would have been impossible. Not my theories, but his facts make it worthy of your consideration.

REFERENCES.

1. Wood. Lymphatic drainage of the faucial tonsil. Am. Jour. of Med. Sciences, August, 1905.
2. Robertson. Certain facts concerning the faucial tonsil. Jour. of Am. Assoc., November 24, 1906.
3. Edmunds, A. Glandular Enlargements. London, 1908.
4. Wood. Laryngoscope, Dec., 1907.
5. Wright, J. New York Med. Journal, Sept. 26, 1896.
6. Hodenpyl. Am. Jour. of Med. Sciences, March, 1901.
7. Calmette and Guerin. Revue Scient., 5, p. 259, September, 1906.

XXVII

THE DIAGNOSIS OF TEMPORO-SPHENOIDAL LOBE ABSCESS WITH SPECIAL REFERENCE TO ITS SURGICAL TREATMENT.*

By W. Sohier Bryant, A. M., M. D.,

New York City.

The complications of otitic infection have of late years attracted particular attention in the field of surgery. While rapid advances have been made in the management and operative treatment of temporo-sphenoidal lobe abscess, this most serious complication of middle ear infection still remains almost a terra incognita—a disease with most obscure symptoms and often fatal results.

ETIOLOGY.—Temporo-sphenoidal lobe abscess is now recognized to be due to some infective process which has invaded the cerebral tissue either by metastasis or by direct extension. Our experience leads us to the conclusion that metastatic conditions are extremely rare. A connection with the primary source of infection can be demonstrated in all recent cases. It is only in the abscesses of long duration which have become enclosed in a heavy capsule that all trace of connection with some more external preexisting infection has entirely disappeared. The cause of temporo-sphenoidal abscess may, therefore, generally be considered to be a middle ear infection which has penetrated into the cerebral cavity.

PATHOLOGY.—As we have seen from the etiology, sphenoidal lobe abscess is an infection which has extended into the brain. Its entrance into the brain from its original focus may be by direct extension through the tissues, or by the extension of phlebitis. The first stage is infiltration; the second stage is necrosis; the third is the stage of softening and suppuration; and the fourth stage is encapsulation and resolution. There is

*Read at the meeting of the Southern Section of the American Laryngological, Rhinological and Otological Society, February 13, 1909.

a final stage which may appear at any time after the first stage—this fifth stage is rupture, either outwardly or, more commonly, into the ventricle. a complication which is soon followed by death.

The bacteriology of sphenoidal lobe abscess is the same as that of the parent ear infection. In the order of frequency, streptococci, pneumococci, diplococci, staphylococci are found in the abscess. Abscesses of long duration may be sterile.

SYMPTOMS AND COURSE.—The initial event in the course of temporo-sphenoidal abscess is infection of the middle ear. For the formation of a temporo-sphenoidal abscess it is not necessary that the infection of the middle ear should cause perforation of the drum membrane, or even cause mastoiditis, but it is necessary that the infection should extend through the upper walls of the drum cavity and infect the cerebrum.

This infection from the middle ear may spread to the brain tissue in four different ways. In the order of frequency, these are: (1) by extension of phlebitis, (2) by ulceration, (3) by coagulation necrosis, (4) by the spread of infection through the tissues.

When silent areas of the brain are involved in a case of sphenoidal lobe abscess, the symptoms may be reduced to a slight earache and somewhat more marked headache, complicating otitis. But when the abscess is located in the active areas and occupies the anterior part of the auditory center it is accompanied by sensory aphasia; if the infection extends to the more posterior part of this region, there will be some evidence of motor aphasia and disturbance of ocular movements. If the abscess has extended to the motor area along the fissure of Rolando, symptoms of motor impairment will follow. The febrile reaction of uncomplicated sphenoidal abscess is always mild.

Brain abscess may not be suspected until rupture, with resultant meningitis. if the abscess ruptures outwardly; or by pyocephalus or cerebrospinal meningitis if the abscess ruptures into the ventricle.

The symptoms of brain abscess are often obscured by the concomitant fulminating symptoms of meningitis and sinus thrombosis; or they may be so mild as to escape observation. In either case, the brain abscess is not suspected until operation or autopsy reveals the true condition.

The course of the brain abscess which has been cited has
been that with the more obscure symptoms. Fortunately the
symptoms of the abscess are not usually as obscure as the above
data would indicate.

There are usually constitutional symptoms of infection, a
slight rise of temperature, and rapid pulse. The effect of
intracranial pressure caused by the abscess gives a paradoxical
symptom of rising temperature and falling pulse rate, which
is pathognomonic of cerebral abscess. The polynuclear leucocyte percentage is sometimes increased. Together with these
symptoms, the fundus oculi occasionally shows choked disk
with neuroretinitis. In doubtful cases daily retinoscopic examinations are desirable for the detection of the rapid changes
which often occur. Symptoms of cerebral irritation may be
absent or marked, from a slight irritability of the patient to
delirium and coma. Brain abscess is usually associated with
increased tension of the dura mater, which is demonstrable by
palpation after exposure through the calvarium.

The course of the abscess, if without treatment, varies with
the extent and virulence of the infection. In the mild case of
infection, a small, or moderate sized abscess is formed with
thick enveloping capsule, which in a few cases finally becomes
cicatrized or calcified. More often the mild infection remains
encapsulated for an indefinite time or until lowered constitutional resistance can no longer oppose the spread of the infection. Meningitis soon follows, with extension, ending
finally in death. In the virulent infections, the area involved
rapidly spreads, often progressing too rapidly for pus formation. Cerebrospinal meningitis soon develops and death
quickly follows.

DIAGNOSIS.—The diagnosis of temporo-sphenoidal abscess
is positive in cases where there is aphasia with middle ear
suppuration. It is presumptive in cases of middle ear inflammation if there are symptoms of intracranial pressure and constitutional symptoms of infection which are not explained by
the presence of meningitis or thrombosis.

In some cases the diagnosis of the existence of temporo-
sphenoidal abscess cannot be made until the dura mater has
been inspected after an operation for mastoiditis when the
conditions found have required the exposure of the dura. In
these cases, if the dura mater shows a fistulous opening or

suspicious circumscribed patches of granulations, the presumptive diagnosis of temporo-sphenoidal abscess can be made, but the abscess cannot be definitely established until it has been located by puncture.

If, when local convalescence has followed a successful mastoid operation, the patient still has lingering headaches and slight constitutional symptoms of infection, with or without demonstrable intracranial pressure symptoms, and without aphasia, we may safely conclude that either meningitis or brain abscess is present. With meningitis, the symptoms are more marked and the disease runs a shorter course than with brain abscess, which usually has obscure symptoms and progresses very slowly.

There are on record cases of sphenoidal abscess which were found without the presence of any middle ear infection. The diagnosis of such cases intra vitam is very difficult. If there are intracranial symptoms referable to the cerebrum in any way suggesting brain abscess with normal tympani, the history of the case is of extreme value, since a history of suppuration, even though it be a long time previous, is a strong presumptive proof of the presence of temporo-sphenoidal abscess.

·TREATMENT.—The treatment of temporo-sphenoidal abscess consists in surgical drainage, and removal of the infected tissues.

TECHNIC.—The mastoid operation should precede the intracranial operation, in order to more conclusively confirm the diagnosis of intracranial abscess, which follows the discovery of fistulous tract and intracranial extension of necrosis. The mastoid operation serves also to remove the peripheral cause of the central infection and to open the route of drainage.

When we determine that drainage from the lowest part of the wound will be necessary, we can dispense with a trephine opening or an osteoplastic flap in the temporal fossa.

This lower drainage is obtained through the aperture in the skull made by the extension of the mastoid operation, and if we enlarge this cranial opening we obtain all the advantages of upper and lower openings, with the addition of a simplified technic. The best technic for opening the abscess is to continue to extend the primary mastoid operation and uncover a large area of dura mater over the location of the abscess.

This gives opportunity of placing the drainage in the most dependent part, which will give better results than an osteoplastic flap at a higher level.

After performing the mastoid operation we follow the route of infection, open the cranial cavity and enlarge the opening along the floor of the middle fossa by removing the tegmen, the upper wall of the external meatus, and as much of the adjacent squama as is necessary to uncover the seat of the abscess.

The next move is to locate the abscess. In some cases the abscess can be located by focal symptoms; in others, by fistulae or necrotic areas, and if these two methods are insufficient, by the use of an aspirating needle and syringe, testing the temporo-sphenoidal lobe in all directions for pus.

When finally the abscess is located, it must be evacuated by an x-cut in the dura mater, sufficient to expose the whole area of the abscess. The cut is carried throughout the outer wall of the abscess with a sharp knife.

Great care must be taken to sterilize the wound before opening the dura mater with a sterile knife. The best method of sterilization is by careful syringing and mopping with salt solution.

In the early stages of the abscess, before the formation of pus, there is little to be evacuated; in more advanced abscesses, the pus will be forced out through the free opening by the intracranial pressure.

The next point is the maintenance of drainage. In the serous and necrotic stages of the abscess, and before the formation of the capsule in the suppuration stage, sufficient drainage is accomplished by thoroughly exposing the infected area. There are two great difficulties in obtaining drainage of a brain abscess: (1) The tissue is of a very soft consistency, and is, therefore, liable to be injured by any resistant drain. For this reason it is better to use soft tissues such as rubber tissue or gauze, and to avoid packing. When the great depth of the wound demands more collapsible drainage, decalcified bone tubes are the best. (2) The tissues, because of their soft consistency, have a tendency to collapse and to close the wound too readily, thereby obstructing drainage. For these two reasons, the best results are obtained by making large exposures and extensive incisions. Under these circumstances, less depth of drainage is necessary since the surface drainage is more effective.

In old abscesses, with thick encapsulating walls, the contents must be evacuated before drainage can be inaugurated. The thick contents of these abscesses can be extruded only through the wide incision of the external wall, and the cavity is cleaned with peroxide of hydrogen and lightly packed with gauze, which is placed so as to widely distend the opening.

The post-operative care of the wound requires scrupulous antisepsis to prevent the spread of the old infection and the entrance of new organisms. In order to assist drainage, the wound may require two or three dressings daily. The wound should be kept open as long as possible to maintain drainage to the utmost. Even after the wound is completely healed, the patient is still in great danger of recurrence, and should therefore be very careful in his habits, especially avoiding the increase of blood pressure and cerebral congestion. The patient should be kept under observation for a year or more, in order that the least unfavorable symptom may be noted.

The question of brain hernia always has to be considered in connection with operations on brain tissue. The occurrence of hernia suggests increased intracranial pressure, which it tends to relieve. If hernia occurs, effort should be made to have it extrude the abscess. To accomplish this, compression is applied over the exposed brain, leaving the outer wall of the abscess unprotected.

PROGNOSIS.—From the author's experience, the prognosis for cases taken early in the brain infection is recovery for over 50 per cent: for complicated cases, and for those seen late, the mortality is very high. Without operation, the disease is almost always fatal.

The prognosis for perfect recovery and regeneration of cerebral function is good for the cases where the functional impairment is due simply to pressure or to inflammation, but bad for cases where the functionating areas are destroyed by necrosis or suppuration. The general health and cranial condition are not good for several years after convalescence, even in the best cases; in some cases, the patient may remain an invalid.

Causes of death from brain abscess are meningitis, septicemia and intracranial pressure.

SUMMARY.—The diagnosis of temporo-sphenoidal lobe abscess is often obscure, but suggestive symptoms are always present, and confirmatory ones can always be found on careful search. The treatment is operative drainage. The technic of the operation is directed to extensive exposure and incision of the infected area, to allow free drainage, with economy of drain. The tympanic route for drainage is selected because of its technical convenience and because of its dependent position.

XXVIII.

REMOVAL OF THE TONSIL (COMPLETE) IN ITS CAPSULE.

A Description of the Technic of the Operation, Position, etc. (Illustrated).

By Frank C. Todd, M. D.,

Minneapolis.

Surgery of the ear, nose and throat was slow to take its place in the advance with general surgery. Only very recently has it stepped into the front ranks with the latter. No wonder then that many continue to practice in the old-fashioned way.

The main reason rhinologists and laryngologists have lagged so far behind their brother surgeons, is that they began wrong. Specialists in ear, nose and throat diseases at first were not surgeons, but physicians treating diseases of those organs. Had they begun with the proper knowledge of the principles of surgery, they could not have failed to see the mistake they were making in attempting to cure a mastoid abscess by incomplete and improper drainage or chronic suppuration of the middle ear with necrosis, by medication. Certainly they could have appreciated that the slicing of a portion of a diseased tumor from between the pillars of the fauces was poor surgery. Such practice upon any other such tumor existing elsewhere in the body would be condemned.

This apology for the tardiness in the advance of our surgical work seems necessary. A further discussion as to the advisability of doing a complete tonsil operation, however, would be to admit the present existence of this failing, for to-day the man who does not attempt to remove the entire diseased tonsil manifests poor and antiquated surgery.

Having finally agreed upon this principle, it remains for each of us to determine what would seem to be the best method of accomplishing the desired results. The removal of the entire tonsil in its capsule leaving intact its bed of muscular tissue and the faucial pillars uninjured, gives the best ultimate results. But if the muscle tissue is torn or otherwise materially injured, or the pillars are greatly dam-

aged, or portions of the tonsil remain to form adhesive
bands between the pillars and to continue the disease process, then the results are not the best that can be secured
and may even bring about such cicatricial contraction as
to interfere with the normal action of the muscles thereby
causing discomfort and disturbance. And yet it is evident
that considerable traumatism to these structures may take
place and the results be good, even though not ideal. As
throat surgeons, however, it is our duty to try to bring
about ideal results and to so perfect our technic as to
accomplish this end.

As early as 1897 the writer became convinced of the
advisability of the removal of the entire tonsil. At first an
attempt was made to bring this about by the use of forceps,
drawing the tonsil into the tonsillotome. Difficulty arose
from the resulting hemorrhages, which were not lessened
upon substituting various forms of scissors. Removal by
cauterization, after trial was abandoned for obvious reasons. Early attempts were made to remove the tonsil in
its capsule by the use of a dull periosteum elevator, with
success only in those cases where the tonsil was very firm.

During this process of evolution tonsillotomy was gradually eliminated from the practice of the writer and the
technic changed until the method described below was
worked out. The operation of complete removal of the
tonsil has been practiced by the author many times and is
here described for whatever it may be worth.

METHOD OF OPERATION.

Position:—When done under local anesthesia, the patient
may remain upright. The tonsil may often be anesthetized
by wiping cocain with cotton tipped probes well into the
crypts. Under a general anesthetic the patient should be
placed in such a position that the blood can not flow into
the larynx, for this, I believe, is practically the only danger
of this operation.

The position which is used by the writer during general
anesthesia as applied to this operation was so far as he
knows original with him (See figures 1, 2, 3, 4 and 5). It
has been in use for eleven years. The patient (No. 1) is laid
upon his back on a flat table and the head bent backward
and downward at a right angle over the edge, the inverted

face looking directly at the surgeon. The nurse (No. 2) sits upon a low stool (about six inches high) on the left side of the patient, holding the jaw forward to facilitate breathing, it being found that when the tongue depressor is inserted breathing is sometimes obstructed. The anesthetist (No. 3) stands by the side of the patient's body (on the left side), administering the anesthetic, watching the patient and assisting in holding the jaw forward, while the surgeon's assistant (No. 4) stands upon the right side of the patient, near his body, holding the tongue depressor in his right hand and being ready with his left hand to swab out whatever blood collects.

It will thus be seen that the head is in such a position that whatever bleeding takes place must run out of the nose or into the roof of the mouth, but can not run up hill into the larynx. The table being properly placed, daylight may be utilized, shining directly into the mouth from above on each side of the operator (No. 5), who sits upon a stool in front of the patient's face. The Whitehead mouth gag is used because it stays in place and is always out of the way. In this position with assistants also placed as described, a splendid view of the field of operation is secured and quite a number of observers may stand behind the operator and view the operation, while the operator is secure in feeling that he will not choke his patient and he can work with celerity.

Technic:—With a pair of dull serrated forceps (Figure 6) the right tonsil is grasped (these ring forceps do not tear through the tonsil as is the case with pronged forceps, though the latter are better if the tissue is very soft), the dull dissector, shown in Figure 7, is then used to peel the tonsil out from its bed at the upper angle, in front, and below. By pushing the pillars back the tonsil will leave its bed and the separator can even be used with facility in suitable cases to completely remove the tonsil in its capsule.

The snare is next introduced over the right tonsil, the tonsil again grasped with the tonsil forceps and pulled out into the snare. Being really attached only by a pedicle to the posterior pillar it can be readily removed as the snare is slowly brought through, care being taken before closing the snare to so thoroughly sponge the blood and secretion away as to allow a good view, because of the possibility of accidentally engaging the uvula in the snare.

Hemorrhage:—It will thus be found that excessive bleeding does not take place in this operation, because dull instruments are used exclusively and care is taken not to injure the pillars. If bleeding however does take place it may come from one vessel; search should be made for the bleeding point which should be grasped with the artery forceps, usually a twist will be sufficient to stop it, though it is not a difficult matter to tie it off. More commonly the bleeding is a general oozing; if so, it may be quickly stopped by pressing a sponge-holder grasping a piece of moistened gauze, covered with tannic acid powder, against the bleeding surface. If necessary this procedure may be repeated several times.

Usually no delay is necessary, especially if the operator has been careful in his technic, and he may proceed at once with another snare already prepared and remove the remaining tonsil. No further anesthetic being necessary, he quickly proceeds to the next step which consists in performing adenectomy. The operator (No. 5, figure 5) standing, places his left forefinger in the mouth pulling the pallet forward and feeling the adenoids and the structures of the postnasal space with that finger. He then inserts a (right) curette (Figure 8), the blades of which are slanting to more effectively cut and with one clean sweep severs the mass. Following this the other (left) curette is inserted, this going back into the posterior portion of the nares on the other side. A dull ring side scraping curette (Figure 9) is then used to scrape the remaining remnants in the vault and in the fossa of Rosenmueller, the operator still using the left forefinger as a guide to determine whether or not more adenoid tissue is present. Finally a piece of gauze wrapped over the right forefinger is inserted into the vault and the whole area rubbed with this rough gauze. The position of the head during the adenoid operation remains the same, the nurse holding the jaw in place with the assistance of the anesthetist, and the surgeon assistant holding the patient, who at this time may be struggling, though insensitive to pain.

The operation now having been completed the patient is turned on his face, the head allowed to drop some over the end of the table until bleeding has ceased.

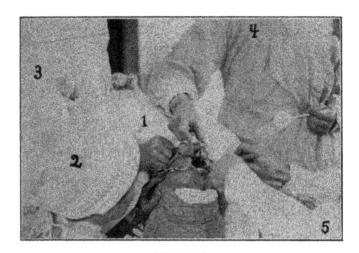

FIGURE 3.
Dissecting tonsil.

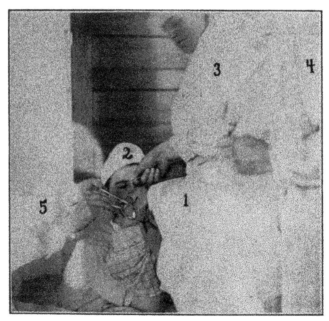

FIGURE 4.
Side view during dissection of tonsil.

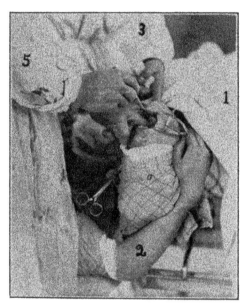

FIGURE 5.

Removing adenoids, left forefinger pulling
pallet forward and feeling adenoids.

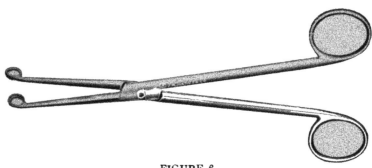

FIGURE 6.

Author's Serrated Ring Tonsil Forceps

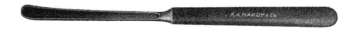

FIGURE 7.

Author's Dull Tonsil Dissector.

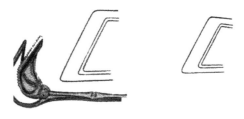

FIGURE 8.

Author's Adenoid Curette with Toothed Clamp
(made in rights and lefts).

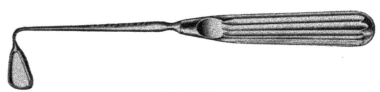

FIGURE 9.

Krause's Dull Ring Adenoid Curette.

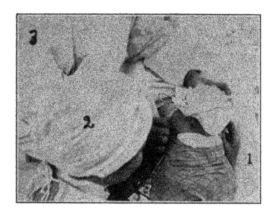

FIGURE 1.

Administering the anæsthetic.

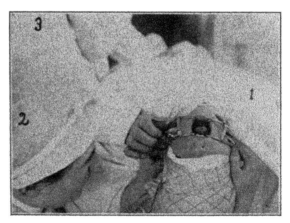

FIGURE 2.

Mouth gag in position, nurse holding angles of jaw forward.

XXIX

A METHOD OF PRECISION FOR INFLATING THE TUBE AND TYMPANUM.

By Thomas Hubbard, M. D.,

Toledo.

Politzerization has been practiced for more than half a century and the original method is still quite unanimously approved by otologists. For purposes of diagnosis and treatment the air bag is probably the most commonly used article in our armamentarium. It has survived most of its contemporaries, and chiefly because of its harmlessness as well as simplicity of construction and operation. I wish to impress the conviction that any safe and successful method of tympanic inflation must embody the essential features as described by Politzer in 1863. There is, however, opportunity for improveing certain mechanical deficiencies of the original apparatus without verging on the impractical or sacrificing the feature of safety. This brings me to mention some of the defects of the ordinary method. The volume of air is small and the act of inflation so brief that the operator has scant opportunity for utilizing delicacy of compression and is rather compelled to depend on the natural safety valve, the velum, to guard against producing too high tension in the nasal cavity and tympanum. Some prevent overtension by releasing the fingers holding the nostrils. Every practitioner must have had the impression that the method would be more effective if he had a larger volume of air under compression. The larger the volume the greater the elasticity and the more positive and effective the inflation with comparatively less tension. The lower the tension the better opportunity for delicacy of manipulation. One might make comparison with the use of large and small syringes for aural irrigation. With a large syringe the operator can control and use a gentle current more effectively than with the high pressure current from the small syringe.

A strong hand can compress the Politzer bag up to about two-thirds of an atmosphere, but as a matter of fact only one-tenth to four-tenths of this tension is applied within the nares and tube. It is evident that there is scant opportunity for exercise of delicacy of touch when there is such disproportion between force exerted and the actual applied tension. It scarcely requires further argument to prove that with a large volume of air having the features of elasticity and reserve, the same dilating and cleansing force can be applied with greater delicacy and precision than obtains with the ordinary method, and that too with a lower degree of tension.

This must not be considered an endorsement of the method of using the air direct from the compressed air tank for inflation. In fact I wish to express a caution against this procedure. It is too much like attempting to modify the street current for purposes like electrolysis. The method which I advocate may be compared to the storage cell system, the compressed air for inflation being drawn directly from an intermediate reservoir of definite known tension.

The purposes of inflation are three-fold: (1) To restore normal tension, (2) to restore anatomical relation, (3) to cleanse tube and tympanum of accumulated secretions. In acute conditions the establishing of normal air tension is chiefly trophic as to therapeutic effect. Incidentally sound transmission is improved, and drainage and absorption of inflammatory exudates encouraged. The degree of resistance to inflation is in this condition an unknown factor. It depends largely on the tubal congestion and amount of mucus at the mouth of the tube. It is certainly irrational to assume that it is safe to use the maximun of force, that is, as much as the safety valve (the velum) will permit, in these acute conditions. Painful Politzerization is not justifiable. It often means an acute exacerbation of inflammation. The indications are to inflate with the least possible pressure, and thus restore physiological conditions. In subacute and chronic states the object of inflation is to restore normal tension, to break up adventitious adhesions, relieve venous and lymphatic stasis and encourage absorption and drainage. If there be a perforation it is obvious that a sustained air current through the tube is indicated. The popularity of the catheter method can be ascribed in part to the fact that ordinary Politzerization is not effective for this purpose.

With these indications clearly in mind: gentle inflation in, or rather following, acute otitis; carefully regulated sustained or intermittent pneumo-massage effect in subacute or chronic conditions, the problem is to so modify the Politzer method as to meet the requirements.

In 1893, in *Archives of Otology*, I described this apparatus. It does not seem to have made much of an impression and I venture to call attention to it again with increasing confidence in its practicability and precision.

DESCRIPTION OF APPARATUS.—The *regulator* controls the tension of the air delivered at the *cut-off*. Twenty to twenty-five pounds is a fair working pressure. Between the *regulator* and the *pressure gauge* is an *air-filter* packed with cotton containing camphor-menthol crystals. The *clamp cut-off* (wrapped in gauze) is held in the same hand with the *Politzer air bag*, which latter and also the *nasal tip* is connected by tubing with the *air reservoir*. The *manometer* registers the maximum degree of tension in the whole system and when in actual use it must record the maximum pressure in the nares and tympanum. There is an uncertain factor of resistance at different points of the system and the operator cannot determine the actual tension within the tympanum during a momentary inflation, but he can be certain that it is not greater than the manometer indicates. As a rule the inflation is prolonged sufficiently to give an accurate reading of actual tension within the tube and tympanum, and further by intermittent pressure of air bag an effective degree of pneumo-massage can be applied. The Politzer airbag held partially compressed in the hand is the safety valve of the apparatus and can be manipulated with a delicacy of touch adapted to degree of resistance, and special indications, such as the age of patient and stage of inflammation.

The essential features of this apparatus are, sterile air under known tension, a reservoir (2 liters) with manometer attachment insuring the proper degree of elasticity in the volume under compression, and the cut-off and Politzer air bag under perfect control of the hand.

The special points to be observed in construction are that the cut-off must be one permitting the passage of a generous flow of air, the old fashioned clamp type being the best, and a free calibre of tubing and connections must obtain throughout the system. The large bulbous nasal tip of size adapted to the age of the patient is advised.

Clinical experience impresses me that the usual estimate of pressure applied in inflation is rather high. A degree of tension represented by 4 to 10 inches of mercury in the manometer is the ordinary pressure used, the same being about one-eighth to one-third of an atmosphere, or 2 to 5 pounds.

I have purposely omitted mention of the use of medicaments as this paper is concerned chiefly with the physical problems. It is very easy to impregnate the air with camphor-menthol or antiseptic vapor such as formaldehyde, and further, the air in the reservoir can be heated to a definite temperature by the insertion of an electric lamp of low candle power.

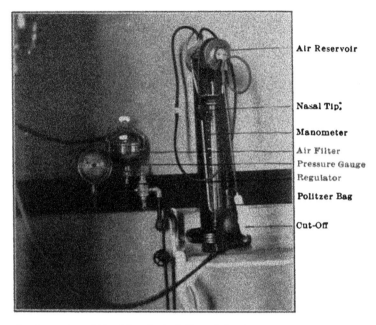

Air Reservoir

Nasal Tip.

Manometer

Air Filter
Pressure Gauge
Regulator

Politzer Bag

Cut-Off

An Apparatus of Precision for Inflation of the Tympanum.

XXX

METHODS OF OPENING THE MAXILLARY AN-TRUM, WITH PRESENTATION OF A . NEW INSTRUMENT.*

BY JOHN O. ROE. M. D.,

ROCHESTER.

It is a well recognized fact in medicine that the more obscure the etiology of a disease, the more intricate the diseased structures. and the more complicated their anatomical relations to other parts, the more numerous and varied will be the remedial measures proposed for its relief or cure. This is very well illustrated in the varied medical and surgical measures that have been brought forward for the treatment of accessory sinus diseases. It is a matter of daily observation that when the exciting cause of a disease is removed the disease itself often speedily disappears—*sublata causa tollitur effectus.* Nature effects a cure if the normal. functions of the part are not too seriously interfered with. This restorative tendency, this vis medicatrix naturae, is to be observed in the case of diseases of the maxillary antrum as well as in diseased conditions of any other part of the body. This is due to the fact that diseases of the antrum are almost invariably secondary to diseases of the associated structures in the nose that obstruct its ostium and interfere with its normal functions and cause infections to extend to its cavity.

It is, therefore, of the utmost importance before attempting an operation on the antrum itself for the cure of an empyema, to carefully investigate the structures in the immediate vicinity of the hiatus semilunaris and the infundibulum. that may be regarded as the gateway to the different sinuses. This region has been appropriately termed by Ballenger "The Vicious Circle," although, as there is no circle involved, I think the term vicious center would be a name quite as appropriate for

*Read before the American Laryngological Association at its thirteenth annual meeting, held at Montreal, Canada, May, 1908.

this region. This is a particularly vicious center, for there is no region of the body in which the anatomical conformation is subject to such infinite variations as the cellular structures of the nose. It is this variation which accounts for the fact that a disturbance in the same location will in one case produce most serious results, while in other cases the effects will be but slight.

Moreover on account of these great anatomical variations, the direction of the drainage of the different cells is by no means constant, and, consequently it may be very readily-diverted from its proper channel. It has been shown by Zukerkandl, Logan Turner, Wright, Myles, Cryer, Killian, Jansen and others that obstruction of these channels, and particularly of the infundibulum, may divert the discharges from the frontal sinus or ethmoidal cells directly into the antrum. It is, therefore, readily seen that in case of disease of the frontal or ethmoidal cells the antrum may become the innocent receptacle of infectious discharges. When the antrum has been so long a reservoir for such discharges as to become the seat of an independent disease, which nature is unable to cure on the removal of the exciting cause, irrigation and medication through the ostium maxillare should be resorted to. If these measures fail, the opening of the antrum becomes a necessity.

The four well-known routes by which such an opening is made are through the alveolar process, the canine eminence or canine fossa, the hard palate and the naso-antral wall.

In those cases in which the exciting cause of the antral trouble is a diseased tooth penetrating the floor of the antrum, the extraction of the tooth and the free opening of the antrum through the tooth socket, through which opening the antrum can be thoroughly irrigated and medicated, will, in many cases, if the disease has existed for but a short time, speedily cure the affection. In all such cases, however, in which the disease does not speedily yield, other methods should be employed. The very old and common practice of inserting a permanent canula through the maxilla to drain the purulent discharge into the buccal cavity is not only ill advised, but can not be too strongly condemned.

The opening through the roof of the mouth is only advisable in certain cases for the removal of growths which are so located as to make this route the most direct method of reaching them.

In making the opening though the anterior wall of the antrum the Küster operation, which consists in taking away a sufficient portion of the wall to permit a free examination and exploration with the finger, and the Denker operation, which is simply an enlargement of the Küster, opening forward to the anterior angle of the sinus so as to render this portion of the cavity entirely accessible, are those commonly employed.

In those cases in which the entire chain of cells is diseased, the antrum, the ethmoidal cells, the frontal sinus and in many cases the sphenoidal sinus also, Jansen has proposed the extensive external operation of laying open the entire chain. This operation is only called for and only warranted in extreme cases in which the cavities are the seat of myxomatous or other growths. In all ordinary cases of empyema of the antrum and ethmoidal cells, associated with nothing more than a degenerated condition of the mucous membrane that has resulted from a prolonged maceration in pus, these external operations are, in the opinion of the writer, unnecessary, for the reason that diseased conditions of the maxillary sinuses, and also of the ethmoidal cells which are commonly associated with an empyema, can be successfully treated by the nasal route. I simply mention these methods for the purpose of comparison, in order to emphasize the advantages of the nasal route over all other methods in the treatment of such conditions.

As a combination of the external and internal routes, Caldwell, of New York, in 1895, described a new method by which an opening is made into the antrum through its outer wall sufficiently large to inspect the cavity and to remove any growths that may be found. When this is done the opening is then continued through the naso-antral wall into the nose, through which the subsequent cleansing and treatment of the cavity is carried on, the external opening being immediately and permanently closed. Two years later Luc, of Paris, without a knowledge of Caldwell's operation, performed and described exactly the same procedure and so strongly advocated the operation that it has since been called "The Caldwell-Luc Operation."

This same operation is also advocated by P. Watson Williams; but instead of using a chisel for making the opening through the different bones, he employs a "six-penny trephine" with a gimlet-pin, making an opening into the antrum corresponding to the canine fossa. A circular opening is then made with the same trephine through the naso-antral wall just behind the anterior end of the inferior turbinated body close to the antral floor, removing at the same time the corresponding portion of the inferior turbinal. Through this opening the necessary treatment of the antrum is applied, the buccal opening being allowed to close at once.

Various methods of technic are employed by different surgeons for opening the antrum through the nose, an operation which was first proposed by Gooch and Réthi, and also advocated by John Hunter. The simplest method is by puncturing the wall with a Krause trocar and canula, an instrument which is sometimes used in this manner merely for the purpose of diagnosis. With it the antrum can be washed out and this is often sufficient, in recent or subacute inflammations, to effect a cure.

Vail proposed making a circular or oval opening by means of curved saws after having punctured the bone with his perforator, which process necessitates at the same time the removal of the anterior half of the inferior turbinated body.

Ballenger's operation consists in cutting out a portion of the wall either square or of any desired shape or dimension with his right angle knife. His method he describes as follows:

"The knife should be introduced through the naso-antral wall at the posterior limit of the antrum near the floor of the nose; then make an upward cut, a forward and downward cut. The upward and forward cuts are made with the blade of the instrument at right angles to the naso-antral wall. When the forward cut is made the blade should be turned down, parallel with the naso-antral wall and pulled through it. The inferior incision remains to be made, and is done with the reverse knife, the knives coming in pairs. The knife is introduced into the posterior perpendicular incision at the floor of the nose and drawn forward along the floor of the nose to the anterior perpendicular incision, thus completing the removal of the naso-antral wall. Should the knife fail to remove the thickened lower portion of the wall it may be removed with the Grünwald or other bone forceps."

It has not been the experience of the writer to encounter naso-antral walls so readily pared away with the knife as has been my friend's experience, judging from the above description ; on the contrary, a large majority of naso-antral walls are very firm below the attachment of the lower turbinate and require, in many cases, considerable force to puncture with a drill or chisel.

The success of the operation by the naso-antral route in the treatment of chronic empyema of the antrum depends upon the freedom of the opening, which should allow perfect drainage into the nose and free access to every portion of the cavity for thorough medication. For this purpose I have devised a pair of cutting forceps (vide cut) with sufficient strength to meet the requirements in every case, however firm and resistant the bony wall may be found.

Roe's Antrum Punch Forceps.

These forceps are made in two forms. One with the male blade entering the antrum, the other with the female blade entering the antrum. The former is preferable when the floor of the antrum is above, the latter when the floor of the antrum is below the floor of the nasal passage.

The technic of my operation is as follows: Owing to the great variation in the size and position of the lower turbinate, it being frequently attached very low down or enlarged or curled so as to greatly limit the space between it and the floor of the nose. It becomes necessary in such cases to remove the lower anterior portion of this body in order to make room for the operation. This is done with a slender, probe-pointed knife introduced beneath the turbinate along its attachment, cutting downward and inward toward the septum so as to catch the scroll as it rolls outward, or with

a pair of scissors or a pair of Grünwald's cutters.   A small
angular or curved pointed knife is now introduced and an incision made through the periosteum down to the bone from
behind forward, covering the entire length of the antrum, and
as close to the attachment of the lower turbinate as possible.
By examining the conformation of the jaw, assisted in doubtful cases by the x-ray, we can judge quite accurately as to
the position of the antrum and its forward projection, at
which point the puncture through the bone should be made.
At this point the incision through the muco-periosteum is
turned downward to the floor of the nose, the incision at the
posterior end being also carried downward to the floor.   This
flap is then raised from the bone, carrying the periosteum with
it throughout this subturbinal portion of the wall, and rolled
and turned into the center of the nostril out of the way of injury.   An opening is then made into the anterior portion of the
antrum as close to the floor of the antrum as possible.   This
opening may be made with a curved drill, a trocar, or a chisel.
The most satisfactory instrument I have found to be one of
Myle's curved antrum gouge chisels, particularly if the bony
wall is very thick.   A chisel may be used of the size we wish
the preliminary opening to be, or if a small opening is made it
can be afterward enlarged with a gouge or chisel sufficiently
to admit the blade of the punch forcep.   This instrument is
now introduced one blade through the opening and the whole
wall below the turbinal attachment is removed by nipping it off,
a piece at a time.   It is quite important that the lower stump
of the wall be leveled off so that there shall be no projection
between the floor of the nose and the floor of the antrum.
Should it be desired to remove a portion of the anterior border
of the wall of the antrum, this can be most easily done with
Wagener's forward cutting antrum punch forceps.   When the
lower portion of the wall has thus been completely removed,
the cavity is carefully explored and any growths that may be
found removed.   The cavity is then thoroughly irrigated and
carefully dried out.   The periosteum and mucous membrane
that has been raised from the inner wall is trimmed if necessary and turned down over the stump of the wall and carefully
held there by thoroughly packing the entire antrum and also
the nasal cavity with iodoform gauze.   It is unnecessary to deal
especially with the upper border of the incision, as it is thin,

drains freely and readily heals. By thus covering the lower stump of the wall with mucous membrane we have left a uniform mucous surface and a perfectly free opening into the antrum making it practically a recess of the nose. We can now deal with any growths or abnormal conditions which may be present and medicate the cavity as we would any other diseased mucous surface. This conversion of the antrum into a portion of the nasal cavity is never followed by any ill effects nor the slightest discomfort. The practice of vigorously curetting the antrum and destroying its mucous membrane so often recommended in the treatment of empyema of the antrum cannot be too strongly condemned. It is an operation that should only be done as a part of the radical operation of obliterating the antrum by the complete removal of its anterior wall and its lining membrane.

In several cases which I have recently operated upon in the manner above described, the lining membrane of the cavity had become degenerated from long maceration in muco-pus until it was a boggy mass and in many places the bone had become denuded. By giving the antrum free drainage, keeping it clean by frequent irrigation, and stimulating solutions, such as nitrate of silver, the tissues have regained their tone, the periosteum and mucous membrane have become restored, and at the end of four or five weeks the patients were well.

The advantage of this method over other methods is the freedom and ease with which the cavity can be irrigated and medicated, the patient being very readily taught to do the washing himself. Moreover, perfect drainage is maintained by providing a permanent and free ostium to the cavity at its most dependent point. The danger of a recurrence of the empyema is thereby prevented regardless of the infection to which the cavity may be subjected. Finally the necessity of an external operation is avoided except in the case of growths so large as to require the most radical measures for their removal.

XXXI

REPORT OF A PROBABLE CASE OF SARCOMA OF THE SPHENOIDAL SINUS WITH REMARKS.

By Dunbar Roy, M. D.,

Atlanta.

W. W. C., age 56, traveling man, consulted me in March, 1904, on account of some deafness in the left ear which came on during the month previous, as the result, so he thought, of a severe cold. This impairment in his hearing disappeared very slowly. At the time of the cold he was treated by an aurist in another city, but in the physician's endeavor to pass the eustachian catheter into the tube on the left side, so much pain and bleeding was occasioned that the patient ceased the treatment and allowed it to continue as it was until he came under my observation. His past history presented no unusual symptoms. He had always enjoyed good health and had never suffered from any severe spell of illness. In 1885 he suffered from inflammatory rheumatism but that passed away in a short time. He is a moderate smoker and drinker. Absolutely no history of syphilis. During the last winter he contracted a very severe cold and the left ear became affected as stated above. On examination I found the following conditions: His pharynx showed the usual smoker's throat, with the soft palate exceedingly relaxed, so much so, that it was impossible to make a post-rhinoscopic examination without the aid of a palate retractor. The nasal cavity showed nothing abnormal except the membrane over the inferior turbinates was corrugated and thickened. There seemed to be no difficulty in nasal breathing. The catheter was easily passed into the eustachian tube on the right side and that was perfectly free and open. On the left there seemed to be some obstruction in the naso-pharynx which rendered the passage of the catheter rather difficult. However it was used from day to day with some benefit to the middle ear although the sounds were never clear. The right ear appeared normal In the left the drum was retracted and the malleus very prominent. Tuning fork heard longer by BC than AC. This was true for all registers. Hearing diminished one-half. The patient was treated for several days with only slight benefit at the end of which time he was compelled to leave the city. I did not see him again until May 1st, two months later, when he again consulted me with the following history: On April 23rd he noticed some weakness in the left eye and on the 25th he began to see double, wh'ch symptom has remained constant ever since. He also has been suffering with severe neuralgic pain in the eye and over the left side of the face and head. Some roaring in the left ear.

Right eye is apparently normal. Vision equals 20/40, with + 1s equals 20/20. Left eye, vision equals 20/40, with + 1s equals 20/20. There is almost total paralysis of the external rectus of the left eye with a consequent homonymous diplopia. Pupil reacts to light and accommodation. The ophthalmoscope shows no change in the disc. In the lower outer quadrant of the fundus there is a small hemorrhagic spot. The veins appear a little larger than normal, but there are no signs of a papillitis. This eye appears to be more normal than the right, as far as its ophthalmoscopic appearances. By shrinking the tissues in the left nasal cavity, the naso-pharynx can be seen and at this point there is a decided bulging, especially as you look towards the vault. On touching this swelling with a probe it appears firm and bleeds very easily. It does not however interfere with nasal respiration. It is practically impossible to pass the eustachian catheter into the tube on this side. The patient was placed upon large and increasing doses of potassium iodide and all smoking and drinking interdicted.

May 5th there was a decided exophthalmos and total paralysis of the external rectus muscle. Pain in and around the eye has been quite severe. There is a slight ptosis. The urine was examined and found to contain albumen and some hyaline casts. The patient was now placed in the hands of a neurologist and I continued to see the case in conjunction with him. About May 12th the patient was placed in a hospital where he could have better attention. This change was found to be of no benefit, as he began to have marked mental hallucinations almost amounting to a raving, inability to sleep and absolute dread of his surroundings. Consequently he was removed to his daughter's house where he was satisfied to be nursed by an old colored servant whom he had known in his childhood. The exophthalmos increased, the facial nerve on that side began to be affected, his memory failed and nights were made hideous by these delusions. He was gradually growing weaker and at no time was there any further fundus lesion and his vision seemed to remain good. Under treatment his kidneys became more active and the albumen disappeared entirely from his urine. Pain continued to be severe deep in the orbital cavity. There is no apparent change in the naso-pharynx. During all this time he was taking as high as 75 grains of the iodide three times daily. The neurologist was under the impression that there was possibly a tumor on the posterior part of the orbital plate, extending backwards and upwards into the frontal convolutions. He advised an exploratory craniotomy. Accordingly this was done by Dr. Nicolson about the middle of June. Absolutely nothing pathological was found although Dr. Nicolson explored with his finger all the upper surface of the orbital plate. Patient rallied well from the operation and for a few days seemed to improve, probably due to the lessening of the intracranial pressure. The pain was much reduced. At no time was there any trouble with the proper functions of the bladder and bowels. There was no paralysis or paresis in any other portion of the body. No difficulty in deglutition. His appetite was poor and the patient gradually became weaker. His mental symptoms, while not so marked as previous to the operation, were decidedly noticeable. One week after the operation the patient died in convulsions which were diagnosed as uraemic. Unfortunately no post-mortem could be obtained. The history of this case is exceedingly interesting and at the same time somewhat obscure. Two facts are clear: (1) There was evidently a tumor (probably sarcoma or epithelioma) at the base of the brain involving at least the body of the sphenoid and encroaching upon the inner extremity of the orbital cavity. (2). There was also present symptoms of a chronic nephritis. Whether the simultaneous occurrence of these two conditions were accidental or stood in some relationship to each other we are in no position to deny or affirm. Both conditions being recognized about the same time, it was naturally impossible to say which originated first.

In this case all the most prominent symptoms could be referred to a sphenoidal growth and in fact these were the symptoms complained of by the patient, the renal trouble seemingly produced no inconvenience as far as could be elicited by the history. The first real symptom complained of by the patient was a roaring and difficulty in hearing out of the left ear. This he attributed to a severe cold and was so treated by an aurist who however was unable to pass the eustachian catheter on that side. This in itself was suggestive of the beginning of the growth in the sphenoidal cavity, pressing downward and to the left against the eustachian tube. Not improving, the patient consulted me one month later for the roaring and deafness in the left ear. A bulging in the naso-pharynx was then noticed and also the impossibility of passing air through the eustachian tube either by the catheter or the Politzer method.

On May 1st the patient returned with no relief in the ear symptoms with a paresis of the external rectus and exophthalmos of the left eye. Five days later there was complete paralysis of the left external· rectus, some paresis of the facial nerve on the same side, marked exophthalmos, bulging more marked in the naso-pharynx, bleeding easily when touched and also severe pain around the left orbit and the same side of the head. A sarcoma or epithelioma in the sphenoidal sinus would produce just this train of symptoms. The sixth nerve comes from the medulla, bends over the posterior end of the pons and runs along in an exposed manner for some distance. For this reason neurologists tell us that this nerve is the one most frequently affected after traumatism and from the pressure of tumors at the base of the brain. The fibres of the seventh are very close to the sixth and close to this are fibres of the eighth, or auditory nerve. Slight pressure on both of these would produce some paresis of the muscles on the same side of the face and some tinnitus in the left ear from the same cause. The tumor also encroaches upon the apex of the orbit as was manifested by the exophthalmos, not however involving the optic nerve nor any other of the motor nerves of the eye. This latter symptom led me to the conclusion that the tumor originated in the sphenoid cavity as a center rather

than in some portion of the brain, since clinical and pathological observation has shown that even sphenoidal and posterior ethmoidal cells may be the seat of an adventitious
growth and yet the optic nerve show no symptoms of involvement.   On the other hand, a tumor of the brain substance is
more than likely to show some papillitis or stasis in the appearence of the optic disc, and this nearly always bilateral.   As an
aid to making a diagnosis of the brain tumors from the appearance of the fundus, Dr. Byrom Branwell, in his book on Intracranial Tumors, has this to say: "The absence of double optic
neuritis does not necessarily exclude the presence of a tumor;
but the fact that there is no optic neuritis does suggest doubt;
and unless very clearly defined, or unless the physician
feels satisfied that there is no condition present except a
tumor which could reasonably be expected to account for the
phenomena of the case, he will be wise, in the absence of
double optic neuritis, to hesitate before committing himself
to a positive diagnosis."

In this case there was absolutely no changes in the disc and
vision was as perfect as in the other eye.   There was a small
hemorrhage in the outer inferior quadrant and this was probably due to the atheromatous condition of the blood vessels on
association with renal disease.

In June, 1904, issue of the *American Journal of the Medical
Sciences*, Dr. Chas. A. Oliver, of Philadelphia, has a very interesting report of a case of "Cerebellar Neoplasm in a Subject
with Renal Disease."   The growth proved to be a sarcoma,
and while it was situated in the cerebellum, it nevertheless extended down into the pons varolii and medulla, and in this
way involved some of the nervous structures which were affected by the growth just as in my own case.   In Oliver's case,
as was to be expected from an intracranial growth, there was
a neuro-retinitis in both eyes but more pronounced in the left.
In describing the eye symptoms of this case when first seen,
Dr. Oliver has this to say: "A medium degree of paresis of
the left external muscle together with a slight paresis of the
corresponding orbicularis muscle could be determined both
objectively and subjectively.   There was imperfect action of
the muscles which were supplied by the left oculomotor and
pathetic nerves."   In giving the gross findings at the post-

mortem, Dr. Oliver says the apex of the growth was nipple shaped and projected forward to a point which was situated slightly anterior to the middle line of the pons varolii and reached within 1½ cm. of the origin of the left crus cerebri. Laterally towards the median line, the growth pressed upon the medulla, while on the left side it rested upon the posterior part of the pons varolii. ` The seventh and eighth nerve trunks on the right side appeared to be in good condition, while the corresponding left ones were swollen and indistinct. Dr. Oliver remarks that this case is of interest because the cerebellar growth developed in a patient suffering with renal trouble, and although the macroscopic examination showed marked destruction of the nerve elements m the neighborhood, and although complete blindness supervened with very bizarre ocular palsies, yet the cause of the patient's death was evidently uremic coma. In my own case the cause of the death was evidently uremic, as manifested by the lethal convulsions. In both of these cases a very important point arises as to what effect the growth had upon the renal disease and vice-versa what effect the renal trouble had upon the increase of the adventitious growth. Was the condition of the blood vessles and circulation damaged to such an extent by the renal disturbances as to afford good food for the propagation of a malignant growth?

In the *Annals D'Oculistique* for June, 1896, there is an artiele by Dr. V. Morax, entitled "Ocular Disturbances Observed in a Case of Epithelioma of the Sphenoidal Sinus." in this case the malignant growth extended much more rapidly from the sphenoid sinus into the contiguous cavities than in the case reported by me, consequently there was a considerably more destruction of the surrounding parts and more marked subjective and objective symptoms. The case reported by Dr. Morax is certainly interesting and instructive enough to allow here an abstract of the same: M. V., 53 years old, presented himself at the clinic May 12. 1893, complaining of complete blindness of several days' duration. The commencement of the ocular trouble dated back to the beginning of 1893. Examination of the patient showed that the ocular movements were normal. The pupils were unequal and reacted neither to light nor accommodation. The fundus of the eye showed no lesion. Visual perception abolished

in both eyes. He had severe and continuous headaches.
Later slight optic neuritis, then atrophy of the disc.   In
the beginning no naso-pharyngeal disturbance, later purulent discharge from the nose and appearence of pedunculated
tumors on the pituitary membrane.   Paralysis of the oculomotor nerves.   Ptosis, exophthalmos from intraorbital tumors.   Death one year after the commencement of the affection from broncho-pneumonia.   Autopsy: Primary epithelioma of the sphenoidal sinus with dilatation of the sinus. Invasion by the neoplasm of the body of the sphenoid, of the
optic nerves, and of the chiasm. Neoplasmic prolongation
into the orbit, the maxillary sinuses and the ethmoidal cells.
Invasion of the orbital surface and the frontal convolutions.
Broncho-pneumonia.   As will be seen, there were several
symptoms somewhat analogous in this case to the one reported by me, and I doubt not that if the uremic condition
had not intervened and caused death the tumor in my own
case would have extended and produced very much the same
chain of symptoms. It is also noteworthy that death in Dr.
Morax's case was attributed to broncho-pneumonia and not to
the tumor itself. Morax also refers to a case of carcinoma
of the sphenoidal sinus described by Albert in his Lehrbuch
der Chirurgie, in which he says: "Affections of the sphenoidal
sinus are not commonly manifested by the recognizable signs.
I once saw the sphenoid sinus completely filled with a decomposing carcinomatous mass without the slighest symptom
having been observed during life." Morax thinks that this
case was nothing more than an empyema of the sphenoidal
sinus and he closes with this significant remark: "We see,
therefore, that documents are completely lacking and we must
be content to record cases until a sufficient number are
brought together to enable us to sketch the principal clinical
symptoms which will lead to a recognition of neoplasms originating in the sphenoidal sinus."   The question as to the involvement of the sphenoidal sinus with an abscess or adventitious growth without at the same time affecting the optic
nerves, is an exceedingly interesting question, especially since
of late years more attention has been given to the pathological involvement of this sinus by both oculist and rhinologist.
Considerable original work on this question has been done by
Onodi and Eversbuch in Germany. In a very extensive ar-

ticle accompanied by anatomical plates, Professor Onodi has gone very thoroughly into this question and has published the same in the December, 1904, issue of the *British Journal of Laryngology*. I shall take the liberty of quoting freely from this monograph.

In this article, Prof. Onodi has undertaken to show the close anatomical relationship between the optic nerve and the posterior accessory sinuses, especially the sphenoid, and also from this anatomical relationship any disturbance of vision is likely to occur when these sinuses are the seat of very severe pathological changes, such as abcesses, adventitious growths, etc. In numerous dissections Prof. Onodi found that there was a great variation in these relations and has thus summarized his findings:

1. The optic canal may be formed on both sides by the sphenoidal cavities.

2. The optic canal may be connected on both sides with the most posterior ethmoid cells only.

3. The optic canal may be formed on one side by the sphenoidal cavity, on the other by the most posterior ethmoidal cell.

4. The optic canal only on one side may be related either with the sphenoidal cavity or with the posterior ethmoidal cell.

5. The optic canal may be related on one side both with the sphenoid cavity and with the posterior ethmoid cavity.

6. The optic canal may be related neither with the sphenoid nor with the posterior ethmoid cavity.

From this summary it will be seen that the optic canal when seen in the close relationship with the sphenoidal cavity or the posterior ethmoidal cells, is always in imminent danger of injury with a consequent involvement of the optic nerve should these sinuses become affected. However, it must be borne in mind that it takes very gross pathological lesions of these sinuses to cause injury to the optic nerve, and fortunately when such lesions or abscesses do occur, they always have a tendency to drain themselves through their natural openings into the naso-pharynx and nose rather than to empty themselves above, forward and outward into the orbital cavity.

Berger and Tyrmann have published a monograph on the connection between diseases of the sphenoid cavity and blindness. Up to 1886 they had collected 23 cases only from the

literature, and Onodi remarks that "since that date very little
has been written in text-books of the eye and nose, as to the
diseases of the spheno¦dal cavity, producing by its close relationship with the optic nerve, blindness and nasal defects."
The important fact was establ¦shed by Berger and Tyrmann in
the¦r stat¦stics that "no defect in vision has been shown in a
number of cases, during the whole course of the affection of the
sphenòidal cavities, in caries or in the growth of a tumor, up
to the death of the patient." Consequently in making a diag-
nos¦s of the involvement of the sphenoid cavity with some
pathological condition we should never wait until the optic
nerve has become involved, as that always shows an extension of the process to a point where treatment will prove of
but little avail.

Should the optic nerve become involved as the result of
such pathological conditions, it is usually an optic neuritis
and that too unilateral.

Lapersonne has this to say: "Optic neuritis is rarely seen
in inflammation of the frontal sinus, more often in inflammation of the maxillary or ethmoid, but is produced, if at all,
by inflammation of the sphenoid sinus. A chief characteristic of neuritis due solely to sinus inflammation, is that it is
unilateral. Although strictly speaking both nerves may be
affected in the optic canal by the inflammation of both sphenoidal sinus, a double edematous neuritis ought rather to
make one think of an intracranial process."

It is not surprising that in the case here reported by me, the
optic nerve was not involved although there was marked exophthalmos, protrusion into the naso-pharynx, etc., because the
post-mortem examinations findings in other similar cases show
the rarity of such an involvement. For instancé, Onodi says
"Post-mortem examinations show that tumors in the region
of the body of the sphenoid leave the optic nerve intact."
Reinhardt has reported that in case of cancer of the upper
jaw, the bones of the cranium being greatly thinned by caries,
the body of the sphenoid being so softened that it could be
cut away with a knife, the post-mortem findings showed
that the optic and olfactory nerves were normal.

Ponfick mentions a case where "a sarcoma had originated
in the body of the sphenoid, and the optic nerve, though involved in the tumor, was normal." Onodi says that he and

Schmidt-Rimpler have reported cases which show that "in cases of sarcoma of the sphenoid, both optic nerves may remain intact."

Even cases have been reported where severe suppuration of the sphenoidal cavity has occurred with the simultaneous destruction of the bone, and yet there was no disturbance of vision.

Baratroux describes a case in which a large part of the sphenoid was extruded through the nose without any consequent interference in vision. Hajek saw in several cases, considerable syphilitic affection of the anterior wall of the sphenoid cavity without any special optic nerve symptoms. Flatau records 26 cases of empyema and caries of the sphenoid cavity, but mentions no interference with the sight.

Foucher also describes a case of a girl 15 years old, where necrosis of the turbinate bodies and sphenoids were found, where the patient died and yet the vision was not affected. Dr. Hinkle has reported 20 cases of sphenoidal empyema treated, where there was no involvement of the eyes.

In studying the literature of diseases of the sphenoidal sinus, it would seem to be the exception for the eyes to be involved even in the most severe pathological conditions.

This subject is certainly one of great importance and the study of it still in its infancy, so that we must have a report of every pathological condition which will aid us in the elucidation of this subject. As Prof. Onodi says in concluding his article from which I have freely quoted: "I have put together on the basis of my investigations, all the material at my disposal, to explain the present day position of the question, to point to this question waiting for solution, to draw general attention to this interesting and important subject. Whilst I commend these questions to the special attention of the ophthalmologists, I shall hope that the joint rhinological and ophthalmological study of this subject, in many respects still unknown, will lead to successful enlightenment."

ABSTRACTS FROM CURRENT OTOLOGIC, RHINO-LOGIC AND LARYNGOLOGIC LITERATURE.

The Operative Treatment of Purulent Meningitis Following Inflammation of the Labyrinth.

WITTMAACK, Jena (*Münch. med. Wochenschr.*, No. 47, 1908), shows that all cases of meningitis following inflammation of the labyrinth are not necessarily fatal if properly dealt with. In two of his cases where the diagnosis was confirmed by spinal punction, the Neumann labyrinth operation, followed by a free incision of the cerebellar dura from the sinus to the porus acusticus, resulted in recovery. Great weight is laid upon early diagnosis, spinal punction, radical operation and incision of the dura.

Horn.

The Use of Pyocanase in Acute Suppuration of the Middle Ear.

LEUWER, Bonn. With this new preparation, here in Germany so widely experimented with as a treatment for angina, diphtheria, etc., Leuwer found that his results were not better than by the usual methods with boric acid. Complications were not prevented and cases came finally to operation in the usual number.

Horn.

The Treatment of Traumatic Defects of the Lobe of the Ear by Means of Plastic Methods.

SCHMIEDEN, Berlin (*Berlin. klin. Wochenschr.*, No. 31, 1908). In the case of a boy with entire loss of the external ear the author successfully built a new ear by the following series of operations, fourteen days apart:

1. Excision of cartilage from the right ribs and free implantation under the skin of the breast.

2. Enveloping the cartilage with the skin of the breast, in the general form of the ear.

3. Formation of a long flap with the base in the region of the clavicle. The flap was then turned up and sewn in place.

4. The base of the flap was cut through and the breast scar made smaller.

Horn.

Rosenmueller's Fossae and Their Importance in, Relation to the Middle. Ear.

FRANCIS P. EMERSON, Boston (*Boston Med. and Surg. Jour.*, April 23, 1908). A further study of one hundred cases in adults, showing the relation of Rosenmueller's fossae to diseased conditions of the middle ear, confirm the conclusions, **viz.**:

1. Pathologic amounts of lymphoid tissue are present in Rosenmueller's fossae in a large number of cases of chronic secretory and suppurative ears.

2· This cannot be detected with certainty by posterior rhinoscopy alone, even where a good view of the vault is obtainable.

3. In every chronic case there should be a routine digital examination.

4. Where much tissue has been found and removed, the process of healing should be watched that no fibrous bands form.

5. It is possible in a large majority of cases to predict the involved ear by the condition of the corresponding fossa.

6. Results, where after-treatment is followed, are particularly good in removing abnormal sensations, restoring uniform hearing without fluctuations in the partial or complete relief of tinnitus, and in the prevention of recurring salpingitis.

7. If directions are given to blow one side of the nose at a time and carefully, the affected tube is no more apt to be infected later than its fellow.

Outside of the cases of otitis media suppurativa chronica, the symptoms are associated with chronic secretory ears having the following definite symptoms: Stuffiness, fluctuating hearing, low pitched tinnitus and recurring unilateral salpingitis. There is no age limit, and under the above conditions it is almost invariably present.

Richards.

The Treatment of Acute Catarrh of the Middle Ear.

WALB, Bonn (*Deutsch. medizin. Wochenschr.*, No. 47, 1908). In the course of a paper on this subject, the author drives another nail into the coffin of Bier's method of the treatment of purulent ear disease and mastoiditis by means of passive hyperemia. Based on the study of twenty cases, Professor Walb is at one with almost every other specialist in Germany, that the rubber cravat in this condition is about as safe as a stick of dynamite in the hands of a child. Keppler, who was a surgical assistant of Bier's and not a trained otologist, published the first paper on the subject, and was followed by Eschweiler of Bonn, who also in his first, but more especially in his latest paper, led the otologic world to believe that in the treatment of mastoiditis the knife was to be relegated to the ash-barrel, and that the millennium in the treatment of th's disease had been reached by the use of the elastic neck-band.

It soon appeared that in other parts of Germany, men uninfluenced by local conditions, were unable to obtain any such brilliant results, and reports of deaths from thrombosis of the sinus and unfavorable operative conditions followed one other in rapid succession. Not until the present paper appeared was it shown that these twenty cases studied in Bonn during 1905-06 were as unfavorable as the others, and on account of the dangerous conditions which followed this method of treatment the author suggested that it should only be carried out in a hospital under trained eyes.

Horn.

Purulent Inflammation of the Inner Ear.

UFFENORDE, Göttingen (*Medizin. Klinik.*, No. 39, 1908.) In a clinical lecture he reviews clearly the diagnostic difficulties of varying grades of inflammations in the cochlea and semicircular canals. He claims that labyrinth inflammations occur in 1 per cent of all middle ear inflammations or more commonly than sinus phlebitis, meningitis and brain abscess together. The paths of infection in the order of their commonness are the prominence of the lateral semicircular canal, the oval window, the round window and the promontory. He believes that in one case the Fallopian canal acted as the path of the infection. The experience of the last ten years seems to have settled beyond a doubt that the cochlea alone is concerned in the perception of sound, while the vestibular apparatus concerns itself with the ataxic function alone. The physiologist Hensen alone clings to the old theory that the vestibular apparatus is connected with the function of hearing. He casts some doubt on the methods of Barany, claiming to have had cases of undoubted defects in the semicircular canal system, where he was able to produce caloric rotary and galvanic nystagmus. (See ANNALS for Dec., 1907,

Barany. "Methods of Examination of the Semicircular Canals.") The diagnosis of purulent inflammation of the labyrinth is of very great importance. The mortality from non-operated cases is very high. If in these cases the symptoms of labyrinth irritation do not quickly disappear by conservative methods, we must proceed at once to operation. The mere determination, however, of a labyrinth inflammation is not in itself an indication for the labyrinth operation, or even the radical operation. A local inflammation can take place in one part of the labyrinth and be cured without involvement of the whole structure. His indications for labyrinth operation are when meningitis serosa, deep-seated extradural abscess, or cerebellar abscess complicate the labyrinth inflammation. A purulent meningitis determined by the lumbar puncture is not now a contraindication. The invasion of the internal ear by a cholesteatoma or a tuberculous process is a distinct indication. In other cases our individual experience and the results of the previous radical operation must determine the course of events. In closing he gives his own method of total ablation of the labyrinth by means of a preliminary laying bare of the facial nerve in its Fallopian canal.

Horn.

The Modern Methods of Investigating the Vestibular Apparatus and Their Practical Meaning.

BARANY, Wien (*Mediz. Klinik.*, No. 50, 1908). In the ANNALS for December, 1907, this well known investigator described, for the first time in English, his newly discovered methods of examining the labyrinth. In the present paper he lays more weight on the side which appeals to the general practitioner and shows how a careful observation of eye nystagmus, in cases where dizziness, vomiting or nausea seem to arise from a genital trouble or a stomach complaint, might save the physician from making a terrible mistake and sacrificing the life of the patient. The value of the method in medico-legal investigations is also shown and how a proper use of the same would exclude all simulated dizziness on the part of the patient. For a full elucidation of this most important subject, the reader is referred to the original monograph. "Barany—Physiologie und Pathologie des Bogengang-Apparates." Faanz Deuticke, Wien. Price, Marks 2.50. (Bound in paper.)

Horn.

II.—NOSE.

The Operative Treatment of Nasal Septum Deformities.

KRETSCHMANN, Magdeburg (*Muen. med. Wochenschr.*, No. 41, 1908), proposed, at the last annual meeting of the German Otological Society, to substitute for the ordinary submucous septum operation, a proceeding of such surgical magnitude, that the paper was not regarded at all seriously. By gaining access to the nose through the mouth, that is by making a long incision under the upper lip, raising up the periosteum to the apertura pyriformis, making a circular incision of the mucous membrane in both nostrils and with a strong retractor pulling this portion of the face up over the nose, the author claims to have a freer access to the septum than is possible even by the Freer submucous method! A claim that hardly anyone would deny him. That a general narcosis must be used, that "usually severe hemorrhage takes place," to be controlled, as the author recommends, by a combination of artery forceps, compression, $H_2 O_2$, and various astringent powders, as well as adrenalin, are mere details. The author found the intubation narcosis, of Kuhn, with a tight tampon in the nasopharynx the safest and prevented the aspiration of most of the blood. The cut is carefully sewed up, rubber drains are inserted in both nostrils and the patient remains, under favorable conditions, in bed for "3-4 days." There is a severe swelling of the face and eyelids in a few days, the patient keeps a stiff upper lip for some time, but the end result is satisfactory.

For additional details, we refer the reader to the original.

Horn.

Methods of Transillumination of the Sinus Frontalis and Antrum of Highmore.

VOHSEN, Frankfurt (*Berlin. klin. Wochenschr.*, No. 28, 1908), describes his new transillumination lamp, which contains a rheostat in the handle. In comparing the two sides, he first investigates the healthy sinus and noting the amount of current necessary for a clear outline, uses the same amount of current for the other side. If now a clear outline is not obtained and more current is necessary, he is in a position to look with suspicion on the darkened sinus. His technic seems to_be a_ distinct–advance over the ordinary happy-go-lucky methods which has thrown such discredit on the value of transillumination.

Horn.

The Use of Potassium Iodid in Diseases of the Accessory Cavities.

HEMPEL (*Berlin. med. Wochenschr.*, No. 39, p. 1769, 1908) has had good results in acute as well as in chronic cases by the use of potassium iodid. Its value in these conditions, although perhaps but little noted in the literature, has long been known, and it is by no means new.

Horn.

The Value of the X-Rays in Rhinology.

SCHEIER, Berlin (*Deut. med. Wochenschr.*, No. 41, p. 1767, 1908). In a paper read before the International Rhino-Laryngological Congress in Vienna, 1908, the author shows the place the Röntgen photography holds in the diagosis of diseases of the accessory sinuses. Unfortunately, with other authors, he belittles the value of transillumination, and fails to mention the fact that such a thing as a suction apparatus exists. Surgeons were able to diagnose fractures before the advent of the X-ray; and rhinologists, who are not always in a position to have a photograph made, are still able to recognize the absence of a frontal sinus, without an unnecessary operation.

Horn.

The Relation Between Diseases of the Nose, With its Accessory Cavities, the Nasopharyngeal Cavity and the Eye.

KUHNT, Bonn (*Deut. med. Wochenschr.*, No. 37, 1908). In the International Laryngo-Rhinological Congress at Vienna, last year, the author of our present methods of radically combating the pyogenic diseases of the frontal sinus and ethmoid labyrinth, discussed, under the above title, a subject of vast importance, and shows how closely bound together is the work of the rhinologist and laryngologist. It is impossible to here review in detail all of the interesting points brought out in this long paper; the mechanical and circulatory disturbances of the eye, with its changes in conjunctiva and cornea; the inflammatory intraocular diseases; the influence on glaucoma; on Basedow's disease; the retinal changes, especially retinal detachment; the remarkable changes in the field of vision for red and green which occurs in almost every case of acute and chronic accessory sinus disease, are matters which deserve most careful study.

Horn.

The Diagnosis and Treatment of Suppurative Conditions of the Accessory Sinuses.

MARTENS (*Deutsche medicinische Wochenschrift,* January 28, 1909). The experience of the physician in regard to the frequency of diseases of the accessory nasal sinuses differs very decidedly from the pathologic findings at autopsy. At autopsy diseased conditions of the sinuses are found much more frequently than was suspected during life. One reason for this is that many suppurative processes of the sinuses cause so little suffering that the patient does not seek the advice of a physician. In certain cases also the diagnosis presents many difficulties.

Aids to the diagnosis of affections of the accessory sinuses have increased very much during the past few years. Transillumination and skiagraphy are of the greatest service. Trial punctures of the antrum of Highmore are made, and the nasofrontal duct is made more patulous so that pus in this region can be more readily detected.

The ethmoid cells offer the greatest difficulties to intranasal manipulations.

In ethmoid disease, unless pus can be seen coming directly from the cells, repeated examinations may be necessary to make a diagnosis, and if the patient and physician lack the necessary amount of patience, many cases of ethmoiditis may be overlooked.

The subjective light reflex, and skiagraphs may point to the disease, but after all, the surest indication is the presence of pus in the nose.

In cases in which no pus can be found on nasal examination the suction method, which has been advocated by certain authors for years, will draw out even the smallest quantity of pus. This is particularly true in disease of the ethmoid cells.

The writer recommends for this purpose the use of a specially constructed pump with a vacuum meter, with which a uniform pressure can be maintained.

He has been able to demonstrate the presence of pus in certain cases in which absolutely none could be found in the nose before the suction pump was used. It is particularly useful in disease of the posterior ethmoid cells and sphenoidal sinus, conditions often presenting great diagnostic difficulties.

It is also of great value in the treatment of suppurative affections of the sinuses. The main object of the treatment in acute cases is to get the pus out of the sinuses; and this, the author states, can be readily accomplished with the suction pump.

Theisen.

The Sphenoidal Sinus; a Study Based on the Examination of Eighty-five Specimens.

JAS. A. GIBSON, Buffalo (*Jour. A. M. A.*, December 19, 1908). The transverse diameter is slightly greater than the antero-posterior: when the expansion of the air chamber takes place in the anterior direction, it usually does so as enlarged posterior ethmoid cells. The average antero-posterior diameter of 81 specimens was 23.25 mm (24/25 inch); transverse diameter of 70 specimens was 29 mm (1 3/16 inch): vertical diameter of 75 specimens was 18 mm (3/4 inch). Thickness of anterior wall averaged .25 to .50 mm (1/100 to 1/50 inch): the roof varies from .25 mm to 1 mm and over, rarely 2 mm: the floor is usually thicker than either of the other boundaries, being always thickest posteriorly and ranging from .25 mm to 9 mm (1/100 to almost 1/3 inch). The thickest part of the posterior wall is always found on the same level as the floor: this wall varies in thickness from .25 mm to 10 mm (1/100 to 2/5 inch). The anterior wall of the sinus usually projects in front of a plane drawn vertically through the hamular processes. The bony wall between the optic foramen and the sinus is very thin, varying from .25 mm to 1 or 2 mm. In eighty specimens the distance between the anterior wall of the sinus and the anterior nasal spine varied from 45 mm to 71 mm, the average being 57 mm (2 1/2 inches).

The lamina separating the two sinuses may be displaced either to the left or right and is frequently obliquely placed: no communication was found between the sinuses. The least distance from the anterior nasal spine to the posterior wall of the sinus is 57 mm (2 1/8 inches). An instrument may be inserted to this distance without fear of entering the cranial cavity.

Richards.

The Present Status of The Radical Operation for Empyema of the Sphenoid Sinus.

Ross HALL SKILLERN, Philadelphia (*Jour. A. M. A.*, December 19, 1908). A modified hook for opening the ostium sphenoidale and a modification of the Hajek bone forceps are used. After cocain anesthesia with 20 per cent solution and adrenalin the posterior half of the middle turbinate is removed with scissors and cold snare: the posterior ethmoid cells are then broken through with Hajek's ethmoid hook, the debris being removed with a conchotome or similar instrument. The ostium being visible, the evulsor is introduced and the ostium opened 8-10 mm. in diameter. The bent forceps of Hajek are now used and as much bone removed as is necessary to ensure a permanent opening, which should reach to the floor of the sinus. Granulations, if present, should be let alone for two weeks, when if they have not subsided under free drainage they may be curetted, but never on the superior and lateral walls.

Richards.

III—LARYNX.

Isolated Paralysis of the Musculus Rectus Externus With Purulent Middle Ear Disease on the Same Side.

PEYSER, Berlin (*Berlin. klin. Wochenschr.*, No. 26, 1908). Based on a study of his own case and others gathered from the literature, the author comes to the conclusion that paralysis of the abducens takes place from the purulent middle ear disease, per contiquitatem, by way of the soft parts.

Horn.

Fundamental Principles in the Treatment of Laryngeal Tuberculosis.

BOURACK (*Archives Internationales de Laryngologie*, July, 1908, to January, 1909) begins by speaking of the number of articles which have appeared upon this subject in the last five years and of certain new procedures which have to a certain extent taken the place of the older methods. He refers to the teach'ng of only twenty-five years ago, that laryngeal tuberculosis was an incurable infection. The surgical treatment has been bitterly opposed and for a long time practiced by only a few men. Today, with more or less restrictions, it is employed in the majority of clinics. There are indeed even partisans of exo-laryngeal methods, "laryngotomy, laryngectomy, partial or complete, and .tracheotomy." In the last few years there have been repeated in the foreign press new, skeptical views on the treatment of laryngeal tuberculosis. Today there is certainly neither the doubt and despair of 1870 and 1880 nor the enthusiasm of 1890 on the subject. One can now make his examination without partiality. Above all we can actually assert as proved the view that laryngeal tuberculosis ought to be treated energetically as a local affection and that we ought not to confine ourselves to treatment of the lungs, nor to a belief that a physico-dietetic treatment is sufficient. Great attention should be paid to the condition of the lungs. The observations of the last ten years show that pulmonary tuberculosis, especially fibroid forms, can be healed; nevertheless the lesion of the larynx is an independent one as is shown by the fact that we can get healing here while the disease in the lungs advances. This destroys the argument of those who say all that is required is to get the pulmonary condition better. It must not be forgotten that laryngeal affection left to itself has a tendency to progress and spontaneous healing is a great rarity. In the majority of the most important clinics of the world the choice of medical or surgical remedies varies with the condition in the particular case. Medical treatment is, however, insufficient, as we do not know of any medical specific against it. No one has any longer the faith in lactic acid, menthol, etc., which he formerly had. Krause, the discoverer of lactic acid, today recommends intravenous injections of betol. While energetic applications of lactic acid, 50 or 75 per cent or even pure, or of para-chloro-phenol or phenol-sulforicine or the mixture of Bonain have at times produced healing, at other times they are entirely powerless. There are today few opponents of the surgical treatment of laryngeal tuberculosis, if one can judge from literature. The difficulty is to determine the precise indications for its employment. We can say, however, in general, that the cases where operative intervention is to be employed are more limited than was the case ten years ago. The debut of laryngeal tuberculosis presents itself under such a variety of forms that no general system of treatment can satisfactorily be established, each case requires its own particular line of treatment. Authorities now insist upon one feature which cannot be overlooked—the *healing tendency* of the organ—it is due to this that the curette or galvano-cautery are a benefit at times with extensive infiltration and at other times are powerless against infiltration or against ulceration which does not appear extensive.

It is on account of this that indications for operative intervention are, according to the most recent authorities, fixed in such an uncertain manner. In general, however, the limits have, in the last years, been notably changed compared with those given by Krause. For example, Imhofer does not regard an advanced general condition and a pronounced local process as a contraindication to operation, because, according to his opinion, laryngeal tuberculosis is curable in the advanced stages. Kuttner operates even when the laryngeal lesions are extensive.

Bezold formerly operated for a bad general condition particularly with the aim of relieving the patient when suffering from dyspnea and dysphagia, but after a number of failures he has become more prudent in the choice of his cases; he no longer operates when the erosions are of slight extent, if the infiltrations are not ulcerated and if the process does not present any signs of rapid advance. On the other hand, he hastens to operate in cases where the infiltration shows a distinct ulceration and is commencing to advance, if there are ulcerated indurated borders and if there is a tubercle under the ulceration. Contrary to Mermod and Grünwald, he does not use the galvano-cautery except rarely, never when the infiltration and inflammation are extensive. From his experience as director of the Sanitorium of Falkenstein, he has no confidence in tracheotomy and believes all exo-laryngeal methods involve too much risk.

Gleitsmann announced in 1903 the following indications for curettage: First—primary laryngeal tuberculosis. Second—limited infiltration and ulceration. Third—indurated infiltration of the interarytenoid space and infiltration of the arytenoid cartilage and the false vocal chords. Fourth—in the initial stages of pulmonary affection. Fifth—in advanced pulmonary tuberculosis with dysphagia, the result of inflammation of the arytenoid.

Heryng in the first years of his enthusiasm operated even upon the most advanced cases, but in recent years he has become more circumspect and gives the following indication for operation: First—tubercles of the epiglottis. Second—chronic infiltrations of the posterior wall. Third—chronic tubercles upon inflamed tissues resisting other methods of treatment. Fourth—affection limited to one region of the larynx.

Krause operates also in cases of diffused infiltration of the false vocal chords, posterior wall and epiglottis and in extensive ulceration when there are extensive lesions in the lungs.

The Vienna school is in general more conservative than is the Berlin school.

Hajek does not operate except when there are very small ulcerations and the general condition is satisfactory.

At the meeting of the Laryngological Society of London, the majority of those present expressed themselves in favor of the endo-laryngeal methods in the treatment of laryngeal tuberculosis.

Semon regards perichondritis of the arytenoid and edema as contraindications, and that success is less likely where there is general inflammation.

Levy uses curettage in cases of limited ulceration and not alone in cases of ulceration which show a tendency to advance. He advises excision in cases where one can hope to be able to entirely remove the diseased part and the galvano-cautery in cases of superficial ulceration of small extent. Tracheotomy can be employed in others, but never total resection.

Finder and Alexander, from the clinic of B. Fraenkel, recommend curettage particularly in tubercles and ulceration of limited extent and they regard advanced pulmonary trouble as an contraindication. They never touch indurated infiltrations on the posterior wall. The best results, according to Finder, are obtained by the use of curettage where there are ulcerations of the false and true vocal chords of epiglottis. Exo-laryngeal methods have not been received with great favor.

Blumenfeld reported fifty-four cases of laryngotomies performed for tuberculosis.

Gluck, out of two hundred and fifty cases, has done thirteen for tuberculosis; in eleven of these there was a good result obtained.

Exo-laryngeal methods are recommended by many authors

in cases of laryngeal tuberculosis in cases of pregnant women. Contrary to the usual impression, such a condition in pregnancy is not rare; almost all the patients die after confinement.

Tracheotomy has rarely had a favorable action, probably because it was practiced too late.

Authorities differ about the advisability of performing an abortion. Tracheotomy has been recommended as a therapeutie means in laryngeal tuberculosis since 1868.

M. Schmidt in 1897 gave the following indications for tracheotomy: First—laryngeal stenosis. Second—grave lesions of the larynx if the lungs are not seriously affected in the absence of stenosis. Third—the rapid progress of the disease before the appearance of dyspnea. Later, Schmidt does not insist upon the indication furnished by the lungs.

Chiari believes an early tracheotomy has a favorable effect not only upon the evolution of the laryngeal affection, but also upon the pulmonary affection. Nevertheless in adults, in spite of the great authority of Schmidt, tracheotomy plays an inconsiderable role in the treatment of laryngeal tuberculosis. The operation has been condemned by MacKenzie.

Krause, aserts that by immobilization of the diseased organ, one can hope theoretically to obtain improvement in the local condition, he has, indeed, witnessed two favorable actions. These favorable results are, however, rare as a rule when the condition of the lungs is advanced. Generally when employed, after the operation the expectoration becomes more abundant, the disease advances and the suffering of the patient is, at times, greatly increased.

Mermod is also opposed to tracheotomy, especially as he has observed two cases of extensive ulceration around the tracheal wound. The other methods, *electrolysis, cauterization* and *incision* are of much less importance.

Mermod was at one time enthusiastic in the use of electrolysis but he has now abandoned it, except in advanced cases on account of the time necessary. He employs the monopole cathode introduced into the larynx with a current of fifteen to twenty milliamperes and also employs it in the case of voices of professionals when redness or slight infiltration of one of the vocal chords exists. The *incision* is also very little employed today. The most frequent form of surgical treatment is the *curette*.

More recently the employment of the galvano-cautery has come forward.

Grünwald, in a recent article (1907), recommends warmly, deep cauterization for the purpose of destroying morbid tissue, thus avoiding, as far as possible, any reaction in the tissues and without destroying, without definite object, the mucosa in order not to give a channel for the spread of the affection. Where the lesions are well defined, and particularly when situated in the interior of the larynx, he practices laryngo-fissure. In affection of the vestibule of larynx, and especially in the lower portion of the pharynx, he practices subhyoid pharyngotomy. If there is perichondritis, he practices a partial resection. If there is grave stenosis, he practices tracheotomy.

Mermod makes use of cauterization in many hundreds of cases, even in those with grave complications.

He has abandoned curettage since he had two severe cases of hemorrhage. One advantage of the galvano-cautery over the curette and cutting instruments is its small diameter. In his opinion it is necessary to destroy all the diseased tissue which is accessible to the eye and instrument. It makes no difference to him whether the infiltrations are ulcerated or not. Many months are often necessary because long intervals have to elapse between treatments. He believes that the indications for its use should be enlarged to the greatest possible degree. He has, indeed, obtained good results in cases which seemed to be most desperate. He does not give any precise indications, but takes into account, as do Finder and the others, the healing tendency. In short, he often fixes the indications ex juvantibus et nocentibus. If the operation increases the trouble, there is little probability that one can obtain success; but in the sluggish cases he believes in energetic local treatment not only with the aim to heal, but at least to relieve the suffering of the patient. He has observed ten cases where the laryngeal affection remained for a long time the only manifestation of tuberculosis. Out of 280 cases treated by galvano-cautery 60 have remained healed for a year after the operation; 40 for more than two years; 17 for more than three years; and one has had no return in 16 years. In recent years attention has been turned to *photo-therapy, x-ray and radium.* The results, unfortunately, do not allow us to form any opinion at present as to their value.

As a conclusion of the foregoing we can say that up to the present time we have no method which is a sure cure for laryngeal tuberculosis. Nevertheless we can not question that energetic treatment often obtains good results where expectant treatment would allow the patient to perish. In our treatment the patient should be placed under the most favorable climatic and hygienic conditions, employing the best surgical means at our disposal, generally curettage or galvano-cautery. Sur-alimentation is of the greatest importance and to that end all the functions of the stomach and intestines should be looked to. Constipation should be avoided; proper breathing through the nose is essential. All of these measures can be more easily applied where the patient can receive the constant attention of a physician and is subject to a regular régime. This can be best done in a sanatorium. The climatic conditions of the sanatorium play an important role. It is, then, of the first importance to take into consideration the form of the affection when one advises a removal to a particular altitude. This will depend upon the form of the affection—whether it is torpid, the cough dry or the expectoration abundant. First—we have a choice of treatment by pure air. Second—treatment by the sun's rays. Third—treatment by elevation and altitude. Fourth—by sea air and sea baths. Air rich in ozone is desirable, humid air is to be avoided. The patient should be protected from the cold north winds and placed where cloudy days are not frequent nor changes in temperature sudden. The importance of solar baths is today admitted. Authorities differ regarding the advantages of mountainous airs for patients with febrile symptoms and affected with congested form of laryngeal tuberculosis. It is a fact that dry mountainous air has a good effect on patients who suffer from abundant expectoration, while sea air is much more desirable for patients who have a dry cough. The sea air is badly borne by those who suffer from congested forms. Chronic and pronounced laryngeal catarrh, which is often found, ought to make us think of the possibility of tuberculosis, especially in those of an early age. With these general measures it is important to employ local treatment. From a critical study of the various published works and from my own personal observations, we should proceed as follows: During the first few weeks no operative intervention should be undertaken. The patient can employ at home, many times a day, disinfecting and inhalation treatments. Further, we can use injections or cauterizations by using lactic acid or formalin or a mixture of lactic, chromic and formalin or a mixture of lactic, formalin and phenic acid or by methelyne blue.

It is important to recommend to the patient to avoid all fatigue from voice use.

Körner has, in a recent communication, recommended iodide of potassium. If this medical treatment does not answer and if limited infiltrations should have a tendency to ulcerate, especially when they are located on the true vocal chords or in the arytenoid space or upon the epiglottis, the employment of the curette is indicated. This should be used with confidence and energy after thorough anesthesia. Such an operative treatment should not be undertaken when we are dealing with congested forms if the pulmonary lesions are deep, but we should not be stopped by this contraindication. In cases of granulation, which precede stenosis, we must not wait too long. When it is possible we should remove the granulation with cutting forceps. In the case of superficial infiltrations upon the epiglottis or the vocal chords, especially if diffused on the free borders, and if the affections are found below the vocal chords, the curette is insufficient. It is necessary then to employ the galvano-cautery. Nevertheless, when one knows how to make use of the curette it can also be used when the process is largely extended, when for example there are large ulcerations of the epiglottis, false vocal chords and the arytenoid space. In the case of large and profound infiltrations we can attempt the destroying of them by deep cauterization. Vegetations of the posterior wall of the larynx, which, as we know, often proceed for a long time without ulcerating, ought, by preference, to be left alone, at least if they do not show any tendency to break down and if the functional troubles resulting do not become more severe, producing loss of voice and painful dyspnea. If the operative intervention is badly borne it will be necessary to abandon it. When there is danger of suffocation as a result of the infiltration and granulation, tracheotomy will have to be performed if the physician is opposed to curettage.

Harris.

BOOK REVIEWS.

De Krankheiten Der Oberen Luftwege.

By MORITZ SCHMIDT AND EDMUND MEYER. Fourth Edition.
Published by Julius Springer, Berlin. Price, bound, 22
Marks ; postage, 2.10 Marks.

A new edition of this most popular of all German text books
on the Diseases of the Nose, Throat and Upper Air Passages,
will be greeted with pleasure by its old friends and is certain
to make many new ones.

The recent death of Moritz Schmidt led us to fear that the
former edition would be but an insufficient monument to his
name. Prof. Meyer, his friend and pupil, has undertaken the
editing of the new volume, which while retaining the general
form of the old, has given us a strictly modern text book.

Moritz Schmidt's original aim was to put a book into the
hands of the general practitioner, which would enable him not
only to appreciate the close relationship between diseases of
the upper air passages and general diseases, but also to recognize what he could himself properly treat and what should be
sent to the specialist.

A clear and convincing style, a wealth of practical details
in treatment, and the personal experiences of this great
teacher, characterizes the work. It seems hardly fair to select
any one chapter for review, as they are all good. The chapter
on Syphilis is especially fine. A clear and lucid explanation
of the Wasserman's serum reaction, an acceptance of the
Spirillum as the causative factor in the disease and a general
survey of the often clouded symptomology, is given.

Leukemia, Gout and many other of the rarer diseases of
the upper air passages are fully treated, and special attention
is given to the new growths of the larynx and trachea.

For the laryngologist, the chapter on the Nervous Diseases
of the Respiratory Tract is of especial importance. One gains
at once a comprehensive view of the entire subject and the
lesson is so clearly taught that it remains forever in the
memory.

Many have said that the book reads like a novel and truly
one finishes the 700 pages with a sigh of satisfaction, for one
feels that it is possible to compile an encyclopedic text book
and still have it interesting.

The illustrations are all from the well-known hand of the artist Helbrig, and the press and binding leave nothing to be desired. Horn.

Beiträge Zur Anatomie, Physiologie, Pathologie und Therapie des Ohres, der Nase, und des Halses.

Herausgegeben von A. Passow und K. L. Schaefer. Published by S. Karger, Berlin, Carlstrasse, 15.

The reviewer of this important contribution to the current literature of the anatomy, physiology, pathology and therapy of the ear, nose and throat, has taken the liberty of waiting until two volumes have appeared, before passing judgment on the new journal. Under the above title, Passow, the director of the Charité Clinic in Berlin, and Professor Schaefer, well known for his work on the physical and mathematical side of the physiology of the ear, nose and throat, have undertaken the direction of this journal, which seems to fill a place unoccupied by any of the other journals now in existence. It covers the more scientific and technical side of our specialty as concerns especially physics and physiology, as well as various important practical contributions regarding operations, new methods, etc.

Two volumes appear during the year, containing about 500 pages. The subscription price is twenty marks or five dollars per volume, separate numbers of which appear at irregular intervals of about six weeks.

The following selection from the list of titles well indicates what a wide range of subjects is covered by this journal and shows the importance of the scientific side of our specialty:

Band I. Über Stellung und Bewegung des Kehlkopfes bei normalen und pathologischen Sprechvorgängen. Von Priv. Doz. Dr. H. Gutzman, Berlin.

Band I. Beiträge zur Submukösen Fensterresektion der Nasenscheidewand. Von Dr. Gustav Killian, Freiburg i. Br.

Band I. Das Satyrohr eine intrauterine Belastungsdifformität. Von Priv. Doz. Dr. Carl Springer, Prag.

Band II. Die Prognose des otischen Hirnabscesses. Von Prof. Dr. B. Heine, Königsberg i. Pr.

Band II. Beiträge zur pathologischen Anatomie der Otitis externa beim Hunde. Von Dr. R. Imhofer in Prag.

Band II. Über die Wahrnehmung der Schallrichtung. Von Dr. Kurtz Münnich in Berlin. Horn.

Larynx Tuberculosis and Pregnancy.

SOKOLOWSKY, Königsberg (Sammlung aus dem Gebeite der Nasen, Ohren, und Halskrankheiten., Band IX; Heft 6.

In an exceedingly interesting and important article the author shows what a problem confronts the general practitioner and specialist, when out of 230 pregnant women, who had at the same time a larynx tuberculosis, 200 died in pregnancy of that disease, while in the 18 cases where an artificial abortion was made, 14 of these were saved.

His conclusions, with which nearly all the authorities who have studied this subject agree, are:

1: Pregnancy complicated with larynx tuberculosis, leads almost always to death. In the few that survive, 70 per cent of the children are tubercular.

2. Tracheotomy as a therapeutic measure is of little value.

3. Early artificial abortion is always indicated in pregnancy complicated with larynx tuberculosis.

Three exceptions to this rule are to be noted:

    a. In the case of tuberculous larynx tumors.

    b. Where the larynx tuberculosis appears in the last few weeks of pregnancy.

    c. Where the condition of the patient is palpably hopeless.

4. Every married woman with tuberculosis should be warned of the dangers attending conception.

HORN.

Physiology of Voice and Speech.

BY PROF. H. GUTZMANN, Berlin. Published by Friedr. Vieweg & Sohn in Braunschweig. Price, unbound, 8 Marks; bound, 9 Marks; Postage, Mark 0.50.

Prof. Gutzmann, in the present work, has brought together much of the important matter appertaining to the Physiology of the Voice and Speech, which was formerly only to be found in his scattered monographs. The book is a survey of recent advancements in this branch of science and is not directed alone to the physician, but to the Physiologist, Phoneticer, Linguist, Specialist for Disturbances of Speech and the Teachers of the Deaf and Dumb.

The matter is explained in the author's clear and lucid style and the 200 pages of text are all solid information. The presswork is of the best and many well selected pictures, diagrams and tables illustrate the work.   HORN.

The Proceedings of the "Vereins Deutscher Laryngologen" for 1908.

A. Stuber's Verlag, Würzburg.   Price, Marks 7.50.

The latest developments of rhinologic and laryngologic science, as brought out in the annual meeting of the German Laryngological Society, seldom find their way into the current literature.   Some very important papers were read, a detailed review of which would be here impossible.   Prof. Killian in his paper on the "Diseases of the Accessory Sinuses in Scarlet Fever" brought up a subject of extraordinary interest.   Von Eichborn's demonstration of the latest method of treating carcinoma of the mouth and throat by means of "fulguration," which briefly stated is the use of electrical currents of enormous tension and frequency, has led us to hope that some progress has been made in the battle against this dread disease.   The other papers were of equal interest and a copy of the proceedings should find its way yearly into the library of every German-reading specialist.

HORN.

The History of Laryngology at the University of Heidelberg.

By PROF. A. JURAZ.   Published by A. Stuber's Verlag, Würzburg.   Bound in paper; Price, Marks 3.00 ($.75).

To the friends and students of Prof. Juraz and others interested in the historical development of laryngology this little brochure lets one into the secret of local conditions in this famous old university, and shows how, even in Germany, politics play an important role even at the expense of science.

HORN.

ANNALS

OF

OTOLOGY, RHINOLOGY

AND

LARYNGOLOGY.

VOL. XVIII.   SEPTEMBER, 1909.   No. 3.

XXXII.

PROGRESS OF LARYNGOLOGY AND RHINOLOGY SINCE THE INVENTION OF THE LARYNGO-SCOPE, WITH SPECIAL REFERENCE TO THE PARTICIPATION OF AMERICA IN THIS PROGRESS.

By John Sendziak,

Warsaw (Poland).

Mr. President and Fellows of the American Academy of Oph-thalmology and Oto-Laryngology:

It is first my pleasant duty to express to you my sincerest thanks for the great honor of inviting me to come to America and deliver an address at this meeting.

I have accepted this invitation with greater willingness in that it gives me the opportunity, as a representative of the Polish nation, of expressing my gratefulness to your great country which has so generously and appreciatingly recognized the merits of my countrymen, Kosciuzko and Pulaski, who

*An address delivered before the American Academy of Ophthalmology and Oto-Laryngology, at the meeting in New York City, October 4 to 6, 1909.

joined in the fight for its freedom. And I feel thankful too for your country's hospitality and generosity towards my people who are forced by grievous conditions to seek in another hemisphere means of earning their daily bread.

Before passing to the subject proper of my address, the development of laryngology and rhinology since the invention of the laryngoscope, with special reference to the participation of America in this development, allow me to honor the memory of the distinguished representatives of our specialty in America who have been called away by the common foe from their great activity. I shall mention here only the names of Elsberg, a pioneer in American laryngology; O'Dwyer, Morgan, Hooper, Jarvis, Thorner, Mulhall, Lincoln, Daly, Asch, Dickerman, Glasgow, Shadle, etc., all of whom have achieved a permanent place in laryngologic literature.

Let me, also, as a representative of European laryngo-rhinology, salute the great body of our fraternity in America, among the most eminent of whom are those who are here assembled.

In preparing the paper which was written for the fifty-year jubilee of the invention of the laryngoscope, and published in the *Centralblatt f. Laryngologie* last year, upon the development of laryngology and rhinology in the individual countries, I was struck by the uncommon strength and number of the papers written by our American colleagues.

It is sufficient to state that one-third of all the literature on laryngology and oto-laryngology comes from America.

It is worthy of note that here in New York where this meeting takes place, the first general laryngological society was founded in 1873, more than thirty-five years ago. The first German society, however, was organized in 1877, four years later, as the oto-laryngological section of the Association of German Naturalists and Physicians. In other countries, such societies were founded much later.

In general, oto-laryngology and ophthalmology, often associated together, did not attain the recognition in any European country as in America.

Already in 1861, soon after the invention of the laryngoscope, the great Elsberg, who died alas too soon, was teaching his specialty in the New York University. Since that time special chairs of oto-laryngology have been established in all the American universities, more than one hundred in number.

In this regard and with respect to special hospitals devoted to oto-laryngology and ophthalmology, old Europe remains considerably behind her younger sister.

There are quite a number of special oto-laryngologic journals (six) in America, about one-sixth of all publications of this character. It is worthy of note that the *Archives of Laryngology* was established in New York in 1880, nearly thirty years ago. It was unfortunately only continued for three years. Only two European journals were founded before this, the *Monatsschrift für Ohrenheilkunde, etc.*, in Germany in 1867, and the *Annales des Maladies des Oreilles, etc.*, in France in 1875.

The tremendous development of American laryngo-rhinology is strikingly shown in the immense number of papers published, 13,000, more than one-fourth of those in the literature of laryngo-rhinology during the past twenty-five years. In this respect America occupies the first place among the nations of the world.

Of these, about 1300 of the American publications are general in character; there are fifteen manuals of laryngology, rhinology and otology, about one-sixth of the total of such publications.

Several of those have passed through a number of editions, testifying to their value, for instance, Solis Cohen, Seiler, Sajous, Bosworth, Coakley, Braden Kyle (four editions of this excellent treatise have been published). One of the first treatises on diseases of the upper-air passages was published in America, that of Horace Green, in 1840, in prelaryngoscope days. The first was published in Germany in 1829, by Albert of Bonn. One of the best histories of laryngology came from the pen of your very distinguished fellow-citizen, Jonathan Wright.

The exceedingly important relation between laryngo-rhinology and general medicine, to which attention was called first by Loeri of Buda-Pesth in 1885, and later by Friedrich of Leipzig, and Semon of London, has been the subject of many valuable papers by Americans, viz., Goodale, Goldsmith, Freudenthal, Johnston. Mayer, Simpson, Harris, Stucky, Levy, Stein, Bryant and many others who have discussed the relation of diseases of ear, nose and throat to nervous and mental diseases, rheumatism, gout, diabetes mellitus, lues, tuberculosis and diseases of the digestive and circulatory systems. All but Simpson came to the conclusion that a causal relation undoubtedly exists between them.

The relation between diseases of the nose, especially those of the accessory sinuses, and the eye, to which attention was called in Europe by Ziem, Jonas, Onodi, etc., has been, of late, carefully studied by American specialists: Pierce, Cutler, Griffin, Holmes, Hoople, Murphy, Johnston, Halstead, Pooley, Hastings, Posey, Brawley and Loeb (anatomic research). Flatau and Gutzman in Germany have written many special articles on the voice and its culture and speech defects; in America, Hudson Makuen, Scripture, Miller, Solis Cohen, Holbrook Curtis and many others.

In the realm of anatomy, histology, pathologic anatomy, bacteriology and physiology of the upper-air tract, in which Zuckerkandl, Onodi and Hajek in Austria, B. Fraenkel, Kuttner, Heymann and Klemperer in Germany, Semon and Horsley in England, Dmochowski in Poland and Broeckaert in Holland have distinguished themselves, I may mention the very valuable papers, in America, of Loeb, Ingersoll, Bryson, Delavan, Holmes, Wood, Ballenger, Jonathan Wright, Pierce, Hooper and many others.

I pass on to the methods of examination of the upper-air passages. As an auxiliary to laryngoscopy, which was introduced more than fifty years ago by Garcia, Tuerck and Czermak, there have been added a number of methods, especially autoscopy by Kirstein of Germany, high and low tracheoscopy (this latter was first applied by my compatriot, Prof. Pieniazek of Cracow), bronchoscopy, the famous work of Killian of Freiburg, esophagoscopy (Stoerk in Austria, Mikulicz in Poland, Hacker and Rosenheim in Germany), transillumination of the accessory nasal cavities (Vohsen of Frankfort on the Main and my compatriot, Heryng) and radioscopy, the application of the Roentgen rays, minutely described at the first international congress of laryngology at Vienna by Burger of Amsterdam, Ferreri of Rome, Gradenigo of Turin and Killian of Freiburg.

All of these methods have been described in detail in America. Above all, Chevalier Jackson, of Pittsburg, who wrote an excellent monograph, the first in English, on tracheobronchoscopy, esophagoscopy, and gastroscopy, then Halstead, Chisholm, etc. French brought photography into the service of laryngology, Beck stereoscopy and stereopticon color photography and Bleyer the phonograph.

Levy made studies of the newer diagnostic methods, such as tests for tuberculosis (ophthalmoreaction of Calmette) and the Wasserman reaction for syphilis (Smithies, etc).

Passing on to the remedies and therapeutic methods which have enriched our field since the advent of laryngoscopy, partly collected in the excellent pharmacopea of Lefferts (2d edition, 1885), I must in the first place cite cocain (eucain, alypin, etc.), introduced in 1884 to laryngology by Jellinek of Vienna. The introduction of the specific serum simultaneously by Roux of Paris and Behring of Berlin was of the greatest inportance in the treatment of diphtheria, as well as the use of intubation in laryngeal diphtheria, which was the contribution of the eminent American physician, O'Dwyer.

Phototherapy (sunlight, ultra violet rays, Finsen's method), Roentgen rays and radium, the latest discovered by my compatriot, Sklodowska (Currie) of Paris, have been utilized for different diseases of the upper-air passages, especially lupus and malignant disease; likewise electricity, galvanocautery and electrolysis have been utilized in Europe (Gradenigo, Ferreri, etc.) and in America (Freudenthal, Scheppegrell and many others).

Solis Cohen has written an excellent monograph on inhalations, the principal exponent of which in Europe is Heryng of Warsaw.

Other methods which have been tried in minute detail in America are paraffin injections, first applied by Gersuny of Vienna, for malformations of the nose (nez de mouton, etc.) and Bier's hyperemia, regarding which there is still difference of opinion. The former is sometimes dangerous (cases of sudden blindness, Semon, Davis, Smith).

Among the most important remedies applied with more or less success in diseases of the upper-air passages, I must mention orthoform, introduced as a therapeutic agent for laryngeal tuberculosis by the distinguished American specialist, Freudenthal, and adrenalin for making nasal operations almost bloodless.

Many of the new or modified instruments for the diagnosis and treatment of diseases of the upper-air passages were invented by Americans: Jarvis (snare), Bosworth (saw), Richards, Curtis, Allen, Pierce, Stein, Beck, Ballenger, Freer, etc.

Rhinology, a younger sister of laryngology, has shown a remarkable development during the past twenty-five years,

especially with reference to the accessory sinuses. The literature comprehends more than 11,000 papers or publications,
about one-fourth of the entire laryngo-rhinologic literature, of
which 4500 or 40 per cent are American. The investigations
of Thomson and Hewlett of England, of Wurtz and Lermoyez
of France, and Schousbone of Denmark, showed that the
healthy nasal secretions are free from bacteria and possess
bactericidal properties. As to the cause of atrophic rhinitis
some authors in America, such as Rice, regard it as due to a
special organism (Loewenberg-Abel diplococcus), while others, for instance the well-known specialist Kyle, do not.

Beck among others in America opposes Grünwald's theory
of the simultaneous causal connection between atrophic rhinitis and affections of the accessory nasal cavities. As to the
treatment of this obstinate disease most of the writers in
America, for instance Richards, are pessimistic. On the contrary, Brown of Triest, and Laker of Graz consider vibratory
massage as most efficacious (Weightman in America), but the
method has not come into general use. The same thing applies to electrolysis by Belgian authors (Cheval, etc.) and
antidiphtheritic serum by Italian writers (Belfanti, Della Ve-
dova, etc.).

Hypertrophies of the turbinates are best treated with galvanocautery, less so by resection. Stucky in America is not
favorable to operations on the middle turbinate, a view with
which I concur.

Deviations of the nasal septum have of late been made the
subject of many papers in America, by Jackson, Ballenger,
Swain, Rhodes, Hurd, Sheedy, etc. Killian in Europe and
Freer in America almost simultaneously devised the submucous resection operation, now generally adopted.

Braden Kyle proposes the V shaped resection and Price
Brown the H shaped. (This latter is simply a modification
of Asch's well-known method.) Beck has recently written
a valuable paper on the surgery of the external deformities
of the nose. Freudenthal has, among others in America, contributed a paper on bleeding from the nose, Gleitsmann,
Mosher and Thrasher on tuberculosis, Donelan, Lincoln and
John Mackenzie on syphilis and Jonathan Wright, Cobb, Levy,
Price Brown, Wishart, etc., on malignant neoplasms.

As to the so-called reflex neuroses of nasal origin (asthma,
hay fever, headaches, cough, enuresis nocturna, epilepsy, etc.)

it should be stated that since Hack's publications appeared the boundless enthusiasm has given way to a more rational opinion to the effect that there is undoubtedly a causal relation which, however, is by no means so frequent as certain writers such as Jonas in Germany still maintain; at that, sometimes, but not so very frequently, the removal of the cause by appropriate surgical operation on the nose is followed by the disappearance of the nervous symptoms. Wendell Phillips of New York, on the contrary, is somewhat skeptical of this point.

It should be mentioned that more recent publications suggest new methods of treatment of asthma by bronchoscopy (Nowotny from the clinic of Pieniazek in Cracow), and of hay fever by serum (Loeb), by submucous injections of alcohol (our esteemed President Stein) and by immunization (Curtis).

In the main, it should be stated that in recent literature the abuse of nasal operations may be noted, to which Semon justly drew attention in Europe and John Mackenzie in America. This pertains especially to the use of the galvanocautery, the resection of the turbinates and operations on the nasal septum.

Above all, the development of our knowledge of the accessory nasal cavities and their pathologic process has been marvellous during the past twenty-five years. Beginning with Ziem's clinical investigations on the antrum of Highmore and the anatomic research of Zuckerkandl, the subject has been carried forward by such men as Killian, Grünwald, Gerber and Uffenorde of Germany, Hajek and Onodi of Austria and Oppikofer of Basel, all authors of the newest and most exhaustive monographs on the subject.

In America there have been many valuable papers written on the subject, anatomic and physiologic by Loeb, Chisholm and Ingersoll, clinical by Lothrop, Coffin, Myles, Coakley, Cobb, Richards, Ingals, Jackson, Curtis, Roe, Holmes, Theisen, Ballenger, Kyle, de Roaldes, Johnston (empyema) and by Gleitsman (tuberculosis).

In general, it may be stated that skiagraphy occupies the final position in the transillumination of the accessory cavities for diagnostic purposes.

So far as the nasopharynx is concerned the greatest attention during the past twenty-five years has been devoted to the so-called adenoid vegetations, although the pathologic condition had been described in 1868, more than forty years ago, by the Danish otologist, Wilhelm Meyer, in honor of whom the laryngologic world erected a monument in his native town, Copenhagen.

One of the best monographs on the subject was written by Gradenigo of Turin. Many valuable papers have been published in America, among others, by Braden Kyle, Paz, de Roaldes, Legurd, Richards, as well as Freer, who proposes the operation through the nose, an old method suggested by the father of adenoids vegetations, now generally abandoned in Europe for Gottstein's or Beckmann's curettes, applied through the mouth, without general narcosis (except in England).

Roy has written a paper on Tornwaldt's disease, bursitis nasopharyngealis, and Makuen on nasopharyngeal tumors.

The oral and pharyngeal cavities have been made the subject of many papers during the past twenty-five years—about 13,000, of which 3,500, more than one-fourth, have come from America. Among these are the anatomic as well as physiologic papers of the distinguished American specialists, Wood, Pierce, Ballenger, etc.

The nature of the so-called follicular angina and its relation to diphtheria have been the subject of many papers. Most of the writers (B. Fraenkel, myself and others) on bacteriologic grounds regard it as an independent pathologic process having nothing in common with true diphtheria, staphylococci, streptococci and pseudodiphtheritic bacilli being constantly found in follicular angina. De Roaldes and Ward have written, among others, on this point.

An enormous literature exists upon diphtheria and its treatment with the Roux-Behring antidiphtheritic serum, both in Europe and America, about 6,000 papers, of which 1,500, one-fourth, are from America.

The results are generally favorable—for instance Martin in America reports only 9.7 per cent of deaths. The treatment of croup by intubation, now adopted in Europe, is of everlasting credit to the American physician, O'Dwyer.

Cobb, Fitzwilliams, Holmes and others have written on tonsillar, peritonsillar and retropharyngeal abscess. Chevalier Jackson advises tonsillectomy instead of tonsillotomy, for hypertrophied faucial tonsils, an opinion with which Richards concurs. It is, however, difficult to agree with this view.

Hypertrophy of the lingual tonsil, to which attention has been drawn in Europe only in more recent times (Michael's of Hamburg excellent monograph), has been discussed by many writers in America, Gleitsmann, Oppenheimer, etc.

Vincent's angina, but lately described as due to the haeillus fusiformis (Plaut-Vincent), has been described among others by Buhlig in America, but the pathologic process itself requires still further investigation. The same requirement exists for the pneumococcus infection of the throat described recently by Semon.

Bryson Delavan, Newcomb and Chevalier Jackson in America have written on tonsillar and peritonsillar bleeding.

Myles, Gibb, Mayer, etc., have written on diseases of the salivary ducts and glands and Stein and Shoemaker on leucoplakia buccalis.

Many of our American colleagues (Richardson, Brown Kelly, Braden Kyle and Wood) have written on mycosis tonsillaris benigna, a disease described under this term for the first time by B. Fraenkel of Berlin in 1873, and afterwards by Heryng of Warsaw (mycosis leptothricia pharyngis). They all adhere to Siebenmann's theory that it is not a proper mycosis, but a hyperkeratosis of the epithelium, the leptothrix buccalis being only accidental. With reference to the so-called black tongue (lingua nigra) which some authors, especially in Poland, Cionglinski, Hewelke and myself, as well as Schmiegelow of Copenhagen, hold to be mycosis (mucor niger, the cause), Johnston and others in America regard it as hyperkeratosis of the lingual papillae.

Robertson, Gleitsmann, Johnston, Levy, Mosher and Danziger have contributed papers on tuberculosis of the oral cavity and pharynx, Bulkley on extragenital syphilis (syphilis in the innocent, 1894) and Goodale, Ross, Freer, Goldstein, etc., on malignant disease.

Tremendous development is shown in our knowledge of the larynx and trachea. The total number of papers reaches about 10,500, of which America has contributed 2,500, almost one-fourth.

Our understanding has attained the highest efficiency in two of the pathologic processes, thanks to the laryngoscope, tuberculosis and malignant tumors of the larynx. Both had been regarded as incurable, as something in nature "noli me tangere." In the first place Moritz Schmidt of Germany in the year 1880 and Heryng of Poland in 1886 proved that laryngeal tuberculosis, a most frequent disease (affecting about one-third of all cases of pulmonary tuberculosis), is undoubtedly curable and that the rational treatment of the disease is surgical. I must say, however, that the enthusiasm in this respect was later greatly diminished (Semon, Schroetter, Chiari in Europe and Jonathan Wright, Robinson, White, Pierce, Casselberry, etc., in America).

It is noteworthy, however, that Bryson Delavan in America already in 1875 wrote an excellent monograph on laryngeal tuberculosis and that Gleitsmann of New York is one of the most earnest enthusiasts in presenting the matter at the international congresses.

Lactic acid, introduced by Krause of Berlin in 1885, has had its advocates up to the present time (Heryng in Europe, White, Coakley, etc., in America).

I appreciate most highly the orthoform treatment of laryngeal tuberculosis recommended first by Freudenthal and applied successfully by Stein, White, etc., especially in cases of dysphagia (best, per se).

Attention, very justly I think, is being drawn to absolute silence as a best curative agent in these cases, especially when combined with climatic treatment in sanatoria. (Semon in Europe and Levy and Freudenthal in America.)

Until we find a specific remedy for the cure of pulmonary tuberculosis, it will be rather fruitless to speak of the radical cure of laryngeal tuberculosis, an opinion which I expressed already in 1889 in my monograph on this subject- (*Jour. of Laryn.*).

As to the relation of pregnancy to laryngeal tuberculosis, Freudenthal and others in America agree with Kuttner of Berlin, that artificial abortion is indicated in such cases.

I pass now to the second important disease, cancer of the larynx, which has become a living question, particularly since the time of the German Emperor, Frederick III.

Before Billroth's time, cancer was likewise considered in the light of "noli me tangere."

With the first laryngectomy performed in 1873 by Billroth, begins the rational, i. e., surgical, treatment of this disease.

It should be stated that in 1864, soon after the introduction of the laryngoscope, the efforts in this direction were made by Elsberg in America, the author of the excellent monograph,

"Laryngeal Surgery in the Treatment of Laryngeal Tumors," by the endolaryngeal route, the method later spread abroad, especially by B. Fraenkel of Berlin. The first two laryngotomies (laryngo-fissure) were performed by American physicians, Buck in 1851 and Sands in 1863. This method is now regarded as the most efficacious in the treatment of the disease, thanks particularly to Semon of London.

It must also be stated that the first lasting result (twenty years recovery) was attained by this method by the Nestor of American laryngologists, Solis Cohen; the best general results being those of Semon of London (80 per cent recoveries) and Chevalier Jackson of Pittsburg (78 per cent).

In my paper prepared for the First International Laryngological Congress, held in Vienna in 1908, entitled "Die Frage der Radikalbehandlung des Larynxkrebs in den letzten 50 Jahren" (1858-1908), I succeeded in collecting from the literature, a tremendous number of cases of laryngeal cancer operated on by the different methods, namely, 1,002. I stated that laryngofissure gave the best results, about 50 per cent of recoveries, endolaryngeal methods 46 per cent, presenting, however, much less security as to relapses, partial laryngectomy 22.8 per cent, and total laryngectomy, 21.6 per cent. The best results from laryngectomy, total and partial, were obtained by von Bergman and Gluck in Germany, Kocher in Bern, Novaro in Turin, Cisneros in Madrid, and Solis Cohen and Hartley in America.

In the main, laryngotomy (laryngofissure) has the greatest number of adherents, including besides Semon and Jackson, already mentioned, von Bruns of Tübingen, Pieniazek of Cracow, Chiari of Vienna, Moure of Bordeaux, and Schmiegelow of Copenhagen.

In addition to Jackson, Bryson Delavan has written in a pessimistic vein upon the subject, and also Stein, Watson, John Mackenzie, etc.

Edematous processes involving the larynx (laryngitis submucosa acuta, erysipelas and abscessus laryngis) have been subjected to considerable elaboration, especially by Kuttner of Berlin in 1895, Massei of Naples in 1885, Hajek of Vienna, 1898-1900, and Semon of London, 1890-1895. The last authority regards acute laryngeal edema or laryngitis submucosa acuta, Massei's erysipelas of the larynx, Senator's acute infectious phlegmon, and angina Ludovici as identical processes, i. e., acute septic infections of the pharynx and larynx.

The American authors who have written on this subject include Pierce on laryngeal phlegmon, and Richardson. Bryson Delavan, among others in America, has written on laryngitis hypoglottica acuta, an affection of the cricoarytenoid articulation, to which Semon drew attention in 1880.

The stenotic processes of the larynx, so admirably described by my compatriot, Pieniazek, have been considered in many valuable papers in America, among others, Price Brown, Fisher and Rogers. Knight, Miller, Casselberry and many others have written upon the etiology, pathology and treatment of vocal nodules (chorditis cantorum), to which Chiari drew attention in Europe.

Roy and Parker advise tracheotomy and thyrotomy in the treatment of papilloma in children. Most European specialists, with Rosenberg of Berlin at the head, favor intralaryngeal operations in such cases.

The greatest progress in our work has been in the domain of nervous diseases of the larynx. This includes the discovery of the phonatory and respiratory centers of the larynx by Krause of Berlin in 1889, and by the English writers Semon and Horsley in 1890, and Risien Russel in 1895, the so-called Semon's law (properly Rosenbach-Semon's) as to the greater vulnerability of the abductors of the larynx in organic paralysis, although the cause of this and of unilateral cortical paralysis is not as yet determined, and the origin of the motor nerve of the larynx, which most authors now believe to be in the nucleus of the vagus.

To the names already quoted of those who have distinguished themselves in this field must be added those of Onodi of Buda-Pesth, Klemperer and Grabower of Germany, Hooper of America, Masini of Italy, and the youngest Broeckaert of Holland.

Recurrent and abductor paralysis was made the subject of discussion at the annual meeting of the American Laryngological Association in 1908 by Gleitsmann, Bryson Delavan, Casselberry and Clarence Rice.

The laryngeal disturbances (paralyses in tabes dorsalis) so minutely described by Burger of Amsterdam, as well as by myself (*Klin. Vortraege. a. d. Geb. d. Otol., etc.,* 1899) have been considered in many papers by American writers, Stein, Freudenthal, Freer, Friedberg, etc. Coolidge has written upon foreign bodies in the larynx, and Emil Mayer of New

York upon scleroma, so well described by the Europeans, Schroetter, Stoerk, Juffinger in Austria, Pieniazek and Bauro-wicz in Poland, and Gerber in Germany.

The diagnosis and treatment of diseases of the trachea and bronchi has also shown great development in the last few years. In this connection, I must mention the new method of tracheo-bronchoscopy introduced by Killian of Freiburg, which permits of the removal of foreign bodies from the trachea as well as from the bronchi. The excellent monograph by the very distinguished American specialist Chevalier Jackson is especially noteworthy in this regard. In addition to this, Newcomb has written an excellent paper on the anomalies, hemorrhage, inflammation and infections of the trachea, Theisen on tumors, Simpson on stenoses, and Coolidge and Mayer on foreign bodies.

Three thousand papers have been published on the thyroid gland during the past twenty-five years, of which more than 700 (about one-fourth) come from America.

Semon of London showed (1883-1884) that the so-called Kocher's cachexia strumipriva seu thyreopriva and the myxedema of the English writers, cretinism and tetany occurred as the result of one and the same pathologic cause, the suspension of the function of the thyroid gland, and Horsley, also of London, proved that these conditions could be successfully treated by thyroid preparations (thyreoidin), which gave the basis for the organic treatment of this disease.

Sajous of Philadelphia has lately written (1908) on the adrenothyroid center (glandula pituitaria). Tuholske, also of America, has lately drawn attention to the importance of the parathyroid gland (after its extirpation tetany and death result). Halstead and Richards have also written upon this subject. Wilson, Barker, Stengel, Halstead and Solis Cohen have discussed exophthalmic goitre. The last is not inclined to favor the surgical treatment of the disease; however, Kocher's clinic in Bern showed good results, 3½ per cent of deaths and 83 per cent recoveries. Crile's (America) are not so good—6 per cent of deaths. At any rate the older methods of treating goitre by parenchymatous injections of tincture of iodin and iron are almost entirely abandoned, the surgical treatment being regarded as the most rational one.

Barker adds a fourth symptom to the trinity of symptoms of this disease, exophthalmus, goitre and palpitation of the heart, viz., muscular tremor. He maintains that tachycardia and exophthalmus are wanting in one-third of the cases. Lesonon has written on the thymus.

The literature of the esophagus and its diseases is relatively small, 1,700 papers, of which America provides 500, nearly one-third. Still much progress can be noted in the more recent times, especially along the line of esophagoscopy and gastroscopy, in which regard there is in America one of the leading exponents, Chevalier Jackson. This method and the application of the Roentgen rays have given the greatest aid to the diagnosis and treatment of certain conditions of the esophagus, foreign bodies, diverticula and neoplasms.

Myer, Mersbach, Halstead, Guizez have written in America on esophagoscopy, Lange on Roentgen ray examination, Schroeder and Ruth Adams on stenosis, Lercher and Huber on dilatations, Farlow on spasms, and Elsner, Seelig and many others on carcinoma.

Mr. President and Fellows of the American Academy of Ophthalmology and Oto-Laryngology: In this short and therefore inadequate resumé, I have endeavored to show the enormous development of our specialty, laryngo-rhinology and otology, since the discovery of the laryngoscope, especially, however, during the past twenty-five years. We have seen that America has taken an important part in this development. Allow me, therefore, as a representative of European laryngology, in conclusion, to express to the progressive medical profession of America my sincere wishes for the continued fruitfulness and greater glory of our specialty.

VIVAT, CRESCAT, FLOREAT OTO-LARYNGOLOGIA ET OPHTHALMOLOGIA AMERICANA.

XXXIII

NASAL OBSTRUCTION: EXPERIMENTAL STUDY OF ITS EFFECTS UPON THE RESPIRATORY ORGANS AND THE GENERAL SYSTEM.*

By Willis S. Anderson, M. D.,

Detroit.

The object sought in the experiments outlined in this paper is to determine what effect, if any, follows the complete or partial closure of the nostrils of animals. Guinea pigs, rabbits and dogs are the animals employed. Two methods of closure of the nostrils have been used: First, cotton and collodion; second, denuding the surface and suturing, while the animal was under ether. The first method is applicable to small animals, where it is desired to close one or both nostrils for not to exceed three or four days; the second method, for all work upon dogs, and upon rabbits and guinea pigs where prolonged closure is desired.

There are certain anatomic differences between the throats of animals and man that ought to be considered. The nose, throat, larynx and trachea are more nearly on a straight line in the lower animals. The larynx is placed higher in the throat, and the epiglottis is readily seen in the dog and rabbit by holding the mouth open. The most important difference, from the standpoint of my experiments, is the relation between the soft palate and the epiglottis.

The soft palate of the guinea pig (Fig. 1) forms a curtain which completely separates the buccal from the nasopharyngeal cavity. This muscular curtain is perforated by a small opening, which is closed in the passive state. The opening of the larynx, with its rudimentary epiglottis, is directly behind the perforation in the soft palate. It is evident that during the act of swallowing this sphincter like opening in the soft

*Read before the American Laryngological, Rhinological and Otological Society at Atlantic City, June, 1909.

palate relaxes, and the base of the tongue, which has a raised surface, presses the food through the opening. When the nose is entirely obstructed swallowing is necessary in order to get air into the respiratory passages.

The soft palate of the rabbit (Fig. 2) forms a curtain similar to that of the guinea pig, but the opening into the nasopharynx is larger. The epiglottis is well developed, lies in front of the soft palate and covers the opening connecting the buccal with the nasopharyngeal cavity. The relations of these structures in the dog more nearly approaches to that of man (Fig. 3). The curtain of the soft palate is not complete, as in the guinea pig and rabbit; the epiglottis is large and projects up in front of the soft palate. Except when the dog swallows there does not seem to be normally any communication between the buccal and the nasopharyngeal cavities. When the nostrils are closed, and the dog is compelled to breathe through the mouth, the current of air apparently passes through slits on either side of the epiglottis, but there is little evidence to show that normally mouth breathing is practiced.

Very early in my experiments certain changes were found in the lungs of the rabbits and pigs. The question arose whether the changes were due to interference with breathing, or whether the ordinary laboratory animal had frequently pathologic conditions in the lungs. In order to ascertain these points I examined the lungs of fifty guinea pigs supposed to be normal. Macroscopic examination showed one positively diseased, and several others with small abnormal areas. Microscopic examination of a small number showed the lungs to be regularly normal. I do not doubt if a number of sections were made from each lung, and carefully studied, the proportion of diseased lungs would be increased, but from the standpoint of my experiments, the changes regularly found in the lungs, following closure of the nose, cannot be attributed to preexisting disease.

Rabbits have frequently a catarrhal discharge from the nostrils, accompanied by changes in the lungs. Such animals were not used except as mentioned. The examination of a small number of lungs showed that a larger proportion were diseased than in the case of pigs, but the conditions observed were not comparable with the regular changes found in the animals experimented upon.

The observations upon animals with artificially obstructed nostrils will be considered in the following order: First, the effect upon guinea pigs and rabbits; second, the more extended observations upon dogs; third, the histologic changes; and fourth, an attempt will be made to correlate the facts obtained, and to draw such deductions as seem warranted.

The effects upon guinea pigs when both nostrils are closed are shown in Table 1. Those that lived over 48 hours breathed some through the nose. This is notably so in numbers 2, 3, 8, 19, 22, 23, 24 and 137. It is exceptional for a pig to live more than 36 hours with the nostrils tightly closed. Distention of the abdomen, due to swallowing the air, is noticeable, and frequently becomes marked within an hour after closure. This peculiar gulping in of the air is made necessary by the relation of the soft palate as mentioned above. The distention is more marked when the intestines are filled with food, and can be lessened by fasting the animal. It seems to be a contributory cause of death, but not the essential factor, as in some instances the pigs died quickly without distention. Pig number 25 died within two hours after both nostrils were closed, and the stomach was found to be ruptured. Number 27 also died within two hours, but the abdomen was not markedly distended, nor was the stomach ruptured.

The effect upon guinea pigs with one nostril closed is illustrated in Table 2. Of the 15 pigs twelve had the right side closed and three had the left side. Two lived eight months with one side entirely closed. (Numbers 1 and 9.) Two died within 12 hours. (Numbers 66 and 67.) Probably the left nostril was accidentally filled with collodion, as the pigs appeared similar to the ones with both nostrils closed. Eight died on an average of 9 3/4 days. Three lived thirty days, but in each instance the closed side partially opened. Number 92 lived only five days, but the resistance of this pig was probably lowered by a previous attempt to close the nostril.

The effect upon rabbits with one nostril closed is shown in Table 3. Seven had the right side closed and four the left. The longest duration of life is 113 days (No. 72); the shortest, 4 days (No. 57); the average duration was a little less than 45 days. Number 57 developed a catarrhal discharge from the left nostril, which undoubtedly interfered with the breathing through that side. As the right nostril was closed by operation, the rabbit had to breathe largely through the mouth. The distended abdomen was evidently due to swallowing the air. As there was a marked congestion of the upper lobe of the right lung, it is probable that an acute infection hastened the death of the rabbit. Number 60 developed an abscess on the right side of the neck, which may have been the cause of death. It is noteworthy the uniform loss of weight of the rabbits with one nostril closed. Death resulted when about one-half of the weight was lost. Distention of the abdomen is usually not present in rabbits. A few rabbits that lived for months developed noisy breathing, suggestive of asthma.

It is clear that there is a causative relation between nasal obstruction and the death of these animals, as the number experimented upon is too large to attribute the deaths to accident. The determining cause of death is not clear. The length of time the animals live, and the symptoms do not point to asphyxiation, nor to carbonic acid gas poisoning as the cause. There are two factors that seem important in explaining the cause of death: First, infection as the result of lowered resistance; second, acute dilatation of the heart (Fig. 4). There are a certain number of guinea pigs and rabbits that show evidences of infection. The lungs are involved, and the lesions noted are intense congestion and areas of bronchopneumonia. The pulmonary condition is sufficient to account for death in some instances, but not in all. In my early examinations the condition of the heart was not closely studied, but with added experience I began to notice what was apparently a dilated condition of the heart. To determine this point it is necessary to have control animals of the same weight as the animals experimented upon, for the size of the heart is proportional to the weight of the animal. When the hearts of the pigs and rabbits experimented upon were compared with the animals of the same weight, it was found that dilatation regularly took place in the animals that lived 24 hours to two or three days. As the right ventricle was the portion involved, it would seem as though some mechanical impediment to the pulmonary circulation was the cause of the dilatation, and that the phenomenon was comparable to acute dilatation of the heart in poorly trained athletes, after excessive exertion.

The effect of nasal obstruction upon dogs, as outlined in this report, is based upon the study of 18 with partial closure of the nostrils, and upon 24 puppies born of mothers with nasal obstruction. A study of the breathing and pneumographic tracings of normal dogs has been made, and the condition of the lungs noted in a number of instances. Several years ago in another laboratory the nostrils of two dogs were closed, but the results were similar to the ones reported in the present series, so they will not be further considered.

Ether was used in all except No. 11. The orifice of the nostril was denuded and sutures were inserted. It is comparatively easy to close one nostril, but difficult to close the second. The effort of the dog to breathe tends to pull the sutures out, and the unavoidable infection of the parts leads to sloughing in some cases. Two-thirds, or more, of the opening of the nostrils were closed on an average. We will consider first, the changes noted in all of the dogs; and second, the special features that are of peculiar interest.

Labored breathing is a constant symptom, and is in a general way, proportional to the degree of obstruction, although an occasional dog seems to have but little dyspnea in spite of marked obstruction. The breathing is characteristic of asthma and emphysema; there is an apparent enlargement of the chest, and retraction of the intercostal spaces in the more marked cases. Pneumographic tracings of the breathing of dogs is shown in Fig. 5. The upper tracing, A, is from a normal dog; the middle, B, is from a dog (No. 11) with nasal obstruction. It shows the irregularity of the breathing as compared with the normal. The lowest tracing, C, is from a dog with cough, dyspnea and a peculiar, long, slow inspiration and a quick expiration. The dyspnea is increased on exercise. When both nostrils are closed the dogs have to breathe through the mouth, but if even one-fourth of the space remains they will draw air through the narrowed opening rather than breathe through the mouth.

The hair as a rule becomes shorter, thinner and lighter in color. This thinning of the hair usually commences over the abdomen and along the legs, then over the back and neck. A dandruff like scurf is noticed, but scabbing is not the rule unless the parts become excoriated. With this change in the hair there is a peculiar wrinkling of the skin in some instances. (Figs. 6, 7 and 8.)

The general nutrition, as measured by the body weight does not seem to be affected in the animals that live for a number of months, but a certain proportion of the dogs, more often the younger ones, as a result of lowered resistance, die from infection. They had abundance of wholesome food, and were under similar conditions. No attempt was made to weigh the food ingested, or to estimate the excretions.

As regards the resisting power, we can divide the dogs with nasal obstruction into two groups (Table 4): The older dogs that live for months and gradually develope dyspnea, suggestive of asthma and emphysema; and the younger ones that are prone to infections. Those that die of infection usually have a mucopurulent discharge from the nostrils, emaciate, grow gradually weaker and die within three months. The determining cause of death seems to be bronchopneumonia. One of the younger dogs shown in the table (No. 104) lived 8 months and was killed because of a parasitic skin lesion. This apparent exception is explained by the fact that the nose was opened, and the increased space was followed by marked improvement in the breathing and the general condition. The number of young dogs experimented upon is too small to be positive as to just what influence age has upon the resisting power.

The effect of nasal obstruction upon the progeny is interesting. Twenty-four puppies have been born of mothers with about one-third of the normal breathing space (Table 5). Of these, two were found dead and three died within twenty-four hours. Eleven died at intervals from 31 to 93 days, under the best of care and with suitable food. One died of distemper on the ninety-ninth day. Three pups were used for other purposes, and from them no conclusions can be drawn. Two had their nostrils sewed up when they were five and one-half weeks old. The only conclusion that can be drawn from these two is that they both died sooner than is usual when pups of this age are experimented upon. (See Table 6.)

The two that are alive at present—48 days old—are not developing as normal dogs should. It is doubtful if they will grow to maturity.

The mothers seemed to have plenty of nourishment for the pups during the period of lactation, and later the puppies were given warm, fresh milk and other suitable food. I have no data as to the quality of the mother's milk. At birth the puppies appeared normal and developed fairly well for a few weeks, but they were less active than normal dogs, gained less in weight and gradually showed evidences of malnutrition. The hair as a rule became thinner, lost its natural gloss, and in one litter it was almost entirely gone. With this loss of hair there was a peculiar wrinkling of the skin similar to the mother. Macroscopic examination of the organs did not reveal the cause of death. A detailed study of one litter, in connection with the mother, will be given later. The point to be emphasized at this time is that interference with the normal nasal breathing of dogs has a marked deleterious effect upon the progeny. In some instances the male parent had obstructed breathing. We have also a few observations where the male had obstructed breathing and the female was normal. So far our observations seem to show that it is through the female that the weakened vitality of the progeny occurs, but perhaps further observations over a longer period will show that the influence of the male is also a factor.

The effect upon the offspring of rabbits is based on a very limited experience. It is very difficult to breed rabbits with nasal obstruction, and several attempts have failed. One rabbit a month after the right nostril was closed had four bunnies. They were all very small and died within a few hours. About thirteen months later she had a litter of five. One found dead; one died on the twelfth day; one died on the sixteenth day; one on the twentieth day; and two alive on the twenty-seventh day (May 24).

We will next consider the resistance of normal pups as compared with those of the same age born of mothers with nasal obstruction (Table 6).

Four puppies, each five and one-half weeks old, were used; two were normal and two abnormal, that is, born of a mother with about one-third of the normal breathing space. The nostrils were closed in each instance. The table shows that one normal dog lived 38 days, the other 8 months with obstructed breathing, while the abnormal ones under similar conditions lived 18 and 15 days respectively. In one instance (105) both sides of the nose of the normal dog were not closed at the same time; but on the other hand one of the abnormal dogs (107) had more breathing space than the normal, yet lived less than one-half as long. One of the normal dogs (104) was peculiarly resistant for a young dog, but this is partially accounted for by the fact that the nose was opened for a few weeks prior to the death of the animal. This dog will be considered later.

The conditions under which these dogs were experimented upon were so nearly the same that, taken in connection with other experiments, the conclusion is warranted that there is a marked difference in the power of resistance between normal dogs and those born of mothers with obstructed breathing.

There are some interesting observations that have not been brought out in the study of the above tables. The history of two dogs will illustrate many of these points. Male puppy (104), five and a half weeks old is shown in Fig. 6, weight, three and a half pounds; born of healthy parents, was used for the following experiment: Under ether both nostrils were closed on July 27, 1908. Dyspnea was noticed from the first, and it soon became apparent that the dog was not developing as he should. On September 13, the dog seemed sick. He had a temperature of 105° F., but on the 29th it had dropped to 101° F., and the dog seemed much better. In November it was noticed that he was losing his hair on the abdomen. This grew more marked until there was but little hair on the abdomen, legs and tail. Dyspnea increased, with shallow breathing and forced expiration, suggestive of asthma and emphysema. While the dog was gaining in weight it was not the gain that a normal puppy should make; the increased weakness and dyspnea became more and more evident, until death seemed imminent. On January 5th, I opened the nose so that the dog could breathe freely. There was an improvement in the condition; the hair commenced to grow and was more normal in gloss; the dyspnea almost disappeared and the dog appeared lively. Early in March he unfortunately became infected with the follicular mange, and it seemed best to kill the animal on March 30, 1909. Macroscopic examination of the lungs, liver, kidneys and spleen revealed nothing abnormal.

This dog illustrates what I have observed in other animals, that the reopening of the nose is immediately followed by improvement in the breathing and the general condition. It is to be regretted that he became infected with the mange, as further observation would have been desirable.

The history of the next dog is the most interesting of the whole series. Female (11), weight about 25 pounds. She was lively, healthy looking animal with long, reddish, curly hair of normal gloss. On October 31, 1907, I sewed up the right nostril. As healing took place, a small opening remained. On December 13 the left nostril was closed, and upon healing no opening remained. In spite of the labored breathing which followed, the air was drawn through the narrowed nasal opening and not through the mouth. The dyspnea gradually increased, the chest assumed a more barrel shaped contour, the hair was noticed first to become shorter and thinner, then bare places appeared over the rump, legs and abdomen (Fig. 7). The weight did not vary to any extent, but the dog was less lively than formerly. About five months after the nostrils were closed, the loss of hair had extended to the neck and head, wrinkling of the skin was very evident and the dog was weaker and had an old and decrepit appearance (Fig. 8). The breathing was strongly suggestive of asthma and emphysema. The first week in June, 1908, she suddenly appeared better. Examination showed that the left nostril had torn open, and the increased breathing space accounted for the improvement noted. The hair commenced to come over each hip, and she appeared livelier in every way. The breathing space on each side was still narrowed. About this time it was noted that she was in heat for the first time since she was under observation. On August 31, 1908, she had eight puppies; one was found dead. All seemed normal in development. The seven that lived were apparently properly nourished by the mother, and were weaned at the usual time. About the time they were weaned it was noted that the hair of all the pups was growing thinner, and a peculiar wrinkling of the skin similar to the mother developed. Their growth was not normal, they commenced to emaciate, they were less lively and had a dried up, wizened appearance that reminded one of a child suffering from hereditary syphilis. Besides the loss of hair they had a dandruff-like scurf. The condition was suggestive of scurvy, but it could not have been due to the lack of suitable food, as they had plenty of fresh milk, meat, bread, etc. The last few days of their life they were separated into two groups, and special care was given to the feeding of one group. This made no difference in the length of time they lived.

I am indebted to my colleague, Dr. Buesser, for the following report as to the condition of the blood of the mother and puppies: "The hemoglobin estimate was made by the Tallqvist color scale. Two normal dogs for control showel 100 per cent each; mother, 60 per cent; four puppies, 50 per cent each; one, 45 per cent; and one, 60 per cent. The mother and the puppies show an anemia as compared with the two normal dogs used for controls. The leucocytes were somewhat increased in the mother, and markedly increased in the puppies; the red cells were smaller, showed signs of destruction by irregularities in shape, and contained less hemoglobin. The general picture indicates a secondary anemia."

The length of time the puppies lived is as follows: One, found dead; one, 57 days; one, 60 days; and five, 61 days. Post mortem examination of the puppies failed to reveal the cause of the peculiar condition which led to their death. The macroscopic changes in the organs were very slight. The lungs were more or less congested, but inflated readily. Some congestion of the liver was noted in several.

On November 10, 1908, the mother of the pups was killed by chloroform, and an examination of the organs made. This dog had had obstructed breathing for a year. On the day she was killed the following observations were made. Respirations 22 per minute, very labored, with retraction of the intercostal spaces. Post mortem: Body warm. Skin over the abdomen and chest almost hairless, very smooth and soft, with no dandruff or scabbing. There were some short hairs over the back and legs; over the exposed parts the hair was very thin, with some irritation and scabbing. The skin of the face and neck was very wrinkled, that of the body to a less degree. The lungs collapsed when the chest was opened. No adhesions or fluid in the pleural cavities. Inflation of the lungs showed them to be comparatively normal. Kidneys slightly congested. No enlarged mesenteric glands.

It is claimed that unilateral nasal obstruction in man predisposes the lung of the same side to disease. Chauvet in a recent article concludes, from a study of unilateral closure of the nostrils of six rabbits, that the lungs of the side corresponding to the nasal obstruction is the more often diseased; that scoliosis and deformity of the chest occur; and that changes in the sinuses follow nasal obstruction. (*Revue Hebdomadaire de Lary. d'Otol. et de Rhin.*, March 20, 1909.)

From records of nearly one hundred animals experimented upon I found no evidence that disease of the lung bears any relation to the side obstructed, nor did I find the deformities of the chest pictured by Chauvet.

A mucopurulent accumulation occurs in the nostril obstructed, due probably to interference with drainage, but marked macroscopic changes in the turbinals, or sinuses, were not observed. It would be natural to expect changes to take place in the development of the bones in young animals with nasal obstruction, also that histologic changes would occur in the nose as the result of the long continued contact of the mucous membrane with the mucopurulent discharge, but on these points I have not sufficient data to warrant conclusions.

Many histologic changes have been noted in the lungs of the animals experimented upon, but the marked pathologic condition of some lungs and the comparative freedom from disease in others have made the interpretation of the findings somewhat difficult. The complete closure of the nostrils in the smaller animals is followed by definite changes in the lungs. In the pigs that die within 24 hours there is usually an intense congestion, edema sometimes with hemorrhagic areas. If they live a little longer there is a peribronchial infiltration, or distinct evidences of a bronchopneumonia. If the animal lives several days we may find extensive hemorrhagic areas; dilatation of the vessels; interstitial infiltration of blood; atelectasis, with collapse of the bronchi; and emphysema. The bronchi may be normal, or show evidences of inflammation; empty, or filled with blood, mucus or desquamated epithelium. If the pig lives a number of weeks the inflammatory changes are less marked, but the emphysema is more extensive. While the lesions observed are varied, there is a certain harmony observed that is suggestive of one of two causes: First, inflammatory changes, the result of infection, due to the lowering of the vitality of the animal; and second, mechanical changes, the direct result of the interference with normal breathing, which leads to collapse of the bronchi, areas of atelectasis, and emphysema.

The study of the lungs of dogs with obstructed breathing may, in a general way, be divided into those where the inflammatory lesions are prominent; and those where the mechanical, or emphysematous changes, are predominant. The lowering of the resistance, noticeable in the younger dogs, predisposes to infections; so we naturally find bronchopneumonia, seropurulent pleurisy and other inflammatory lesions as evident causes of the comparatively prompt death of the animal. On the other hand, if the dog has sufficient vitality to withstand infection, the mechanical obstruction to breathing leads to gradual changes, of which emphysema is the type.

A number of sections from the lungs of the dog (No. 11) whose history was detailed above have been studied. We must remember that as a result of a year of difficult breathing the dog had developed all of the symptoms of a chronic asthma with emphysema besides certain peculiar nutritional changes, referable to the hair and skin. We might expect under such circumstances that there would be marked changes in the structure of the lungs, but macroscopically they seemed normal and even the microscopic changes though significant, hardly seemed commensurable with the clinical symptoms. We found evidences of a chronic bronchitis, increase of interstitial tissue, bronchopneumonia, and distinct areas of emphysema.

The dilatation of the right ventricle and the weakening of the heart has an important bearing on the changes in the lungs. The cardiac failure would naturally lead to intense congestion and dilatation of the vessels as an early symptom, and brown induration and increase of interstitial tissue later.

We cannot transfer the results of experiments upon animals to man without certain reservations, but our clinical experience, in a general way, is in harmony with the results as outlined above. Patients with nasal obstruction usually have a lowered general resistance, are more susceptible to colds and other infections, and there seems to be a causal relation between that syndrome of symptoms commonly known as "Catarrh," and imperfect nasal breathing.

Obstructed nasal breathing has long been recognized as a factor in the etiology of asthma. As long as the underlying cause of asthma is not known, and the pathology indefinite, it would seem that experiments upon animals offered a fruitful field for the study of this disease.

The following conclusions are suggested by the results of the experiments outlined above:

1. That nasal obstruction leads to death, or serious impairment of vitality.

2. That the lowered resistance predisposes to infections.

3. That local disease of the respiratory tract is induced.

4. That obstruction of the nostrils leads to dilatation of the heart.

5. That changes in the skin and the blood of the dogs occur.

6. That symptoms resembling asthma and emphysema may be induced in the lower animals.

7. That emphysema of the lungs can be demonstrated histologically.

8. That reopening the occluded nostrils is followed by prompt disappearance of the symptoms.

Table showing the effect upon thirty pigs.

Both Nostrils Closed.

The nostrils of the first two pigs where sutured. All of the others were closed by cotton and collodion.

Lab. No.	Wet wt in gms.	Duration of ...		Remarks.
2	......	6 Days.	...	... wollen ... first 24 ... ... ar a little air through nose.
3	......	12 Days.	... partl dly ... ... B.	
7	......	18 Hours.	... entirely led.	
8	......	3½ Days.	... di ... at first, ... through the nose.
15	......	36 Hours.	... ttrely cl d. ... di ...
16	......	36 Hours.	... ttrely cl ed. ... di ...
17	......	15 Hours.	... ttrely cl ed. ... di ...
18	......	4 Days.	... nt entirely cl ed.
19	310	4 ...s.	... entirely ed. ... nt di ...
20	310	2 Days.	... ply nt entirely ... within an ...
22	300	3 Days.	... nt entirely cl d. ... ... nt ...
23	300	3 Days.	... nt entirely cl ed. No dist ... ... after closure or 48 hours. No distention.
24	300	2 Hours.	... ... Stom ... ruptured ... ... in ...
25	302	2 Hours.	... nt ...
27	300	30 ...s.	... ...
28	302	12 Hours.	... fed morning of ... ... filled.
30	290	12 Hours.	... ed morning of ..., r ... ... rte. ... wel fid.
31	300	12 ...s.	... ed morning of operation, r ... marked. ... wel filled.
32	300	12 Hours.	... fed morning of ..., nor ... Not ... ... wel filled.
33	290	52 Hours.	... ed morning of operati n, nr for 24 hours afterwards. Not di ... Not
34	305	24 Hours.	... ... in ...
75	950		Not ... At nd of 23 hours lively. Put an extra dressing of cotton and collodi n.
			Did within 45 minut e.
77	853	36 Hours.	Di ...
78	800	60 Hours.	Di d. ...
79	753	36 Hours.	Not ...
119	550	18 Hours.	Mely dist ...
120	520	18 Hours.	Mely dist d.
121	440	18 Hours.	ately dist ...
136	300	16 Hours.	Not ... ...
137	260	56 Hours.	Very little Mon. Breathed a little through nose.
138	255	36 Hours.	Dist ... ...

TABLE No. 2. GUINEA PIGS.

One Nostril Closed.

No. 36 closed by Cotton and Collodion. All others closed by suture while animals were under Ether.

Lab. No.	Weight in gms.	Nostril closed.	Duration of life.	Remarks.
1	-----	Left.	8 M.	Wt. March 27·'08, 320 gms. At death 265 gms. No distention.
9	-----	Left.	8 M.	Wt. Mar 27·'08, 300 gms. At death 305 gms.
36	270	Left.	10 Days.	No distention. Wt. Dec. 23·'08, 250 gms.
42	255	Right.	6 Days.	No distention.
44	360	Right.	14 Days.	No distention.
45	290	Right.	10 Days.	No distention.
46	310	Right.	10 ?s.	No distention.
47	305	Ri gt.	15 Days.	No distention.
48	300	i gt.	30 ?s.	No distention. Right nostril opened up about ¾.
49	310	Ri gt.	30 ?s.	No distention. Right nostril opened up about ½.
50	300	Right.	30 Days.	No distention. Small opening.
63	375	?gt.	8 ?s.	No distention.
66	290	Right.	12	Marked ... Probably pig did not breathe through either nostril. (See No. 67.)
67	270	Right.	12 Hours.	Very ?le distention. Probably pig did not breathe through either nostril. (See No. 66.)
92	365	Right.	5 Days.	Diste tio n. This pig had ...sen closed before, but opened up. Resistance ...bably ...ered.

TABLE No. 3. RABBITS.

One Nostril Closed.

The nostrils were closed by sutures and Collodion dressing while the rabbits were under Ether. The first weight was taken at the beginning of the experiment, the second after the death of the animals.

Lab. No.	Weight in gms.	Nostril closed.	Duration of life.	Remarks.
57	......	Right.	4 Days.	Some distention. Catarrhal discharge from left nostril, which interfered with bathing. Right side entirely closed.
60	3000	Right.	62 Days.	Emaciated. Swelling the size of small orange right side of neck (abscess).
68	2175 / 1010	Right.	45 Days.	Right nostril entirely closed.
69	2000 / 999	Right.	49 Days.	Right nostril entirely closed.
71	2100 / 900	Right.	47 Days.	
72	2175 / 1060	Right.	113 Days.	Right nostril entirely closed.
95	1620 / 860	Left.	44 ?	
96	1235 / 623	Left.	30 Days.	
97	1550	Left.	19 Days.	Left nostril entirely closed. Emaciated, wt. 11 days after closure of nose, 1340 gms.
98	...... / 1600 / 925	Left.	23 Days.	Left nostril opening size of pin head.
130	2035 / 1200	Right.	57 Days.	Right nostril opening size of pin head.

TABLE No. 4.

Difference in Resisting Power Between the Old and the Young Dogs with Nasal Obstruction.

Older Dogs.

Lab. No.	Average weight.	Degree of obstruction.	Duration of life.	Remarks.
11	30 lbs.	Two-thirds.	1 year.	This dog had ast rha nd emphysema, with loss of hair and wri kling of skin. Killed.
81	24 lbs.	Three-fourths.	8 months.	dai edh, otherwise phly vold ahe l fed for mhs.
65	20 lbs.	Two-thirds.	10 months.	dai edh, otherwise phly vold ahe lived for mhs. This dog st younger kn ost of his group.
61	21 lbs.	Two-thirds.	al ie.	This dog has hed since eb., 1908, wth nasal obstruction. At sent rell t hel.
64	26 lbs.	Three-fourths.	14 months.	dai adh, otherwise phly would hve lived for mhs.
82	22 lbs.	Four-fifths.	alive.	This dog has hed since ath, 1908, wth nal obstruction. (hce of
99	25 lbs.	One-half.	alive.	This dog lved sne Jne, 908, with nasal obstruction. Some Dyspena, but well und.

Younger Dogs.

Lab. No.	Average weight.	Degree of obstruction.	Duration of life.	Remarks.
12	12 lbs.	One-third.	Nt uite 3 days.	Did f om te i tin of he lungs. Congestion, nd Coli tin of yn Lungs.
73	16 lbs.	Less than ⅓.	19 days.	Mt rge fm hd areas. tid (right) stril. I he conges- tin of lungs nd
95	7 lbs.	Four-fifths.	48 days.	5½ vas dd wn nt sal tis. Lung On vry marked. Seropurulent fld in pl jgd ad ali- dd.
104	9 lbs.	Four-fifths.	8 mnths.	This dog ne id wth fol rije, nd vas kill d. Na nd tha hd nd dd wn e pri nt ws æt. 5½ ves dd Eally resi nt dr pg dog.

(Remarks: Note how much more susceptible the younger dogs are to infections, and how they die after a few months, while the older dogs live for many months. The lungs are regularly involved in the younger dogs, while the older ones develop asthma and emphysema, without evidence of infection.)

TABLE No. 5.

The effect upon the Progeny when the Mothers have about Two-thirds of Their Nasal Breathing Obstructed.

Mothers		Puppies			Remarks
Tab. No.	Wt. lbs.	No. in litter	Wt. oz. Found	Days lived. dead. / Alive	
11	33	8 — 1	7.66	57	At birth they appeared normal. Before death they were emaciated, scurvy-like, with hair mostly gone and skin wrinkled. They had plenty of fresh, wholesome food. They resembled the mother at the time of death.
		2	10.66	60	
		3	8.25	61	
		4	9.33	61	
		5	9	61	
		6	6.12	61	
		7	8.66	61	
65	20	4 — 1	-----	-----	All very small. One was found dead, the other the died in ab[out] 24 hours. ...ition, hair ...th Wt. at d[eat]h, 4.75 lbs. Sewed up the nostrils of ...when 5½ weeks ld. ...ree used for other purposes. ...ttle thinning of ...r, progressive ...ss and emaciation. No cause of death ascertainabl ...ein the first three. The fourth died of distemper.
65	25	1	9.20	93	
6?	22	5	-----	-----	
61	25	4 — 1	8	44	
		2	7	39	
		3	8	31	
		4	8	99	
82	24	2 — 1	4.50	Alive.	Neither of the puppies are developing as normal ones ho[u]ld. Age, 41 days. No. 1 l sin[g] wt. No. 2 slight gain.
		2	5.50	Alive.	

...[Summ]ary: Of the 24 pu[p]s, two were f[o]und d[e]ad; fort[h] ...died u[n]der the best of care; one died f[ro]m dis-[tem]per; three were used for ...ther purposes and from ...m no conclusion ...an be drawn. The longest any li[v]ed was 99 days. M[o]st of ...m died within two months, or less. [W]o had both nostrils cl s ... when 5½ ...ks old. The only conclusion that ...an be drawn f[ro]m t... s[he]two is that they b[o]th died s o ...than is u[su]al ...wn pups of this age are ...xper[i]...nd upon. The two that are alive after 41 ... show diminished res[i] ...te.

TABLE No. 6.

Resistance of Normal Pups as Compared with those of the same age Born of Mothers with Nasal Obstruction.

Abnormal.

106. Wt. 2 lbs. 7 oz. Age, 5½ weeks.
  Sewed up both nostrils.
  Lived, 18 days. Wt. at death, 18 1/3 oz.

107. Wt. 2 lbs. 6 oz. Age, 5½ weeks.
  Sewed up both nostrils.
  Lived, 15 days. Wt. at death, 18½ oz.
  Pin head opening right nostril.
  Left has a little larger opening.

Normal.

105. Wt. 5¼ lbs. Age, 5½ weeks.
  Sewed up left nostril, and 11 days later sewed up the
   right nostril.
  Lived, 38 days. Left nostril pin head opening, right
   entirely closed.

104. Wt. 3½ lbs. Age, 5½ weeks.
  Sewed up both nostrils.
  Left nostril entirely sed, right ab ut three-fourths
   closed.
  Asthma and emphysema developed.
  Became infected with thar age and was killed
   afr living eight months.

(Remarks: Note that the ages of the four dogs were the same; that the normal dogs lived 38 days and eight months respectively, while the abnormal ones lived 18 and 15 days respectively. In one instance (105) both sides of the nose of the normal dog were not closed at the same time; but on the other hand, No. 107 (abnormal) had more breathing space than the normal (105), yet lived less than half as long. No. 104 (normal) was peculiarly resistant for a young dog.)

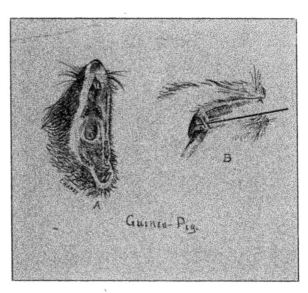

FIGURE 1.

A. Anterior view of guinea pig's throat. showing fauces, soft palate with sphincter-like opening. B. Lateral view, showing probes through opening in soft palate.

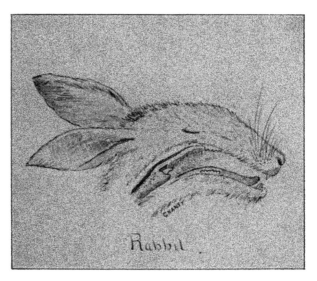

FIGURE 2.

Lateral view or rabbit's throat.

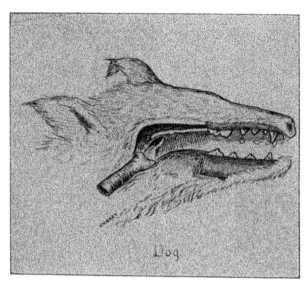

FIGURE 3.
Lateral view of dog's throat.

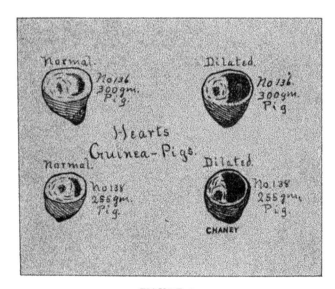

FIGURE 4.

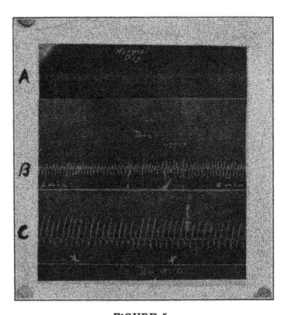

FIGURE 5.

Pneumatograms. A. Normal dog. B. Dog with nasal obstruction. C. Dog with dyspnea.

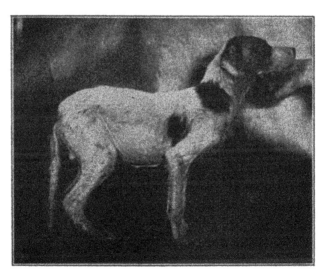

FIGURE 6.

Dog No. 104. Showing loss of hair with nasal obstruction.

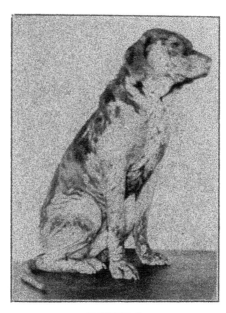

FIGURE 7.

Dog No. 11. Showing loss of hair and wrinkling of skin following nasal obstruction.

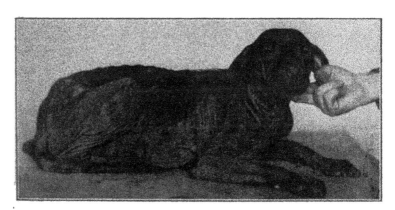

FIGURE 8.

Dog No. 11. Showing loss of hair and wrinkling of skin following nasal obstruction.

XXXIV

THE PHENOMENA OF VESTIBULAR IRRITATION IN ACUTE LABYRINTHINE DISEASE, WITH SPECIAL REFERENCE TO THE STUDIES OF DR. BARANY OF VIENNA.

By Philip D. Kerrison, M. D.,

New York.

However interesting the earlier experiments and hypotheses may have been as bearing upon the physiology and function of the semicircular canals, we must now recognize the studies of Flourens in 1824 to 1828, and the later experiments of Prof. Ewald of Strasburg, as the basis upon which our present clearer understanding of the phenomena of vestibular irritation mainly rests.

Ewald's Experiments (Fig. 1).—Ewald[1] experimented separately upon the three semicircular canals of pigeons after the following method: Having exposed the selected canal, a small hole is drilled into its most prominent presenting part. A second opening between the first and the small or smooth end of the canal is bored, and into this a lead mass is introduced, completely obliterating its lumen at this point. Into the first opening is introduced and secured a small cylinder, open at both ends, within which a minute, movable piston rests. To the outer end of the cylinder is attached a piece of rubber tubing, the opposite end of which communicates with a rubber ball or bulb. Obviously compression of the bulb will drive the piston further into the cylinder and cause displacement of the endolymph in the canal experimented upon; and since this canal is closed in the direction of its small end, it is evident that the endolymph movement must be toward its ampulla. It is equally clear that if we begin with a partially compressed

---

1. Ewald. Physiologische Untersuchungen über das Endorgan des nervus octavus. 255-266.

bulb, we may by release of pressure induce an endolymph movement in the opposite direction, i. e., away from the ampulla and toward the small end of the canal.

These experiments gave in the different canals the following reactions:

Right External, or Horizontal Canal.—Compression of bulb (causing endolymph displacement toward ampulla) was followed by strong, gradual movement of the head, exactly in the plane of the canal, to the left. Coincidently with this head movement, the eyes were moved, also in the plane of the canal, to the left. On release of pressure the head and eyes quickly regained their normal position.

Suction (i. e., endolymph movement in right horizontal canal toward small end of canal) gave rise to gradual movement of head and eyes, always in the plane of the canal, to the right. But this latter movement to the right caused by suction was much less forcible than the opposite movement caused by compression.

Right Posterior Vertical Canal.—Compression (i. e., endolymph movement toward ampulla) was followed by gradual movement of the head, exactly in the plane of this canal and toward its ampulla, i. e., to the right. Suction gave rise to movements of the head and eyes in the same plane but in the opposite direction, i. e., to the left. But in this canal, suction was followed by much stronger movements than those produced by compression.

The reactions of the anterior vertical canal are similar to those of the posterior vertical, varying only in accordance with its different plane.

It is worthy of note that in the case of the horizontal canal the strongest head and eye movements followed displacement of endolymph in the direction of the ampulla, whereas in the posterior vertical and anterior vertical canals the strongest movements were those which followed displacement of endolymph toward the small ends of the canals. In each canal, however, the strongest movement produced was toward the opposite side.

Vestibular nystagmus is always composed of a quick movement in one direction and a slow movement in the opposite direction. It must be borne in mind that in the experiments above described the gradual movement of head and eyes, caused by either compression or suction, corresponds to the slow component of vestibular nystagmus, and represents therefore a nystagmus in the opposite direction.

Ewald's experiments established definitely the following important facts: (a) Excitation of a single canal can produce nystagmus only in a plane corresponding to the plane of the canal; (b) by reverse movements of the endolymph in any single canal we can produce a reversal of the direction of the induced nystagmus, and (c) the strongest nystagmus which can be induced by irritation of a single canal is always in the direction of the ear experimented upon.

For any one who has the position and plane, and the relative positions of the ampullar and small ends, of each canal clearly fixed in memory, the writer suggests the following simple rule, based upon Ewald's experiments, by which the reactions following endolymph movements in the different canals may be easily recalled, viz.:

Displacement of endolymph in any particular canal gives rise to nystagmus in which the eyes move in a plane parallel with the plane of the canal, and of which the slow movement is always in the direction in which the endolymph moves.

Remembering that the direction of vestibular nystagmus takes its name from the direction of the quick eye movement, and that the gradual head and eye movements of Ewald's experiments correspond to the slow component of vestibular nystagmus, the wording of the above rule may be reversed and abbreviated as follows:

Nystagmus induced by endolymph displacement in any particular canal is in a plane parallel with the plane of that canal, and in the direction opposite to that of the endolymph displacement.

Character of Vestibular Nystagmus.—To establish a claim to vestibular origin a nystagmus must present the following characteristics: (1) It must be composed of a quick movement in one direction and a slow movement in the opposite direction. (2) It is increased usually in rapidity and always in length of excursion when the eyes are turned voluntarily in the direction of the quick movement. (3) It becomes weak, or may disappear wholly, when the eyes are turned in the direction of the slow nystagmic movement.

The above are invariable characteristics of nystagmus of vestibular origin, whether produced by experimental irritation or in the course of acute labyrinthine disease.

Vestibular nystagmus may be horizontal, oblique, vertical or rotary. The nystagmus caused by acute labyrinthine disease is practically always rotary.

The Caloric Reactions.—The so-called caloric tests, the technic and significance of which were first established by Dr. Barany of Vienna, depend upon the following easily demonstrable facts:

(a) If we irrigate either ear of a normal person with water at body temperature, no objective or subjective phenomena result.

(b) If we repeat this experiment with water appreciably below blood temperature we shall observe the following evideuces of vestibular irritation, viz.: (1) rotary nystagmus toward the ear not irrigated; (2) the patient experiences vertigo, and (3) exhibits marked disturbances of equilibrium.

(c) If we substitute in this experiment hot water, or water considerably above blood temperature, we shall induce exactly the same phenomena with these differences, viz.: (1) The quick nystagmic movement will be toward the ear irrigated, and (2) the ataxia will exhibit certain differences in accordance with laws to be referred to later.

Barany's Theory As to the Causation of the Caloric Reactions[2].—We must regard the whole labrinthine cavity as a vessel containing fluid of temperature probably identical with that of the blood. If now we bring cold or hot water in contact with one wall of this vessel, the specific gravity of that part of the contained fluid nearest this wall will be increased or reduced, and will sink or rise according to the physical laws governing fluids of different specific gravity.

The parts of the semicircular canal system nearest the surface of the inner tympanic wall are (1) the anterior part of the horizontal canal, and (2) the external, or ampullar, third of the anterior vertical canal which points almost directly downward (Fig. II). Syringing the ear with cold water would therefore influence the temperature first at these points. With the head in the upright position, however, endolymph movement in the external canal would be prevented by its horizontal position. On the other hand, sudden cooling of the ampullar end of the anterior vertical canal would by condensation of the endolymph at this point give rise to an endolymph movement downward toward its ampulla. That this experiment in normal persons is invari-

---

2. Barany. **Physiologie und Pathologie des Bogengang-Apparates beim Menschen.** 27-29.

ably followed by rotary nystagmus toward the opposite side is in exact accord with Ewald's experiments. This theory of the causation of caloric nystagmus is further supported by the fact that if the head is quickly inverted so that the top of the head is directed downward toward the floor, the direction of the nystagmus is reversed, i. e., is now toward the ear irrigated. That the use of hot water, which by reducing specific gravity would cause an endolymph movement in the opposite direction, invariably gives rise to rotary nystagmus toward the ear irrigated, lends further support to this view as to the causation of these phenomena.

The value of these experiments depends upon the fact that after the vestibular apparatus has been destroyed, either surgically or by disease, no reaction follows the application of heat or cold. The caloric tests are therefore invaluable as a means of determining impairment or loss of vestibular function.

Rotation or Turning Experiment.—When a normal individual, seated with head erect upon a revolving chair, is turned fairly rapidly in either direction,—let us say to the left,—a horizontal nystagmus is set up with the quick eye movement in the direction in which he is turned, i. e., to the left. When the rotations are suddenly arrested, the nystagmus is reversed, the quick eye movement being now to the right.

Barany's experiments with a large number of supposedly normal persons showed that 10 fairly rapid rotations produce a maximum reaction, and that the average duration of the nystagmus following this experiment is 40 to 45 seconds. This describes the average, with great variations in individuals.

Explanation of Rotational Nystagmus In Accordance With Ewald's Experiments.—The mechanical influence of sudden turning of the head in the horizontal plane upon the fluid in any particular canal depends upon the relation which the plane of this canal bears to the horizontal plane. Thus, with the head erect the two horizontal canals are approximately in the horizontal plane. When the head is suddenly turned in either direction—let us say to the right—the fluid in these canals by reason of its inertia at first lags behind, i. e., suffers an initial displacement in the opposite direction. This initial endolymph movement in the right horizontal canal is toward its ampulla, while in the left horizontal it is toward the small end of the canal. Now according to Ewald's experiments, these are precisely the endolymph movements which in these canals, give rise to nystagmus to the right, and this phenomenon is always present during 10 rotations to the right. When, however, the rotations are suddenly stopped there occurs, again by reason of its inertia, an endolymph displacement in the opposite direction with the result that the direction of the nystagmus is reversed, i. e., rotation to right is followed by nystagmus to left.

During rotation about a vertical axis it is evident that the endolymph movement in any canal is at its maximum when the canal lies in the horizontal plane, and becomes progressively less as the plane of this canal is changed and the angle of extension between its plane and the horizontal plane is increased. Finally when the plane of the canal becomes vertical, i. e., is at right angles to the plane of rotation, no appreciable endolymph movement results from rotation in the horizontal plane. Obviously, therefore, during rotation with the head erect, the influence of the two vertical canals is practically eliminated. When, however, the head is bent directly forward or directly backward to an angle of 90° with the vertical, the posterior vertical canals are brought more into the horizontal plane and rotation gives rise to a rotary nystagmus due chiefly to endolymph movement in these canals.

Rule for Determining the Form of Nystagmus Which Shall Follow Rotation[3].—Sitting erect upon a revolving chair a person revolves about a vertical axis. If now we imagine his eye cut through in a horizontal plane, i. e., by a plane at right angles to the axis about which he revolves, it is evident that this section will describe a line upon the cornea which will vary according to the position of the head. This line will indicate the form of the nystagmus (Fig. 3).

Thus, with head erect, the horizontal plane in bisecting the eye will form a line passing horizontally across the cornea, and produce a horizontal nystagmus (Fig. 3, A). With head bent laterally toward the shoulder so as to form an angle of 45° with the vertical, a horizontal section will be indicated by a line passing obliquely across the cornea, and produce an oblique nystagmus (Fig. 3, B). If the head is bent fully toward the shoulder so as to form an angle of 90° with the vertical, the eye will be bisected in a plane at right angles to its transverse diameter, and give rise to a vertical nystagmus (c). With the head bent forward so that the face looks directly downward, the horizontal plane would divide the orbit so as to re-

---

3. Barany. Ibid. 12-13.

move a segment which would include the iris. It should, therefore, be indicated by a circular line about this iris. The character of the nystagmus, however, is indicated by the points of contact at which the horizontal plane enters the orbit, and not by those at which it cuts its way out. With the head bent directly forward, therefore, a horizontal section is indicated by a curved line above the iris, and turning to the right will be followed by rotary nystagmus to the left (d). With head bent directly backward so that the eye looks upward, a horizontal section describes a curved line below the iris. With head in this position, rotation to the right is followed by rotary nystagmus to the left. But in this case the concavity of the nystagmic curves is directed upward (e).

This rotation experiment is therefore particularly instructive since it enables us to induce at will different forms of nystagmus, and to study the accompanying variations of vertigo and ataxia.

Vestibular Symptoms In Acute Suppurative Labyrinthitis.— We must now revert for a moment to the clinical side of labyrinthine disease. In this we shall have to confine ourselves to a very brief synopsis of the symptoms referable to vestibular irritation.

Let us assume that the patient is suffering from a chronic suppurative otitis media of the right ear, from which the infection has spread to the inner ear. Shortly or immediately after invasion of the labyrinth, he experiences distressing vertigo, which usually forces him to go to bed. Examination of the eyes reveals marked rotary nystagmus toward the left (sound) side. The nystagmus is at this time present in whatever position the eyes may be turned, but is aggravated when they are turned toward the left (i. e., in the direction of the quick nystagmic movement), and is minimized when they are voluntarily held in the opposite direction. The vertigo is of rotary character, surrounding objects seeming to rotate about him in bewildering fashion. If supported in the upright position, objects seem to rotate in a vertical plane usually from the right (diseased) side toward the left. Occasionally they seem to rotate in the opposite direction. When lying upon his back, the plane of seeming rotation is changed from the vertical to the horizontal. With eyes closed, he has the impression of himself rotating. If able to stand, he is markedly unsteady, and with eyes closed falls, or tends to fall, toward the right (i. e., diseased) side. At the onset, nausea

and vomiting are very frequent, if not invariable, symptoms.
All these symptoms are of lessened severity while he lies
quietly in bed. He usually maintains voluntarily, therefore,
a quiet position in bed.

Course of the Disease.—All of the above symptoms usually
subside fairly rapidly and in a somewhat regular order. That
is to say, the vertigo and ataxia regularly disappear before the
nystagmus. By the end of the first week, the vertigo may have
ceased to distress the patient as he lies quietly in bed; while
the nystagmus may be still very marked. Sudden or violent
head movements may, however, induce recurrence. From the
end of the second to the end of the fourth week, not only the
vertigo and ataxia, but also the spontaneous nystagmus, may
have completely disappeared. The patient is now free from
subjective symptoms referable to vestibular disturbance, and
may be able to walk or move in all normal ways without discomfort. He has now entered upon the stage of the disease
in which it is of the greatest importance to gauge the amount
of injury to the labyrinth by means of the caloric test.

Deductions To Be Drawn from the Caloric Reactions.—
(1) If irrigation of the diseased ear with hot or cold water is
followed by normal reactions, we may assume with confidence
that the labyrinth has been the seat of a comparatively mild
lesion which has undergone resolution, leaving the vestibular
structures intact and functionating. Prognosis good.

(2) If, on the other hand, after irrigation, with heat or
cold, persisted in from three to four minutes, no caloric reactions are induced, we may conclude that the labyrinth is the
seat of a suppurative process which has either destroyed the
vestibular structures, or at least has resulted in injury sufficiently severe to have annulled vestibular function or irritability to thermal stimuli. This condition describes the so-
called latent stage of suppurative labyrinthitis, in which the
ultimate prognosis is grave.

In the minds of many Barany's name seems to be associated
chiefly with the caloric tests. To my mind the value of his
studies depends equally upon the fact that they have enabled
him to establish certain more or less definite, constant relations between vestibular nystagmus and the attendant phenomena of vertigo and ataxia. If we can accept his hypothesis that the same laws govern the spontaneous nystagmus
of labyrinthine disease and the induced nystagmus of experi-

mental vestibular irritation, it is evident that we may resume our studies of labyrinthine disease with a surer hand.

Barany's studies have led him to formulate the following laws as governing the spontaneous vertigo and ataxia of vestibular disease:

(a) Spontaneous vertigo of vestibular origin is always accompanied by spontaneous vestibular nystagmus, and is always increased when the eyes are voluntarily turned in the dircetion of the quick nystagmic movement.

(b) Vestibular ataxia is always accompanied by vestibular nystagmus, and is always influenced by the position of the head.

(c) A person having vestibular nystagmus tends to move in the plane of the nystagmus and to fall in the direction opposite to the quick nystagmic movement.

If, as Barany believes, these are constant relations between the three components of the symptom complex characteristic of acute labyrinthine disease, it is obvious that we have control tests by which we may gauge the value of single symptoms. Thus vertigo which is not accompanied by nystagmus even when the eyes are turned strongly in the direction away from the suspected labyrinthine lesion, and which is not influenced by the position of the eyes, has little value as pointing to labyrinthine disease. Disturbances of equilibrium which are not influenced by the position of the head, can hardly be assumed to be of vestibular origin.

Let us re-state briefly the laws governing vestibular ataxia, and test their value as applied to the ataxia following the rotation, or turning, experiment.

1. Vestibular ataxia is always influenced by the position of the head.

2. A person exhibiting vestibular nystagmus tends to move within the plane of the nystagmus and to fall in the direction opposite to that of the quick nystagmic movement.

It seems to me that we shall obtain a clearer understanding, and avoid apparent contradictions, of the latter rule, if it be made to read as follows:

A person exhibiting vestibular ataxia tends to rotate within the plane of the nystagmus and in the direction opposite to that of the quick nystagmic movement.

This tendency to rotation is about an axis passing through the patient's head, and he falls or tends to fall only as this rotation, modified by his contact with the earth, throws his body in one or the other direction.

Let us now observe a person who, seated with head erect, has been turned ten times to the right. When the rotations are suddenly stopped, he exhibits well marked horizontal nystagmus to the left. He also experiences vertigo. Let him at once stand and, with head still erect and feet closely approximated, close his eyes. The nystagmus being in the horizontal plane, the reaction movement should be, not falling, but gradual turning in the horizontal plane to the right (Fig. 4). This, however, may not be demonstrated, i. e., he may stand quietly. Let us investigate the first rule which declares that vestibular ataxia must be influenced by the position of the head. Direct him to bend the head forward to an angle of 90° so that the face looks directly downward. The plane of the nystagmus is now changed from the horizontal to the vertical, and the nystagmus being to the left, the head tends to rotate in the opposite direction, i. e., toward the right shoulder. This, however, throws his body to the left. That this contradiction of the rule that the patient usually falls or moves in the direction opposite to the quick nystagmic movement, is apparent rather than real, is made clear by the accompanying diagram (Fig. 5).

If he had bent his head directly backward to an angle of 90°, instead of forward, he would inevitably have fallen in the opposite direction, as shown by Figure 6.

Another example may be cited in the rotary nystagmus following the caloric tests, or that occurring in acute labyrinthitis. Here the plane of the nystagmus being vertical rather than horizontal, the patient standing with head erect, falls in the direction opposite to the quick eye movement. And since in suppurative labyrinthitis the nystagmus is almost invariably toward the sound ear, it is perfectly correct to say that he falls usually in the direction of the diseased ear. It must not be forgotten, however, that in certain forms of circumscribed, irritative labyrinthitis, the nystagmus is in the direction of the diseased ear, in which case the patient would of course fall, or tend to fall, in the direction of the sound ear.

The other contention of Barany,—viz., that vestibular vertigo and vestibular ataxia are invariably accompanied by some degree of vestibular nystagmus,—is of decided clinical importance. So far as the phenomena induced by the rotation and caloric tests may be relied upon, this contention is substantiated. In my experience these experiments have in normal persons been invariably followed by vertigo and ataxia, usually pronounced, and by nystagmus, and in no case have the vertigo and ataxia been found to persist after the nystagmus has disappeared. I have personally never seen a case of labyrinthine disease in which vertigo and ataxia have persisted after disappearance of the nystagmus.

Naturally where one has so often to deal with hysterical and neurasthenic patients suffering from intercurrent aural disease, one may meet with apparent contradictions to any law dealing with subjective symptoms (e. g., vertigo) or with objective symptoms which may be under the unconscious influence of the will (e. g., disturbed equilibrium). It is now an established fact that many neurasthenic patients exhibit under certain conditions certain peculiar, uncontrollable eye movements which are not of vestibular origin and in no way resemble vestibular nystagmus. In like manner, it is obvious that vertigo and apparent disturbance of equilibrium may in neurasthenic patients depend wholly upon functional disorders of the general nervous system.

The far-reaching influence which Barany's theories, if accepted, must exert upon our conception of labyrinthine disease is emphasized when we consider their points of divergence from the theory and practice of von Stein. Barany holds that disturbance of equilibrium is characteristic only of the acute stage of labyrinthine diseases, and that it regularly disappears as the lesion advances either toward resolution or toward destruction of the vestibular structures. This view is supported by the fact that vestibular ataxia as a subjective symptom rapidly disappears after surgical destruction of the labyrinth. Barany therefore attaches little importance to disturbed equilibrium as a diagnostic sign in the latent or chronic stage of suppurative labyrinthitis.

Von Stein has elaborated exhaustive methods of eliciting symptoms of disturbed equilibrium requiring according to his own statement one or even three hours for the thorough examination of a single patient. Since such an examination would be quite impossible in the acute stage of suppurative labyrinthitis, it is clear that von Stein regards his tests as appropriate to the later, or chronic, stage of the disease.

Barany believes that in the chronic stage of suppurative labyrinthitis, the vestibular apparatus is in the great majority of cases no longer responsive to the usual stimuli (i. e., that its function is abolished), and that it is therefore illogical to expect disturbance of equilibrium as a result of disease localized in an organ which is not essential to static or dynamic equilibrium, and which, moreover, is no longer irritable.

Von Stein apparently believes that at no stage of suppurative labyrinthitis are disturbances of equilibrium absent; and that while these disturbances may not interfere with the patient's ability to walk or stand normally, they may be clearly demonstrated by requiring him to perform certain acts in which he is not practiced by daily custom, e. g., jumping or hopping with eyes closed, standing alternately on one and the other foot, standing on an inclined plane, etc, etc.

A possible error in all such tests lies in the fact that different individuals, depending perhaps on differences of age, muscular strength, general physical condition or, if you please, upon physiologic variations in the normal power of static or dynamic control, may when called upon to perform any unusual muscular feat, exhibit apparent disturbances of equilibrium which can not properly be referred to any organic lesion.

It is now generally conceded that vestibular ataxia is a symptom induced by vestibular irritation, acting either upon the diseased labyrinth, or by ablation of its function through disturbed balance of the unopposed healthy organ; and further that it disappears as a subjective symptom after the diseased labyrinth has been destroyed surgically, or its function (i. e., irritability) completely annulled. If, therefore, von Stein's tests elicit a veritable vestibular ataxia in the chronic stage of labyrinthine suppuration, we must assume that it is due, not to irritation of the diseased and non-functionating labyrinth, but to excitation of the sound labyrinth which is no longer balanced by an opposed healthy organ. But if von Stein's tests give positive results only by reason of ablation of function in the diseased labyrinth, why should we resort to so uncertain and exhausting an examination when far more definite data may be obtained by so simple a procedure as the caloric test?

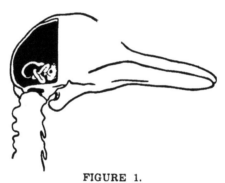

FIGURE 1.

Horizontal semicircular canals of pigeon (after Ewald).

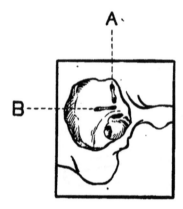

FIGURE 2.

A, Anterior vertical canal. B, Horizontal semicircular canal.

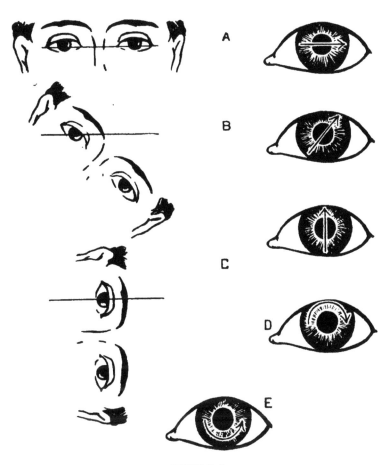

FIGURE 3.

Showing various forms of nystagmus following rotation. A, horizontal; B, oblique; C, vertical; D and E, two types of rotary nystagmus.

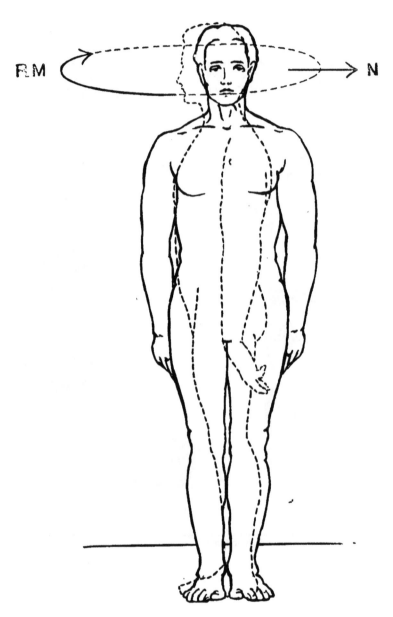

FIGURE 4.

Illustrating ataxia, or reaction movement, accompanying vestibular horizontal nystagmus, the head being held in the erect position.

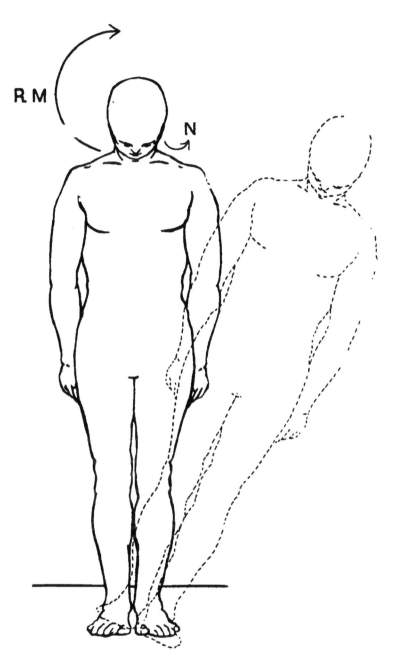

FIGURE 5.

Illustrating ataxia and reaction movement accompanying horizontal vestibular nystagmus, with the head bent directly forward to an angle of 90° with the vertical.

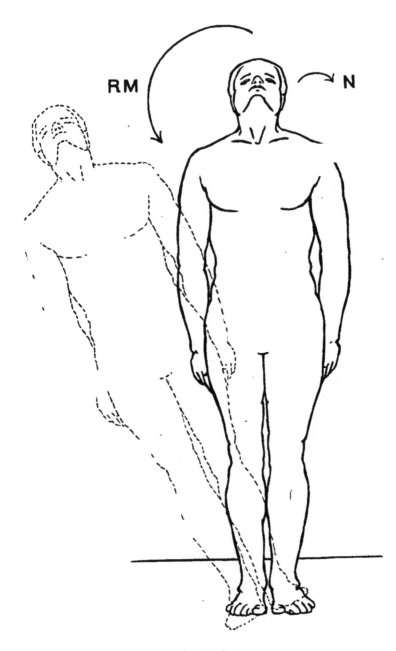

FIGURE 6.

Illustrating the reaction movement—i. e., direction of falling—
accompanying horizontal nystagmus, the head being bent directly
backward to an angle of 90° with the vertical.

XXXV

NECROSIS OF THE COCHLEA—REPORT AND ANALYSIS OF A CASE.*

By Alfred Michaelis, M. D.,

New York.

At the outset it must be said that necrosis of the bony labyrinth of the ear is a condition not very frequently cncountered. Up to the year 1886 Bezold had been able to collect records of but forty-one cases from the world's otological literature. Theophile Bec, in 1894, published a brochure at Lyon—"De la necrose du Labyrinth"—in which the number of cases collected was but sixty-five—still a very measurable number. Albert Oesch, in 1898, collected and discussed all reported cases of necrosis of the labyrinth, within the limits of an inaugural dissertation published at Basel. This also indicates no very great addition to the figures of Bezold and Bec.—(78.)

A survey of the literature in the last decade since Oesch's collation is productive of a very small increase in the number of reported cases. Gerber, in 1904, added twelve cases, some observed by himself and the rest being cases reported by other aurists. Since then there has been no great increase to Gerber's list of ninety cases. Reports of local hospitals indicate the same infrequency.

It seems worth while to report to you this case of necrosis of the labyrinth, or to be more specific, necrosis of the cochlea, not only on account of rare occurrence, but also because of the questions which such cases have invariably raised—questions dealing with the physiology of the internal ear, and about which some observers are still at odds. Foremost among these is the question of the auditory function in cases of necrosis of the labyrinth.

ETIOLOGY.

Necrosis of the labyrinth is almost without exception, a consecutive condition. There are on record two or three cases of primary necrosis, but doubt has been cast on the

* Read before the Otological Section, New York Academy of Medicine, January, 1909.

genesis of even these. That it is necessarily a slow process cannot be gainsaid. It may be set down as a pretty well fixed rule that chronic purulent otitis media usually precedes and accompanies necrosis of the labyrinth; and it is furthermore conceivable that when this chronic purulent otitis has had indifferent treatment, or possibly none, conditions are established which predispose to extension of the middle ear disease to the labyrinth.

The improved methods of treatment of middle ear abscesses on the one hand and the growing regard of the laity for the gravity of this aural disease, will no doubt make for an even rarer occurrence of necrosis of the labyrinth.

SYMPTOMS.

There are certain symptoms arising in the course of a chronic purulent otitis which point to the invasion of the labyrinth. They are vertigo, facial paralysis, pain, a fetid discharge, and the rapid growth of granulations and polypi. Increased deafness is usually not noted, because the hearing has suffered before from the middle ear disease; and the graver symptoms of the invasion of the internal ear draw away attention from this symptom, especially if the other ear is normal.

It is perfectly possible to have some of these symptoms in the course of a middle ear abscess without any lesion of the labyrinth. After all, the thing that certifies the diagnosis is the extrusion of some part or all of the bony labyrinth. Destruction and sequestration of the entire labyrinth is rare, and seems to have been encountered in children only. In adult life the sequestrum consists most frequently of a portion of the inner framework of the cochlea, usually the first one or two turns. Cases of exfoliation of the semi-circular canals, or of the vestibular portions of the bony capsule are also recorded, however. The preponderance of cochlear sequestra over other portions has led Bezold to conclude that the most common points of invasion of the labyrinth are below—namely, the round window, or via the variable cells on the floor of the tympanic cavity below the promontory.

It is needless to add that such an invasion of the labyrinth at all times constitutes a grave menace to the life of the patient. The wonder is that the mortality for the cases recorded was not greater, only 16 or 18 per cent having succumbed to meningitis, brain abscess, etc.

Prefaced by these brief and elementary remarks, we come now to the consideration of the case:

F. K., a vigorous young man of 26 years, was referred to me for treatment about two years ago. His own history and that of his family was good. At the age of 14 he had diphtheria, which was followed by discharge from his left ear. He has no recollection that the right ear was also involved at that time. Two years ago he discovered that the right ear was also discharging. As he lived in a small community near New York, the aural condition received scant attention. His hearing had been poor all these years. A week or two after the right ear began to discharge he began to have intolerable pain on this side. The pain radiated to the temporal and supraorbital regions, and completely disabled the patient. The intensity was undiminished for three weeks. This attack compelled him to seek relief and he was told he had a growth in his ear. The local physician made some attempts at removal.

At this point the patient came under my care and observation. He came for relief from the pain on the right side. In view of the more urgent symptoms his hearing was not tested at this time. The physical examination of the right ear disclosed this condition: Canal almost filled with granulations and polypi, with ill-smelling pus oozing from the interstices between the polypi. According to regional origin there seemed to be three groups of polypi— an anterior, a superior, and a posterior group.

The left ear was also discharging foul pus quite freely. There were no granulations or polypi, and the entire drum was destroyed with the exception of a narrow falciform border above. The denuded malleus handle, not adherent, projected downward into the cavity. The mucous membrane lining of the tympanic cavity was greatly thickened, and pus proceeded from the spaces above the cavum tympani.

Cleansing and curative treatment was instituted for the left ear, and the work of removing the granulations and polypi from the right side was begun at once. Since the patient lived at some distance he was seen but once a week, and hence the work of removal extended over five or six weeks. The anterior and superior groups were entirely ablated during this time. It could then be determined that the anterior group of granulations originated at the lower end of the malleus handle. The upper group sprang from the epitympanic space posterior to the malleus. The posterior group proceeded from the inner wall of the tympanic cavity in the promontorial region. The last mentioned group resisted treatment. What seemed to be the base of the growth was removed in as many weeks. At each examination a growth of considerable size was found to have recurred. It was crater-like in appearance. When removed for the third time the entire base was cauterized with chromic acid. Roughening of the underlying bone could be felt at this time. The ear was clear of all growth, and the discharge had diminished noticeably. No recurrence of growth was observed when the patient returned a week later. Discharge had almost ceased and a whitish mass the size of a small pea could be seen lying on the floor of the cavum tympani. It was easily lifted out and proved to be a fragment of carious bone, which from its conformation was plainly a portion of the cochlea. There was a depression now where the base of the recurring polypus had been. It felt soft and boggy to the probe. All this time the pain had diminished in intensity and by the time the ear had been cleared of growth it had disappeared entirely.

The appearance of the right ear was as follows: The malleus was dislocated downwards and adherent to the inner wall. The drum anterior to the malleus was preserved but also adherent. The posterior half of the drum was gone. The prolapse of the malleus and the adhesions around its neck and head had almost entirely shut off all access to the accessory spaces above. There was only a pin point opening posterior to the malleus, and a slender probe could be inserted only for a limited distance. On the inner wall, in the promontorial region, there was a boggy depression still raw looking. The long process of the incus was gone, and the other parts of that ossicle could not be discovered through the small orifice leading up. Dry treatment was instituted, and for six months after this the patient had no further trouble. Discharge on the left continned in spite of treatment.

At the end of the six months the right ear began to discharge again. The pus proceeded from the small opening above, and there was a tendency to granulation at this point. Treatment was again resumed and at the present time the ear is absolutely dry, and the epidermization of the tympanic cavity is complete. The fossa rotunda is visible, and 3-4 mm. anteriorly is a pit marking the point of exit of the sequestrum.

THE SEQUESTRUM.

The sequestrum consists of that part of the modiolus cochlearis of the first cochlear turn. The basis modioli with its central canal for the cochlear branches of the auditory nerve may be seen, and the lamina ossea spiralis is also present. The two scalae are plainly visible. Height 2 mm., and the greatest width is 4 mm.

AUDITORY TESTS.

Hearing tests were conducted immediately after this unexpected exfoliation of a part of the cochlea. The tests were made with Hartmann's series of forks, and were entirely qualitative.

	Right Side.			Left Side.	
	Air.	Bone.		Air.	Bone.
C 32	Neg.	....	C 32	Neg.	....
C 128	Neg.	Pos.	C 128	Pos.	Pos.
C 256	Neg.	Pos.	C 256	Pos.	Pos.
C 512	Neg.	Pos.	C 512	Pos.	Pos.
C 1024	Pos.	Pos.	C 1024	Pos.	Pos.
C 2048	Pos.	....	C 2048	Pos.	....
Watch	Neg.	Pos.	Watch	2½ cm.	Pos.

Weber's Test: Conducted with C 256 yielded lateralization to the right side distinctly, accompanied by a "buzzing sound," to use the patient's language.

It was discovered by accident whilst testing with C 256 that the patient could hear this fork on the right side when applied quite lightly even, to any part of the external ear. The bone conduction for the watch was better on the left than on the right side. Further tests conducted about six months later, in the main confirmed the original results. The patient again lateralized to the right, and again the tone of C 256 was accompanied by a buzzing sound.

C 128 heard when applied to auricle.

C 256 heard when applied to auricle.

C 512 heard when applied to auricle.

Galton, 1.06—both sides.
Koenig's rods—41,000.
Loud voice, 25 cm.
Acumeter, 2½ cm. right, 65 cm. left.
Final hearing tests were made last July, with the following results:

	Right.			Left.	
	Air.	Bone.		Air.	Bone.
C 26	Neg.	.....	C 26	Neg.	.....
C 128	Neg.	Plus.	C 128	Plus.	Plus.
C 256	Neg.	Plus.	C 256	Plus.	Plus.
C 512	Plus.	Plus.	C 512	Plus.	Plus.
C 1024	Plus.	Plus.	C 1024	Plus.	Plus.
C 2048	Plus.	.....	C 2048	Plus.	.....

Lateralization again to the right side, together with a "buzzing sound."

C 512 ⎫
C 128 ⎬ all heard on the right side when lightly applied
C 256 ⎭ to auricle of that side.

Right.	Left.
Watch—Air, neg.	Watch—Air, 5 cm.
Watch—Bone, plus.	Watch—Bone, plus.

Watch heard louder on the left by bone than on the right.

Speech: Some words spoken in middle voice were heard at 2 meters. Loud voice 3½ to 4 meters. This applied to both sides.

On testing bone conduction for duration, the following resulted:

Right.	Left.
C 256 ...... 14 seconds.	C 256 ...... 16 seconds.
C 512 ...... 22 seconds.	C 512 ...... 28 seconds.
C 1024 ...... 12 seconds.	C 1024 ...... 16 seconds.
Galton whistle, 2.5.	Galton whistle, 1.2.

ANALYSIS.

Let us revert to the symptoms of necrosis of the labyrinth stated at the beginning of this paper. The presence of pain has been noted. The occurrence of profuse and fetid discharge was also mentioned in the history. The polypi and granulations recurred rapidly after each removal, and this fact has been noted in many of the cases on record. There remain but two symptoms stated at the outset, of which no mention was made in detailing the history of the case—vertigo and facial paralysis. It is evident that these two symptoms could not have been very prominent, or were wanting entirely, since no allusion has been made to them. The patient does not remember to have had trouble with his face at any time. On the other hand, he remembers to have had three or four transitory attacks of vertigo, at about the period of the subsidence of the pain. The vertigo ensued when he picked up some weighty object, and there was a slight tendency to fall toward the right. There never was any actual fall, however.

It seems, then, that with the exception of facial paralysis present in 80 per cent of all cases, all the symptoms commouly noted were present. The patient dated the onset of his trouble on the right side only two years back. It is not unlikely, however, that the purulent middle ear disease was present long before this. Certainly the polypi could not have developed to so great an extent in the two or three weeks between the onset of the pain and the examination of the ear. We have to deal here undoubtedly with a neglected middle ear abscess.

Thus the conditions of chronicity and an antecedent middle ear suppuration are satisfied. There is no way of determining when the invasion of the labyrinth took place. In any event the death and sequestration was not a rapid process.

When we review and analyze the results of the tests for hearing we arrive at the most interesting and important feature of this report. Most observers have come to the conclusion that an ear whose cochlea has suffered destruction, even in part, as in this case, has lost its power to hear.

The consensus of opinion is that the sound ear does all the hearing, and that it is impossible to exclude this ear from participation when the side whose labyrinth is destroyed is tested. Failure to recognize this fact has led some observers to ascribe hearing power to ears whose labyrinths were destroyed.

If we refer to the last tests made upon the case here reported we note, taking up the question of air conduction first, that the voice was apparently heard up to four meters by the right and left ears when tested separately. Both ears were now closed and the right side tested again, and again the right side apparently heard the selected words at four

meters. Thus by means of this test, known as the Denert-
Lucae test, one·proof is adduced that speech could not have
been independently heard on the right side.

The same test was employed when air conduction was
tested with the tuning forks. The forks were heard just
as well when the right side was closed.

It will be noted that the higher notes, C 512, C 1024 and
C 2048, were heard by air conduction on the right side.
This, of course, is contrary to all experience, and contrary
to the accepted fact that in nerve deafness, of which this is
an example, the higher tones are not heard. But we know
that all the treble tones whose wave lengths are short have
greater penetration and are harder to shut out from the
untested ear. In this way we may explain what seems a
departure from accepted laws for determining auditory
nerve involvment.

When we come to analyze the tests made for bone conduction we must recall to mind that if it was difficult to
exclude the sound ear in air conduction, it is impossible to
exclude it from participation when bone conduction is
tested.

Weber's test, which at the best is not always conclusive,
yielded rather mystifying results. The patient with great
positiveness referred the preponderance of sound to the
right side, stating that it was a "buzzing sound." He also
claimed to hear all the forks that were applied to the right
mastoid bone at the point of application, and not on the
other side. The writer was particular to elicit this information. The patient was very positive in his assertion.
If we add to this the fact that some forks were heard on
the right side even when placed lightly anywhere on the
right auricle, our conclusions appear to be still more confused.

The phenomenon of the "buzz" which the patient claims
to have heard when the lower forks in the series were applied to the mastoid or vortex seems almost to fortify the
theory maintained by some that the labyrinth has sound
perceiving and organs other than the cochlear ones. The
theory that the maculae acusticae of the vestibule have the
function of perceiving noises seems to gain support by the
assertion of the patient, that a buzz was heard with or instead of a tone.

It does not need to be emphasized that tones or even

noises other than the tonal vibrations enter into the sum total of sound of most forks and particularly those of the lower and middle register. In other words, there is a mixture of essential tone and adventitious sounds and noises. Bearing this fact in mind and also recalling that in this particular case, both from the symptoms and pathology, there was apparently no involvement of the vestibular part of the labyrinth which contains the maculae acusticae, we might reasonably conclude that the maculae had exercised their supposed noise-perceiving function when the forks were applied. The perception of the pure tonal vibrations was, however, eliminated since Corti's organ was destroyed. This deduction would seem justified both by the macular theory and by the nature of the case described. In the light of the still unshaken theory of Helmholz this deduction, whilst fascinating, is purely fanciful.

There is little question that the delicate membranous labyrinth, and especially the cochlear contents, cannot possibly survive when the bony envelope or framework is destroyed, and most physiologists are agreed that the cochlea is the sole tone-perceiving and tone-analyzing portion of the membranous labyrinth.

The only tenable conclusion is that the sounds which are seemingly perceived on the side whose labyrinth is destroyed are only the expression, in a diminished degree, of what the opposite ear is able to hear.

That this is so Bezold was able to prove by tests for duration of hearing by bone conduction, and the results obtained, when this case was tested for duration, support his conclusions. The duration in seconds on the right side was less than on the left side. The lesser duration on the right is due to loss by penetration to the opposite side. The improvement in hearing on the left side which was noted at each successive test also gave rise to an apparent improvement on the right side. That the patient referred sound perception to the right side in all of the bone conduction tests can only be explained by his inability to localize the sound.

XXXVI.

SUPPURATION OF THE LABYRINTH.

By Lafayette Page, A. M., M. D.,

Indianapolis.

The labyrinthine capsule, containing the delicate and wonderful mechanism for the perception of sound, combined with the equally wonderful organ of equilibration, is well adapted for protection against the invasion of disease. The fact that the labyrinth is so rarely invaded by the purulent process, which is so often present in the tympanic cavity, bathing its outer wall in pus and the products of decay, is evidence that nature has afforded unusual protection for these organs. Bezold estimated that the labyrinth is involved in the necrotic process in the proportion of only one case in every five hundred of chronic purulent otitis media, while Friedreich estimates the proportion to be one in every one hundred. The percentage of involvement is probably greater than either of these estimates. Since the great majority of cases of labyrinth suppuration occurs during the first decade of life, many of them pass unrecognized. Until quite recently our knowledge of this affection has been in a very chaotic state. The symptomatology has been ill defined. The difficulty which the investigators have encountered in ascertaining the physiologic functions of the cochlea and the vestibular apparatus with their disturbed functions in pathologic processes has rendered diagnosis uncertain. The recent and concentrated effort among otologists to master these difficult problems of diagnosis has been well rewarded. We now feel that we can base our diagnosis on tests and well defined symptoms and outline the treatment or surgical procedure with a degree of certainty that places this subject well within the realm of exact science.

MODE OF INVASION.

The most vulnerable points in the labyrinth wall are the horizontal semicircular canal, the fenestra ovalis and rotunda and the pars promontoria; and from within, the porus acusticus internus is the most frequent avenue of infection. The fenestrae present the greatest structural weakness to invasion. The horizontal semicircular canal is regarded by Jansen as the most frequent site of infection. This is due to the close relationship of the attic, the chief seat of pathologic activity in chronic middle ear suppuration. Friedreich emphasizes the importance of the oval window as an exceedingly vulnerable point, owing to the frequent granulomatous changes about the foot-plate of the stapes, destroying the annular ligament. The intimate vascular connection between the lateral and petrosal sinuses and the labyrinth render infection possible along these venous channels by metastasis, without producing fistulous openings in the outer capsule (Richards). The accumulation of septic material about the oval and round windows and the horizontal semicircular canal from pathologic processes in the middle ear, producing granulomatous changes and gradual erosion from without, is the most common mode of infection of the labyrinth. When the infectious process has once gained entrance to the vestibule or cochlea, the destructive changes are rapid, and the spread of the disease to the brain is easy along the course of the facial and auditory nerve sheaths, and the saccus endolymphaticus.

SYMPTOMS.

Marked or well defined symptoms of labyrinth suppuration are present only in those cases of rapid or sudden invasion. When the process of crosion takes place slowly, the vestibular functions are gradually accommodated to the changes, so that manifest symptoms are not always observable. In a large percentage of cases in which the labyrinth is extensively destroyed, there are no characteristic symptoms to direct our attention to the labyrinth, as the seat of disease. Such symptoms as nausea, vomiting and disturbed equilibrium are not sufficiently characteristic to more than suggest involvement of the labyrinth. They may all be present in intratympanic disease, cerebellar abscess or cholesteatoma. Any affection from without, disturbing the intralabyrinthine pressure, may produce these symptoms, as we have all observed. Profound deafness, occurring suddenly, is always suggestive of involvement of the cochlea in the purulent process; tinnitus and the various hallucinations of sound are suggestive symptoms. Bezold and Friedreich both regard disturbed equilibrium as the most constant symptom in this affection. Nystagmus, with nausea and vomiting, they consider very transient phases of the disease. In the active diffused form of a purulent involvement of the labyrinth, the symptoms which are usually present are nausea, vertigo, nystagmus, headache, slight fever and coated tongue. If the patient attempts the upright position, disturbances of equilibrium are very manifest, especially when standing with eyes closed and feet together. Having these symptoms, including profound deafness and tinnitus, we can feel quite sure of labyrinth involvement (Jansen). In the typical cases the diagnosis is obtruded upon us, but in the large percentage of chronic cases, in which the process is circumscribed and latent, we may be caught unawares.

Barany has recently discovered, by numerous tests, that in every man possessing a normal vestibular apparatus, on syringing the ear with cold water there is produced a distinct nystagmus, which lasts from one-half to three minutes. If the right ear is syringed with cold water, the head being in the upright position, there is produced a rotary and horizontal nystagmus, directed toward the left side and is best observed when the patient looks to the left side. If the water is of the temperature of the body, no nystagmus is produced. If water of a temperature higher than of the body is used in syringing, the nystagmus is reversed; that is, the nystagmus is directed toward the ear which is being syringed. This test reveals the normal reaction of the vestibular apparatus to heat and cold. Now if the semicircular canals are destroyed, syringing with cold water produces no nystagmus, so the reaction is negative. In a circumscribed labyrinth suppuration, canals not destroyed, such as fistula of the labyrinth, the nystagmus is to the diseased side. In an acute diffused labyrinth suppuration, in which the functions of the labyrinth are suddenly paralyzed, syringing the diseased ear produces no nystagmus. Spontaneous nystagmus is to the sound side. In old cases of diffused labyrinth suppuration the reaction from cold is negative, and there is no spontaneous nystagmus.

Barany calls our attention to the number of reported cases of death from meningitis following the simple radical mastoid operation—patients who were strong and healthy, except perhaps for an occasional attack of vertigo. The post-mortem of such patients always showed the presence of an undiagnosed labyrinth suppuration, which after the radical operation produced fatal meningitis. He further says that when the diagnosis is clear, every case of such suppuration should be operated on radically and the labyrinth itself opened at the same time. This test is a great contribution to our diagnostic methods. Its value is not confined alone to the diagnosis of suppuration of the labyrinth, but is of great value in cerebellar abscess and acoustic tumor.

The equilibrium tests are of decided diagnostic value in some cases. To state them briefly: "First, standing with open and then closed eyes, to note the unsteadiness of position; second, walking with open and then with closed eyes, noticing a tendency to ataxic gait or divergence from a straight line, a tendency to walk in a curve generally; third, jumping, feet and knees in apposition and eyes closed, to ascertain any tendency to fall toward the affected side; fourth, the rotation test, by turning the patient rapidly on a revolving chair and suddenly stopping. The rotation should first be toward the sound side, and then toward the diseased side. The sensation of giddiness is most marked when turned toward the affected side."

These tests are not of so much practical value in clinical practice as the caloric test. Our patients are not usually willing to submit to these undignified gymnastics called for in equilibrium tests, especially if they happen to be suffering from the unpleasant symptoms of the disease. The galvanic test is rarely used at the present. The tuning fork tests are generally conceded to be of doubtful value in the diagnosis of this affection. Bone conduction is usually impaired; the range of audition is greatly reduced; the upper tone limit is lowered, and the lower tone limit is elevated. The Weber test is lateralized in the normal ear. Rinne is negative.

The value of many of these tests depends largely on the personal equation. The difficulty of using these tests for diagnosis in very young children is obvious.

Barany says the life of the patient may depend upon an accurate investigation of the functions of the labyrinth, and the experience of all those who have operated on these cases would verify this statement. In testing the hearing of those who have had the labyrinth partially or completely destroyed, one of the most difficult problems which we have had to encounter is in successfully eliminating the hearing in the normal ear. With all the devices which have been contrived for this purpose, it has been practically impossible to occlude the good ear. Professor Voss, of Frankfurt, Germany, in the current number of the *Beitraege*, describes a device which seems to successfully occlude the hearing in the normal ear. Without fully detailing this test, it consists in directing a current of compressed air against the drum membrane of the normal ear, while we are conducting our hearing test in the affected ear. The compressed air forces the drum and stapes inward, increasing the intralabyrinthine pressure to the point of producing total deafness in the good ear. It remains to be demonstrated if this is an absolute test.

PROGNOSIS.

The prognosis of suppuration of the labyrinth is not so utterly hopeless as the location of the purulent process would lead us to expect. In spite of extensive necrosis, approaching very near the dura, the internal carotid and the jugular, complications producing death are comparatively rare. Nature is ever on her guard, erecting barriers around sequestra and osseous fistulae, preventing the advance of the disease with proliferations of connective tissue and osteosclerosis.

"Fatal termination is usually due to the extension of the carious process to the facial canal, the cranial cavity and the venous sinuses, resulting in death from meningitis, abscess of the brain, sinus thrombosis and phlebitis. Erosion of the walls of the carotid canal and lateral sinus may terminate in fatal hemorrhage or general pyemia."

INDICATIONS FOR OPERATION.

To determine the necessity for operation in these cases requires the best surgical judgment. We should hesitate to invade this dangerous region until the indications become imperative. Richards has well defined the proper surgical attitude in these cases, in the following statement: "Considering, however, the doubtful value of symptoms as indicative of actual invasion of the labyrinth, the difficulty of eliminating cerebellar disease, the unreliability of tuning forks in differentiating, in this class of cases, middle ear from labyrinthine lesions, the practical certainty that we will destroy the organ for the purpose of useful hearing, the actual danger to life should we commit the error of opening a normal labyrinth to an infected cavity—the correct surgical attitude is not to enter the labyrinth upon symptoms, etc., alone at the primary operation, unless there is direct evidence that the labyrinth is involved."

These words were written before the Barany method of testing the functions of the labyrinth were perfected. While this advice would probably be modified in some degree from the light thrown on this subject by the very recent discoveries, yet it indicates the proper course, even now, for those who have not had wide experience in operating on these cases. Reckless exploration of the labyrinth certainly endangers life. Jansen says that the labyrinth operation is permissible in every diffused infectious disease of the entire labyrinth or of one of its two portions, especially of the vestibule. He also emphasizes the necessity of operating in all cases of accidental luxation of the stapes, following currettment, in which the following symptoms develop after twenty-four hours following the radical mastoid operation: rise of temperature, coated tongue, increasing nystagmus and equilibrium disturbance.

Jansen represents the most extreme radicalism in surgical treatment of this disease. For those who do not possess such skill and wide experience, the more conservative course is the wiser.

METHODS OF OPERATION.

As has already been pointed out, many cases of suppuration of the labyrinth are not discovered until the radical mastoid operation reveals fistulous openings in the outer labyrinthine capsule. The primary step in every operation on the labyrinth is the complete exposure of the tympanic cavity and horizontal semicircular canal, by the radical mastoid operation. If the vestibule or cochlea are to be opened, the widest exposure possible within the limits of safety is necessary. Owing to the great variations in the anatomical relationships of the labyrinth to the facial canal, the sigmoid and petrosal sinuses, the jugular bulb and the carotid canal, our course must be modified to suit these varying structural relationships. Every operator must choose his course to suit the anatomical variation. After the tympanic cavity has been thoroughly exposed, the wound should be packed with gauze, soaked in adrenalin, until the field of operation is perfectly clear of blood. If it is discovered that the canals are the seat of the carious process, they are removed by gradually shaving away with chisel or burr as far as the ampullary openings into the vestibule, keeping in mind all the time the close relationship of the horizontal canal to the facial nerve. By this method the vestibule is opened from above and behind the nerve. If the vestibule is found to be involved, a counter opening is made through the oval window, which is enlarged downward, exercising great care to avoid fracturing the inner wall of the vestibule. Often it will be found necessary to remove the horizontal canal. This will be found comparatively simple and easy. In other cases, a complete exenteration of the canal system is necessary when they are found to be perforated with fistulous openings and contain granulations and pus.

The Bourguet method of opening the labyrinth consists first, in the radical mastoid operation, thoroughly exposing the tympanic cavity and curretting the tympanic end of the eustachian tube, then introducing the Bourguet· protector into the oval window, so as to protect the facial nerve from injury. The bridge of bone between the oval and round windows is chiseled away ·with a delicate chisel, thus exposing the vestibule. This opening may be enlarged, so as to expose the interior of the cochlea. The cavity is then gently cleansed of granulations and pus, a wick of gauze placed and the mastoid wound lightly packed with gauze.

I have only indicated the merest outline of the operative technic. There are several modifications of these two methods of entering and exploring the labyrinth.

The following cases will illustrate some of the very interesting phases of this affection:

CASE 1.—E. B., aged nine years, consulted me December 6, 1906, on account of headache, tenderness and swelling over the mastoid and discharge from the left ear. The discharge began six months previous, following an attack of measles, and had persisted since, without pain. In examining this little girl, I was attracted by her intelligence and patience, which enabled me to make a thorough and satisfactory examination. There was a large perforation of the membrana tympani, which was filled with protruding granulations. I could easily detect a necrotic area about the promontory with a fine probe. Loud conversation was apparently heard with the normal ear closed. Weber lateralized in the normal ear; Rinne negative. Nystagmus, vertigo and nausea were entirely absent and had been so from the beginning of the discharge. (The Barany tests were not known at that time.) A radical mastoid operation was performed two days later. There was extensive destruction of the mastoid cells and the tympanic cavity was filled with granulations. After removing the necrotic ossicles and granulation, the cavity was packed for a few minutes with adrenalin gauze, so that the outer wall of the labyrinth could be carefully explored.   A large fistulous opening was found in the promonotory, close to the fenestra ovalis, which led into the cochlea.   The outer shell of the cochlea was chiseled away with a small gouge.   The interior of the cochlea was filled with granulation and pus and the modiolus with the osseous lamina was found to be completely detached, and was removed en masse as a sequestrum.   The cavity of the labyrinth was carefully mopped out with gauze and wick drainage was placed, and the operation completed in the usual way.   This was followed by an uninterrupted recovery, and there has been no discharge of pus from the ear since.

We should naturally expect a complete destruction of hearing in this ear, since the cochlea was so extensively removed. Yet, with all the known devices for eliminating the normal ear, such as herpetic sealing, creating a vacuum with pneumo-massage, there was apparently a certain degree of hearing in the affected ear for loud conversation.   This was also the conclusion of others, who verified the tests.   Recently I have used the Voss test for eliminating the normal ear, and find the defective ear completely destroyed for hearing.

CASE 2.—Mrs. L., aged thirty-two, consulted me May 2, 1907, on account of distressing vertigo, headache and high-pitched noises in the left ear, which had been continuous for the past few months.   The symptoms had become so annoying of late that she was unable to attend to her household duties.   She could not fix the exact time when the discharge began, as it was not accompanied by any marked acute symptoms.   She thought she had trouble with that ear in childhood, and that it had been quiescent for several years, with slight tenderness, until discharge began, about three years previous to my examination.

On examining the ear, I found the tympanic cavity, mastoid cells and antrum filled with a very extensive cholesteatomatous mass, the full extent of which I could not fully determine. The membrana tympani was completely destroyed, and pus was flowing all about the deeper portions of the mass.

The radical mastoid operation was advised and performed three days later.   After chiseling through a thick mastoid cortex, a large cholesteatomatous mass was exposed, which extended deep into the posterior cranial fossa, near the internal auditory meatus and surrounding the canal system. There was an epidural abscess, and the posterior and horizontal canals were necrotic and in communication with the abscess cavity. The cholesteatomatous mass and granulation tissue were cleared away and the semicircular canals were completely removed as far as their ampullary openings in the vestibule. The Panse flaps were used for lining the cavity and gauze wicks were placed. Equilibrium disturbances were annoying for a few weeks after the operation. Recovery has been complete. Two years have elapsed, without any sign of return of the cholesteatoma or other disturbance of equilibrium.

CASE 3.—On May 16, 1906, Mrs. J., aged fifty-three, consulted me, on account of severe pain about the left eye and a purulent discharge from the nose.

Examination revealed the middle turbinates greatly swollen and pus flowing from the anterior and posterior ethmoid cells of the left side.

One week later, on the 24th, I was called to see this patient, at her home, on account of distressing pain in the left ear and a facial paralysis on the same side. Finding the drum distended, a free incision was made at once, which was followed by a bloody serous discharge. She was sent to the hospital the same day, as marked mastoid involvement was already present. The facial paralysis continued, and on the following day the mastoid was opened and found to be extensively involved in a very active purulent process. The usual simple mastoid operation was completed. Two days later the right ear became involved, with all the symptoms of an active invasion of the labyrinth. Swelling over the mastoid, nystagmus, nausea, vertigo on rising in the bed, profound deafness and high-pitched noises were present. The radical mastoid operation was performed, thoroughly exposing the outer wall of the labyrinth. The region of the oval window and the horizontal canal were examined, for fistula, but the point of invasion of the pyogenic process could not be found, so the operation was completed without opening the labyrinth.

The healing process in both mastoid wounds was slow, and it was with the greatest difficulty that I succeeded in stimulating the granulating process. The facial paralysis of the left side gradually abated, and at the end of two months both wounds had completely healed.

The results have been total deafness in the right ear, while the hearing in the left ear returned to normal. The nystagmus and vertigo persisted for several weeks after the operation. Considering the great virulence of the infection and the poor vital reaction in this patient, the results have been most satisfactory.

CONCLUSIONS. ·

Recently most exhaustive tests have been applied to these cases to determine if the labyrinth of the affected ear was in any way functionating. The Barany tests were negative in all three cases for the operated ear. The hearing tests were uncertain. Until the Voss test for eliminating the normal ear was used, it was impossible to determine if a certain degree of hearing did not exist in the operated ear of all these patients.

I am now of the opinion that all reported cases in which it is claimed that any degree of hearing remains after removing a part of the cochlea is a mistake, and if the Voss test for eliminating the normal ear is applied in these cases it will convince the operator that complete destruction of hearing always follows the removal of any part of the cochlea.

These cases have been presented and examined by several members of this section.

REFERENCES.

Barany. New Methods of Examination of the Semicircular Canals and Their Practical Significance.

Ballenger. The Surgery of the Vestibule.

Blake. Purulent Affection of the Labyrinth Consecutive to Disease of the Middle Ear.

Canfield. Diagnosis and Treatment of Suppuration of the Labyrinth.

Friederich, E. F. Die Eiterungen des Ohrlabyrinths.

Jansen. Surgical Treatment of Infective Labyrinthitis After Fifteen Years' Experience.

Politzer. Diseases of the Ear.

Reik. The Symptomatology and Diagnosis of Labyrinthitis Consecutive to Purulent Otitis Media.

Richards. Treatment of Purulent Affection of the Labyrinth Consecutive to Disease of the Middle Ear.

Voss, Prof. Dr. O., in Frankfurt a. M. Ein neues Verfahren zur Feststellung einseitiger Taubheit. Beiträge zur Anat. Physiol. Path. und Therap des Ohres der Nase und des Halses, Bd. II, Hft., 34, p. 145.

XXXVII

SLOUGHING FIBROMA OF THE NASOPHARYNX.*

By Henry L. Swain, M. D.,

New Haven, Conn.

Some years ago our distinguished Fellow, Dr. E. Fletcher Ingalls, made to the association a brief statement which was of the utmost comfort and support during the many trying hours which a certain case of sloughing fibroma gave me. The hope given in the statement that I might carry my patient through years enough until he finally outgrew the tendency to recurrence, was so helpful in the dark hours of almost sure defeat, that I consider it to be my bounden duty to briefly chronicle what happened to my patient, supporting as it does what Dr. Ingalls had said. I hope hereby to doubly fortify some other much to be pitied colleague who may have resting upon him the freighting of another life to a safe and sound state of health.

Dr. Ingalls stated, as most of you will remember, that there came to him, after years of absence, a man who, when last seen, had been given up to die from the ultimate results of a recurring fibroma of the nasopharynx. All that the skill of our versatile colleague and friend could accomplish had been exhausted. Radical and conservative measures alike failed. At some certain period the growth ceased to enlarge, shrank, and finally disappeared, leaving desolate and empty the enlarged nasal chambers which it had so completely filled in the past. Other than the evident deformity of one side of the face and his dreadful experience, the young man had nothing to show of all that he had been through.

On the 28th of October, 1899, there came to me a young boy of thirteen years, whose brother I had treated for adenoids some years previously. The general idea which the mother had of the case was that her son had nothing more the matter with him than had ailed his brother, only that the obstruction

---

*Read at the thirty-first annual meeting of the American Laryngolical Association, in Boston, May 31st to June 2nd, 1909.

which seemed to have come in h's nose was worse than in the older boy. She had, however, had a dream that the present patient had been suffering from tumor in the nose, had had a dreadful operation, and had died as a result of it, and it was this spectre in the background which colored and shaped the future clinical history, as will appear in the subsequent statements. I found that the young man was suffering from a rather typical appearing, firm, round, nasopharyngeal tumor, which I took surely to be of the fibromatous type, which had its base quite typically at the upper part of the lateral wall of the nasopharynx of the right side.

Various attempts were made in the subsequent few weeks to remove the growth with a snare, but all of them failed because the young man had not then learned the amount of self-control which he later developed to a remarkable degree.

On the first of January, there seeming no other way to get around the difficulty, and mindful of the splendid work of Dr. Lincoln and Dr. Delavan with electric currents, I conceived the idea that it might be possible to shrink this mass down by ignipuncture, exactly as we are so often able to accomplish with even quite firm tonsils, and was much pleased to find that I was able to produce thereby a considerable slough.

On the 15th of the month the patient was very desirous of trying again to have the growth removed by the snare, but the attempt failed because of the bleeding which was started up, and which was quite severe and lasted an hour. It was then evident to me that, unless it was by cauterizing (ignipuncture), further attempts at removal had better be stopped, and Dr. Wm. H. Carmalt, of New Haven, who had been called in consultation in the case, felt also that perhaps the slower method would be the better one. We considered radical removal under an anesthetic, but this the family objected to.

From that time until the first of May, once every week or ten days, the portions of the tumor which presented in the nose which could be reached from in front were freely cauterized, the aim being to attack the pedicle of the tumor as much as possible with the idea that the subsequent cicatrization might, by including the nutrient vessels, cause a loss of nutrition and subsequent decrease in the size of the tumor. The patient had begun to bleed quite freely whenever the slough, which sometimes was considerable, came away from the cauterized area. Also various attempts were made from time to time to cauterize the nasopharyngeal surface by passing the

electrode up behind the palate. These were not wholly successful. So much bleeding took place later from the nasopharyngeal surface of the tumor, that he was given a powder
of ferripyrin and tannin, equal parts. The insufflation of this
into the nasopharynx would usually stop the bleeding.

On the 26th of May the patient began having a good deal
of odor to the breath, and this was accompanied by some
swelling of the tumor. On the 31st the patient bled, according to the statement of the mother, a full quart. Allowing it
to be a pint, it was surely a very considerable hemorrhage. I
being out of town at the time, the patient was brought on a
mattress in a fainting condition to Dr. Carmalt's office. The
effort and the physical exertion, or something, had so stopped
the bleeding that when they got to his office, Dr. Carmalt
merely swabbed the nasopharynx out with some tannic acid
and antipyrin solution and sent the boy back home again.

We again talked the matter over as to whether radical
operation was not advisable, and also brought in the opinion
of Dr. Delavan, and supported by him, all our views concur-
ring, we continued to wait for the electricity to accomplish
what it could before resorting to such measures. No serious
hemorrhage took place, and considerable slough kept forming.

Not much was done during the summer months, and the
growth seemed to have ceased to enlarge. On the 7th of September, a large slough came away, and as this slough had
formed after an interval of a month or six weeks, during
which time nothing had been done in the cauterizing line, it
occurred to me that the sloughing was really the result of
natural processes rather than entirely the outcome of my own
efforts at cauterizing. The slough which now came away was
of a considerable size, and following its removal a half a tea-
cupful of blood was lost. As a result the tumor certainly
began to shrink somewhat, and we were much encouraged.
One could see through below the tumor and see the posterior
wall of the nasopharynx below the growth, a thing that had
not happened since the start.

On the 23rd of November the tumor was again markedly
swollen as though about ready to slough, and for the first
time it was evident that the growth was tending to advance
into the nose rather than to grow lower down into the pharynx.
Again following the release of a large slough the growth contracted. and this time the upper and medium part seemed to
have shrunk.

With varying fortunes, the growth on the whole apparently somewhat increased, and a very bad bleeding spell took place upon the 29th of April, 1901, as the result of the coming away of a very foul-smelling scab, and he bled in spurts for two hours. I found him practically exsanguinated, pulse hardly palpable at the wrist, and so weak that it seemed every moment as though he must pass away. A little powder up into the nasopharynx seemed to stop the bleeding, and the pulse tension was immediately raised by the dropping of an adrenalin solution, 1 to 500, under the tongue. Giving him plenty of water and using the adrenalin, we finally restored his pulse to something like a commendable volume, and he pulled through the difficulty with the tumor very much smaller than it had ever been.

Having satisfied myself that direct ignipuncture surely was insufficient, and having for the purpose installed a suitable electric controller, on November 1st, I attacked the tumor again as soon as it started to enlarge by the bipolar electrolytic method, using a Casselberry electrode. We used as strong currents as the patient could possibly bear, and applied the electrolysis as frequently as it seemed at all possible, and the result was that the patient was very little different, if any, by the first of December.

It having occurred to the mother that during both summers we had had less trouble than during the winter, we thought it might be wise to avoid the extreme cold weather, and the query was whether a milder climate might not help to keep the patient from having these dreadful sloughing times. As another sloughing period seemed imminent, as judged by the odor, at my advice they went to New Orleans and came under the care of Drs. De Roaldes and King. His description, as taken from Volume XXV of our own transactions, page 147, will indicate the condition in which the patient arrived in his care:

"The tumor was an exceedingly vascular fibroma, attached to the nasal wall with a nasal prolongation occupying and dilating the right mucosa. It had already reached the sloughing stage, and several abundant hemorrhages had weakened and exsanguinated the patient. When he first came under our observation surgical interference was not considered advisable on this account, but under the influence of our mild climate, a nourishing diet, and tonic medication, his state of health improved so much in two months that we felt justified in attempting radical removal of the growth, and so advised the parents. The tumor had greatly increased in size, until the nasal portion reached anteriorly to within half an inch of the vestibule of the nose. In the right cheek could be seen and felt a rounded movable tumor about the size of a walnut, apparently independent in its development of the post-nasal growth. Parental consent being finally obtained for operation, I decided to attempt its removal with Doyen instruments, under cocain anesthesia."

The attempt resulted in failure, and a microscopic examination showed the growth to be a telangiectatic fibroma.

Another attempt was made under an anesthetic on the 6th of May, after the patient had recovered from the bleeding which had thoroughly exhausted and exsanguinated him, following the former attempt. Again I will quote: "Operation, May 6th. The carotids were exposed by Dr. Parnham, the right external was tied, and ligatures were passed under the common carotids on both sides to make compression, if necessary, when the tumor was being cut through. I then performed tracheotomy, transfixed the tongue with a strong ligature, tied the palate forward with a rubber catheter passed through the left nasal cavity, inserted a mouth gag, and placed the patient in the Rose position. While compression was being made on the free arterial trunks, I attacked the growth with the scissors as in the preceding operation, and by vigorous efforts cut through the fibrous mass close to the attachments and brought it out through the mouth. In spite of all our control of the arteries, the hemorrhage was almost overwhelming for the patient, and when controlled by gauze packs, saline infusion had to be practiced immediately. This was skillfully done by Dr. E. D. Martin, whose valued assistance we had also obtained. The patient responded well to the infusion, and as the bleeding into the pharynx had ceased, the tracheal wound was closed." Examination after the patient recovered from the effects of the operation showed that the septum was displaced completely over to the left side, and the right nasal cavity was enormously dilated. A small part of the base remained attached to the body of the sphenoid in the posterior part of the nasal fossa. In addition to this the tumor had spread to a broader base, including nearly half of the nasopharyngeal wall.

On the 4th of June, the patient having returned to New Haven, we were sorry to have to chronicle the fact that the growth seemed to be returning in what might be called the middle part of the base, i. e., tending to grow into the nose rather than into the nasopharynx.

On the 17th of July the nose was partly filled up by the growth, and especially in the region of the middle fossa of the nose, it was certainly growing rapidly. The facial part of the growth was much enlarged.

The patient was then referred to Dr. Sprenger for x-ray treatment. These treatments were given to him as often as he could stand them until the 15th of November, the only effect appearing to be to make the facial and more superficial parts of the growth a little smaller, but the back part of the growth towards the nasopharynx increased rapidly in size. Then the usual sloughs began to appear, and with them the hemorrhages.

On the 4th of December the patient had an enormous, sudden hemorrhage which inside of fifteen minutes had brought him nearer to the grave than at any of the previous occasions. He was kept completely plugged behind and in front for a week, and when the plugs were finally safely removed, it was found that the facial tumor, which during the packing had swollen up considerably, went down as though a large abscess cavity had emptied itself, and both it and the internal tumor decreased enormously in size. By the time the shrinkage was over the whole mass was scarcely one-third the size which it was previous to the formation of the sloughs and the fearful hemorrhage. It was evident that the tumor on the face connected with the antrum and that the nasal wall of the antrum had atrophied by pressure, and that the whole antrum and nasal cavity were united into one irregular space. The patient also ran a temperature at this time and succeeded in getting up a middle ear infection upon that side. During the time of quiescence, which followed this tremendous change and destruction of tissue, the patient's physical condition gradually returned to somewhere nearly normal. For a month immediately following this episode he could scarcely be moved from his bed.

In the late spring, apparently with the return of the full vitality of the patient, the growth started once more to recur, and feeling that the patient ought to have the benefit of all the resources that we could command, I referred him to Dr. Delavan, of New York, to see if electrolytic treatment at his hand might not be of more benefit than it had been at my own. During the latter part of the spring and throughout the summer Dr. Delavan, and later Dr. Harris, gave the patient electrolytic treatment to the anterior part of the tumor, and into the nasopharyngeal part injections were made of trichloracetic acid. Later the electricity was omitted altogether.

Early in September, this being the year 1903, a sloughing spell came on, during which he was taken to New York and remained at the Manhattan Eye and Ear Infirmary. The sloughs came away without any terrible hemorrhage, although he had to be plugged for twenty-four hours on one occasion owing to the severity of the bleeding.

In the third week of September he developed a severe attack of erysipelas, which nearly cost him his life. Having recovered from that, the tumor presented a smaller, hollowed-out appearance on the anterior and under surface. It still extended into the nose, so that it was almost as far front as the anterior end of the inferior turbinate, and behind extended well down toward the palate. Later on the growth gradually began to shrink away; it disappeared from the anterior and inferior portions within the nasal cavity, making its last stand in the nasopharynx.

. During the next year the patient had more or less of the same treatment. He had one or two serious bleeding spells, but none of the extent and terrible force of the former experiences. He spent the two subsequent winters in Pasadena and California in that neighborhood, during which time he had only one slight sloughing spell. He developed a fistula in the external part of the face which apparently connected with the parotid gland so that he had continuous flow of at first matter and finally only clear fluid. for over two years. This is still open and in the two years just past has been kept continually packed with gauze.

The last three winters he has spent at home, and at the present writing there is nothing but scar tissue to be seen in the vault of the pharynx where the tumor masses had come and gone. His nasal cavity is filling in somewhat. There is a partial attempt at restoration of the inferior turbinate, but the middle turbinate and the nasal wall of the antrum have disappeared by pressure, as has the posterior half of the nasal septum. His chief difficulty now lies in keeping the nostril clean, because, as it often happens in atrophic rhinitis, it is difficult in a dilated nose to keep the mucus from inspissating and giving odor to the breath and otherwise disturbing the patient. He has not had any hemorrhages to amount to anything for the last two and one-half years, and apparently, then, has fulfilled the hope that, through all his distressing history I have held up to him, that he might be another case like Dr. Ingalls'. His present age is twenty-two, so that I feel he has lived beyond the probability of recurrence and well-nigh the possibility of it.

Dr. Harris, in replying to a recent letter which inquired as to his views of this particular case, closed his letter with a statement so admirably worded to express my own views that I reproduce it as the closing sentence of this brief chronicle of the most remarkable instance of nasopharyngeal growth which my experience has included. He said:

"Viewing it in the light of subsequent events, with a desire to give all credit to the treatment, I must confess that today I am skeptical as to the real benefit derived. It has seemed to me that the history of this remarkable case, while it was under my care, conformed entirely to the periods before and after and that we were dealing with a neoplasm which possessed the peculiar power of sloughing away and then recurring.

"It is gratifying to learn that the history here conforms to the history of other similar cases, namely, that if the patient can be kept alive for a number of years, the growth will of itself disappear. In all my reading and clinical work I have never known a case of such severity where the ultimate outcome has been so satisfactory."*

---

*Since writing this history early in June, the patient, while eating some ice cream in a drug store, was suddenly attacked with violent bleeding from the nose and before it could be stopped an enormous amount of blood was lost The druggist who furnished the receptacles for receiving the blood asserts that at least two quarts were lost. The patient finally fainted and at that time the nose was plugged anteriorly and posteriorly. Some bleeding also took place from the fistula in his cheek, which was also packed tightly at that time. He was taken to a private hospital and remained there two weeks, having during that period no recurrence of the bleeding. Just previous to this hemorrhage he had been having some slight bloody oozing following the removal of inspissated mucus which had latterly bothered him more than usual. Twice during the previous month he had been obliged to pack the nostril anteriorly owing to bleeding of some amount. Whether this was all due to the fact that he had been having an attack of rheumatism and had been taking considerable doses of the salicylates is not quite clear to me, although it is quite possible. In any case, this last event adds another peculiar incident to this long struggle, coming, as it does, so soon after the writing and reading of this paper and after a period of three years of practical immunity.

XXXVIII.

REPORT OF A FATAL CASE OF STATUS LYMPH-ATICUS OCCURRING IN A PATIENT OPERATED ON FOR TONSILLAR HYPERTROPHY UNDER COCAIN-ADRENALIN INFIL-TRATION.*

By Thomas J. Harris, M. D.,

New York.

I desire to report briefly a fatal case of tonsillectomy. Such accidents are, unfortunately, too frequent where a general anesthetic is employed, but so far as we can learn they are exceedingly rare where, as in the present case, only a local anesthetic was employed. The patient was a Russian Jew, aged thirty. He presented himself in my service in the Post-Graduate Hospital, complaining of repeated sore throats. Examination revealed large tonsils of the socalled submerged variety. According to the house surgeon's notes, he was admitted to the hospital at 11 a. m., April 22, 1909. His appearance was that of a short, muscular, workingman. A fluid lunch was given and at 1:15 p. m. 1/60 gr. of sulphate of strychnine was administered by the mouth. One-half hour later the patient was sent to the operating room and had a 1/5 of 1 per cent of cocain hydrochlorate in a normal saline solution containing two drachms of 1/1000 adrenalin-chlorid injected into the tonsils. The solution was freshly prepared before the operation. The tonsils were very cryptic and the contents of the first syringe containing 1 1/2 drachms entirely escaped and was expectorated. A second syringeful was injected. Of this at the outside not more than thirty minims could have been retained. There was, then, in all approximately 1/12 of a grain of cocain retained and from eight to ten minims of a 1/1000 solution of adrenalin-chlorid. After the first injection the patient complained of feeling badly, vomited and had a slight convulsive seizure, presenting the appearance that

*Read at the Thirty-first Annual Meeting of the American Laryngolical Association, Boston, June 1, 1909.

we often see where cocain has been employed locally for a nasal operation. His head was lowered for a moment and he sat up again and permitted the injection of the second syringeful.

Anesthesia was prompt and I immediately without difficulty enucleated both tonsils with the cold wire snare. No bleeding followed. During the removal of the tonsils the patient's head was supported by an assistant. The operation could not have consumed more than two minutes. At the completion of the operation I was at once struck by the pallor of the patient and discovered that he was unconscious. He was at once placed upon the operating table with the head in the Rose position. At this time respiration was plainly visible, but I was unable to get any pulse at the wrist, although there was a peculiar fluttering or tremor at times. Morphin was administered hypodermically followed by whiskey and strychnin and oxygen and artificial respiration were employed for more than an hour before we desisted in our attempts at resuscitation.

An autopsy was performed by the coroner, assisted by Drs. Palmer and Beck of the house staff, the same afternoon. I am indebted to the latter for the following notes made at the time: Nothing abnormal was discovered in the lungs. When, however, the pericardium was opened it was found that the right auricle was swollen. The right auricular appendage was dilated with fluid blood until it was five times as large as the left. The right ventricle was also swollen, but not so much as the right auricle. The auricle showed a peculiar power of contractility, a wave of contraction passing over the entire auricle and sometimes returning when the auricle was stimulated by a blow of the instrument. The muscle wall of both sides of the heart looked normal. The left side of the heart was rather undersize in proportion to the size of the man. The valves were all normal except the tricuspid, which must have been opened due to the dilation of the right side. The thymus gland weighed eighteen grammes and was bunched up in the top of the sternum. The distance from the sternum to the body of the vertebrae was one inch. The trachea and bronchii contained a little blood and mucus. The stomach contained dark-colored mucus. The glands of the axilla and groin were slightly enlarged. The kidneys were normal.

The pathologist of the hospital, Dr. H. T. Brooks, examined the thymus gland and reported that the most striking feature was that it showed no atrophy, which in a person of this age is to be regarded as abnormal. The patient died in all probability, of an overdilated right ventricle, due to the enlarged thymus with its action on the trachea and recurring laryngeal, with the cocain-adrenalin injection acting as exciting cause.

During the last few years a great deal of interest has been taken in the subject of the thymus gland, and recently a symposium was held in the New York Academy of Medicine on status lymphaticus. One of the most complete articles on the subject is to be found in "Osler's System of Medicine," by Aldred Scott Warthin, Ph. D., M. D., from which I take the liberty of quoting at some length.

"Atrophy of the lymphoid tissue with its replacement by adipose and fibrous connective tissue takes place gradually from the second year to the advent of puberty and more rapidly after this time, so that in the adult the thymus comes to be replaced by a mass of fibrous tissue and fat containing small nodes of lymphoid tissue.

"Numerous cases occurring in the literature of the last several years have proved beyond all doubt that such a compression of the trachea does occur as the result of thymic enlargement, even when the increase in size does not far surpass the limits ordinarily regarded as normal.

"All thymic enlargement may be regarded as relative or absolute. The weight in different individuals varies greatly. In general it may be said that any thymus weighing fifteen grammes or more is hyperplastic. Increase in the thickness is of far greater importance than an increase in any of the other dimensions.

"Thymic enlargement occurs as apparently an independent condition or in association with the status lymphaticus, tonsillar hyperplasia, adenoids, etc.

"In thymic death all symptoms point to suffocation resulting from tracheal stenosis and secondary laryngeal spasm as the chief, if not the only, cause of the fatal termination. To a reflex spasm of the glottis may be added a reflex cardiac paralysis, or the latter may alone be the direct cause of death in those cases of sudden death in which all signs of tracheal compression or laryngeal stenosis are wanting.

"The compression of the great vessels lying beneath the thymus may cause disturbance of blood pressure, cardiac dilatation. We must, therefore, conclude that the immediate cause of death varies in thymic enlargement, but the general picture is that of a convulsive attack of thymic asthma of the severest type. The muscular spasm closes, the face becomes ashy, then intensely cyanotic, reflex irritability is lost, there is rapid cardiac failure and death suddenly ensues. The reported cases of thymic death tend to show that its occurrence is often apparently induced by a number of factors that have no effect on the normal individual. Sudden death from fright or intense emotional excitement during trivial surgical operations has in too many instances been associated with enlarged thymus. It is probable that a large proportion of deaths occurring in surgical anesthesia are due to this condition. An enlarged thymus has been found in many of the sudden deaths associated with slight operations, such as the removal of teeth or adenoids and tonsils."

The foregoing conforms very largely to the conditions in our case. The patient had an enlarged thymus, eighteen grammes, which while not excessive is sufficient to account for all the symptoms produced. There was the convulsion with pallor followed by the intense cyanosis. There was, however, no tracheal stenosis, and the death, as shown by the autopsy, was undoubtedly of cardiac origin. How important a role the local anesthesia played it is difficult to say. From what authorities on the subject say, the slightest agency, as fright or excitement, is sufficient to serve as an exciting cause. We cannot conceive that the small quantity of cocain, 1/12 of 1 per cent, freshly prepared, to have contributed largely to the fatal result. Whether the amount of adrenalin (eight to ten minims of 1/1000 solution), with the possibility of more having been absorbed through the stomach from .the first syringeful (although it is our firm belief that this was all expectorated), can be considered a more weighty factor, is open to question. While it has been employed very largely in this form, we recognize that a number of warnings have been given regarding the possibility of accident, especially where there was a diseased condition of the heart or blood vessels, which in our case was not present. We have not had an opportunity to thoroughly examine the literature, but in a hasty survey we have not been able to discover any reported case of death from cocain-adrenalin infiltration. We have heard, however, of one such case occurring in Baltimore within the last few months, where a Schleich solution was introduced for the removal of the tonsils. Here, we were informed, the patient died three hours after the operation. Two cases have recently occurred in New York City, one where a strong solution of cocain-adrenalin was introduced into the nose on cotton in a young healthy adult, and the other where a strong solution was painted over the tonsils of a boy for tonsillectomy.

XXXIX.

NERVE DISTRIBUTION IN RELATION TO NERVE REFLEXES SIMULATING LOCAL INFLAMMATION.*

By Arthur Ames Bliss, M. D.,

Philadelphia.

The development of painful sensations within the upper respiratory tract and ear, as well as through the head, at points more or less distant from the site of an inflammation, produces a class of patients in whom diagnosis and treatment present many elements of uncertainty and doubt. Over this wide area, "reflex" irritation depends largely upon the distribution and intercommunications of the fifth and eighth pairs of cranial nerves, the trifacial, pneumogastric, glosso-pharyngeal, and spinal accessory. There results a complicated network of sensory, motor, and sympathetic fibres, each one a possible track for short circuiting or deflecting nerve impulses, by each fibre, in terms of its own function, to areas remote from the causative lesion. And the mere "reflex," alone, is rendered, in many instances, more complicated by the intensity of the suffering produced and the need for relatively prompt relief. The trifacial nerve, perhaps the chief offender, has four ganglia which form the whole of the cephalic portion of the sympathetic system. Its first and second divisions are sensory nerves, the ophthalmic and superior maxillary, with the ophthalmic and spheno-palatine ganglia. The third division, inferior maxillary, connects with the otic and submaxillary ganglia. The interlacing of fibres between these three divisions and the ganglia is direct, and their communication, also, with the sympathetic plexus of the cavernous sinus and with the carotid plexus. Emerging from the distal source of this great nerve, the Gasserian ganglion, fibres go to the tentorium cerebelli and the dura of the middle cranial fossa. Its ophthalmic and superior maxillary divisions

---

* Read at the meeting of the American Laryngological Association, held in Boston, May 31-June 2, 1909.

are closely associated with fibres which bring the spheno-palatine ganglion and nasal nerve, and naso-palatine nerve, in intimate relation, by means of the ciliary nerve, with the iris and ciliary muscles. The trifacial is the great sensory nerve of the cranium and face. By its ophthalmic division, it gives sensation—and pain, as well—to the frontal sinus region, fore-head, and the scalp as far back as the occiput. The course of its three main branches lies between the ocular muscles, and they supply the corrugator supercilii occipito-frontalis, and or-bicularis palpebrarum muscles with common sensation—too frequently, with uncommon sensation. The ophthalmic's nasal branch, the nasal nerve, is distributed over the very area, on the side of the nose and inner angle of the orbit, exterior to the anterior ethmoidal cells, supplying, also, the conjunctiva, lachrymal sac, and caruncle lachrymalis. The superior max-illary connects its anterior dental nerve with its Meckel's ganglion. This ganglion, itself, sends that most sensitive nerve of the nasal chambers, the naso-palatine, or nerve of Cotunnius, out below the opening of the sphenoidal sinus, and across the nasal septum within constant reach of the pressure of a swollen middle turbinated body. The posterior branches of this Meckel's root of many nasal evils, this spheno-palatine ganglion, are the vidian and the pterygo-palatine nerves, con-necting it with the nasopharyngeal region and the carotid plexus of the sympathetic. Over this track pass the reflexes that produce asthmatic attacks of purely nasal origin. To make matters worse and more confusing, as stated before, Meckel's ganglion is in relation with the ophthalmic ganglion. The inferior maxillary branch of this troublesome fifth nerve is a nerve of three functions, sensory, motor, and special sense for the tongue. Its otic ganglion brings it in close relation with the external auditory meatus and canal, by the auriculo-temporal nerve, and, with the chorda tympani, by fibres from the gustatory or lingual nerve, as well as from the submaxil-lary ganglion. At several critical points this trifacial nerve is in relation, by communicating fibres, with the facial nerve.

In a state of health it is, doubtless, proper to regard the tri-facial nerve with considerable admiration, for its purpose to control so many and varied activities, but, when coryza devel-ops and the special poisons of grip establish their cycle of symptoms, this remarkable nerve can become the originator of much suffering for the patient and perplexity for the phy-sician.

I think that we are too apt to regard the very complex tangle of anatomy constituting the nasal chambers, as a simple architectural structure of bony boxes, rather apart from the functional activities that are inherent in all vital tissue. We look at them from the standpoint of a mechanic, and develop the habit of regarding morbid activities within them, as prone to follow the very definite course of inflammation, hypersecretion, and suppuration. So, when pain develops within the region which they control, we tend to the belief that this pain is due always to the existence of pressure by occlusion or retained secretions. So resort must be had to methods of carpentry and plumbing. It is well to remember that a neuritis or a neuralgia of the fifth nerve, and of its separate branches and ganglia, can occur, as with any nerve, and may occur from any of the causes that produce neuroses elsewhere, from autointoxication, or from direct inflammation, as in the complex of symptoms which we call grip. With the onset of rhinitis, there develops, at once, a vicious circle; for irritation of sensory fibres of the ophthalmic and superior maxillary react on the sympathetic plexuses, and we have vasomotor irregularities, which, in themselves, increase the irritability of the sensory nerves. The fifth nerve now rises to the occasion, and the whole area of its distribution may be involved in a general mass of misery. The streaming eyes avoid the light, and movements of the ocular muscles are painful. The head aches from the face to the back of the neck, and the teeth are sensitive. The ears are sore and aching, and the tensor of the drumhead and the stapedius muscle vibrate in quivering, spasmodic movement. The frontal sinus region is excessively tender to the touch; so, also, is the area over the anterior ethmoid cells. There may be a contraction of the orbicularis muscle, forming a thickened body over the eyebrow, which we may fancy to be true swelling over the frontal sinus. Of course, these areas are painful under even light pressure, and the bony box idea of the nasal chambers favors the happy thought that the frontal sinus is full of pus; so, too, the ethmoid sinuses; "*anyhow,* something must be stopped up, inside, that ought to come out!" Now, for drills, chisels and rongeurs!

Well, in the majority of attacks of an acute rhinitis, there is no pus in these sinuses. It is doubtful if any exudate exists there. I am convinced that, more often than not, the mucous lining is not even swollen. The pain is a neuralgia or neuritis of the wretched fifth nerve. The best results will come from the simplest and most gentle treatment of the nasal chambers, and full attention to the patient's general condition, of which the nasal discomfort is merely a local expression. Then, too, in this class of cases, it is not so very difficult to cause a real infection of the sinuses by overanxiety to probe into them. Once infected, of course, you have a surgical state of things, and some aggressive minds would be delighted with a certainty, now, for the need of carpentry and plumbing. I believe that a safe guide for the real need of surgical interference is found, as in acute mastoiditis, in the temperature range, the duration and continuance of real pressure symptoms, and in the mental state of the patient. We cannot ignore the fact that the ophthalmic vein and cavernous sinus are related closely to the frontal sinus regions. The lymph vessels, also, may be carriers of infection to the meninges. In cases, even, of true sinusitis, we have, also, the elements of a neuritis of the associated nerve tracts. The wise physician must consider the data at his command, and, while not deceived by a nerve irritation, which, in most instances, is the gist of the situation, be on the alert for manifestations of what may be a grave condition within the nasal sinuses, demanding surgical treatment. When an acute influenza complicates a case of chronic sinusitis of any one or more of the nasal sinuses, there is less reason for giving too much weight to the question of nerve irritability, alone, in a desire to avoid surgical procedures. But, in these cases, the clinical conditions are apt to be presented with a frankness that leaves little doubt as to the requirements for relief.

In purely acute cases, aggressive surgery is almost never needed. In chronic cases with acute infection added, the necessity for it is not infrequent. In chronic cases, alone, free from any acute exacerbation or infection, the question of operative treatment must be decided by the judgment of the physician, based upon a study of the conditions presented by each patient, alone. No one can state bluntly that, as a rule, every chronic case of nasal sinusitis must be attacked by gouge, chisel, and curette, or that, on the other hand, it must be treated only by irrigation and antiphlogistics.

The glosso-pharyngeal branch of the eighth cranial nerve, by its tympanic branch, Jacobson's nerve, from the petrous ganglion, is distributed to the fenestra ovalis and fenestra rotunda. It has communicating branches to the greater and lesser petrosal nerves, and, by the latter, to the otic ganglion. I saw a lady, on one occasion, who had been distressed for many months by a peculiar cough. After a long course of fresh air and forced feeding treatment, she had been urged to try the climate of Southern California. No one had examined this patient's ears. Her cough was peculiar, and was of a character that always should excite suspicion of a "reflex." It was "dry," hacking, ineffective, at times paroxysmal, and with gagging. One could say, too, that this patient had laryngitis, for the vocal cords were pinkish, and the mucosa of the larynx reddened, from the irritation of coughing. This patient's ears were filled with impacted cerumen over a bed of hard, desquamated epithelium. The hearing was not affected to an extent that was noticeable. The very simple matter of clearing the external aud'tory canals ended the patient's long term of hacking cough, forced feeding, and medication. The "reflex" irritation had gone over the track of the otic ganglion, inferior maxillary, glosso-pharyngeal, and pneumogastric nerves to the pharynx, larynx, and trachea.

The existence of aural pain, simulating that of an acute otitis media, coincident with dental caries, eruption of the teeth, and irritation of the dental nerves, is so well recognized as to need merely a passing notice. Less frequently noted is the persistence of discomfort, and even pain, over the mastoid region and back of auricle, which has led to the trephining of the mastoid cells, in the belief that the cause might be intracellular inflammation. The auricular branch of the pneumogastric, Arnold's nerve, joined by filaments from the glosso-pharyngeal, reaches the surface between the mastoid process and the external auditory meatus. This distribution is well to remember in cases of vague mastoid aching, where all evidences of mastoiditis are wanting. A case occurred in my practice, during the epidemic of grip this winter, where the patient, a man of middle age, suffered intense pain within the ear, over the corresponding mastoid process, down the neck, and over the temporal region of the same side. He had a persistent temperature, well above normal, lasting many days. The drumhead was quite red, but without distension, reddened by the instillation of drugs to relieve the pain. Hearing was normal. The pain was spasmodic, and was not developed by pressure on the mastoid process. It was a case suggestive of a possible otitis media, with mastoid involvement, but the cycle of symptoms overreached itself in its efforts to deceive. The distribution of the painful areas, the character of the pain, itself, all pointed to a neuralgia, and yielded to salicylates and aspirin. Reference has been made to aural cough; but we have, also, a reflex cough that is distinctly "nasal." In some individuals any irritation along the course of the naso-palatine nerve, but, especially, opposite the posterior half of the middle tubinated body, will develop this "reflex." It may become a very annoying feature of attacks of rhinitis, paroxysmal in type, of vasomotor instability; or, it may be caused from pressure from structural defects in the nasal chambers. Such coughing is not laryngeal or tracheal. It is nasal in origin, and will not yield to sedative medication.

The glosso-pharyngeal nerve, by its pharyngeal branches, uniting with filaments of the pneumogastric, goes to the pharyngeal plexus, uniting there with the external laryngeal and sympathetic nerves. It has a branch to the tonsils, going, also, to the soft palate, anastomosing with the palatine nerves. Elongated uvulae that flap about the fauces, sticking to the pharyngeal walls or to the tonsils, can thus produce coughing, quite as well as by tickling the larynx. Inflammation of the tonsils, especially enlargements of these masses, with retention of caseous substance, hyperplasia in the form of fibrous bands binding down such swollen tonsils, can all be productive of "reflex" coughing, which might lead a careless observer to suspect laryngitis, tracheitis or bronchial catarrh. For many chests will give suggestions of abnormalities in percussion and auscultation that are not due to lesions, but, rather, to structural idiosyncrasies. Taken in connection with a purely "reflex" cough, they can suggest to the examiner's mind a causative element, although harmless in themselves, thus producing uncertainty and errors in diagnosis.

The sensory nerve of the interior of the larynx, including the vocal cords, is the pneumogastric's superior laryngeal nerve. Its course, along the side of the pharynx, behind the internal carotid artery, brings it into association with the deep chain of cervical lymphatic glands, and pressure from an enlarged gland, even without the added element of suppuration or caseation, may induce "reflex" coughing. A child, eleven years of age, having enlarged glands in the left side of the neck, was annoyed by a persistent and very distressing cough, most noticeable at night. The patient had hypertrophied faucial and pharyngeal tonsils, but was free from any other lesions. I excised the tonsils and adenoids, thus obtaining relief from mouth-breathing. The cough continued, however, until the cervical lymphatic glands were completely removed by a very thorough dissection of the neck. As the superior laryngeal nerve and the pharyngeal branches of the pneumogastric are associated closely, a simple condition as hypertrophy of the mucous follicles in the pharynx, especially in the lateral chain, behind the posterior faucial pillars, can excite a reflex in the form of a so-called laryngeal cough.

Pressure on the recurrent laryngeal nerve is more apt to be attended with changes in the patient's voice, or interference with respiration, rather than with reflex coughing. I note, in passing, the well-known fact that an aneurism at the aortic arch, or in the right subclavian artery, is revealed, very often for the first time, by the picture of a laryngeal paralysis reflected in the laryngeal mirror, and this is the case, also, where tumors exist in the mediastinum. Equally well known, in these days, is the development of right-sided laryngeal paralysis from an infiltration at the right pulmonary apex, within the pleura or overlying lymphatic glands. But the relation of laryngeal lesions with affections of this motor nerve of the vocal cords is too well developed in medical literature to justify a further discussion of this subject. This mere sketch in outline of the distribution of the fifth and eighth pairs of cranial nerves may explain a puzzling class of patients, whose subjective symptoms are intensely distressing, and yet whose recovery is rapid, under internal medication or very sedative local treatment. It may indicate, also, the need for care to avoid unnecessary surgical interference in this class of cases, especially in subjects where the pro and con are uncertain as to the need for opening into any one or more of the nasal accessory sinuses. Exact diagnosis is of great importance in these cases, where it is often most difficult to make. The X-ray and transillumination are, indeed, most helpful, but are far from being infallible guides. With all our modern mechanical aids, we must still depend, very largely, on personal and direct observation, aided by clinical experience. Errors in these cases are made easily. Aggressive operators may be led astray by their surgical zeal and the apparent, although not real, need for its exercise. Thus, much unnecessary suffering may be inflicted by an undue surgical interference, the evil results of which, it is true, may not be revealed to anyone, unless to the conscience of the operator.

XL.

TAKING COLD.*

By D. Braden Kyle, M. D.,

Philadelphia.

The expression "taking cold," as so frequently used by patients, and sometimes by medical practitioners, is in so many
cases a misnomer, that I have purposely used the term to call
attention to this particular fact. The practitioner of special
medicine so often sees the individual with a condition resembling a cold in which there is no history of exposure nor usual
systemic phenomena, and yet, to all intents and purposes, the
patient is suffering from a cold in the head, or has taken cold.

Let us first, then, divide the condition of taking cold into
three classes: First, actual cold; taking cold; acute rhinitis.
Second, an underlying systemic condition which produces some
local manifestation and irritation in the mucous membrane,
predisposing the individual to taking cold. Third, an underlying systemic condition in which the patient has not taken
any cold, but the symptoms produced in the mucous membrane
are those of a cold.

The first condition is a separate and distinct process, a simple acute rhinitis. The second is a compound process, a systemic condition and a local process. Just what particular function is wrong is to be determined by the practitioner, but the
systemic condition predisposes the individual to cold; in other
words, it lessens the vitality of the mucous membrane and
lowers its resistance. And in the third condition—let it be
neuroses, let it be a circulatory, a vasomotor, or chemic, or
an organic, or systemic lesion which is locally manifested in
the mucous membrane of the upper respiratory tract—the irritation thus produced in this local manifestation produces a
lesion identical with that of having taken cold. In other
words, a patient may have every symptom of cold in the head,

---

* Paper read before the Southern Section of the American
Laryngological, Rhinological and Otological Society, Richmond, Va.,
February 12, 1909.

and yet have not been exposed; in fact, it is likely that he may have been seated before the fire in a comfortable, well ventilated room, free from draughts or exposure.

It is with the second and third classification that this paper deals, although the subject is that of taking cold. The first classification of simple cold, we will omit, and deal entirely with the second and third classifications, as given above.

Taking cold, then, implies more than a local condition. It may be dependent on constitutional conditions, either original or acquired. Certain individuals, under varied conditions, are more susceptible to cold at one time than another. At certain times a person may be exposed and not take cold, yet at another time, without any apparent rhyme or reason, he takes cold. This cannot be explained on any other basis than an individual systemic or constitutional condition.

The lithemic condition, where the patient without any exposure whatever may suddenly develop a severe cold, is also classed under the ordinary term of "cold." This, however, is due to the faulty chemistry of the secretion, where the glands of the mucous membrane, in pouring out their normal secretion (this secretion having been perverted), produce an irritating mucus, which in turn inflames and irritates the nasal mucous membrane, causing every symptom of a severe cold in the head. Individuals with rheumatic, gouty, or lithemic diathesis are especially predisposed. Such individuals, with necessarily sensitive mucous membranes, would certainly have the so-called chronic cough.

Contagious and infectious diseases also render the mucous membrane sensitive and predispose the individual. This is illustrated by the catarrhal conditions following all the infectious diseases of childhood, and, in fact, all infectious fevers. Frequently, following the recovery from the original lesion, the patient is for several winters very susceptible to cold, and usualy has a slight, hacking cough.

Digestive disturbances, torpid liver, constipation, faulty elimination due to a lesion of the genito-urinary tract, may be a systemic underlying etiologic factor.

Fatigue, either physical or nervous, renders the individual very susceptible, and, while this should be classed under constitutional conditions, yet the individual's general health may be good, but at the time of exposure his physical or mental exhaustion renders him more liable to take cold.

Nasal irregularities and obstruction, rendering the mucous membrane sensitive, are also predisposing factors.

Persons with sensitive skin or sensitive areas are also very susceptible. Interference with the function of the skin, which may be due to chilling of the surface when a person is warm or overheated, may predispose the individual to taking cold. When a portion of the body, especially the back of the neck or head, or the extremities, is exposed to draughts, the person is very likely to take cold.

Sudden changes of temperature and climatic conditions may act as local and systemic predisposing factors; also sudden changes of temperature, from a hot to a cold room, or the reverse, are equally predisposing factors.

Over-ventilated or poorly ventilated rooms, especially in school buildings, where the individual is exposed to a draught by poor ventilation, may predispose to cold. Individuals living and especially sleeping in rooms heated by means of registers, in which there comes from the furnace dry heat charged with dust and irritating gases, owing to the irritating effect on the nasal mucous membrane, are rendered more susceptible to cold.

Certain seasons render individuals more susceptible to taking cold than others. The spring of the year, when the individual is likely to change from heavy clothing to a lighter weight garment, is a decided predisposing factor. In certain sensitive individuals, the exposure of the ankles or wrists to draughts predispose that individual to taking cold; yet, after all, many of these so-called predispositions or sensitiveness on the part of the individual are due to a systemic condition which renders him susceptible to taking cold.

Occupation may predispose an individual to taking cold. The mucous membrane of the upper respiratory tract, owing to the constant irritation from extraneous material, is in a constantly susceptible condition. Colds and cough follow, and the individual is constantly exposed to a serious infection.

Irritating vapors may cause the mucous membrane to become sensitive and render the individual much more susceptible. Dust and smoke may also be classed as predisposing factors.

The automobile is an exciting factor. Individuals exposed to dust and facing strong wind suffer with faceache, conjunctival irritation, and nasal congestion; this continued congestion blocks up the accessory cavities and tends to congestion of the nasal mucous membrane, lessening its resisting powers and interfering with normal functions, thus predisposing the individual to taking cold. The same condition has been observed in railroad engineers and individuals who test the speed and vibration of engines.

In many of the above mentioned predisposing causes the process known as "taking cold" may be arrested in the early stages, if the cause can be removed before the congestion passes into the second stage of the inflammatory process, saving the patient from the cough necessary to the resolution stages.

In the various forms of rheumatism and gout is frequently observed the irritation of the mucous membrane of the upper respiratory tract, especially the nasopharynx and larynx. The same is true of the lithemic individual with the excessive alkaline or the excessive acid secretion, or a neutral secretion containing irritants.

The nasal congestion of puberty, due to hyperemia, or the nasal congestion of middle or old age, or the menopause period, in which the congestion is a cyanotic or sluggish one, all give rise to a condition similar to a cold in the head.

Nervous excitement, shock, nervous tension, constant worry, through their effect on the nervous system and general perversion of the secretion, will cause constant irritation of the mucous membrane and give rise to symptoms identical with those of a cold in the head.

The irritating effect of the nasal and nasopharyngeal secretions on the mucous membrane, as an exciting factor, can be clearly demonstrated by changing the chemistry or the reaction of the secretions, by internal medication, and you will find that the cold in the head will clear up as suddenly as it came, showing that it was nothing more than a local manifestation of a systemic condition — a faulty chemistry — the secretion either coming to the surface as an irritant, or, when coming to the surface, undergoing chemical changes, producing an irritant.

It is a well-known fact that in certain individuals the actinic rays produce congestion of the nasal mucous membrane and also the conjunctiva. Some individuals, when exposed to the actinic rays, especially when associated with the glare from water, will develop in a few minutes an irritated condition of the mucous membrane almost identical with a sudden and acute cold, or probably more resembling the condition known as hay fever. All the forms of hay fever, rose cold, horse fever, rye fever, ragweed fever, and similar conditions, no matter by what name known, are in many if not all cases due to the irritating effect of the secretion, either direct or in combination with some extraneous material, but the symptoms produced are very much the same as the ordinary cold in the head.

Frequently children suffer from so-called cold in the head, often due to exposure and carelessness. There is a tendency on the part of some practitioners, parents and nurses, to do what they please to term "hardening the child," by cold baths. In many instances this is fatal. Certain individuals do not react from the cold bath, while in others it is an excellent tonic to the circulation and may serve to prevent the individual from taking cold. It is purely a personal equation, and it is simply folly to endeavor to harden the child who is suffering from some systemic condition which irritates his mucous membrane, by the cold bath process. I have several cases in mind in which this cold bath was insisted upon, and, to be sure, the child now does not take any cold, but is quietly resting out in Cedar Hill (Cedar Hill being one of our largest cemeteries).

It narrows the matter down to a question of personal or individual equation, and the individual and personal study of every case as to why the child or individual takes cold, as to what form and course this so-called cold pursues, and why on one occasion without exposure he takes cold, and on another occasion after being exposed he does not take cold.

Nasal congestion, causing mouth breathing and continual symptoms of cold in the head, as observed in boys and girls at the age of puberty, we all know is due to a physiological process. It is in reality a physiological hyperemia of the erectile tissue. Why, then, sacrifice this membrane? Why cauterize, cut or burn this perfectly normal tissue? Local treatment does practically no good, but in the course of a few months, or when the individual has passed through the age of puberty, you will find that this tendency to take cold in the head, or the chronic condition of cold in the head, has disappeared, and instead of having a scarred and irritated mucous membrane you now have a perfectly normal and healthy tissue.

The same is true in regard to local treatment and surgical interference in a vast majority of conditions as described in this paper. To be sure, sometimes sedative local treatment may give a certain degree of comfort to the patient. and the nasal congestion may be so marked as to threaten involvement of the Eustachian tube and middle ear, or of some of the accessory cavities. Then and only in such cases where the threatened danger would be greater than the loss of a certain portion of the tissue, should operative interference be offered. In many instances where the local condition is really a local manifestation of a systemic condition, solutions and treatments applied locally only aggravate the already irritated tissue, and the treatment should be directed medically toward the removal of the underlying cause; in other words, the application of the old surgical teaching. "Remove the cause."

Reviewing, then, these systemic conditions which bring about irritation of the mucous membrane which resembles taking cold, it certainly shows that in a large percentage of cases of so-called cold in the head, no one remedy could be applied, and that the individual must be studied as carefully for the predisposing cause or underlying element as though typhoid fever or a beginning pneumonia were suspected. In other words, every individual case should be studied from an individual standpoint. The individual study of cases enables the physician to scientifically apply his remedial agent and not empirically prescribe a cold remedy. My own experience has been that out of one hundred persons presenting themselves for relief of what they call a cold in the head, or having taken cold, or frequently taking cold, at least eighty per cent belong to the class of the systemic condition, either constitutional, organic, or chemic.

XLI

LARYNGEAL PARALYSIS AS EARLY INDICATION OF SYSTEMIC DISEASE.

By George T. Ross, M. D., D. C. L. (Hon.),

Montreal.

Virchow is quoted as saying that "no medical specialty can flourish which separates itself completely from the general body of medical science; no specialty can develop usefully and beneficially if it does not remain in relationship with other specialties and drink ever and again from the fount of general medical knowledge, thereby preserving for science, even if it should not be necessary for practice, that unity upon which the position of specialism rests intrinsically."

Our knowledge of the intimate relationship of ear, throat and nose diseases to internal medicine has been greatly advanced in the past twenty years, but there are many inexact conditions constantly facing us in this specialty, proving that the field of this relationship has as yet been only superficially explored, and I venture to predict that during the next decade morbid states in the region of human anatomy which we specially cultivate and their correlated symptoms to general medicine will be surprisingly extended, because of further discoveries in pathologic research.

The nervous system being almost entirely inaccessible to direct observation, with trifling exceptions, the state of this system can be ascertained only by the manner in which its work is done; and morbidity reveals its presence here in some cases only by derangement of the normal physiologic function. This disordered function being our only guide to diagnosis of certain affections in the larynx, the necessity for close study and early recognition of any divergence from the normal is self-evident, especially when such divergence is possible without any manifestation of subjective signs.

Although many diseases of the larynx exist which are strictly limited to that organ and are essentially local, yet a larger and more important number of laryngeal affections for which the aid of the specialist is sought, is only part and parcel of systemic disease for which constitutional treatment is mainly required. Local lesions may exist where the trained hand of the special surgeon is called for, but to that extent only his art is called upon in many diseases of the general system. Again, cases occur in which without any anatomical change existing in the larynx very unpleasant sensations and painful states are found in that organ, all of which are relieved by systemic treatment alone, such as general anemia, periodical disturbances of the circulation, general plethora, nervous excitability, gout, rheumatism, etc. These ailments are now fairly well understood, but what is not so well known is the raison d'etre of those actual organic lesions, as well as disordered functions occurring in this organ which are indicative and symptomatic of grave general disease and are forerunners of it.

The elucidation of these laryngeal symptoms is difficult as well as interesting, because many intricate questions in neurology, both physiologic and and pathologic, present themselves and take the laryngologist often beyond the sphere of his specialty.

Discussion of general laryngeal paralysis opens up too large a subject for this short paper. I would only, therefore, venture to briefly call your attention to the earliest recognizable paretic state of the cords or of one cord, as being of practical value in establishing diagnosis; for if the paralysis be unilateral it may in no way proclaim its existence subjectively, and must be sought for if one does not wish to miss the opportunity of making early diagnosis. While cord inaction may be due to local conditions, it may, on the other hand, indicate future trouble, and be simply a silent storm signal of the coming grave event. A patient may present himself with complaints which have not apparently any direct bearing on laryngeal disease, but by following a routine practice of making thorough examinations we sometimes are rewarded by lighting upon a unilateral posticus paralysis unexpectedly. No perceptible change being evident in our patient's vocalization, he assures us there is nothing wrong with his throat, and the ordinary laryngeal functions being unembarrassed his statement seems reasonable. When we have found it we cannot say, however, that the faulty state of one cord is pathognomonic of any approaching particular disease, since it may arise from some trivial local lesion or surface irritation. For instance, an enlarged lymph gland may by pressure cause a paretic cord lasting for years, thus a guarded prognosis is called for where a graver lesion is not discoverable. In no other organ of the body is disease so dependent on the general condition of the system as the larynx, and conversely the finding of certain signs in the larynx throws light on latent or obscure processes in the entire system. The recognition, therefore, of the earliest indications of trouble cannot be overestimated.

That state of unilateral abductor paralysis wherein we notice the fixation of a cord in the so-called cadaveric position, causing a cracked, raucous voice to a degree which gives discomfort to the patient and he realizes that something is wrong; as well as that state of partial laryngeal stridor, which sometimes ushers in unilateral abductor paralysis, was most ably delineated to the profession in May, 1908, at Montreal, by Gleitsmann, Casselberry and Delavan, and little reference will now be made to these conditions in this connection. In such cases of tangible laryngeal symptoms which are both subjective and objective, the laryngologist turns at once, or at least should do so, to the vital phase of the question and searches for constitutional disturbances, which when found reveal the pathologic cause or causes of the trouble. But of a more problematic character is the question of primary simple posticus paralysis, wherein one cord is fixed in the median line with the free border taut and with phonation remaining normal. The median posticus position is caused by the early failure of the abductors (Friedrich), thus illustrating Semon's law, that the abductors are the most vulnerable in the event of any arising morbidity. The first step in the further progress of this posticus paralysis is relaxation of the taut border, which then becomes concave towards the median line and bows outwards, going on to complete recurrent paralysis.

Regarding the three cases that I noted where the early phenomenon of abductor paralysis occurred, I am compelled, unfortunately, to speak from memory alone as regards two of them, which, of course, militates against my observations, since they are now unsupported by clinical data which I formerly possessed. This loss was due to the confusion incident to our moving into a new hospital building over a year ago. The old records after removal were found to be so chaotic and disarranged that reference to them was not feasible.

CASE 1.—A. B., aged 50, a laborer, was treated at the Western Hospital-- for chronic nasopharyngitis and unilateral abductor paralysis for six months. His voice was natural during this time and no peripheral irritation existed beyond a catarrhal state of the laryngeal mucosa. His mode of life was very precarious and when opportunity offered he stimulated freely. No personal history of luetic infection; his family history was unreliable, which indeed, might be said of his entire statement. After six months' irregular attendance at the clinic he developed pronounced symptoms of tabes dorsalis. The patient later left the city and was lost sight of.

CASE 2.—J. B., male, aged 40, in fair general health, claimed to have drank enough beer to float an ocean steamship, attended the clinic complaining of dry throat (perhaps because he had not had his usual daily allowance of moisture). Only symptom present, unilateral abductor paralysis. No sensory signs referable to this organ. His attendance at the out-door clinic was very irregular, but my recollection is that on and off, for the greater part of a year, he appeared occasionally, when signs of tabes dorsalis arose and I was pleased to send him to another clinic.

CASE 3.—J. G., aged 37, came to the hospital complaining of nasal stenosis. Examination of his larynx showed unilateral abductor palsy without subjective laryngeal symptoms. In three weeks bilateral paralysis ensued and he entered hospital for treatment. During his two weeks in hospital his inspiratory stridor was such as to necessitate constant preparation for tracheotomy, but in that time the cords relaxed and breathing became easier. In four months later typical ataxic symptoms were in evidence. In this case I have the exact data, having lectured on it and exhibited the patient to students at the clinic 12 years ago. I retained an extract of the lecture. On reviewing this lecture I notice that many facts then referred to as bearing on laryngeal paralysis were quoted in the symposium upon this subject at the Annual Meeting of the American Laryngological Association in May, 1908, wh'ch goes to support Dr. Delavan's statement on that occasion, viz.,—"of late years not much has been advanced on this subject and that little has not been illuminating." If, however, we take the comparison a little further back, the discoveries and advances due to pathology and bacteriology have been very distinctly illuminating.

Thus far I have referred only to those cases of paralysis in which there is no accompanying peripheral inflammation

locally, or at most only a small area of such around the arytenoids and not a general laryngitis, but in estimating the
value or significence of cord palsy, unilateral or otherwise,
we have to bear in mind other possible causes of this phenomenon, where both objective and sensory signs are very
pronounced. Rosenberg (Berlin) gives a record of three
cases which he found very anomalous, and although due apparently to peripheral conditions they failed to yield to suitable
extended treatment and hence the suspicion of latent constitutional disease was unavoidable. These cases lasted three
months, eight months and thirty-two months respectively, and
the last one had not entirely recovered when he made the
report. They were all cases of unilateral cord paralysis in
conditions of acute and chronic laryngitis, which is different
from the ordinary experience of laryngologists, for in such
cases the paralysis is commonly bilateral from the general
surface inflammation. These cases were well worthy of study
from their stubborn nature in yielding to the treatment of a
specialist of high standing, and where the patients had the
great advantage of good social status, and all that pertains
to it, in change of climate, sea voyage, etc. In such unusual
cases where the cure was unaccountably protracted the natural
tendency would be to think of tubercle, syphilis or cancer, but
all these people eventually recovered normal cord functions.
Should similar cases as these occur in the out-door clinic of
any hospital, where the individual was deprived of the social
advantages mentioned, the treatment would have been still
more protracted, in all probability. Indeed, the case would
be remarkable for possessing sufficient faith in any physician,
who in a fractional part of the time stated did not by his
remedial measures demonstrate the practical advantage of
continuing under his care.

CONCLUSIONS.

The brevity of this paper necessarily excludes many other
pathologic causes of early laryngeal palsy, such as bulbar
lesions, aneurism, insular sclerosis, syringomyelia, etc., all
of which, however, generally have some accompanying sensory signs. The object of this article will be accomplished
if I succeed in directing attention to the great necessity there
exists for further and closer investigation into physiology and
pathology as applied to laryngeal disorders similar to these
cited herein. At the present day it is impossible to interpret

and foretell the exact significance of, and give a definite prognosis in, such anomalous cases as I have quoted, and I think a very careful record should be kept of all similar cases and reports made from time to time to enlighten us on what is thus far, to some extent at least, a terra incognita. I doubt if I would ever have reported these few cases had not discussion arisen between a neurologist and myself on this question, who maintained that the literature on unilateral cord palsy as related to tabes dorsalis was very meager, and if my experience could be established it would spell "originality." Perhaps one reason why unilateral cord paralysis has so often been attributed to hysteria, when there did not exist any other discernible lesion, is the infinite variety of forms which hysteria causes in what we term "nervous" subjects, and we may be inclined to fall back on this diagnosis when otherwise at fault, since the word "idiopathic" is no longer tenable. To prove of any value these silent cord palsies must be followed to a finish, and we all know how difficult it is to keep patients under observation who have no tangible evidence to themselves of the necessity for carrying it out. Herein lies the chief obstacle to establishing data in such cases, and of course these few instances quoted of the trouble in question are comparatively valueless, for it requires an extended series to prove any unusual records. In estimating the value of this objective sign we must also remember that many subjects of tabes have had syphilis, some authors maintaining that the one disease entails the other, or indicates the other, so that a true luetic palsy may coexist with tabes.

XLII.

NASAL MYXOSARCOMA IN A CHILD OF THREE YEARS.

By George T. Ross, M. D., D. C. L. (Hon.),

Montreal.

Emile Lalonde, aged 3 years, of French-Canadian parentage, born in Montreal, was brought to the Western Hospital, with a history of obstructed nasal breathing for six weeks past. It was impossible to obtain much reliable information from the parents, who had not noticed anything specially wrong until epistaxis begun. There was no account of injury or hereditary cancer. Child was never ill before present complaint. His appearance was normal except anemia, not very pronounced. Recently there was marked obstruction to nasal breathing, especially at night. No cough, but the voice had a socalled nasal tone. Epistaxis very frequent.

Examination of the nose showed right side practically normal. In vestibule of left naris a greyish yellow mass was seen, blocking it entirely. This was found to be of soft consistency with pus covering it. It was encapsulated, very friable and bled at the slightest touch. No fetid odor or excoriating surface of the upper lip.

Operation.—Under general anesthesia I removed the growth with forceps scissors and electric cautery. It was found diffusely attached to the septum at the bony and cartilaginous junction. The resulting hemorrhage was severe, but easily controlled. In two weeks the tumor recurred, but was much less in size. This recrudescence was controlled by operation every two or three weeks, each time the growth being smaller. After the fifth operation the child was not brought back to the hospital.

PATHOLOGIST'S REPORT.

Pathological Laboratories,
Western General Hospital, Montreal.
Growth from Nasal Septum.   13th November, 1908.
       Baby Lalonde.
Material for examination consisted of small snippings and one or two round nodules, which on section were of a white

homogeneous appearance. Microscopically one of these larger nodules showed at one side a loose reticulum with some stellate and pointed cells, with here and there scattered round cells, having one or more nuclei; the single nucleus was often in a state of division and occasional nuclei were fragmented. At the margin there was a uniform matting together of round cells, having deep staining single nuclei or nuclei in process of fragmentation. The section gave the appearance of a myxoma or a hypertrophied nasal mucous membrane which had undergone sarcomatous transformation. Diagnosis—Myxo-Sarcoma.

A. G. NICHOLLS, M. A., M. D.,
Associate Professor of Pathology, McGill University.

Remarks.—The child's condition did not seem to suffer much during operative treatment notwithstanding the severe hemorrhage from time to time. The difficulty of treating a child of 3 years and keeping the wounds clean after operations, can be best appreciated by those who have done it. In this case the mother declined to allow the child to remain in hospital and so the home care was inefficient and consequently detrimental. Several specimens were sent from time to time to the pathologist who found such examination confirmatory of previous opinions. No glandular involvement. Half a year after the last operation I examined the little patient and found the left naris normal except the scar tissue on the septum, showing the site of former growth. The parents reported the child's health perfect.

Price Brown gave a statistical report in October, 1906, of results of operations in sarcoma of the nose by various methods generally adopted and these were collated from many authors whose records were thought worthy of citation. He found that operators who had as many as 20 cases did not trouble to keep records of them, being impressed with the hopelessness of the disease in question. The summary of the work referred to, whether operations were done internally or externally, in which patients were observed until final results were obtained, was that out of 51 cases 27 per cent recovered after operations of whatever kind. After intranasal work, however, it was noticed that the recoveries were 31 per cent as against 24 per cent after the extranasal method, while some cases had to be done both ways. Brown's personal record of

4 cases were all treated by intranasal electric cautery, and while three recovered perfectly, the fourth died of sepsis.

Although the results in nasal sarcoma are usually very fatal and recoveries after operation constitute a very small proportion, yet in this case the early destruction of the growth may tend to more favorable outlook, even if this is offset by the disease manifesting itself at such a tender age. Some authors maintain that more than half of these cases are fatal ultimately no matter how they are treated.

XLIII

AURAL COMPLICATIONS IN THE EXANTHEMATA.

By Charles R. C. Borden, M. D.,

Boston.

In the minds of the profession at large, diphtheria is regarded as the first of the three contagious diseases developing
aural complications, scarlet fever next in frequency, and
measles last and least. As a matter of fact, measles is first,
scarlet fever second, and diphtheria is low in the percentage
of ears involved. Statistics vary somewhat with the different
writers, but all agree with the foregoing statement of relative
frequency.

In the Boston City Hospital Dr. McCollom[1] reports 24 per
cent in measles and 18 per cent in scarlet fever. Downie of
Glasgow[2], reports 26.1 per cent in measles and only 12 per
cent in scarlet fever. Caiger[3] reports 11 per cent in 4,015
scarlet fever cases; Burkardt[4] 33 per cent and Finlayson[5] 10
per cent in 4,339 cases of scarlet fever. In a series of cases
observed by the writer, but 1.3 per cent developed aural complications in diphtheria. Thus will be noticed the striking
difference between the three diseases.

Naturally, more complications will arise in severe infections,
in septic cases, and in those having especially acute throat or
nose symptoms. Bronchopneumonia, a common complication of the eruptive diseases, causes not only middle ear inflammations, but many mastoids as well, and profuse nasal
discharges, so common in these diseases, are particular enemies
of the ear.

No hard and fast rule may be given as to the time of onset.
But in a general way it may be said that in diphtheria and
measles, the complications usually occur soon after the acute
symptoms have developed. This is particularly true of
measles. But in scarlet fever, middle ear infections may be
expected any time, from the first to the last day; more frequently late in the period rather than early. Many cases are
seen in the Boston City Hospital from forty to one hundred

days after admission. Of course the complications may arise at any time and do so in each of the three diseases with sufficient regularity to prevent any special rule being made. But in a larger number of cases, the general course will agree with the above statements.

The course of the complications ranges over a wide area. Beginning with the slight earache or simple deafness, they occasionally extend to acute mastoiditis with alarming complications. At the onset there is no means of knowing to what extent they may progress; consequently it is the duty of the attending physician to exert his greatest skill in each and every case.

Diagnosis to skilled aurists is usually easy. It sometimes happens, however, a case is seen which is exceedingly hard to diagnose, and will cause considerable anxiety before the true nature of the condition is decided.

In my experience, more obscure cases of mastoiditis have developed in diphtheria than in either of the other two diseases. As a rule, mastoid involvement in diphtheria is less active in its symptoms and less typical in a general way.

In scarlet fever and measles, the usual pressure symptoms are prominent and unmistakable, and upon operation, free pus is found in quantity. In diphtheria, not only are the symptoms less active, but in some cases, on operation, pus is usually small in amount and occasionally is not found at all. I have seen several cases in this disease, in which diagnosis was made entirely by exclusion, no typical symptoms being present. On operation no pus was found, yet recovery was complete and rapid, the lesion being probably an infective osteitis.

The ordinary course of the aural complications, is to develop a simple middle ear inflammation, to rupture spontaneously, to discharge serum, sero-pus, or thick creamy pus; to persist from a day or two up to several weeks, and to heal without further trouble.

Were this all that might take place, little or no harm would result. Unfortunately, many cases fail to be arrested in the acute stage, but pass on into a chronic process, which occasionally persists for a lifetime.

In measles, mastoiditis usually develops soon after the acute stages of the disease are present. In scarlet fever and diphtheria, especially in scarlet fever, it frequently arises after pital many mastoids have developed from three to ten weeks

the discharge has become chronic. In the Boston City Hos-
after admission, and it is the rule rather than the exception
for them to arise late in the diseases of scarlet fever and
diphtheria.

In both children and adults, aural symptoms differ somewhat from those of other causes, a very prominent and
striking difference being the absence of pain.   Perhaps 80
per cent of the children seldom complain of this symptom.
The majority of cases show the first evidence of middle ear
complication by a spontaneous rupture of the drum membrane
together with a discharge more or less profuse in amount.
At times the first symptom will be a sudden rise in temperature, with no apparent cause.   Inspection will show a bulging
drum membrane of a grayish red color.   Even with a marked
bulging of the tympanic membrane, pain is frequently absent.
Incision of the drum membrane in this case quickly restores
the temperature to normal.   In adults, pain is more frequently
observed, but cases are often seen with bulging drum membranes and elevated temperature who have little or no distress
from pain.   As a rule, when pain is present, it is by no means
as severe as in cases of acute otitis from grippe, pneumonia,
etc.

In nearly every case seen by the writer, spontaneous rupture takes place near the same location.   This is a spot near
the lower margin of the membrane, immediately below or a
little behind the umbo.   The writer has seen few cases rupture far from this location.   This is a very fortunate circum-
stance, and doubtless explains why so many cases recover in
spite of the absence of scientific treatment.   The character
of the discharge varies in the different diseases.   It usually
begins with a thin serous fluid, sometimes tinged with blood.
A few cases continue so for a few days and cease.   The ordinary course, however, is to soon change to creamy pus and
continue for a week or two, gradually becoming less and less,
until dry.   Diphtheria as a rule, causes a thicker discharge and
less in quantity, than the other two diseases. By all means the
most characteristic discharge is seen in measles.   In practically every case there is a profuse. brownish-white fluid with
less of the creamy nature of pus.   The amount is usually
tremendous, and it causes more destruction of the membrane
than any other aural discharge.

In my opinion, when such a condition exists, and daily inspection shows the perforation in the drum membrane rapidly

becoming larger, a mastoid operation should be done at once, without waiting for other symptoms, in order to save the hearing apparatus from further injury. I have performed this operation a number of times for this condition, and have never failed to find the mastoid cavity filled with pus and soft granulations.

In many cases the discharge will be great in amount, yet inspection of the drum membranes will fail to show any redness or bulging of that organ. Such cases usually heal without any special difficulty. Other cases, however, will show redness and bulging, and offer great difficulty to recovery and a greater menace to future hearing. Frequent incisions are sometimes called for and much good accomplished thereby. As a rule, however, when frequent opening of the membrana tympani is demanded in a case, a mastoid operation should be seriously considered, with a view to establish drainage backwards through that bone. Pus from the middle ear is frequently kept active by profuse nasal and nasopharyngeal secretions, and will persist as long as this cause is present. I have frequently performed adenoid operations for the relief of both conditions in scarlet fever and measles, with most gratifying results.

An adenoid operation during one of the infectious diseases would seem at first strongly contraindicated. It may be done, however, when necessity demands, and splendid results follow in scarlet fever and measles. This does not apply to diphtheria, however, as dangerous sequelae have followed the procedure in this disease.

Sudden rises in temperature in the exanthemata, without apparent cause, are usually due to ear complications. Inspection shows a bulging membrane, the color and appearance of which are quite different from the ordinary acute ear. The color is a grayish red and not the deeper red usually seen. The bulging assumes a flattened condition extending over the entire surface, also quite different from the ordinary, and is characteristic in a way of the exanthemata. When incision is performed on this drumhead, a distinct feeling of resistance to the knife is encountered, giving a thick, porky sensation. This thickened, infiltrated condition of the membrane undoubtedly accounts for the color, flattened appearance, and absence of pain.

The temperature seldom remains elevated after good drainage becomes established.

Except in diphtheria, acute mastoiditis is usually prominent and unmistakable.

The absence of pain is frequently noted, and in children it is not the first symptom to excite attention. In many cases, in young children, the first evidence of trouble is a sudden marked bulging forward of the auricle, together with edema and swelling over the mastoid. Tenderness is present on pressure over the swelling, and within the canal are found the typical mastoid symptoms.

One of the most striking features of aural work in the exanthemata, is the alarming frequency of mastoiditis in adult measles cases.

Dr. David N. Blakely[*] has published valuable statistics on this subject. In a series of 341 patients ill with measles, he reports that 14.96 per cent developed middle ear inflammation. Of this number 11.76 per cent of the cases having discharging ears came to a mastoid operation. Of the 6 patients having mastoid operations, five of them were in adults. The sixth occurred as a secondary operation in a child who had previously been operated on in another institution before admission to the Boston City Hospital. He further states that in 81 adult scarlet fever patients, not one had middle ear involvement of any kind.

In two series of mastoid operations of my own, 44.44 per cent and over 50 per cent occurred in adult patients having measles. In these two series of cases no mastoid operation occurred in adults ill with scarlet fever.

Adult scarlet fever patients occasionally develop middle ear inflammation, but mastoiditis among them is comparatively rare.

Thus it will be seen that in measles, adults are in considerable danger from mastoiditis, while in scarlet fever the danger is comparatively slight, even with middle ear inflammation present.

In conclusion I wish to emphasize the following points:

(1). In scarlet fever, children are quite liable to middle ear inflammation which may or may not involve the mastoid cells. Adults are much less so, and rarely have mastoiditis.

(2). In measles both adults and children are very susceptible to middle ear involvements and adults are especially in danger of mastoiditis.

(3). In cases where there is a tremendous aural discharge present for more than two or three weeks, the mastoid operation should be seriously considered as a means of providing drainage, other than through a small pin hole perforation in the delicate membrana tympani.

(4). Occasionally a case will arise, in which the diagnosis may be difficult. If, after carefully ruling out every other possible cause by exclusion and the mastoid remains in doubt, if the symptoms of the patient are at all serious, operate. The danger is greatest from waiting.

(5). If after the acute symptoms of scarlet fever and measles have subsided, pus in the middle ear is kept active by profuse nasal or nasopharyngeal discharges, examine the patient for adenoids. If the growths are present remove them thoroughly. This procedure in the course of diphtheria, however, is questionable.

(6). General practitioners should regard aural discharge as a menace to hearing, and occasionally to life, and not as a more or less common complication without special importance. In a series of 1164 cases previously reported by the author[7] in children up to 16 years of age, having aural diseases, 31.6 per cent had chronic purulent otitis media of long standing.

BIBLIOGRAPHY.

1. McCollom, John H. Laryngoscope, Vol. XV, September, 1905.
2. Downie. Diseases of Infancy and Childhood. Holt, 1897.
3. Caiger. Welch & Schamberg, 1905.
4. Burckart. Welch & Schamberg, 1905.
5. Finlayson. Acute Contagious Diseases. Welch & Schamberg, 1905.
6. Blakely, Daniel N. Archives of Pediatrics, July, 1899.
7. Borden, C. R. C. Annals of Gynecology and Pediatry, September, 1907.

XLIV

NASAL TUBERCULOSIS—A CASE AND REMARKS.

By W. Scott Renner, M. D.,

Buffalo.

The patient, whose case I am about to report, was a robust, healthy looking woman, 28 years of age and weighing 180 pounds. She came to consult me on April 16th, 1908, from a remote country district of western New York.

She complained of complete obstruction of both nostrils, which gave her great discomfort in breathing, interfered with her sleeping and produced a characteristic intonation of the voice. She stated that this condition had been coming on gradually for several months and was accompanied by a profuse malodorous discharge.

Upon examination I found both nasal fossae completely obstructed by a pyriform tumor occupying the position of the nasal septum. My first impression was that the tumor was probably an abscess of the nasal septum, but closer examination revealed the fact that the side of the tumor encroaching upon the lumen of the left nasal fossa, was a marked deflection of the septum to that side, and that the mucous membrane covering it was normal in character and directly in contact with the cartilaginous portion of the septum, where it belonged. The projection into the right nostril was a dark red and somewhat lobulated tumor, completely filling the fossa, whose surface had been more or less altered in appearance by two or three lines of electric cauterization. The tumor was elastic in character, not dense.

I made a provisional diagnosis of sarcoma, removed a specimen for microscopic examination, prescribed a placebo and requested the patient to return in about a week. The pathologist, Dr. Charles Bentz, of the University of Buffalo, returned a report of his examination, stating that the tumor was a characteristic tuberculous growth containing giant cells, etc., and that he had discovered tubercle bacilli in several of the microscopic slides from the specimen.

When the patient next visited me I removed the growth

piecemeal, with snare and curette, until I reached the underlying cartilage and healthy mucous membrane, posteriorly
and at the suture between the bony and the cartilaginous portion of the septum. When I had, in this manner, removed
the growth from the septum, I discovered that the anterior
portion of the lower turbinate of the same side was indurated
and superficially ulcerated. The floor between the two tumors
was likewise ulcerated.

The following day I removed most of the anterior portion
of the inferior turbinate, with scissors. and forceps, until
no more evidence of disease was discernible. At this and at
subsequent visits I thoroughly cauterized the wound surface,
on both the septum and the outer nasal wall, with lactic acid.
I also cauterized the edges of the wound, where the mucous
membrane appeared normal, with an electric cautery. The
wound surfaces were kept separate by packing with iodoform
gauze until the wounds had healed.

This patient has a good family history, free from tuberculosis. She has an old scar in the cervical region, and gives
a history of glandular abscess in childhood. She has four
children, one of whom, she says, has "lung trouble." But I
have never had an opportunity to examine this child.

I referred the patient to Dr. De Lancey Rochester, of Buf-
falo, for an examination of her chest. He reports as follows:
"I find no disease of the lungs here. Heart is not very strong.
There is history of old gland abscess in the neck," etc.

At no time, while under my care, did. the patient have any
rise of temperature. Since her recovery from the local lesion
it has been impossible to carry out any systematic treatment
of the case. However, I prescribed potassium iodide and
recommended tonics and out-of-door life. Had she been able
to visit the city from time to time I should have instituted
tuberculin treatment.*

Whether this should be considered a primary infection of
the individual is questionable. As already mentioned, she
has an old scar, on the neck, of a lesion which was probably
active twenty years ago and may, or may not, have been
tubercular. The nasal infection, I should judge, commenced
as a tuberculoma of the nasal septum and subsequently infected the lower turbinate. The infection may have started
as a "contact infection" of an erosion of the concave cartilag-

---

*This case was seen by the author on May 28, 1909, when no
evidence of a return of the lesion could be detected.

inous portion of the septum, and not by secretion from the patient's lungs. Or, she may have been infected by the secretions from her own child, seven years old, who may have tuberculosis.

This is reported as a typical case of nasal tuberculosis, which usually commences in the cartilaginous portion of the nasal septum, as a tuberculoma. The usual classification of the various forms of nasal tuberculosis is that suggested by Gerber in Heymann's Handbook and adopted by Prof. Gleitsmann in his report at Vienna last year. It includes tuberculous ulcer, diffuse infiltration, tuberculoma and lupus. A simpler division is: true tuberculosis of the nasal mucous membrane and lupus of the nasal mucous membrane.

Tuberculous infiltration and tuberculoma are identical in character. The latter is simply a greater elevation of the diseased tissue above the surface attacked by the infection. Both of these undergo some ulceration in time. These two forms are supposed to be primary in character, and differ, in this respect, from the tuberculous ulcer of the nasal mucous membrane, which is a secondary infection.

Although tuberculosis of the nose is a comparatively rare disease, a sufficient number of cases has been reported, and critically studied, during the past fifteen years, to establish their clinical characteristics and etiological factors. Up to the time that Prof. Chiari wrote his paper, in 1894, on "Tuberculoma of the Nasal Septum," only twenty-one cases, including six of his own, had been reported. Since that time the number of cases reported has rapidly increased and exhaustive articles have been written upon the subject by Gerber, Pasch, Caboche, Gerst, Katz and others.

Authors who come into contact principally with cases of pulmonary tuberculosis, have, with very few exceptions, contributed very little to the literature on this subject; and the cases which they have reported have been those of simple ulceration without any perceptible proliferation of tissue. This is the form of tuberculosis which occurs in the nose in advanced pulmonary conditions which is like that found in the pharynx in advanced phthisis. For instance, Karl von Ruck, in his report on the treatment of pulmonary tuberculosis, in 1903-04, cited eight cases, and, in his report of 1905-06, he reported six cases, all of which were ulcerative in character. Caboche states that of twenty cases of tuberculous ulcers of the nasal mucous membrane, which he collected from the literature, eighteen appeared as the ultimate manifestation of pulmonary phthisis.

The poliferative form of nasal tuberculosis is considered to be primary, and most of its characteristics are illustrated by the history of the case just cited. It occurs, usually, in people of robust health who have no other active tubercular lesions, although evidences of latent tuberculosis may be found in other organs. For instance, the patient whose case I have been considering has a scar on her neck, and may also have some undiscovered latent pulmonary lesion.

The tuberculous tumor, or tuberculoma, is of the type of so-called primary infection of the nasal septum. Its presence is discovered by the symptoms of nasal obstruction. Examination, in such cases, reveals a tumor of variable size, starting from the typical spot on the cartilaginous portion of the nasal septum and varying in color, according to its vascularity, from gray or pale red, to dark red. This description may also apply to any tumor of the nasal septum. Tuberculoma, when not removed, may, in time, undergo coagulation necrosis and, possibly, become an ulcer. The process usually commenees on the cartilaginous septum, and other tuberculous lesions in the nose are the result of infection from it, by contact and continuity of surface; it may thus extend to the floor of the nose, the turbinals, the ethmoid, frontal and maxillary sinuses. Infection may start in other parts of the nose, but rarely. It may also occur on the vomer and extend through the nasal duct to the conjunctiva.

Caboche claims that all primary infections of the nasal septum are lupic in character; and that twenty-nine out of forty-four cases of tuberculoma of the nasal septum, which he collected from the literature, were undoubtedly lupus; and of twenty-one observations of tuberculous infiltration of the nasal mucosa, only four are probably lupus; all the others, seventeen in number, are absolutely lupus. He sums up by saying: "There are only two forms of nasal tuberculosis: miliary tuberculosis and lupus, which comprises tubercular tumors and the majority of tuberculous granulations."

Lupus of the nasal mucous membrane has all the histologic characteristics of other forms of nasal turberculosis and is distinguishable only by the clinical manifestations. Many authors believe that lupus of the face always commences in an internasal lesion from an infection of the nasal mucosa, and that as the lesion produces no symptoms until the skin is attacked, it is first seen by the dermatologist who rarely pays much attention to the interior of the nose until destruction takes place.

The difference between primary tuberculosis and lupus is not always acknowledged by others than dermatologists. Much that is claimed to be lupus by some is called tuberculosis by others. Hajek, Michelson and Zarnico have entirely given up the classification into nasal tuberculosis and nasal lupus, and speak only of nasal tuberculosis. As we have already seen, Caboche and others claim that all primary internasal tuberculosis is lupic in character; while, on the other hand, Moritz Schmidt, and many other authors, devote a seperate chapter to lupus of the upper air passages.

Primary infection of the nasal mucous membrane is more rare than one would expect from its location, because the nose is protected by weapons of defense in the cillary epithelium of the mucous membrane and the bactericidal qualities of the normal nasal secretion. Tubercle bacilli, and other pathogenic germs, have been found in the nasal cavities of healthy people by many investigators, especially in people, such as nurses and attendants, associated with tuberculous patients. Inoculation may then occur through defects in the epithelium, through excoriations and erosions. This part of the nose is also subject to the insults of the scratching finger and to the use of the soiled handkerchief of some infected person. As has already been stated, the tuberculous ulcer is a secondary infection in patients with pulmonary phthisis.

Some authors claim that all nasal tuberculosis is a secondary ascending disease; yet some, on the other hand, assert that every case of facial lupus has its origin in the nasal mucosa. Many cases that are apparently primary in origin, are, in reality, secondary to some latent lesion in the lungs, or some other organ, which cannot be recognized by any means of physical diagnosis. Consequently, it is almost impossible, during life. to make an absolute diagnosis of primary infection, for we know how often latent tubercular lesions are found postmortem. X-ray examination of the lungs is now being practiced and will probably bring to light many undiscovered lesions.

The tubercular nasal ulcer is usually easily diagnosed from its characteristic appearance and from its association with pulmonary phthisis. The proliferative form can be absolutely diagnosed from histologic findings only. It is usually unaccompanied by pain or fever. The diffuse infiltration may resemble a specific infiltration, which is differentiated by the therapeutic test, although the two diseases may coexist.

Tuberculoma is not apt to be mistaken for syphilis. Syphilis rarely produces as large a tumor as tuberculosis. The tubercular tumor may be confounded, until examined histologically, with papilloma, fibroma and sarcoma. Onodi, for instance, diagnosed a case as carcinoma of the nasal septum, from the clinical picture and the microscopic examination of an excised portion. After radical removal of the tumor, it proved to be a tuberculoma. Pasch and Gerst describe cases of infiltration of the nasal mucous membrane, which are not distinguishable from true hypertrophy of that membrane, producing neither defects nor prominences, as illustrative of this condition. Gerst describes, among others, a case of a woman fifty-eight years old, whose right lower turbinate was uniformly enlarged, posterior extremity much enlarged with irregular surface and dark red in color. This turbinate only partially collapsed on application of cocain and adrenalin, the posterior extremity remaining unchanged. The anterior part only partially collapsed and was anemic, showing dark red colored spots prominent and circumscribed. The left lower turbinate also appeared hypertrophied without the posterior extremity being especially enlarged, and it reacted pretty uniformly to the cocain and adrenalin. After that the middle turbinates were visible and unchanged,—septal mucous membrane normal. The excised posterior extremity of the right turbinate was found to be tubercular. After discovering this, the left lower turbinate, and the mucous membrane on both sides of the septum, were removed and found to be tubercular. The only rhinoscopic changes were in the right lower turbinate, yet, the nasal mucous membrane was found to be extensively tubercular.

In conclusion and by way of summary I would say that, clinically, nasal tuberculosis may be divided into three classes:

First. The tuberculous ulcer, occurring in advanced phthisis, which is usually discovered by the specialist in that line who adds to his pulmonary examination a systematic inspection of the upper air passages, as was cited in the case of von Ruck, who reported fourteen ulcerations of the nasal mucosa in five hundred and fifty-four cases of pulmonary tuberculosis.

Second. The tuberculous tumor and infiltration, for which

the patient consults the rhinologist for nasal obstruction.

Thirdly. Lupus, cases of which are usually diagnosed by the dermatologist after the tubercular lesion of the mucosa has extended to the skin of the nose and face.

The last two are primary in origin and are more accurately termed tuberculosis, rather than lupus. In my opinion, the term "lupus" could, with impunity, be dropped from our nomenclature.

BIBLIOGRAPHY.

1. Gerber, Dr. P. H. "Tuberculose und Lupus der Nase." "Handbuch der Laryngologie und Rhinologie," Bd. 3, pp. 901-930.

2. Gleitsmann, Dr. J. W. "Behandlung der Tuberculose der Oberen Luftwege." Archiv für Laryngologie, Bd., 21, 1908, pp. 111-119.

3. Chiari, O. "Ueber Tuberculome der Nasenchleimhaut." Archiv für Laryngologie, 1894, pp. 121-134.

4. Pasch, Ernst. "Beitrag zur Klinik der Nasen Tuberkulose." Archiv für Laryngologie, Bd. 17, 1905, pp. 454-483.

5. Caboche, Henri. "Contribution to the Study of Tuberculosis of the Nasal Mucosa." Archives of Otology, Rhinology and Laryngology, Vol. 17, 1908, pp. 180-242.

6. Katz, Dr. Leo. "Die Tuberkulose der Nasenscheidewand." Die Krankheiten der Nasenscheidewand, pp. 83-100.

7. Gerst, Dr. Ernst. "Zur Kentniss der Einscheinungenformen der Nasentuberkulose." Archiv fur Laryngologie, Bd. 1908, pp. 309-324.

8. von Ruck, Karl, and von Ruck, Silvo. "A Clinical Study of 261 Cases of Pulmonary Tuberculosis," Treated at The Wingah Sanitarium, Asheville, N. C., 1905-6.

9. Same as above for years 1903-4.

10. Onodi, A. Deutsch med. Woch., 29, 1906.

11. Hajek, M. "Die Tuberkulose der Nasenschleimhaut." Internationale Klinische Rundschau, 1889.

12. Zarniko, Carl. "Die Krankheiten der Nase und des Nasenrachens."

13. Schmidt, Moritz. "Die Krankheiten der Oberen Luftwege."

XLV

SOME OBSERVATIONS UPON THE COMPLETE EXTIRPATION OF THE DISEASED FAUCIAL TONSIL.

By Joseph S. Gibb, M. D.,

Philadelphia.

A series of 100 cases of tonsillectomy in an institution in which the comforts and care of a private home were thrown around the patient gave an admirable opportunity for the observation of the after-effects of this operation and also for contrasting it with previous operations of tonsillotomy in the same institution.

This institution, the Girard College of Philadelphia, admits the pupils at the age of 6 years—and they remain until they are 18 years. The boys are given a good education and it is the policy of the management to provide as nearly as is possible a home life for them. Under the will of Stephen Girard, the founder, boys who are orphans or half orphans (having lost a father) are eligible.

Before admission, the applicant must pass a physical examination, which includes an examination of the nose, nasopharynx and pharynx. Cases which are believed to be affected with disease of the latter parts are set aside by the resident physician for a subsequent examination by myself. So that the cases selected for operation are typically healthy boys, save for the secondary conditions engendered by mouth breathing.

Incidentally a fair idea of the prevalence of tonsillar and adenoid hypertrophies among this class of patients is obtained by this rigid entrance physical examination. In a recent class of applicants in 102 boys, 36 were found to have either hypertrophied tonsils or adenoids or both. Only those cases were classed as necessitating operation in which (1) the tonsils were so large as to be evident to a casual observer. (2) Those in whom the tonsils were buried and covered by the pillars. (3) Those in whom the crypts and surrounding parts gave evidence of attacks of tonsillitis.

Of the 100 cases which serve as a basis for these observations, 65 were operated within one week, so that they were all in the infirmary at or about the same time—the remaining 35 were done within six weeks of each other and were practically consecutive. The cases are prepared for operation in the same manner as for a major surgical operation. Admitted to the infirmary the day before operation; purgative the night before, and the usual preparation for anesthesia.

An anesthetic was administered in every case except in a few older boys with simple nonadherent hypertrophied tonsils. The method adopted for the removal of the tonsils is as follows: The tonsil is firmly grasped by a forceps—the forceps which has served me best after trial of a number of varieties is that sold in the shops as the Mikulicz broad ligament forceps—the tonsil is firmly pulled from its bed by an assistant and the attachment to the pillars severed by the Allis blunt dissector. In many cases the attachment is so firm as to cause considerable tension of the surrounding tissues. Rather than exert force to sever these firm adhesions it has been found wise and expedient to effect separation by means of a sharp instrument, either a properly constructed scissors or tonsil knives. Having effected a thorough separation of the pillars, the finger is introduced and an endeavor made to break up the deeper adhesions and to leave the tonsil hanging, as it were, by a shred of tissue. The forceps still in place, a strong wire snare is passed over the handles, down over the tonsil and around the shred of tissue and slowly drawn home.

In most cases this method has been found to be exceedingly satisfactory,—enucleating the tonsil from its bed often with the capsule attached.

In some cases, however, and especially is this so in the socalled buried tonsil, the gland is so adherent to the surrounding parts and its tissue so friable as to make it difficult for the forceps to retain their hold. Many of these will yield, however, by a proper amount of patience—but there are some which will not. In these latter by effecting as free a separation as possible it is a comparatively simple matter to engage the tonsil within the bits of a good punch and complete the removal.

There are still other cases in which owing to frequent inflammatory attacks the tonsil is not only adherent, but so bound down by adhesions as to resist all efforts to separate by blunt dissectors. In these sharp separators are used and the punch employed to complete the operation. The results of these operations have been most gratifying. This method has been employed by me in a desultory way for several years, but no opportunity had arisen to study the effects in a consecutive series of cases until these now reported, presented.

Every laryngologist has been disappointed at times in the use of the tonsillotome. We have all seen cases of socalled recurrences of the hypertrophy, which simply means that in most instances the operation was not a complete one. Again, we have realized what an ineffective instrument the tonsillotome was in the socalled buried tonsils. It seems to me apparent that if it becomes necessary to remove a tonsil at all only a complete extirpation is indicated.

We know that the crypts which are the part of the tonsil singularly subject to diseased conditions, extends down to or near the capsule; therefore, if a piece is sliced off the tonsil we effect only an increased breathing space in the fauces and this at times only temporarily, while the crypts below the incision remain diseased and a possible source of infection.

Whatever function the tonsil possesses is necessarily abrogated by the conditions already enumerated and which we recognize as diseased conditions; therefore, if it is necessary to remove a tonsil, it should be done in as complete a manner as is possible. Of course it is important that care should be exercised in the selection of cases. No tonsil should be removed unless it is diseased and ceases to be a functionating organ.

In my first case by this method I was considerably chagrined by the severity of the reaction, but experience taught me to reduce this to a minimum. One of the first lessons learned was to employ as little force as possible. It is far better to employ a sharp instrument to sever refractory adhesions than to stretch the tissues until they break. By the latter is induced a cellulitis with subsequent infection and prolongation of the post-operative effects. The same may be said of the too strenuous use of the finger in breaking up the adhesions. It is far better to snip the tissues with a curved scissors or depend upon the wire for the severance. Another important matter is that the pillars shall be entirely free and not included in the grasp of the snare when the final severance is effected. However, even where the greatest care is employed the reaction is at times more pronounced than in the use of the tonsillotome.

Let us study the 100 cases: As an evidence of the usual care given the boys in this institution and not because of the necessity, the operated cases were retained in the infirmary from 2 to 7 days after operation. The average time was 4 days. This long stay afforded an exceptional opportunity to study each case. The efficient resident physician, Dr. Trinder, looked after the cases daily and kept careful notes of any departure from the normal. Again, even after the discharge from the infirmary, the boys remained in the institution and have all been seen from time to time since the operation. It is now a year since the first 65 cases were operated.

As to the temperature range: In 90 per cent of the cases the thermometer registered a temperature between 98-101, and in the larger number of these did not rise above 99. In 9 cases the temperature amounted to 102 and over. The first group, namely, those whose temperature remained below 101, were the type of case mainly with simple hypertrophied tonsil and slight attachment to the pillars. There were, however, quite a few in whom the tonsils were submerged and firmly adherent. In this group there was very little faucial disturbance. While the extent of removed tissue was observed by inspection to be more extensive than is usually seen after a tonsillotomy, the subjective symptoms were not thereby increased.

Later, when the effects of the traumatism had entirely disappeared and the boys were about their usual duties, an examination of the throat disclosed a perfectly normal fauces except that there was not a vestige of tonsil remaining.

The group of 9 cases with excessive temperature were those in which the tonsils were firmly adherent to and submerged beneath the pillars. Most of them were cases in which the tonsil had been the site of repeated inflammatory attacks and its tissue was soft and friable—requiring much dissection and the use of the tonsil punch—hence, unusual traumatism. In these cases there was in addition to the systemic disturbance, both objectively and subjectively, marked faucial symptoms. The patients complained of much difficulty and pain in swallowing. In two there was regurgitation of fluids through nose. The fauces were indurated in the region of the half arches, and the tonsillar wound was the site of a superficial ulcer covered by a slough.

All of these cases made a good, though tardy, recovery and subsequent examination revealed a normal fauces except that the tonsil was absent. It is not at all unlikely that much of the disturbance noted in this last group of nine cases might have been avoided had recourse been made to sharper instruments to effect a separation of the adhesions. These were among the early cases and at that time the lesson had not been learned to avoid as much as possible undue traction on the surrounding tissues which the use of dull dissectors and the finger is sure to produce in firmly adherent cases. Many cases as difficult have been operated since with no more disturbance than in the first group recorded.

In contrasting tonsillectomy by the method described, with previous operations, tonsillotomy, the first point to which I would direct attention is the thoroughness of the operation, Tonsillectomy leaves little to be desired so far as complete ablation of the tonsil is concerned.

Tonsillotomy on the other hand effects a complete extirpation only in those cases in which there are no adhesions or in which there is slight attachment to the pillars. In the large class of submerged or buried tonsils this operation effects in some cases only a partial removal which is almost useless, and in others it is impossible of execution.

As to the after-effects of the two operative procedures: It has been pointed out that in by far the larger number of cases, namely, 90 per cent, there is practically no severe symptoms following the tonsillectomy, the fauces clear rapidly and cleanly and leave no permanent injury or disfigurement. This is as good a result as tonsillotomy shows. It is true that in 9 cases there was unusual systemic disturbance and faucial ulceration and edema succeeding the operation. These cases, however, were all of the deeply submerged, adherent type of cases, requiring much dissection to free.

A type of case is familiar to every laryngologist in which it is necessary to grasp the tonsil firmly with the forceps and pull it from its bed to demonstrate the hypertrophy and then frequently to find it surrounded by a tightly adherent, thinned-out pillar or fold. This, then, was the character of the cases in which excessive reaction followed the dissection and removal.

No comparison can possibly be made between the two methods of operating in cases of this nature, for the reason that the tonsillotome is absolutely incapable of removing such hypertrophies, except the adhesions be first separated, the tonsil pulled from its bed and the tonsillotome used to cut off the remaining shred of tissue from the base. In which case, it simply takes the place of the snare used in the latter part of the operation described and is infinitely less satisfactory.

As to hemorrhage: Tonsillectomy has effected a great change in the operation room in these cases. It is rare to see profuse bleeding by this method for the removal of tonsils. In two cases of the group reported, there was an unusual amount of bleeding—in both of which the cause was a spurting vessel, which clamping with a hemostat readily and quickly controlled. The amount of hemorrhage in a given case is largely under our own control—the more rapidly the snare is tightened the greater the liability to bleeding, for it then approaches a knife in incisive qualities—the more slowly it is drawn home the more crushing force it possesses and the mouths of the vessels are closed. It is only necessary to recall the many anxious moments every operator has experienced in the past when he has successfully excised a large tonsil to find the buccal cavity filled with blood and more blood welling up from a large bleeding area, and contrast it with the proceeding under consideration where only a little oozing follows the snare,—to realize the tremendous advantage in this one particular the modern method affords.

The contention then is, from a study of these cases, that:

(1). Tonsillectomy is the proper operation for the removal of diseased tonsils.

(2). That tonsillectomy in the majority of cases results in no more serious traumatism to the faucial tissues than does tonsillotomy.

(3). That in those cases in which marked systemic and faucial disturbance follows a tonsillectomy it results because of the difficulty attending a separation of adhesions and that these latter cases are totally unsuited for the operation of tonsillotomy.

(4). That tonsillectomy is always a completed operation. Tonsillotomy is only occasionally completed.

(5). That hemorrhage after tonsillectomy is slight and largely under the control of the operator. In tonsillotomy, hemorrhage is often profuse, at times serious.

XLVI.

STUDIES CONCERNING THE SURGICAL TREATMENT OF OTITIC MENINGITIS.

By G. Alexander, M. D.,

Vienna.

(from the ear department of the general policlinic, Vienna, G. Alexander, M. D., director.)

Translated with permission of the author from *Archiv für Ohrenheilkunde*, Vol. 75, p. 222, and Vol. 76, p. 1, 1908.

By Geo. E. Davis, M. D.,

New York.

The progress in the surgical treatment of otitic cerebral diseases has necessarily drawn attention to otitic meningitis. Whereas before in this disease the prognosis was considered as absolutely unfavorable, so that any surgical treatment had been dispensed with from the very beginning, we now report quite a number of operatively healed cases. At this time it is our purpose to introduce a methodic operative treatment of meningitis by classifying and analyzing the material. In so doing we have come to the conclusion that we profit only very little from the autopsy of cases of meningitis with regard to the surgical part of the question; indeed, if we were to judge only by the anatomic cases which previously often enough were the only determinative factor, the possibility of a regular surgical treatment would appear a priori doubtful. Authors have repeatedly referred to the fact that the thick exudate between the soft cerebral membranes, extending deep and far into the sulci along the cerebral surfaces, was absolutely inaccessible for drainage. Besides, if we consider the fact that the inflammation in the majority of cases is not limited to the meninges, but also involves the superficial layers of the brain tissue, a surgical treatment appears even less possible. If we therefore consider only those cases of meningitis whose termination we have been able to witness, i. e., those whose severity finally causes death, we should have to negate the question of healing purulent meningitis and be sceptic towards the reported cases of successful healing.

The clinic, however, furnishes a different view. We have known for a long time that in the course of many middle ear affections, meningeal processes of a specially light form may appear that quite frequently disappear after a few days, sometimes even after a few hours, although in some cases healing occurs only after some time. We are aware of the fact that types of meningitis, the purulent character of which has been positively proved, may also heal. The whole question has become confused by calling the light meningeal processes, without any exact clinical examination, "meningeal irritation phenomena" or "meningeal congestion," little attention being paid to them; whereas, on the other hand, our point of view is that in these cases of healed purulent meningitis we meet with microorganisms of low virulence and the co-operation of a series of favorable circumstances unknown to us. Finally, quite a prolonged discussion arose concerning the circumscribed and diffuse forms of meningitis. Stress has also been laid upon the varying degrees of intensity of the meningitis, in which case, however, only the degree of the clinical phenomena could be determined. The lumbar puncture has proved to be a factor, by no means unimportant, for the classification of such cases; yet, we have found at this clinic, also, that a classification of meningitis by the lumbar puncture is not possible for all cases, so that it is unfortunately without decisive importance for the question of surgical interference.

A thorough study of the cases of otitic meningitis observed by me in the course of the last few years enabled me to classify them according to the special form of the causal disease.

The classification is the following:

1. Meningitis with uncomplicated, acute, purulent middle ear inflammation. 2. Meningitis with uncomplicated, chronic purulent middle ear inflammation. 3. Meningitis with otitic cerebral abscesses. 4. Meningitis with otitic thrombophlebitis and extradural abscesses. 5. Meningitis with labyrinth suppurations.

In each of these groups, three different types of meningitis are found to be differentiated: (1) Such types as retain an anatomically visible connection with the ear region, (2) types that do not show such connections, and (3) tubercular forms of meningitis.

Among the circumscribed forms of meningitis, the study of the inflammations of the meninges limited to the side of the diseased ear becomes especially important, since in a great many cases the alterations appear to be limited to the middle or the posterior cranial fossae. Above all, the labyrinthine meningitis belongs to the latter form.

CASE 1. Otitis media suppurativa acuta dextra. Meningitis serosa. Antrotomy, exposure of the middle and posterior skull fossae. Healing. Lumbar puncture showed clear serum; after 24 hours very fine coagulation, considerably increased pressure of outflow.

History: Johann E., of Vienna, 10 years of age, received at the Ear Department of the University of Vienna May 12th, 1907.

Seven years ago otorrhea of the right side, which soon healed. Since then, once or twice a year middle ear inflammation on the right side, finally suppuration for five or six days at the end of January, 1907. Since then, comfortable, good hearing, no secretion.

Two weeks ago the boy had violent pains in all his joints with fever, headache, vomiting and stiff neck. During the night before his reception at the clinic he had fever, delirium, awoke with loud crying from his restless and frequently interrupted sleep. His hearing was reported to be good on either side.

Findings: The left drum membrane was normal. Right drum membrane in posterior-superior quadrant showed a perforation of the size of a hemp seed; moderately moist, but not fetid suppuration. Functional finding of the left side normal. Conversational speech 9 m. on the right side, whispered speech and acumeter 5 m. Weber to the right. Schwabach lengthened; Rinne, on the right, negative; lower limit of tones moderately restricted, the upper one normal, watch heard by bone conduction. No symptoms of a disease of the static labyrinth. The soft tissues over the right mastoid process are moderately thickened, but no pressure pain. Temperature 38.6°, pulse 60. Operation was made by Dr. Alexander in chloroform narcosis. Typical skin incision, exposure and opening of the mastoid process.. Antrotomy. Bones diffusely softened, however, only ā little pus. Exposure of the sinus of the middle and posterior cranial fossae. Deep position of the dura of the middle cranial fossae. Cortex of the skull unchanged. Dura is much stretched, but not changed otherwise.

Lumbar Puncture: Evacuation of about 15 ccm. of clear cerebrospinal fluid under increased pressure, which after twenty-four hours showed very fine string-form coagulation; microscopically scanty mono- and polynuclear leucocytes, no microorganisms and by culture the fluid was sterile.

May 16, 1907. Gradual decrease of fever. Stiffness of neck the same, headache.

May 22, 1907. Change of dressing. Auditory canal dry. Drum membrane closed. Mastoid wound quiet. Lumbar puncture. In the last few days fever up to 38.4°. Patient is apathetic, lying in passive dorsal position, at times unconscious and repeatedly cries out suddenly. Patient passes urine and stools in bed.

May 26. Patient almost totally unconscious for two days, convulsions, pupils wide and not reacting. Pulse 40-60. Patient takes slight quantities of milk by spoonfuls. The ear wound is dressed every other day. Lumbar puncture.

June 5. Temperature now up to normal. Meningeal phenomena unchanged. Somnolence less.

July 10. Gradual decrease of the meningeal symptoms. Patient takes much nourishment. No vomiting. Temperature 36 to 37°.

July 17. Patient leaves his bed at times.

July 20. Patient is dismissed and referred to ambulatory after treatment. Healing of the ear wound without any reaction. Patient took a milk cure, gained considerable in weight, looks rosy, and has no complaint.

In this case, the meningitic phenomena appeared in their severest state simultaneously with the otitis media; that is to say, two weeks previous to the reception at the clinic.

In the above cited case we cannot decide with certainty whether we had to deal with an exacerbation of a chronic middle ear inflammation, or another acute disease. The findings on the drum membrane, the healing with intact drum membrane and good hearing speak for the fact that the last disease was not connected with the former otitis. The history further shows that the middle ear inflammation began with pains in the joints, accompanied by fever, headache, vomiting, stiffness of the neck, outcries during the night and restless sleep. In operating, the antrum was opened, the sinus and the dura of the middle and posterior cranial fossae exposed. A strict localization of the meningitis in the region of the right ear could not be proved. The dura was pathologically distended. In spite of this, the beginning of the meningitis shows that we had here undoubtedly to do with an otitic meningitis, at least a meningitis plus an otitis, rather than one without an otitis. Since local symptoms in the dura could not be established during the operation, incision of the dura was dispensed with. The lumbar puncture which immediately followed the operation and was later on repeated twice, always showed a clear, sterile, coagulating liquor that escaped under highly increased pressure. The severest meningeal phenomena (delirium, convulsions, drowsiness, complete unconsciousness at times) lasted from May 12th to June 18th. The ear wound during that time was at first dressed daily and then every other day. As regards variations of temperature, the patient was received with fever of 38.6°. After the operation, the fever sank within four days to the normal and two days later again rose; then there was continuous fever for four days, up to 38.5°, when it sank again to the normal and after that time the temperature remained normal. From the clinical standpoint, and with regard to the great intervals of no fever, the case had absolutely the appearance of a meningitis tuberculosa. This, however, is contradicted by the violent meningeal phenomena, their simultaneous appearance with considerable increase of temperature, further by the highly increased pressure of the liquor cerebrospinalis, the findings during the operation and finally the findings of the lumbar puncture. In spite of repeated and exact examination, we did not succeed in finding tubercle bacilli in the liquor obtained by lumbar puncture. Also, the acute course and the favorable issue, the robust physique and considerable increase in weight speak against a tuberculous meningitis, so that the diagnosis must read meningitis serosa acuta.

CASE 2. Otitis media suppurativa acuta dextra. Acute purulent mastoiditis. Antrotomy. Meningitis. Lumbar puncture showed gray-yellow, cloudy, sterile cerebrospinal liquor which escaped under increased pressure. Recovery.

History: Oscar D., of Vienna, 7 years of age, received at

the Ear Department of the University of Vienna on May 26th, 1904, Pr. No. 251, Journal No. 11.733. Patient reports otorrhea for eight days, bad hearing, pain in the right ear. Since a few days, spontaneous and pressure pain in the mastoid process, high fever, no appetite and no sleep.

Status presens: A very restless child with high fever (40°). Even on slightly touching the right mastoid process, patient complains of great pain. The auditory canal in its depth is impassably narrowed. The drum membrane is not visible; fetid secretion. Left ear otoscopically normal. The functional findings of the ear could not be undertaken on account of the youthful age and the severe disease.

May 6, 1904. Operation was made by Hofrat Politzer. Opening of the mastoid process and the antrum. The interior of the mastoid was pneumatic, filled with pus; the bone was softened as far as the sinus, which was exposed to the size of a bean. The bone was not changed towards the antrum, the middle and posterior cranial fossa, which were exposed.

Course: From May 6th to 20th, 1904, that is to say fifteen days, the temperature was 38-40° and mostly of continuous type. Only on two days (May 8th and 14th) there were remissions to 37° and 36.6° in the evening.

May 27th. Lumbar puncture; 10 ccm. of yellow-gray, very cloudy cerebrospinal liquor is evacuated under increased pressure. After six hours thread-like coagulation (Dr. Bartel). By microscope and culture the liquor is sterile. Mono- and polynuclear leucocytes.

During the first week after the operation stiff neck, convulsions, delirium, repeated vomiting, at times patient is somnolent, lying in passive dorsal position. During all this time patient only takes slight quantities of milk that are given to him with a spoon.

With the loss of fever on May 20th, the complaints became less and the stiffness of the neck disappeared. The patient takes nourishment with appetite and can sit up. Comfortable.

July 18th. The wound is smaller, and we find sluggish granulations in it. In changing the dressing, a sequestrum about 6 mm. long and 2 mm. thick is removed. Drum membrane intact.

August 12th. Increase of temperature in the evening to 38.7°, otherwise constantly normal temperature and comfortable.

September 11th. Since small sequestra have been repeatedly evacuated from the wound, another operation is suggested to the parents of the child.

Operation is quiet; chloroform narcosis. Skin incision in the direction of the old wound. In the bone cavity several small sequestra and one of the size of a hazel nut, sluggish granulations and pus. Removal of the external part of the posterior bony wall of the auditory canal. Wound dressed with iodoform emulsion. Bandage.

September 26th. Patient is dismissed after a curetting of the wound, without any reaction, and referred to ambulatory after treatment. According to an inquiry after three years (May, 1907) the boy is perfectly well and the ear entirely healed.

The present case is in its phenomena completely identical with case 1 of my material. Here also we have to do with an acute purulent middle ear inflammation which led to purulent mastoiditis and caused a meningitis. In operating no proof could be found for the direct connection between the middle ear suppuration and the inflammatory process in the meninges; the bone there being unaltered, the meninges were simply exposed; that is to say, at the middle cranial fossa above the tegmen tympani and antri and above the sinus and the neighboring region of the dura of the posterior cranial fossa.

The meningeal phenomena lasted for two weeks, during which time there was high fever of continual type varying between 38° and 40°, and showing a temporary decrease on two days. May 22nd, patient had no fever, when the meningeal phenomena disappeared and patient felt comfortable during his long stay in the hospital (patient spent his convalescence at the hospital in want of sufficient care at his home; i. e., he remained until September 26th), with one exception, and this most likely in consequence of a local retention. June 10th, fever of 38.7° suddenly appeared. Finally, it is worth noticing that the acute trouble in the mastoid process was caused by a chronic purulent ostitis. Repeatedly, small sequestra were evacuated and another operation had to be made on September 11th, removing the diseased bone. Prompt healing followed and since then patient has been comfortable. In this case also, taking into consideration the high fever and the violent phenomena, the diagnosis is meningitis serosa. Finally, the findings of the fundus oculi (marked by considerable distended veins) are not without importance for the diagnosis of meningitis. Of special interest remains the finding of the lumbar puncture: Yellow-gray, intensely clouded coagulating liquor, evacuated under increased pressure, in which were found by the microscope mono- and polynuclear leucocytes, no microorganisms.

In both cases (1 and 2) long subsequent observations allow us to state that the meningitis was completely relieved and permanently cured. In both cases we cannot take the meningitis serosa to be a secondary complication of the otitis media. On the contrary, it seems that here from the very beginning, the meninges and the middle ear had been simultaneously attacked by an inflammatory disease, so that we are having here no meningitis serosa from an otitis, but with an otitis. Both patients made good recovery, especially the one operated May, 1907, who gained remarkably in weight and had a rosy appearance.

Certain forms of serous meningitis are, however, by no means rare, especially in children, as a preliminary stage of a tuberculous meningitis, which may not appear for weeks or months after the first attack. I report here, out of my observations at our clinic in the years 1900 and 1901, three characteristic cases belonging to this class, which may be called really tragic. They were children at the age of 4 to 6 with typical acute purulent middle ear inflammation. All three of them were treated by ear specialists from the very beginning of the disease. The acute inflammatory symptoms in the middle ear disappeared, yet there was no decrease in the suppuration; it did not become fetid, though a copious, creamy or more or less watery pus continued to discharge. On the mastoid process were at times periostitic thickenings which rapidly disappeared with the application of "Burow's solution" and rest in bed, but suddenly meningitis, with high, increasing fever and stormy symptoms, developed.

Antrotomy: Bones over the dura unaltered, tension of the dura not markedly increased. Lumbar puncture showed clear liquor under increased pressure, which, after twenty-four hours, did not coagulate. After eight to ten days with gradual decrease of fever, complete disappearance of the meningeal symptoms. The patients were dismissed feeling comfortable. The one case, however, was received again three weeks, the other five weeks and the third nine weeks after dismissal with typical phenomena of meningitis tuberculosa and characteristic lumbar puncture findings (clear liquor, after twenty-four hours, finest coagulations; microscopic, tubercle bacilli). All of these three cases ended with death.

We can certainly not decide exactly whether we did not have from the very beginning a tuberculous otitis and a tuberculous meningitis. The clinical symptoms rather contradict this. In all three cases the otitis appeared with most intense pain and fever. Tuberculous middle ear suppuration has an insidious beginning and frequently the otorrhea will appear without attracting attention, so that later on patient can give only inexact report as to the beginning of the disease. It is very likely that the local inflammatory focus in the ear and in the meninges was from the very beginning not of a tuberculous nature, but yet offered the basis and premises for the appearance of the tuberculous disease that followed later.

The question arises whether a differentiation of such meningeal processes is possible? Such differentiation would perhaps be possible by an exact measurement of the intradural pressure. This pressure is unchanged with meningitis serosa as a preliminary stage of a tuberculous meningitis, whereas it is always considerably increased in the non-tubercular meningitis serosa. In these cases it would be necessary in making the lumbar puncture to measure the pressure under which the cerebrospinal liquor is evacuated; this is best done by means of one of the usual manometers, as, for instance, Sahli's. The pressure in the meningitis serosa which is only a preliminary stage of a tuberculous meningitis will be found to be normal or not essentially increased.

The two cases reported above are of importance also insofar as they show that the findings by lumbar puncture can be different in cases of meningitis serosa with clinical phenomena of similar intensity and duration. In the one case the liquor was clear, while in the other it was yellowish gray and very cloudy.

Serous meningitis as a preliminary stage of diffuse purulent meningitis is surely more frequent than we would expect, judging from the observations and the proofs we have obtained till now. If in such cases the lumbar puncture is made early enough, we will at first have a clear, sterile liquor evacuated with increased pressure and very fine coagulations after twenty-four hours, whereas if the lumbar puncture is made later it will show an infected cerebrospinal liquor. In this respect we shall report a remarkable case, as follows:

CASE 3. George F., 21 years old, of Triest.

Diagnosis: Meningitis purulenta, following otit. med. supp., etc.

Treatment: Radical operation, opening the labyrinth, repeated lumbar puncture.

History: Five years ago patient had scarlet fever and immediately afterwards suppuration of the right middle ear, which was operated on three months later. Since then, patient was well until April, 1906, when he had otorrhea, and after nine days was again operated: however, the otorrhea did not stop.

Therefore patient came to Vienna in July and a curettement was made. At the latter date pains in the right side of head. Otorrhea not diminished.

Left side: Spur on nasal septum. Pharyngitis chronica.

Left ear: Tympanic membrane lightly retracted.

Right ear: Retroauricular fistula leading towards the tegmen antri and a semicircular cicatrix. Auditory canal filled with thread-fibred pus and narrowed by the projecting anterior lower wall as well as by the slight sinking of the posterior upper wall. The remainder of the tympanic membrane, so far as visible, reddened and atrophied.

Right		Left
A. C	Conversational speech...........	8 m.
O	Whisper	3-4 m.
. ...	Weber	
. ...	Schwabach shortened	
—	*Rinne	
—	C_1	
—	C_4	
O	Watch	

Horizontal spontaneous nystagmus to the sound side.

September 7, 1906. Operation under Billroth's mixture narcosis. Retroauricular curved incision into the old cicatrix. Dissection of the fast adherent periosteum, excision of the fistula. After a few strokes with the chisel the sinus was exposed, with severe hemorrhage from the emissarium; after stopping this the radical operation was completed. Hard and

---

*Rinne right—Air-conduction almost disappeared and bone conduction much shortened.

vascular bone, granulations in the tympanic cavity. Plastic according to Panse. The wound was left open, bandage.

September 8. During the night vomiting several times, vertigo, strong rotatory nystagmus to the left on looking to the sound side. Temperature 38.6°.

September 9. Vertigo diminished, no vomiting. Rotatory nystagmus to the left on looking to the left.

September 9. The loud, subjective noises have become less. Long-stroked horizontal nystagmus on looking to the left, decreasing in intensity and amplitude as the object fixed approaches the middle line. The sensation of vertigo does not accord with the amount and intensity of the nystagmus. Whereas the patient complained one day about vertigo in looking towards any direction, without any appreciable relation between the amount and intensity of the nystagmus, the next day he complains of the apparent movement of objects to be the factors annoying him most. However, the patient has at times sensations of vertigo, increasing in intensity when altering his position. Patient in looking to the left sees parallel, crossed, double images of unequal size, and which he projects correctly. Whereas patient up to September 8th could lie only on the sound side, in which position he claimed to have the least vertigo, he is to-day able to assume any position without vertigo. Only when lying on the diseased side or while changing position, is the patient aware of the sensation of intense vertigo.

September 10. Horizontal nystagmus on looking to the left. Sensation of vertigo continues. Patient lies on the sound side. In sitting up the nystagmus is unaltered. With feet together and eyes closed, staggering is only perceptible. In bending the head to the diseased side, patient falls back and to the right. On closing the eyes, the staggering and falling is not increased. Standing on one foot is almost impossible, whereas he can stand tip-toes, with open and closed eyes, though awkwardly and staggering. Hopping with both feet is accompanied by slight staggering. Patient was a good gymnast. All motions are well made, though accompanied by staggering. Diplopia continues. Change of dressing.

September 11. Nystagmus, on looking to either side, stronger to the left. Sensation of vertigo somewhat diminished. Numbness, light hyperesthesia. General condition bad. Temperature 37.4°, pulse 80, sufficiently strong.

On changing the dressing, we find muco-purulent secretion.

Hearing distance about ½ m. for conversational speech, Weber to the right.

Lumbar puncture reveals yellowish cloudy liquor, evacuated under moderate pressure (about 10 ccm.). By microscopic examination of same we find it rich in leucocytes that give positive iodine reaction.

Operation under Billroth's mixture narcosis. Chiselling off the posterior wall of the pyramid with removal of the posterior and horizontal semicircular canals and opening the promontory, penetrating as far as the interior auditory canal. The membrane labyrinth appeared hyperemic. The dura of the posterior cranial fossa was incised in the form of a right angle, whereupon the cerebellum projected. Tamponading. Dressing. Facial paralysis. After operation short-stroked nystagmus to both sides, frequent vomiting and somewhat benumbed. In the evening 1 cgr. morphin.

September 12. Two o'clock at night, entirely conscious, relatively good subjective symptoms, no vertigo, no nystagmus. In the forenoon two lumbar punctures with withdrawal of about 6 ccm. of very cloudy purulent liquor. Highest temperature 39.2°. Pulse moderately accelerated, strong; in the evening 1 cgr. morphin.

September 13. Very restless, sleepless night, continuous vomiting, 8 a. m. temperature 38.2°, pulse 102. Short-stroked nystagmus to both sides, some headache and tenderness of the neck. Very much coated tongue. Vomiting diminished. No diplopia.

September 14. Slept quietly half of the night. Morning temperature 38.7°, pulse 72, strong. Mind clear, vomiting less, mobility of the head restricted. Lumbar puncture; withdrawal of 10 ccm. of less cloudy liquor; however, under great pressure. Tongue very much coated; 8 p. m. temperature 38°.

September 15. Sleepless, restless night, in spite of morphin injection; temperature at 8 a. m. 38.4°, pulse 90. Patient often shrieks out, neck very stiff, comatose. Distinct Trousseau phenomenon. Nutrient enema. Subcutaneous injection of 20 ccm. Marmorek serum. In the evening 1 cgr. morphin. Temperature 38.2°. No nystagmus any more.

September 16. Sleepless night, continuous delirium, temperature 38° 8 a. m. Dry coated tongue, weak, irregular pulse, incontinence of urine and feces. Change of dressing. Widening of the incision into the dura.

September 17. Condition unaltered. Temperature 36.6° at 8 o'clock a. m. In the evening comatose condition.

September 18. 6 a. m., death.

Post mortem result: Purulent internal pachymeningitis and leptomeningitis at the base of the brain, especially within the region of the chiasma, the pons, the under surfaces of both cerebellar hemispheres and the medulla. Fibrino-purulent inflammation of the inner meninges of the spinal cord.

Flattening of the brain convolutions on the surface. Radical operation of the right ear after chronic otitis, with incision of the dura and puncture of the right cerebellar hemisphere. Acute edema of both lungs, enlargement of the kidneys and the heart.

Double vision, stiff neck and convulsions were in this case the first symptoms of a meningitis that had been a complication of and was most likely caused by a purulent labyrinthitis. The lumbar puncture at the very beginning and one four days later showed a yellow, purulent, cloudy liquor evacuated under moderately increased pressure. The liquor coagulated after twenty-four hours; microscopic, leucocytes with positive iodine reaction, no microorganisms, sterile by culture. A later lumbar puncture showed a streptococci-containing liquor. We have here the type of a meningitis to be considered as a stage between a meningitis serosa and an acute purulent streptococci meningitis. Such meningitis is by no means rare; however, only very difficult to diagnose, because the lumbar puncture for the most part is done after the stage of the purely serous character of the meningitis; that is to say, in the stage of purulent meningitis. In operating, brain tissue immediately protruded into the incision of the dura, a sure sign of encephalitis. An inflammatory swelling of the surfaces of the brain also in this case preceded the infectious purulent meningitis.

Moreover, superficial encephalitis seems to represent a typical accompanying phenomena of acute serous meningitis, and I can, according to the material examined by me, fully confirm the opinions of Bönninghaus and others on meningo-encephalitis.

I shall now report two cases of acute meningitis induced by labyrinth suppuration, which recovered:

CASE 4. First reception. Karl H., 30 years old, bricklayer, of Oberkirchen, Austria, received January 28, 1906.

Diagnosis: Otitis media suppurativa chronica dextra. Cholesteatoma. Labyrinth suppuration. Meningitis ex otitide. Fistula of the semicircular canal.

Therapeutics: Radical operation. Plastic after Panse. (Removal of the lateral and posterior semicircular canals, opening of the upper one as far as the vestibulum.)

History: Patient has been deaf in the right ear since a child. Sometimes otorrhea, the present attack lasting one year and a half. Since eight days severe pain within the entire region of the ear. Three weeks ago patient had violent vertigo for six to eight days. Patient also frequently vomited. To-night nausea, vomiting, severe pain so that patient could not sleep.

Left ear: Clouded retracted tympanic membrane.

Right ear: Slit shaped auditory canal on account of sinking of the posterior upper wall; fetid, abundant secretion.

Right		Left
9 m	Speech	5 m.
6 m	Whisper	at ear
	Weber to the left.	
—	Rinne	Bone conduction slightly shortened, air conduction very much shortened
+	C_1	
+	C_4	
+	A	

January 29, 1906. Radical operation in quiet inhalation narcosis. Exposure and opening of the mastoid process, sinus moderately forward and exposed to the size of a lentil. Tympanic cavity and antrum filled with finely stratified cholesteatoma reaching as far as the sinus. On the lateral semicircular canal a fistula 5 mm. in length and corresponding to the diameter of the semicircular canal, discolored contents of the semicircular canals. Removal of the lateral and posterior semicircular canals, as well as opening of the upper one as far as the vestibulum, which was filled with disintegrated, discolored masses (cholesteatoma) that were removed with the sharp curette. Plastic according to Panse. Wound dressing. Bandage.

February 5. Second change of dressing. Wound granulating well.

February 7. Change of dressing. Fetid secretion from the bottom of wound. No vertigo. No vomiting. Head aches on the operated side.

February 9. Patient has pains in the right iliocecal region. Retention of urine. Increase of temperature.

February 10. Patient is transferred to room 54 of Hochenegg's clinic for operation.

February 15. Laparotomy in Hochenegg's clinic February 10th on account of acute appendicitis. Since February 14th violent headaches, and to-day vomiting so that the patient is again referred to our clinic.

Patient very feeble, sense of localization destroyed, complains of severe, right-sided frontal headaches. Medium rigidity of the neck, and active motions of the head and the cervical portion of the vertebral column are carefully avoided. Moderate fetid pus secretion from the wound cavity. No disturbance of coordination. Long-stroked nystagmus more frequent to the sound side than to both sides.

Operation under quiet Billroth's mixture narcosis. Enlargement of the skin incision of the first operation, at the end of which two incisions are made about 3 cm. long, running horizontally backwards. Elevation and retraction of posterior flaps thus formed. Exposure of the operative cavity. Wide exposure of the dura of the middle cranial fossa and enlargement of the opening in the dura of the posterior cranial fossa, with removal of the basal part of the petrous portion of the temporal bone. Under considerable pressure, extradural pus wells up from below. Dura of the middle and posterior cranial fossa diffusely reddened and strongly injected. The exploration of the posterior cranial fossa negative; that of the middle cranial fossa shows the following: . Brain surface diffusely reddened, moderately edematous.

By lumbar puncture about 10 ccm. of purulent, cloudy, light yellow colored cerebrospinal liquor is evacuated under considerably diminished pressure. Wound dressing. Bandage.

February 16. Patient complains of severe headaches, gets morphin subcutaneously. Restless during night. No vomiting. Slight facial paralysis.

February 19. Patient complains of headaches. Quiet during night. Pulse and temperature normal.

February 21. Very restless night. Most severe headaches.

Ice bag and morphin injection. During day patient is somnolent and lies in opisthotonus, so that the entire body is lifted by the support of the neck.

February 22. Complaints diminished, temperature normal. Patient is lying in quiet dorsal position.

February 23. Patient complains of headaches. Restless night.

February 24. Temperature normal since yesterday. Relatively comfortable with the exception of headaches.

February 26. Fairly comfortable. Headaches less.

March 1. Change of dressing, comparatively comfortable.

March 2. Temperature 39.7°. Sore throat. Aspirin 1.0. Gargle.

March 3. Change of dressing. Relatively comfortable.

March 5. Localized headaches.

March 8. Change of dressing. Comfortable, walks about.

March 11. Patient complains of headaches.

March 13. Patient complains of severe headaches near the right temporal bone.

March 14. Patient complains of the same pains as yesterday.

March 16. Status idem. The wound looks very good.

March 20. Relatively comfortable. Patient has galvanism daily.

March 30. Comfortable. Secondary suture.

April 13. One sequestrum has been evacuated.

May 4. Relatively comfortable. Patient is dismissed and referred to ambulatory after treatment.

Second reception: After May 4, 1906, patient came daily for ambulatory treatment. Otorrhea did not stop. Headaches are still prevailing, though less. Vertigo only on stooping. For two weeks patient complains of an acute pain in his legs as far as the knee.

June 13. A sequestrum came from the ear.

June 19. Two fusiform sequestra 7 mm. long and ¼ mm. in diameter were removed from the ear.

June 25. Condition the same. Patient complains of headaches on the other side. Secretion moderate. In the left side of the nose the posterior end of the lower turbinate and the anterior end of the middle turbinate very much hypertrophied. Operated.

July 5. Patient is dismissed in good condition. Subsequently complete cure.

In this case we have a purulent labyrinthitis with purulent ostitis of the petrous portion of the temporal bone itself in the course of a chronic middle ear suppuration. We cannot establish with certainty how long the labyrinth suppuration existed before patient was received. It is true, it is stated that there was deafness since childhood; however, we know that in chronic middle ear suppuration deafness may occur without the suppurative process involving the cochlea (Kuemmel). In such cases deafness may also have been causel by simple degenerative changes of the nervus acusticus and its ganglions or by atrophy of Corti's organ. Therefore, in our case, the vestibular symptoms are of greater importance. We learn that three weeks before the patient was received he had violent attacks of vertigo, and it is very likely that these indicate the beginning of the labyrinth suppuration.

When operating in the latter part of January a middle ear and labyrinth cholesteatoma was found. After the operation, which consisted in the radical operation, the wide opening of the labyrinth and the exposure of the cranial fossae, vertigo stopped immediately; however, two bad symptoms remained. The wound secretion remained fetid and purulent and the patient complained of continuous headaches, especially on the operated side. These phenomena were suddenly complicated by ileocecal pains. The examination revealed an acute appendicitis, and the patient was referred to the second surgical clinic of Professor Hochenegg and operated February 10th. During the course of an uneventful laparotomy convalescence, sudden symptoms of a severe meningeal disease appeared. High fever, coma and vomiting occurred. The examination immediately on the retransference of the patient to the ear clinic revealed the following: Patient is very weak, at times loss of consciousness, complains of severe right sided frontal headaches, stiff neck, active movements of the head and neck are carefully avoided. No ataxia can be elicited. No disturbance of coordination. Long-stroked nystagmus, more so to the sound side that to diseased side.

The unchanged fetid seeretion indicated a deep seated purulent focus, and in the operation an extensive extradural abscess over the petrosal roof was exposed and evacuated. The dura of the middle cranial fossa was strongly injected, not changed in the posterior cranial fossa. The incision of the cranial fossae revealed in the region of the middle cranial fossa-a diffuse reddening of the leptomeninges. swelling of the temporal lobe, no changes in the cerebellum.

In making the lumbar puncture yellow, cloudy liquor was evacuated under diminished pressure. The violent meningeal phenomena continued for a while, and five days after the operation there was somnolence, strong opisthotonus, and stiff neck. On the eleventh day after the operation, patient first felt tolerably well and the severe headaches also stopped. Three weeks later patient left his bed. During the after treatment small sequestra were repeatedly discharged from the upper petrous portion of the temporal bone. This sequestration undoubtedly caused the chronic headaches, and was also the reason why on the 16th of June the patient had to be taken in again.

June 19. Two fusiform sequestra, 7 mm. long and ¾ mm. thick, were extracted, when all symptoms ceased. Thorough chiselling produced complete healing and patient is perfectly well and able to work.

We have here a case of severe meningitis which, according to its character, has to be classed between the serous and the purulent meningitis. It is distinguished from the serous meningitis by the color of the cerebrospinal secretions (the cerebrospinal liquor was purulent and cloudy) and from the purulent meningitis by the lack of micro-organisms. The infection of the meninges resulted from the labyrinth cholesteatoma, which led to purulent otitis of the petrous bone. It was remarkable that, according to the findings at the operation, the meningitis chiefly involved the middle cranial fossa of the diseased side, and we only learned from the later clinical symptoms the extension of the meningitis to the posterior cranial fossa (strong opisthotonus and stiff neck). The evacuation by the lumbar puncture of the cerebrospinal fluid under diminished pressure might be referred to the fact that before the lumbar puncture the dura of both cranial fossae was incised. Possibly also those causes will have to be taken into consideration to which Frey, Hinsburg. Körner, and Schwartze ascribe the diminished evacuation pressure of the cerebrospinal fluid; viz., meningeal agglutinations at the foramen Magendii or a thick viscid meningitic exudate.

The therapeutics consisted in the removal of the extradural abscess and in the opening and drainage of both cranial fossae. The lumbar puncture was made only once, the incision of the dura was in this case indicated not only by the meningeal symptoms, that clearly pointed to meningitis of the diseased side, especially of the middle cranial fossa, but also by the finding at the operation that likewise indicated a close anatomic relation of the meningitis with the changes in the ear region. There is no doubt that localized meningeal processes are best controlled by a wide opening of the dura. Especially is it indicated in encephalitis (Körner, Manasse), which is manifested by the protrusion of the superficial brain tissue into the incision. We obtain hereby a diminution of the intradural pressure and a reliable drainage. It is only necessary to expose well the region of the necrosed bone and dura and remove thoroughly the diseased portions of the bone. Unfortunately a brain prolapse cannot be avoided.

To this group of circumscribed meningo-encephalitis belong, amongst others, circumscribed meningitis with great swelling of the cerebellar hemisphere of the posterior cranial fossa in the region of the sinus sigmoideus, in cases of infectious thrombophlebitis. With timely and thorough surgical treatment circumscribed meningitis with infectious thrombophlebitis has a rather good prognosis. For illustrating this kind of a disease I may refer to the following case:

CASE 5. Josef C., 19 years old, joiner, of Vienna, received at the Ear Department of the University of Vienna June 30, 1907.

Diagnosis: Otitis media suppur. chronica sinistra, cholesteatoma, extradural abscess of the middle and posterior cranial fossae, thrombophlebitis of the sinus lateralis.

Therapy: Jugular ligature. Radical operation after the removal of the cholesteatoma and thrombus from the sinus lateralis to the bulbus jugularis, opening of the extradural abscess, lumbar puncture.

History: Since his tenth year, suppuration of the left middle ear. Patient's ear was never treated. Three weeks ago patient fell ill with fever, headache and chill and was brought to the clinic since his trouble continued.

Present condition: Strong, well nourished individual, passive dorsal position, active and passive motions of the head and neck considerably restricted. Cutaneous sensibility unaltered, mobility and coordination normal.

Aural findings: Left tympanic membrane destroyed, thin crumby pus in the auditory canal; by the microscope are found many cholestearin crystals, secretion exceedingly fetid. Right tympanic membrane much retracted, clouded.

FUNCTIONAL FINDINGS.

Right		Left
14 m	Speech	1 m.
6 m	Whisper	O.
6 m	Acumeter	O.
	Weber	+
—	Rinne	
Shortened	C_1	Somewhat shortened
Shortened	C_4	Shortened
	Watch	+
	Acumeter	+
None	Spontaneous nystagmus	{ Slow, long stroked, horizontal

With an ear tube conversational and whispered speech are heard on the left side normally.

Fundus oculi unchanged, no morbid phenomena on the part of the other cerebral nerves, no motor aphasia or dysphasia; patient had a chill (41.2°) during night, pulse 108, respiration 24; complains of severe headaches that are localized over the region of the mastoid process and the planum temporale, diffuse swelling of the soft tissues over the mastoid with considerable spontaneous and pressure pain over same and on the throat.

No changes to be found in the abdominal and thoracic viscerae, no pain whatever, nor swelling of the extremities.

July 1, 1907. Operation under Billroth's mixture narcosis. Exposure and ligation of the vena jugularis intern. sinistr. in the middle third of the throat; the moderately filled vein contains fluid blood and is divided through between double ligatures, retroauricular skin incision, 7 cm. long, from both ends of which two parallel skin incisions are made backwards 7 cm.; in separating the posterior cutaneous wall of the auditory canal intensely fetid pus, mixed with colesteatoma, wells forward under considerable pressure; after opening the mastoid process for a short distance, ichorous cholesteatoma masses push forward from the region of the middle cranial fossa under pulsations; radical operation, cleansing the tympanic cavity filled with polypi and cholesteatoma. Curetted the tube; the temporal bone is much necrosed near the middle and posterior cranial fossae, the dura is exposed over the tegmen tympani et antri and over the sinuses the size of a bean. The bone is softened and fetid at the seat of necrosis; lateral sinus wall greyish green, discolored and brittle. The posterior and middle cranial fossae are exposed from the sinus for an area as large as a dollar; exposure of the sinus to and over the knee as much as 4 cm.; downward removal of the tip of mastoid, exposure of the bulbus, splitting and removal of the lateral sinus wall. The sinus is thrombosed corresponding to the entire extent of the pachymeninges; the thrombus is softened in the bulb, and in the lower part, a dark red thrombus reaches far down. After the removal of the thrombi a hemorrhage came from both sides; dressing, fixation of the square cutaneous flaps to the front by means of a suture.

July 2. First change of dressing. Sewing of the peripheral vein ends with two double sutures (jugular cutaneous fistula); change of the bulb drain, ichorous secretion; removal of the strip at the lower end of the sinus, incision of the dura of the posterior cranial fossa ½ cm. to the inner sinus wall; the cerebellum prolapsed some millimeters through the opening, brain surface reddened, evacuation of some drops of cloudy liquor. The lumbar puncture gave a grey cloudy liquor (10 ccm., evacuation pressure unaltered, microscopically many polynuclear leucocytes, no microorganisms).

July 3. Second change of dressing.

Opening of the peripheric vein ends, from which hemorrhagic secretion escapes. The peripheric ends of the vein are kept open by introducing iodoform strips with change of dressing at the bulb.

July 4. Third change of dressing.

Superficial shortening of all strips, change of dressing at bulb and the jugular.

July 5. Fourth change of dressing; much secretion through the peripheric vein end; removal of the drain from the tympanic cavity.

July 6. Fifth change of dressing; fetid secretion in the region of the bulb. H_2O_2 is applied, damp iodoform gauze.

July 7. Change of dressing. Secretion from the peripheric jugular end.

July 8. Change of dressing. Secretion from the peripheric jugular end.

July 9. Change of dressing.

July 11. Patient is comfortable, wound over the jugular free from secretion and granulating. Ichorous pus in the upper part of the wound over the mastoid process.

July 12. Status idem.

July 13. Change of dressing.

July 14. In the upper part the wound seems much inclined to close. Near the sinus still ichorous secretion.

July 16. Change of dressing.

July 17. Change of dressing. Ichorous suppuration.

July 18. Change of dressing. Ichorous suppuration.

July 19. Change of dressing. Ichor near the sinus.

July 20. Status idem.

July 22. Change of dressing. Secretion diminished and less fetid. Granulations arise over the entire surface of the wound.

July 23. Change of dressing.

July 24. Change of dressing. There is no more secretion from the wound of the neck.

July 25. Change of dressing.

July 26. Change of dressing. Unchanged.

July 27. Change of dressing. Unchanged.

July 28. Change of dressing.

July 29. Change of dressing.

July 31. Patient complains of severe vertigo. Rotatory nystagmus to both sides.

August 1. Change of dressing. Secretion scant and not fetid. Rotatory nystagmus less than yesterday, no vertigo.

August 3. Change of dressing. Slight and non-fetid secretion. Rotatory nystagmus to both sides, no vertigo.

August 5. Status as yesterday.

August 7. Plastic.

August 9. Change of dressing.

August 11. Change of dressing. Patient is dismissed and referred to ambulatory after treatment.

August 15. Change of dressing. Brain much prolapsed. Patient has strong nystagmus to both sides. Distinct disturbances of equilibrium, and incoordination on the left side. Left ear deaf.

August 19. After ten turns to the left on the revolving chair rotatory nystagmus to the right, with view straight ahead, for ten seconds. After ten turns to the right rotatory nystagmus to the left, with view straight ahead, for ten seconds.

August 29. Spontaneous nystagmus to both sides; however, more to the right. Upon the revolving chair, after ten turns to the right, no nystagmus to the left with view straight ahead. After ten turns to the left, horizontal nystagmus to the right, with view straight ahead, for twenty seconds. Brain more prolapsed than a week ago.

September 14. Spontaneous, long-stroked, horizontal nystagmus to both sides. After ten turns to the left with head straight, horizontal nystagmus to the right, with view straight ahead, for twelve seconds. After ten turns to the right no nystagmus with view straight ahead.

September 18. Horizontal nystagmus to both sides, strong to the right; however, less than before. On revolving chair: After ten turns to the left, head straight, horizontal nystagmus to right, thirteen seconds. After ten turns to the right, head straight, horizontal nystagmus to left, six seconds. After ten turns to the left, head bent forward, rotatory nystagmus to right, eleven seconds. After ten turns to the right, head bent forward, rotatory nystagmus to left, five seconds.

With the ear tube conversational speech is heard without any mistakes; whispered speech with mistakes.

October 8. The left labyrinth does not react and loud conversational speech is not heard with the ear tube. Further course without any reaction.

The above reported case might be followed by a whole series of analogous observations. We have here to deal with cases of infectious sinus thrombosis with meningeal symptoms. The sinus thrombosis is operated according to the nature of the sinus occlusion, and either immediately after the operation or twenty-four hours later the posterior cranial fossa is opened on the same level as the sinus or in its immediate neighborhood by an incision of the dura. The cerebellum protrudes. On account of the daily change of dressing, the meningeal phenomena will gradually disappear. The lumbar puncture in all of these cases shows a more or less purulent, cloudy, sterile liquor. The meningeal phenomena originate in these cases from the inflammatory change in the sinus wall itself and consist in pachymeningitis externa and interna leading to leptomeningitis and encephalitis. If the incision of the dura is dispensed with or made too late, there is the greatest danger that the circumscribed meningitis, in which, according to the findings of the lumbar puncture, the intradural space is still free of bacteria, will become infected and give rise to a diffuse infectious purulent meningitis. In making the autopsy, we are by no means often able to prove the direct relation between purulent meningitis and sinus thrombosis; sometimes, however, with a diffusely spread purulent meningitis the cerebellar pole especially will appear swollen on the diseased side and covered with much purulent secretion. In two cases a distinct impression of the medial sinus wall on the cerebellar hemisphere could be demonstrated, an indication of great swelling and infiltration of the brain. MacEwen describes and demonstrates an exactly similar case. Spontaneous healing of circumscribed meningitis with sinus thrombosis, without incision of the dura, is certainly rare; at least, it can be seldom proved. In this connection, the report of the following case might not be without interest:

CASE 6. Josef S., 37 years old, of Vienna, received at the Ear Department April 8, 1906.

Diagnosis: Otitis media suppur. chronica. Sinus thrombosis. Pachymeningitis purulenta externa chronica.

Therapy: Jugular excision, radical operation, exposure of the dura. Plastic according to Panse.

History: Patient for eleven years has had suppuration from both ears, with diminished hearing, and was treated for that. A week ago he got headaches and fever. The day before yesterday and yesterday he had chills and vertigo; however, no vomiting.

Left ear: Large perforation in the posterior lower quadrant, little secretion.

Right ear: Auditory canal narrowed and filled with fetid pus. Granulations.

Right mastoid process warmer than the left one. Great sensibility to pressure on the same and the occiput.

Right		Left
4 m	Conversational speech	8-10 m.
1 m	Whisper	5 m.
1 m	Acumeter	5 m.
. . . .	Schwabach shortened	
. . . .	Rinne negative	
Much shortened . . . C₁		+
Much shortened . . . C₄		+
+	Watch	+

No spontaneous nystagmus; nystagmus after turning. caloric and galvanic all normal; no disturbances of equilibrium.

April 8. Operation under Billroth's mixture narcosis. The right jugular is exposed and ligated in the usual way. The jugular contains liquid blood. Radical operation. The mastoid process is slightly sclerosed. Near the sinus the bone is softened and filled with fetid cholesteatoma masses towards the antrum. Plastic according to Panse. Exposure of the middle and posterior cranial fossa and the sinus transversus. The lateral sinus wall is greyish yellow. Extensive purulent pachymeningitis externa. Exposure of the sinus to the region of healthy tissues. After incising the dura, we find strong leptomeningitic adhesions. Opening of the sinus transversus. There is a peripheral thrombosis. Wound dressing. Bandage.

April 9. Patient did not vomit, fairly comfortable.

April 10. Patient has no subjective phenomena and takes some liquid nourishment. Examination of the secretion by the Pathological-Anatomical Institute (April 11, 1906) : Streptococeii in pure culture.

April 16. Secondary suture.

April 19. Comparatively comfortable.

April 25. Relatively slight secretion.

April 26. Relatively comfortable. Daily change of dressing.

May 1. Status idem.

May 7. Status idem.

May 10. Jugular wound healed.

May 11. Patient is dismissed on account of want of room and referred to ambulatory after treatment.

Since then completely healed.

At the time of the operation of the thrombophlebitis, the meningitis had led to a circumscribed adhesion of the pachy- and leptomeninges. Here also the close topographic relation is again observed that exists between the intradural change and those plaques belonging to pachymeningitis externa. Intradural agglutinations may, however, as often represent the beginning as well as the end of a meningitis. In our case they characterized the beginning of the meningitis. Patient never before had shown clinical symptoms of a meningitis. An early incision prevented the intradural infection and the purulent meningitis.

It is striking that with otitic sinus phlebitis, circumscribed meningitis is so frequently found. This may depend upon the fact that the sinus phlebitis is almost always connected with a pachymeningitis externa and not seldom with a pachymeningitis interna.*

From the pachymeninges the inflammatory process may easily progress towards the brain, and especially the pachymeningitis interna involves the danger of a meningo-encephalitis.

Meningitic changes are typically established in case of otitic brain abscess. They seem more frequently to correspond with a diffuse meningeal disease and only seldom show a localization to the diseased side. I may here demonstrate a remarkable observation:

CASE 7. George R. became ill with the symptoms of meningitis and was admitted with that diagnosis into the medical clinic. The examination of the ear revealed a chronic middle ear suppuration. The radical operation was done and, after the removal of the cholesteatoma and the diseased bone, both cranial fossae were exposed. The lumbar puncture which was made immediately showed a clear liquor evacuated under increased pressure. After twenty-four hours, slight coagulation: microscopic, single polynuclear leucocytes, no microorganisms. The symptoms of the disease disappeared and the patient, who was received October 14, 1904, was dismissed December 19, 1904, in perfect health.

Patient was again admitted on January 27, 1905. After his discharge from the hospital, he had felt well, had no headache, no vertigo, slept well and enjoyed good appetite. The wound looked good, little secretion and every other day change of dressing.

January 5. Secondary suture was made. Three days later the sutures had to be removed on account of acute copious and fetid secretion. With it appeared loss of appetite, headaches; however, no vomiting. Patient complained of being very tired and worn out. Change of dressing every day. Suppuration became somewhat less.

There was always slight diplopia, which was very changeable, almost disappearing in the morning, whereas it became more intense toward the evening. In looking upwards, it disappeared and increased the more the patient bent his head downward.

January 27. Sudden headache all over the forehead, especially when patient sat up, nausea and violent, repeated vom-

*Alexander Monatschrift f. Ohrenheilk.

iting during the day. On this account, patient was admitted to hospital.

January 29. Operated under Billroth's mixture narcosis. Lumbar puncture: Purulent cloudy liquor under increased pressure. With the microscope, many polynuclear leucocytes were found, but no microorganisms. Thick coagulum. Exposure of the field of operation was made over the middle and posterior cranial fossae and the sinus transversus by enlarging the opening from the sinus lateralis posteriorly. The sinus transversus was situated remarkably deep; the dura was moderately injected and considerably bulged forward. After the incision, about 100 ccm. of fetid pus was evacuated under high pressure from an abscess in the temporal lobe. A strip of iodoform gauze was put into the abscess cavity, wound dressing and bandage.

January 30. Right facial paralysis, diplopia disappeared.

February 1. Result of ophthalmoscopic examination: Papillae not sharp, somewhat striped on the periphery; the veins are somewhat dilated and tortuous, slight neuritis.

February 3. Change of dressing. Secretion from abscess cavity moderate.

February 5. General condition good, uneventful course. No diplopia. Patient walks about.

February 11. Morning temperature a little above the ordinary (37.2°). No headache, no vertigo, no spontaneous nystagmus.

February 15. Patient is referred to ambulatory after treatment, as the wound looks good and his health in general is also good.

On January 27, 1905, patient was received with the symptoms of an abscess of the temporal lobe and by operation the abscess was evacuated, followed by healing. The original meningeal disease of the patient corresponded to the initial stage of a brain abscess, which has thus been complicated by a meningitis serosa. The meningitis decreased; the abscess entered into the latent stage and became manifest about January 27th. We have repeatedly referred to the importance of finding a cloudy sterile liquor evacuated under increased pressure. (Brieger, Körner, Leutert, Wolff, Alexander.) It might be taken as a characteristic feature of otitic brain abscess. However, cloudy fluid frequently seems to occur only in the manifest stage of brain abscess or immediately before its rupture,*

*In case 11, the puncture made two and one-half weeks before death was still clear.

and meningo-encephalitic changes with otitic brain abscesses have not until now been observed at such an early stage as in **this case.**

Until the last few years, this exceedingly important .character of the cerebrospinal liquid was unknown. Without going into the question of microorganisms, the purulent cloudy liquor was regarded as a sign of purulent meningitis and a contraindication to an operation for the reason of not promising any success. The autopsy revealed a brain abscess! With a timely diagnosis, the patient might have been saved. This point of view, which indeed has never been ours, has been abandoned. But we cannot emphasize sufficiently that, notwithstanding how great the importance of the lumbar puneture may be for diagnosis and perhaps also for **therapeutics,** it is of none whatever as an operative indication, for as long as the clinical phenomena allow an operation, even a purulent liquor containing microorganisms should not stop us from operating.

In connection with the above, I proceed to the discussion of otitic purulent meningitis. A case of healed infectious purulent meningitis is the following:

CASE 8. Otitis media suppurativa chronica dextra. Purulent labyrinthitis with fistula. Extradural abscess. Purulent pachyleptomeningitis.

Radical operation: Removal of the semicircular canals. Opening of the vestibulum and the cochlea. Incision of the dura. Purulent cloudy lumbar puncture. By microscope and culture, gram-positive streptococci.

Hospital report: Anton K., 10 years old, of Inzersdorf, Austria, admitted to the Ear Department of the University of Vienna July 16, 1907.

History: Otorrhea of the right side for four years, which began with pain and stopped at times. In December, 1906, he was operated on at his home; however, otorrhea continued. Since July 13, 1907, severe pains in the ear and head, no **vertigo.**

Present condition: Findings in the right ear: Copious fetid secretion from the fissure-formed, narrowed external auditory canal. Drum membrane not visible, the soft parts over the mastoid process are thickened, reddened, with an operation cicatrix 2 cm. long, in the middle of which we can see a fistula the size of a quill. Granulations in the mouth of the fistula. The sound introduced in the direction of the antrum touches rough bone. Considerable fetid secretion comes from the fistula. Mastoid process is painful on pressure. In the microscopic specimen we find no cholestearin crystals.

Left ear: Drum membrane retracted.

Functional finding: Hearing distance on the left: Conversational speech 8 m., whispered speech 6 m., Weber to the left, Schwabach prolonged on the left, Rinne negative. Perception of high tones normal and of low tones slightly diminished. Watch through the bones positive; there seems to be an apparent hearing distance on the right of 2½ m. for conversational speech and ½ m. for whispered speech; however, the ear tube, 2 m. long, tells us that the patient is entirely deaf on the right.

Vestibular apparatus: Spontaneous nystagmus: Slight horizontal nystagmus to the right in looking to the right. Strong rotatory nystagmus to the left on looking to the left and straight ahead; sometimes also on looking to the right. Caloric irritability on the right diminished. Revolving chair: After ten turns to the right, strong rotatory nystagmus to the left for thirty seconds on looking straight ahead. After ten turns to the left, on looking straight ahead, no nystagmus.

Patient shows pronounced disturbances of equilibrium. Romberg positive. Goniometer: Elevation, facing forwards 8°, facing backwards 6°, on the right and left hand 4° each. Reflexes increased. Babinsky positive. Moderate disturbances of coordination of the right side. Temperature 38.1°. Pulse 50. Patient at present is fully conscious. Movements of the head and neck restricted; slight stiffness of the neck.

July 19. Operation. Skin incision through the scar and fistula. Extirpation of the fistula, curetting the same and exposure of the mastoid process. The latter shows on its lateral surface at the level of the antrum a fistula as large as a quill, in which a rather dry cholesteatoma is visible. Exposure of the sinus and the posterior cranial fossa. The cholesteatoma reaches upward to the dura of the middle cranial fossa. The bony tegmen tympani is completely destroyed. The dura of the middle cranial fossa over the tegmen is covered on the outside with granulations bathed in pus. The cholesteatoma reaches to the inside as far as the labyrinth, forming a fistula 3 mm. long on the front arm of the lateral semicircular canal. Removal of the semicircular canals; opening of the vestibule, in which no flowing liquor is found; also none in the cochlea, which is opened from the promontorium. The incision of the middle and posterior cranial fossae for about 6 mm. each reveals moderate brain edema. Wound dressing. Introduction of gauze strips into the middle and posterior cranial fossae. Bandage. The lumbar puncture showed 15 ccm. of a very purulent cloudy liquor, expelled under increased pressure. With the microscope, abundant polynuclear leucocytes were found, and with the microscope and culture gram-positive streptococci and bacteria coli were found in the pus from the mastoid process.

Course: July 20, 1907. Patient vomited three times in the last twenty-four hours; complains of headaches; rotatory nystagmus to the left less than before the operation; long-stroked horizontal nystagmus to the right; moderate vertigo.

July 21. Nystagmus unaltered; still some vertigo; change of dressing; shortening of the strips.

July 23. Only slight headaches; nystagmus to the right indistinct; rotatory nystagmus to the left; no vertigo; patient is feeling subjectively well. Change of dressing. Since then the course was uneventful.

July 26. Patient leaves the clinic feeling perfectly well with good equilibrium and is referred to ambulatory treatment.

The present case is of interest in several ways. It is, first of all, striking that the microscopic cholestearin test (test for cholestearin crystals) failed, in spite of the large cholesteatoma. This is explained by the fact that the cholesteatoma did not suppurate, but was rather dry, and thus no cholestearin particles were discharged with the pus.* Of functional importance is the relatively considerable apparent hearing distance (2½ m. for conversational speech, ½ m. for whispered speech) of the positively deaf ear. I have repeatedly referred to the fact that in such cases even the examination with an ear tube 1 m. long is not sufficient, and in the present case we obtained the result characteristic for one-sided deafness only by means of an ear tube 2 m. long† (incorrect repetition of whispered speech).

The appearance of intracranial complications without acute suppuration of the cholesteatoms is also unusual. The intra-

---

*See G. W. Mackenzie. Zur klinischen Diagnnostik des cholestea-toms. Monatschrift f. Ohrenheilk., 1908.

†I now use an ear tube 4 m. long, to be had at Rienner, Vienna IX, Van Swietengasse 4.

cranial disease itself doubtless started from the tympanic cavity and the labyrinth; which were diseased some time preceding, and consisted of a meningeal disease within the region of the middle and posterior cranial fossae. Especially in the middle cranial fossa, we found considerable changes; the dura was thickened and covered with granulations; the dura of the posterior cranial fossa was simply injected. The leptomeningitis and encephalitis was indicated by the edematous swelling of the brain, and the infectious character of the disease was definitely established by the lumbar puncture. We can, of, course, only surmise as to the anatomic extension of the pachyleptomeningitis. According to the operative findings, it surely extended over the right side of the middle and posterior cranial fossa, and there were surely changes sufficiently advanced to show an abundance of microorganisms in the purulent, cloudy lumbar puncture liquid. As regards the therapeutics, a radical operation was indicated in consequence of the chronic middle ear suppuration. The vestibule and the cochlea were opened, since the ear was deaf and the static labyrinth not irritable, also since vertigo was present, whereas there was no flowing liquor in the labyrinth. Drainage of the intrameningeal spaces was established by an incision of the middle and posterior cranial fossae, and the course of the intrameningeal processes was shown by the lumbar puncture. which at first was, of course, made for diagnostic purposes. I see a special advantage in the change of dressing on the day after the operation and repeating it daily with gradual shortening and renewing of the strips.

This case is in line with the observations of healed purulent otitic meningitis that have been reported to date. However, this is the first case free of any objections and showing streptococci. Gradenigo, we know, was the first who reported a healed otitic purulent meningitis (staphylococci). In the other cases of Bertelsmann, Brieger, Grossmann, Gruening, Leutert, Maljean, Manasse, Preising, Schenke, Schulze and Sokolowski, we generally had to deal with diplococci. once with bacterium coli, and in a smaller number of cases with staphylococci and pneumococci. The healing of streptococcic meningitis has not as yet been proved, and the present case shows us that, at least in exceptional cases. streptococcic meningitis also may get well. Naturally, the authors endeavored to form an established opinion as to the extension of the healed purulent meningitis, whereby they always made the distinction between circumscribed and diffuse meningitis. However, 't has been overlooked that this distinction is only possible on the cadaver, and then only by microscopic examination. Thus, either party can be contradicted as to the view that the cases of healed purulent meningitis have been circumscribed on the one hand and that they had to deal with diffuse meningitis on the other hand. The diffuse meningitis, a priori, appears to be a dangerous disease, most likely leading to death, and this fact alone must make us think of a circumscribed purulent meningitis when having cases of healed purulent meningitis. Heine has good reasons for stating that the classification into circumscribed and diffuse meningitis is unsatisfactory. Accordingly, in agreement with Lexer, he proposes to entirely abandon the classification of a diffuse meningitis and distinguishes a general meningitis, an encapsulated meningitis and an acute progressive meningitis. The great majority of cases of healed purulent meningitis most likely were of an acute progressive character. Unfortunately, the operative findings do not furnish us any means to judge as to the extension of the process. Indeed, many are inclined to assume that purulent liquor containing bacteria indicates a general purulent meningitis. In certain cases, it may, however, be very difficult to distinguish with certainty between true purulent and purulently clouded liquor, and, therefore, of still greater importance is the fact that in some of the cases observed by me it was determined with certainty that a general purulent meningitis may show only a slightly clouded liquor, which, in some instances, is entirely clear in the beginning. The intensity of the cloudiness is, according to my opinion,' not at all determinative as to extent of the disease of the meninges. I also believe that it is of no special significance as to the question of healing. The virulence of the exciting causes of purulent meningitis is, by all means, a very important factor as to the question of healing. Reference has been made to this fact by all investigators, and it is assumed and admitted by all of them that a favorable prognosis of otitic purulent meningitis depends on a mild degree of virulence. According to the latest investigation, we need go no farther and can assume that we have to deal with only slightly virulent, perhaps disintegrated, microorganisms. Another factor seems to me of equal importance and that is the mode of development of the meningitis. The more acute, the more violent the course of the first symptoms, the worse will be the prognosis. A prolonged initial stage and uncertain symptoms during development render the diagnosis of the case more favorable. I, however, thoroughly believe that we must come to the conclusion that with a favorable issue of a meningitis the meningeal adhesions are of very great importance and benefit, as they encapsulate the meningitis and prevent the appearance of a general meningitis. If these adhesions were so frequent, we should see them oftener. In cases of purulent meningitis that I could follow clinically and anatomically, I have observed them perfectly in only one case (see case 6). According to the idea one gets from the autopsy, I do not believe even if such agglutinations occurred frequently, that they would be able to encapsulate the meningitis indefinitely. In making the autopsy, we frequently enough see circumscribed and localized meningitis, especially at the base of the brain, that remained circumscribed in spite of the lack of any adhesions, and during the autopsy of cases of general meningitis, we observed the little or no effect such agglutinations had.

·I believe that the mode of development of meningitis is indicated by the first attack. Meningitis which originates directly from a local purulent process in the region of the ear usually from the beginning shows the character of an abscess, which it maintains, and remains localized. The more a purulent meningitis represents a remote consequence of the ear disease, the more apt it is to become a general meningitis from the very beginning. From a practical standpoint, we should consider the following: With the same clinical symptoms of meningitis, the findings during operation will enable us to make a probable diagnosis as to the extent of the meningitis. If the inflammatory changes extend from the ear to a circumscribed focus on the dura and into the dura, we will usually have to deal with a partial, encapsulated or a circumscribed meningitis. If the purulent changes do not extend from the ear to the dura, we have a general meningitis.

The favorable issue of the above case 8 must, in the first instance, be traced back to the success of a sufficient drainage. The meningitis, which certainly extended over the middle and posterior cranial fossae, started from the ear, and the drainage was made by an incision of the dura of both cranial fossae, after an extensive opening of the labyrinth. The extensive incisions of the dura made a repetition of the lumbar puncture unnecessary. As in many other cases, the examination of the fundus oculi showed only a dilatation of the veins, but no choked disc.

Cases have been reported above, in which, with purulent meningitis, we obtained by the first puncture a clear, coagulating and later purulent liquor. We can also report a case of purulent meningitis in which the bacteria-holding liquor remained clear and coagulating during its entire course.

CASE 9. Sandor, T., 11 years old, of Trencsin, Hungary, admitted to the Ear Department of the University of Vienna February 1, 1907.

History: Since the age of four, fetid otorrhea from the right side, after measles, until two months ago without any treatment, when a doctor was seen who prescribed syringing the ear. January 22 patient suffered from a headache and violent pains in the ear, acompanied by fever. Patient became apathetic and at times complained a great deal; could not sleep or eat. Three or four days ago the father of the patient noticed the appearance of a swelling behind the ear that grew rapidly and very soon caused an abnormal way of holding the head. This induced him to bring the boy to the clinic.

Present condition: Weak, thin individual. Temperature 38.5°, pulse 88, and volume of circulation good.

Patient can only walk with great effort and lies mostly in passive dorsal position, without noticing anything. The head is bent extremely to the left and held turned, in which position it is firmly fixed by contraction of the left sternocleidomastoideus. Above the right mastoid process was found an oval swelling of the size of a child's fist and the skin over it was reddened and stretched. The swelling is hard and elastic and shows no fluctuation. The auricle is displaced to the front and downwards. From the tumor an edematous swelling extends over the right side of the face. The right eyelid cannot be opened in consequence of the swelling. The skin over the eyelid is slightly reddened. Ankylostomiasis was present. The edema extends backwards over throat and neck down to the vertebral column. Slight rigidity of the neck. The vertebral column is sensitive to percussion, spontaneous and pressure painfulness of the retroauricular swelling. No cutaneous hyperesthesia. Kernig positive. Patellar reflex, left normal, right lost. The tongue is swollen and of raspberry color. Fetid breath.

Findings of the right ear: Auditory canal greatly narrowed by the sinking of the posterior superior wall; fetid purulent secretion; in the pus were abundant cholestearin crystals. The left drum membrane is clouded and retracted.

Functional finding: Left ear approximately normal, the right is totally deaf. No spontaneous nystagmus. Both vestibular apparati are irritable.

February 2, 1907. Operation under Billroth's mixture narcosis. Skin incision over the convexity of the swelling. The soft parts are thickened. Exposure of the mastoid process. From a subperiosteal surface abscess a great quantity of fetid flaky pus is discharged. On the lateral surface of the mastoid process in the fossa mastoidea were two fistulae the size of a quill; in the mastoid process a cholesteatoma the size of a cherry stone extended as far as the antrum. Plastic according to Panse, typical radical operation. Posteriorly, the cholesteatoma reached as far as the lateral sinus wall, which was of a yellowish white color and thickened in consequence of deposited coagulated fibrin. On the prominence of the lateral semicircular canal we find a rough place 2 mm. long. With the puncture of the sinus blood escaped under normal pressure.

Course: February 3. Subjectively well. Temperature 36.6°. Pulse, regular and strong, 84.

February 4-7. Temperature from 37.9° to 39.5°. Vomiting. Patient takes no interest whatever. Change of dressing. The inner ear is thermically not irritable. Cold tampons dipped into perhydrol or ether do not produce any reaction. Repeated vomiting. Movement of the head is painful. From February 8th on, temperature 36.5° to 37.7°.

February 11. Removal of the semicircular canals and opening of the vestibule; removal of the promontorium and curetting the cochlea. Pus fills all the interior of the labyrinth. Opening of the middle and posterior cranial fossae, puncture of the brain. The lumbar puncture evacuated about 20 ccm. of clear liquor under distinctly increased pressure. After twenty-four hours finest dust-like coagulation and no sediment in the clear liquor. Findings by the Pathological and Anatomical Institute: By the microscope in moderately abundant quantities small gram-negative bacilli. The cultures remained sterile.

February 12. Increased rigidity of the neck and stupor. Temperature 36.5°. Pulse 60. Patient died at 10 p. m.

Post mortem findings: Radical operation on the right ear on account of otitis media suppurativa. Cholesteatoma and subperiosteal abscess in the region of the mastoid process. Pachymeningitis externa et interna acuta in the region of the left cranial fossa (on the external surface of the dura mater, we find only granulation tissue during the autopsy, whereas on the inner surface we find a fibrinous purulent exudate), serous effusion into the brain ventricles, puncture of the right temporal lobe and double puncture of the right cerebellar hemisphere (on the inner brain membranes). Calcified tubercles of the apex of the right lung and coalescence of same.

The meningitis surely existed long before patient was admitted, and the history also indicated that for several weeks patient had been listless and remained in passive dorsal position, at times even unconscious. In making the operation, the cholesteatoma was removed and the labyrinth, which was still irritable, at the time was not touched. Not until after the radical operation, and only when the labyrinth symptoms did not diminish and the irritability of the labyrinth ceased, was the labyrinth opened wide and exposed over the pyramid and the posterior and middle cranial fossae; however, the dura showed no changes within this region. The autopsy findings corresponded with those of the operation. The meningitis was decidedly limited to the middle and posterior cranial fossae of the left or sound side. From it we could not trace an anatomic connection; at least, no macroscopic relation with the ear disease; and it consisted essentially of an external and internal pachymeningitis, which is the kind of meningitis that very frequently shows an intimate and distinct anatomic relation with the original ear disease. (Alexander.)

By the lumbar puncture, a clear liquor was evacuated under increased pressure. After several hours the liquor showed finest white stipplings, and the cultures remained sterile, whereas, on the other hand, by the microscope moderately numerous, small, gram-positive cocci in short chains were found, and also scanty gram-negative bacilli. As already mentioned, the remarkable point of this case is the fact that the lumbar puncture liquor remained clear and colorless up to death, which proves the varying condition of the lumbar puncture liquor in purulent meningitis as regards color and transparency.

Cloudy sterile cerebrospinal liquor is characteristic of brain abscess; yet it is found also in some cases of sinus thrombosis and at times with large extradural abscesses. I have, in the above, treated this important chapter of lumbar puncture and referred to the great diagnostic importance of this fact, and yet exceptions are possible, and it is again the purulent meningitis that causes such exceptions.

CASE 10. Josef Lusek, 21 years old, blacksmith, of Vienna, admitted to the Ear Department of the University of Vienna on February 27, 1907.

Diagnosis: Otitis media suppurativa chronica dextra.

Therapy: Radical operation. Opening of the posterior and middle cranial fossae. Puncture of the cerebellum.

History: Since the age of four, otorrhea of the right ear, following measles. It is an intermittent otorrhea, beginning usually with pains and lasting for some days. Three weeks ago otorrhea began again, and since then patient has had violent headaches on the right side; during the last few days, he has had chills, marked vertigo, apparent turning of the surrounding objects, and several times has vomited. For some days, patient has been treated at the ambulatorum of our clinic. Yesterday patient collapsed in the street and was brought in to our clinic by the First Aid Society.

Patient vomited three times during night and once in the morning.

Right   Left

By means of the ear tube conversational speech is heard however incorrectly repeated. } ..Conversational speech.............9 m.

O ....Whisper ....9 m.

O ....Acumeter ....9 m.

  ....Weber ....+

  ....Schwabach shortened ....

  ....Rinne ....+

  ....C_1 ....+

  ....C_4 ....+

— ....Watch ....+

— ....Acumeter ....+

+ ....Spontaneous nystagmus ....+

Typical reaction caloric nystagmus, rotatory, long-stroked; typical reaction galvanic nystagmus, rotatory, long-stroked. Disturbance of equilibrium: vertigo with the slightest motions; with closed eyes considerable disturbance.

Present condition: Strong individual of medium height. Patient stays in bed and, as he states himself, the slightest motion, even that of his eyes, causes vertigo. Patient cannot sit up. Temperature 37°. Pulse strong and regular 78.

Right ear: Fetid pus, cholestearin crystals. Total destruction of the drum membrane; granulations in the tympanic cavity. Left ear normal.

Lumbar puncture yielded a slightly clouded liquor under normal pressure. The microscope showed no microorganisms, but polynuclear leucocytes.

March 1, 1907. Operation in Billroth's mixture narcosis. Typical skin incision. Exposure of the mastoid process. The cortex is hard. The interior is fetid, purulent and soft. In the attic and antrum a fetid, ichorous cholesteatoma was found. Prominence of the lateral semicircular canal was unaltered. Granulations on the base of stapes. Wound dressing. Bandage.

March 3. Patient feels somewhat better, vomited several times. Facial paresis with its phenomena.

March 4. Patient complains of great vertigo. Vomited several times during night. Nystagmus to the sound side; patient complains of diffuse headaches. Temperature normal. **Pulse 52.**

March 5. Patient feels better. No vomiting. Long-stroked rotatory nystagmus to the sound side and some short strokes to the diseased side.

March 6. Vertigo still present. Nystagmus to the sound side. Patient feels better and did not vomit.

March 7. Patient has a severe headache. Increased vertigo to-day. Patient can walk only with support. Temperature 38°; pulse 88. At 6 p. m. operation was made by Alexander. Fetid labyrinth suppuration. Dura of the posterior and middle cranial fossae bulged forward and was injected. Removal of the labyrinth as far as the inner auditory canal. Opening of the cochlea. Function of the cerebellum negative. Wound dressing.

March 8. Patient unconscious. Temperature 36.9°. Pupils wide, unequal and not reacting. Pulse slow (60 a minute).

March 9. 7 a. m., patient died.

Post mortem result: Purulent basal meningitis with special localization of the exudate over the right border of the pons, including the nerve branches running alongside, chronic purulent middle ear inflammation on the right side. Acute edema of the leptomeninges and the brain. Pachymeningitis externa beginning to perforate and fresh internal pachymeningitis in the region of the posterior and middle cranial fossae.

Chronic emphysema of the lungs. Parenchymatous degeneration of the heart and the liver. Acute splecnic tumor. Bacteriologic findings in the smear preparation of the meningeal exudate: Abundant mono- and polynuclear cells; a few gram-positive cocci, as well as gram-negative short rods of the type of the bacillus of influenza.

We have to deal with a basal purulent meningitis with encapsulation of the exudate between the brain surface and the leptomeninges.

On the right edge of the pons and on the nerve branches running along the same, especially along the acoustic and facial, the exudate was heaped up into circumscribed tumor-like masses. This localization explains the peculiar findings of the lumbar puncture. From this suppurative focus, leucocytes entered the cerebrospinal liquid, but no microorganisms, and thus the·lumbar puncture showed. under increased pressure, a cloudy, coagulating liquor without any microorganisms. The meningitis surely existed before patient was admitted to the clinic, as indicated by the history of vomiting and violent headaches. In spite of extensive exposure of the brain and free drainage, we did not succeed in preventing the fatal issue. It was evident at the time of the operation that the vitality of the patient was greatly reduced, also the acute edema of the leptomeninges and the acute brain edema showed that the inflammatory process had already extended from the meningeal suppurative focus to the base of the brain and over the entire meninges and the brain. The hopelessness of this case was demonstrated at the post mortem examination by the pulmonary emphysema, the parenchymatous degeneration of the heart and liver.

CASE 11. Florian G., 24 years old, farmer, of Loich,˙ Austria, admitted November 12, 1906.

Diagnosis: Otitis media suppur. chronica dextra. Cholesteatoma. Chronic labyrinth suppuration. Caries of the temporal bone. Meningitis tuberculosa.

Therapeutics: Radical operation. Plastic after Panse. Opening and removal of the labyrinth. Exposure and puncture of the dura of the middle and posterior cranial fossae.

History: Patient had measles between the age of 4 and 5, influenza between 9 and 10 and typhus when he was 17. In connection therewith he began to suffer with the right leg, having had typhoid fever for six months. After convalescense from influenza, fourteen or fifteen years ago, patient developed right-sided headaches and pains in the ear; two weeks later otorrhea appeared, when the pains in the ear stopped; however, the otorrhea continued with short intermissions. When the otorrhea ceased for a short time, pains in the ear occurred again that lasted until otorrhea began.

The ear discharge was copious in the beginning; later on less, but always fetid. Eighteen days ago otorrhea stopped again and patient again had pains in his ear and head on the right side. For two weeks he had a retroauricular swelling and the pains in the ear and head became so intense that the patient could not sleep. Since then patient often has attacks of vertigo; however, the vertigo was not decided. There is no apparent turning of the surrounding objects, and it is limited to the head. Patient staggers in walking; no vomiting. In spite of having been treated, the headache did not diminish; two days ago otorrhea began again and one day ago a physician in the country cut or punctured his ear, whereupon otorrhea increased and headaches somewhat decreased. Since patient began to suffer with the ear, his hearing is bad, and since eighteen days (i. e., since he has violent pains in the ear and head), patient's hearing is still worse. He had no chill, only when the headaches were specially severe, he became very warm and perspired. At this time patient complains of moderate pains in the ear and head, otorrhea and bad hearing.

Status praesens: Well developed and well nourished individual. No pathologic changes are found in his abdominal and thoracic organs. Temperature 38°. Facialis free.

Left ear: Drum membrane somewhat retracted and cloudy.

Right ear: In the external auditory canal abundant, fetid pus; marked narrowing of the external auditory canal by the sinking of the posterior upper wall; granulations on the same between which pus exudes. In probing this place, we touch soft masses and rough bone. There is a boggy swelling over the mastoid process and the skin is reddened and stretched. The mastoid process is painful on pressure. In washing out the fistula, abundant cholesteatoma masses escape, which contain cholestearin crystals.

FUNCTIONAL FINDING.

Right   Left
With ear tube 2.2 m. . . Speech . . . . .Z. W.
O . . . . .Whisper . . . . .2-3 m.
O . . . . .Acumeter . . . . .8 m.
. . . . .Weber . . . . +
Shortened . . . . .Schwabach . . . . .Normal
Air conduction absent. . Rinne . . . .+
O . . . . .C_1 . . . .+
Greatly diminished . . . . C_4 . . . .+
— . . . . .Watch . . . .+
+ . . . . .Acumeter . . . . +
O . . . . .Spontaneous nystagmus . . . . .O

With cold water, caloric nystagmus, typical reaction; both sides show normal nystagmus after turning.

Standing with closed eyes, patient falls a little backwards and to the diseased side. With closed eyes, patient walks with broad gait and staggers. With eyes open, patient walks well backwards, and also the hopping is good. No ataxia.

November 13, 1906. Operation in Billroth's mixture narcosis. Typical skin incision 7 cm. long. Soft parts thickened. Exposure and opening of the mastoid process; cortex hard. The posterior bony wall of the auditory canal and the interior of the mastoid process are destroyed; in the latter, we find an ichorous cholesteatoma a little larger than a hazel nut, which caused the destruction of the posterior wall of the auditory canal.

The skin of the auditory canal is also partly destroyed. Radical operation, plastic according to Panse. Over the horizontal semicircular canal a small osteophyte of the size of a pea, that caused a narrowing of the antrum. Below the semicircular canal was a discolored bone particle reaching up to the facialis and the fenestra ovalis. Removal of the same. No fistula was found. Wound dressing. Bandage.

After operation: Spontaneous nystagmus to the sound side. Facial paresis in the maxillary branch.

November 14. Moderate headaches on the right side; vertigo; subfebrile temperature. Spontaneous nystagmus to the sound side.

November 15. Moderate pain in the ear and head on the right side. Vertigo less. Nystagmus the same as the day before. Subfebrile temperature. Entirely conscious. Purgative.

November 16. Morning temperature 36.6°. Violent headaches. Faintness. Nystagmus idem.

November 16. 1 p. m., temperature 39°. Violent headaches. Nystagmus to the sound side less than the previous day. 2 p. m., Violent headaches. Vomiting; moderate stupor. 4:30 p. m., temperature 40.5°. Pain also in the forehead. Vomiting; stupor; slight spontaneous nystagmus to the sound side. 5 p. m., labyrinth operation under Billroth's mixture narcosis.

1. Lumbar puncture 20 ccm.; clear liquor containing smallest specks, which is evacuated under high pressure (sterile by microscope and culture).

2. Change of dressing. Long-stroked nystagmus to the sound side, after having exposed the dura of the middle and posterior cranial fossae. Opening and removal of the labyrinth, preserving the facial canal. The cochlea and all labyrinth channels are filled with intense fetid caseous pus. Incision of the dura of the middle and posterior cranial fossae. Puncture of same with negative result. After the operation, violent headaches in the evening. Temperature 40.5°. Ice bag on the head.

November 17. Headaches diminished, owing to the ice bag. Temperature 38°. No vertigo. No vomiting. Faintness, but no stupor. No spontaneous nystagmus. Pupils narrow with slow reaction to light. Pulse slow. Temperature, in the afternoon, 39.5°.

November 18. Very intense headaches. Temperature 38°. ice bag. Otherwise the same as yesterday. Temperature in the afternoon 39.4°. Evening: During day nausea occurred several times. As soon as patient takes some nourishment, he vomits it. In the evening vomiting ceased. Patient takes moderate amount of food. Retention of urine during the entire day. In the evening spontaneous urination.

November 19. Headaches somewhat diminished. Temperature 38.1°. Change of dressing. Shortening of the strips. Slight spontaneous nystagmus to both sides. No vertigo. Temperature in the afternoon 38°.

November 20. Headaches. Temperature 37.1° Herpes. Abducens paralysis on the right. Spontaneous nystagmus to the sound side. Temperature in the afternoon 38.3°.

November 21. Restless night; headache; temperature 37.1°. Afternoon temperature 37.8°. Pyramidon.

November 22. Moderate headaches. Spontaneous nystagmus to the sound side. Temperature 36.8°. Change of bandage. Change of strips. Very little fetid secretion. Temperature 37.8° in the afternoon. No vertigo.

November 23. Moderate headaches on the right side; no other complaint. Takes nourishment very well. Temperature 37°. Spontaneous nystagmus to the sound side. Temperature 39.9° in the afternoon.

November 24. Status idem. Temperature 37°. No vertigo. Nystagmus idem. Temperature 37.9° in the afternoon.

November 25. Slight headaches on the right; otherwise patient feels well. Temperature 37°. Change of bandage. Profuse secretion.

November 26. Status idem. Nystagmus idem. Temperature 37.1°. Temperature in the afternoon 37.8°. Violent headaches.

. November 27. Patient feels well. Temperature 36.8° to 36.9°. Change of bandage. Moderate secretion. Nystagmus idem.

November 28. Patient feels well. Temperature 36.6° to 36.8°. Nystagmus idem.

November 29. Patient feels well. Temperature 36.5° to 36.7°. No vertigo. Change of bandage. One sequestrum was discharged.

November 30. Patient feels well. Leaves his bed for a few hours. Temperature 36.4°. Moderate spontaneous nystagmus to the sound side. Temperature suddenly rose to 40.9° in the afternoon. Faintness. Change of bandage. Moderate secretion.

December 1. Temperature 37.3°. Moderate headaches. Spontaneous rotatory nystagmus to both sides; more so to the sound side than to the diseased side. Temperature 37.5° in the afternoon.

December 2. Temperature 37°. Patient feels very bad. Change of bandage. Abundant secretion. Vomits often during the forenoon. Spontaneous nystagmus to the sound side. Temperature 39.3° in the afternoon. Headaches. Violent vomiting.

December 3. Temperature 40.4° at 8 a. m. Pulse 88. Spontaneous nystagmus to both sides, less to the diseased side.

Restless night; vomited often. Violent headaches. Moderate stupor; no convulsions; no delirium. Stiff neck. Painfulness on pressure on the cervical portion of the vertebral column. Pupils contracted and slowly reacting to light. Change of dressing. Non-fetid pus in the labyrinth cavity, the exposed dura of the middle cranial fossa strongly bulging forward. Puncture negative. Forenoon: Beginning edema pulmon. Somnolence. Retention of urine. Catheterization.

Noon: Status idem. Cyanosis. Pupils narrow. Pulse 120. Injection of camphor. 5 p. m.. beginning of agony. Patient died at 11 p. m.

Post mortem result (Hofrat Weichselbaum): Radical operation had been made on account of chronic purulent middle ear inflammation and formation of cholesteatoma; there was an old abscess in the right temporal lobe. close under the surface and reaching forward to the inferior cornu of the lateral ventricle without breaking into the latter; the abscess was about as large as a walnut and contained thick pus; in correspondence therewith we found a loss of substance on the surface on the temporal lobe, which had a shallow opening; however, in no relation with the abscess cavity; circumscribed, fibrinous leptomeningitis on the convexity of the left frontal lobe and fibrinous leptomeningitis spinalis on the posterior surface of the spinal cord. Hydrocephalus internus acutus. Lobular pneumonia in both lungs; parenchymatous degeneration of the liver and kidneys.

In this case, the same as in the previous one, we have to deal with cholesteatoma and labyrinth suppuration with meningitis. The clear lumbar puncture which was evacuated under increased pressure contained a few very small white stipplings and was sterile. The case is interesting insofar as besides the meningitis, there was also an absces in the temporal lobe. The meningitis extended over the left frontal lobe and the spinal leptomeninges.

This case illustrates the rare combination of a labyrinth suppuration with an abscess of the temporal lobe, originating metastically from the suppuration of the semicircular canal. The meningitis also doubtless was of metastatic origin, as shown by its affecting the side of the sound ear and the vertebral column.

In conclusion, I am going to report on two cases of tuberculons caries of the temporal bone and meningitis with negative findings in the lumbar puncture liquor:

CASE 12. Thomas W., of Aussergefild, in Bohemia, Austria, 39 years old, tailor, admitted November 14, 1905.

Diagnosis: Otitis media suppur. chronica sin.; fistula in the fossa mast.; destruction of the greatest part of the posterior wall of the auditory canal; tympanic cavity filled with granulations. Labyrinth diseased. Softening of most of the petrous bone.

Therapy: Radical operation; removal of the labyrinth and of the entire petrous portion of the temporal bone to the tip; plastic according to Panse.

History: 1904, amputation of the left leg below the knee in consequence of caries. Since June, 1904, otorrhea on the left, beginning with slight pain. Since three weeks a pressure sensation has often been felt in the ear; headaches on the side of the diseased ear; no vertigo; no sensibility to pressure on the mastoid process.

Right ear: Normal drum membrane.

Left ear: Auditory canal filled with polypi and much secretion.

DISTURBANCES OF EQUILIBRIUM.

Right		Left
Normal	Speech	Deaf
Normal	Whisper	Deaf
+	Weber	
+	Rinne	—
Good	C_1	—
Good	C_4	—
+	Watch	—

No nystagmus, no swaying with closed eyes.

November 16, 1906. Radical operation in Billroth's mixture narcosis. Typical skin incision; exposure of the mastoid process. A fistulous opening of the size of a lentil in the fossa mastoidea filled with granulations and cholesteatoma. The sound passes through this into a cavity of the size of a cherry stone, filled with purulent cholesteatoma, at the upper part of the mastoid process. The posterior wall of the auditory canal has been destroyed except the medial portion. After the removal of the rest of the posterior wall of the auditory canal and the lateral attic wall, the entire cavity is seen filled with granulations and pus. The purulent softening and formation of granulations also reach into the labyrinth. The entire labyrinth cavities are filled with pus and granulations. The entire petrous bone and the labyrinth are removed as far as the tip of the former. The latter we let remain in its place since, being elastic, continuing our work with the chisel or the bone forceps might cause a luxation of this portion. It seems that the bony portion that is left is also diseased; at least, that part turned to the wound cavity. In removing the labyrinth, the facial nerve is removed in its entire course through the petrous portion of the temporal bone. The purulent softening also reaches to the sinus, the lateral wall of which is exposed the size of a bean and covered with granulations. Plastic according to Panse. Wound dressing. Bandage.

November 17. In dorsal position; horizontal nystagmus to both sides.

November 18. Rotatory nystagmus to the right with inclination of head to the sound side. Findings of the Pathological and Anatomical Institute of November 21st: Microscope: gram-positive cocci in pairs and gram-negative bacilli. Culture: Staphylococci pyogenes. Anaerobic negative.

November 23. First change of bandage. Removal of strips.

November 24. Secondary suture.

November 29. Removal of sutures.

December 3. Wound closed. Patient without bandage.

December 17. For some days slight increase of temperature; nausea; violent vomiting.

The lumbar puncture reveals a clear liquor under ordinary pressure. After six hours slight coagulation. No microorganisms.

December 19. Since yesterday forenoon unconsciousness. Cheyne-Stokes respiration. Involuntary discharge of urine.

December 20. Patient arouses when accosted and slowly answers questions; complains of headaches; distinct ataxia on the left side; paralysis of the eye muscles.

December 21. Death.

Post mortem result: Acute tubercular leptomeningitis at the base of the brain and to a less degree on the lateral portions of the vortex. A caseous tubercle of the size of a nut in the right temporal lobe.

Chronic tuberculosis with dry caseation of the cervical lmpphatic glands, the trach-bronch., and the bronch-pulm. lymphatic glands; the anterior and posterior mediast., the retroper., the mesent., and the lymphatic glands at the entrance to the liver and spleen; the ing. and axill. lymphatic glands. Chronic tubercles in the spleen and liver. Adhesive pleuritis of the right lung. A cold abscess on the right side of the thorax. Radical operation of the left ear (November 17) on account of chronic otitis and caries of the petrous portion of the temporal bone. Fresh incision wound of the right cerebellar hemisphere.

According to the clinical examinations, the radical operation, as well as the resection of the petrous portion of the temporal bone, the latter being diseased, were indicated. After the resection of the base of the petrous portion and the entire labyrinth, the tip of the petrous portion appeared as a pointed sequestrum, so that its extraction threatened to injure the carotid and was therefore not removed; however, it was hoped that later on the tip would come away spontaneously.

Unfortunately, this hope was not fulfilled. It is true that the condition of the patient was satisfactory for some time. He was even able to walk around. Finally, however, he was attacked by a tubercular meningitis. The post mortem revealed a tubercle in the right temporal lobe, a chronic tuberculosis of almost all the internal organs, a cold abscess, etc. So a cure was a priori impossible. The indication for the mastoid operation was given as a vital indication by the labyrinth symptoms. The course of the case is a type of tubercular labyrinthitis, complicated by tuberculosis elsewhere (lymph nodes, lungs, abdominal viscera, bones and joints).

Ear disease with multiple bone and joint tuberculosis appears less unfavorable prognostically than other forms of tuberculosis. At least, I can report three cases operated for otitis media suppurativa, with multiple bone and joint tuberculosis, which got well after resection of the petrous bone and removal of the labyrinth and have remained well three to five years after the operation.

All other cases—not immediately, it is true, but three weeks to six months after the operation—have died of tubercular meningitis. I remember a case demonstrated by me early this year before the Austrian Otological Society.

Lumbar puncture was performed twice, obtaining a clear liquor each time. It contained no microorganisms, nor could tubercle bacilli be found, even after a long search. It is true that the puncture was made early, four weeks before death.

The following case shows meningitis tuberculosa with negative lumbar puncture findings, taken seventeen days and eight days before death:

CASE 13. Emil Sch., Vienna, 14 years old, student, admitted June 22, 1906.

Diagnosis: Otitis media supp. chronica dextra. Meningitis tuberculosa.

Therapy: Radical operation. Exposure of sinus. Exposure and exploration of the middle and posterior cranial fossae. Lumbar puncture.

History: Patient had scarlet fever when eighteen months old. For five years he has had profuse otorrhea on the right side, slightly fetid. Since two months patient complains of pains in the right ear, which, however, became less lately. Three weeks ago, for the first time, polyps were removed from the ear, and sixteen days ago, for the second time, whereupon the otorrhea stopped. For five days patient complains of headaches; for two days occasional vomiting and more violent headaches. Rest in bed. Patient's hearing is worse on the right side since the beginning of his ear disease. When patient was recieved, he complained of moderate headaches. Patient's physician made attic washings on account of cholesteatoma.

Present condition: Well nourished individual of medium height and weak structure of bones and moderately developed muscles. No pathologic changes in the thoracic and abdominal organs. The skin and the visible mucous membranes are pale. Patient lies in passive dorsal position, most of the time completely motionless and sometimes he makes rapid motions of short duration with his body and extremities. Active movements of the head and neck are avoided; passive motions of same may be made with some resistance. Patient cannot walk about. Reflexes unaltered. Pulse 72, respiration 28, temperature 37.8°.

Left ear: Tympanic membrane normal.

Right ear: Tympanic membrane absent in its greatest portion; only the Shrapnel membrane is present. The stump of the malleus is grown to the inner wall of the tympanic cavity. From the attic and antrum only slight granulations reach into the tympanic cavity, which contains scanty, fetid secretion. The promontory wall in its greatest part is epidermized. From behind and above, with aspiration by means of Siegle's speculum, some pus and cholesteatoma are brought to view. The region of the mastoid process is unaltered. No sensibility to percussion of the skull. No pain by point pressure on the vertebral column.

Right		Left
10 m	Speech	Normal
A. C	Whisper	Normal
+	Weber	
—	Rinne	
Strong stroke + . . .	C_1	Normal
Strong stroke + . . .	C_4	Normal
. . . . — . . .	Watch	
. . . . — . . .	Acumeter	+

Spontaneous nystagmus slight to left side; caloric nystagmus (when in bed) ; applying cold water, very strong horizontal nystagmus to the sound side (left) ; also on looking to the diseased side, afterwards vomiting.

Spontaneous nystagmus slight to left side. Caloric nystagmus (when in bed), applying cold water; very strong horizontal nystagmus to the sound side (left), also on looking to the diseased side; afterwards vomiting.

The patient being stupefied, the examination on the revolving chair and for disturbances of equilibrium cannot be carried out, and for the same reason the functional examination is not free from objections.

Consciousness is so obtunded at times that patient does not even answer quite simple questions, whereas after a few minutes quite often correct and prompt answers are obtained. Patient recognizes and designates properly the objects shown him (watch, key, water glass). He cannot find the name for pen holder; however, when he is asked whether it was a pencil or a tooth pick, he promptly says "No," and when asked: "Is this a pen holder?" he will answer "Yes!" The right nasolabial wrinkle is somewhat obliterated. Facial twitchings can not be observed at this time. Slight paresis of the right abducens. Palpation and temperature examinations reveal normal reaction if made when patient is clearly conscious.

Fundus oculi normal. At 8 :30 p. m., vomiting.

At 9 p. m., June 22, 1906. Operation in Billroth's mixture narcosis. Lumbar puncture: Clear liquor is discharged under high pressure, in which, however, individual, fragile, fibrinous floeule may be seen (by microscope and culture sterile).

Typical skin incision. Chiseling out of the mastoid process. which, in its greater part, was pneumatic. In the cells around the antrum is some fetid pus. After the removal of the posterior wall of the auditory canal, in the upper part of the tympanic cavity and in the antrum was found a suppurating cholesteatoma of the size of a cherry stone, that had destroyed the roof of the antrum. The dura is bare here about the size of a copper and by the removal of the softened bone in the neighborhood is exposed to the size of a quarter. It is covered with granulations. Typical radical operation. Plastic according to Panse. Sinus exposed the size of a lentil, its wall being normal. Incision of the exposed dura of the middle cranial fossa and puncture of the temporal lobe: The edematous brain protruded. Wound dressing. Bandage.

June 23. Horizontal nystagmus to both sides; very strong to the left; very weak to the right.

June 24. Nystagmus to the right (diseased) side no more present; however, very strong to the sound (left) side.

June 23. Patient is lying in passive dorsal position, the eyelids not completely closed. He gives tardy answers to repeated simple questions. Sudden convulsions and moderate facial twitching. Head motions somewhat restricted. Patellar reflex diminished. Temperature 38°. Pulse 100.

June 23, p. m. Vomited twice. Otherwise condition is the same. Temperature 38.5°.

June 24. a. m. Stupor. Patient feels better subjectively; answers more promptly; no restriction of the cervical movements. Temperature 38°.

June 24, p. m. Status idem. Temperature 37.8°.

June 25. Frequent vomiting. Restless sleep; minimum of food taken. Stupor as yesterday. Temperature 37.9°.

June 25, p. m. Status idem. Temperature 37.6°.

June 26. No vomiting. Deep stupor. Temperature 37°. Change of dressing. Removal of the drain. Brain prolapse. Wound dressing. Bandage.

June 26. p. m. Temperature 36.8°.

June 27. No vomiting. Restless; little sleep. Temperature 38°.

June 28, p. m. Subjectively better. Patient spoke only a little with his relatives. Takes nourishment better.

June 29. Increasing stupor. No answers to questions. Sleep restless. Temperature 38.6°.

Change of dressing. A brain prolapse the size of a walnut, red violet. Removal of same. Drainage of the dural opening. Wound dressing. Bandage.

June 29, p. m. Increasing coma. Temperature 38°.

June 30, a. m. Great apathy. No answers to questions. Pupils wide; reaction very tardy. Temperature 36.7°. Pulse, 80, moderately strong. Involuntary passage of urine. Collapse.

With lumbar puncture slightly cloudy liquid escaped with high pressure.

Change of dressing: Removal of the drain. Brain prolapse. Again exploration of the middle cranial fossa, exposure and exploration in front of the sinus of the posterior cranial fossa with negative result.

June 30, p. m. Temperature 38.1°.

July 1. Great apathy; incontinence of urine and feces; minimum of food taken. Temperature 37.6°. Pulse 84 and weak.

July 4. Apathy less. Eats more. Patient seems to recognize his relatives. Change of dressing. Shortening of the drain strips.

July 8. Death.

Post mortem result: Tuberculous meningitis of the base of the brain, the vertex and right hemisphere. Puncture wound of the right temporal lobe, as well as the right cerebellar hemisphere. Suppuration of the puncture channel of the cerebellum. Operative opening of the middle and posterior cranial fossae after the radical operation. Lobular pneumonia. Purulent bronchitis. Calcified lymphatic glands (bronchial glands).

Bacteriologic result: In the pus of the cerebellar exploration wound streptococci.

The question now arises what practical clinical value has lumbar puncture in meningitis? We will contrast importance of the lumbar puncture for the diagnosis, the seat of the disease, and the treatment.

As to the pressure under which the liquor of the lumbar puncture is discharged, we have many variations. Increased evacuation pressure is a sign of increased intrameningeal pressure and always a sure sign of meningitis; in which case, we chiefly have to deal with serous meningitis or diffuse purulent meningitis. Normal evacuation pressure is frequently found with tuberculous meningitis and sometimes also with purulent meningitis, especially with the latter when considerable purulent exudate is present, rendering cerebrospinal liquor less fluid. Such changes can cause the pressure of the liquor, less than normal (Körner). A special apparatus is not necessary for measuring the evacuation pressure. An approximate estimation will do for clinical purposes; with normal pressure the liquor is evacuated in the arc of a circle, with increased pressure in the arc of an ellipse in a strong stream, and with decreased evacuation pressure in an angle with the acupuncture needle or in drops. A negative result of the lumbar puncture is observed in rare instances, when it is a sign of purulent meningitis, with a moderately thick exudate in the posterior cranial fossa and an obstruction of the foramen Machandi, or a sign of spinal meningitis. Finally we cannot see exactly why stress should be laid upon the distintcion between circumscribed and diffuse forms only with purulent meningitis, whereas the serous meningitis is usually a priori looked upon as a diffuse form.

Surely there will also occur cases of circumscribed serous meningitis, especially in cases of labyrinthitis or pyemia (sinus phlebitis), a fact which is of great importance from a therapeutic standpoint.

Rapidly disappearing mild meningitic phenomena are sometimes observed with acute middle ear suppuration. The lumbar puncture reveals in these cases either a clear or cloudy liquor evacuated under increased pressure. This form of meningitis, however, represents sometimes only a preliminary stage of a tubercular meningitis. Finally there are still more chronic forms of purulent meningitis, which, like the brain abscesses, show an initial and latent stage; a manifest and a terminal stage. These stages are known in literature (Brieger, Körner, Voss). Brieger proposed for them the appellation, "chronic intermittent meningitis."

The color of the cerebrospinal liquor is diagnostic from an otologic standpoint. Clear, yellowish liquor is sometimes found with tubercular meningitis; on the other hand, a characteristic color of white or yellow, at the same time cloudy, almost always indicates a purulent meningitis. The transparency is of greater importance. If the normally clear liquor contains very small white dots or threads, accompanied by the clinical phenomena of meningitis, we are likely to have same.

However, we must call attention to the fact that if the suppurative foci are very near to the intrameningeal spaces, considerable cloudiness of the cerebrospinal liquor can be observed; without, however, finding during the operation or perhaps at the autopsy even any trace of inflammatory changes in the meninges themselves (Körner, Voss). As to the microscopic findings, the picture of purulent meningitis is very characteristic, polynuclear leucocytes and microorganisms.

The microscopic examination is not sufficient by which to judge an individual case, as bacteria, that can be easily found by staining, may prove to be sterile by culture or completely innocuous (experiment on animals). In the majority of cases cloudy, grey or yellowish liquor holds bacteria, but my experience has been that even clear liquor may contain bacteria, while a cloudy liquor, free of microorganisms, may represent, on the other hand, typical pathologic changes of the cerebrospinal liquor, of which we shall speak later. Finally, the liquor may be found still clear and sterile with already fully developed clinical symptoms of a purulent meningitis. As to the demonstration of tubercle bacilli in the liquor, we would refer to Breuer's Method.

The appearance of coagulation in liquor that has stood for three to twenty-four hours is of the greatest importance for the diagnosis. Especially in those cases where clear liquor is evacuated by the puncture, this appearance of coagulation indicates a meningeal change, and is thus characteristic for meningitis serosa. Attention must be paid to the fact that the liquor is preserved from any artificial admixture of blood, as such an admixture—even if only in a slight degree—may give rise to formation of coagulation, even in decidedly normal liquor. I, therefore, catch the discharge from the lumbar puncture always in three test tubes, so that in case some blood comes into the needle lumen when making the puncture, it may be received isolated in the first test tube. From the technical standpoint, it may be briefly mentioned that we always make the lumbar puncture by means of an ordinary hollow needle provided with a mandrin, and sucking never is used. The application of a pressure measuring instrument, according to the above statement, therefore, appears to be superfluous, the more, as it may easily contaminate the liquor and cause the unfavorable accident of an infection of the spinal intradural spaces. Especially when examining for staphyloccocci, great care has to be taken, as same may be found in the liquor from external sources.

What diagnostic value, then, has lumbar puncture? We will obtain a good general idea by summing up the several results of examination; i. e., the evacuation pressure, color, transparency, microscopic condition, and coagulability in one table:

	Normal	Meningitis Serosa	Meningitis Tuberculosa	Brain Abscess or Thrombosis (with)	Migitis Circumscripta	Cerebrospinal Liquor Med With Blood	Meningitis Hemorrhagica
Evacuation-Pressure	N.	Incr'd	N.	N.	N.	N.	Incr'd
Color	—	—	—	Incr'd Grey	Increased or dmnshd Purulent yellow	red	red ......
Transparency . .	+	+	+	cloudy	cloudy	cloudy	cloudy
Microscopic Findings	L.	L.	L. Tbc.-bac. +	L. P. M.	L. P. M.	L.	L. P. ......
Coagulability . .	—	+	+ --	+	+	+	+ ......

L=lymphocytes   P=polynuclear leucocytes   M=micro-organisms

Of special importance is the result of the lumbar puncture with purulent inflammatory diseases near the dura, having, however, an extradural course; i. e., with purulent sinus phlebitis and large extradural abscess. Here we always find more or less numerous polynuclear leucocytes in the liquor. Sometimes cloudiness of the lumbar puncture liquor depends upon great numbers of leucocytes, bacteriologically the puncture being entirely sterile.

We find something analogous to the above in non-perforated brain abscesses that are in no direct relation with the intradural spaces. However, the cloudiness in these cases is very strongly pronounced.

I demonstrated such a case in the Austrian Otological Society, October 30, 1908. H. K., 6 years, admitted with symptoms of meningitis and abscess of left temporal lobe (dysphasia, bradyphasia, right hemianopsia, paresis right upper and lower extremities). Admitted October 9. 1905. Otitis media sup. chron. sin.; abscesses lobi temp. sin. The cloudy cerebrospinal fluid contained mono- and polynuclear leucocytes, but no bacteria.

Also the meningitis caused by labyrinth suppuration is of special importance (see Zeitsch. f. Ohrenheilk., 1908).

Even if the polynuclear leucocytes in the liquor do not indicate a purulent meningitis, this finding proves that the meninges are no more normal. That, notwithstanding the result of the lumbar puncture, sometimes no clinical symptoms of a meningeal disease arise and no meningitis is found when making the autopsy, proves nothing. It is positive that for the appearance of clinical meningeal symptoms a certain and by no means low degree of inflammatory changes in the meninges must be presupposed. However, even the macroscopic autopsy finding is not reliable, for, in order to prove the early stage of a meningitis, a microscopic examination of the meninges, and especially of the brain surface, is absolutely necessary. This, however, did not take place in the negative cases reported by Voss.

If we wish to estimate the importance of the lumbar puncture as an indication for operation, it is possible only to take into consideration the results that can be obtained macroscopically in the fresh liquor or by the immediate microscopic examination. It is imperative and long since admitted that if an operation comes into question at all, it must be made immediately. We, therefore, must in no case delay the operation until the formation of coagula and the culture or experimental conditions have been examined. Already here the importance of the lumbar puncture as an operative indication is strongly diminished and is displaced entirely into the background if we refer to the cases of meningitis that healed after operation. The lumbar puncture is of greatest value in a clinical way on account of its rapid and harmless performance. It gives us exact information as to the condition of the meninges at the time of the operation (in case that the lumbar puncture is made immediately after the cranial operation, as I always do), which is of considerable interest. There is no doubt that in earlier times that meningitis which developed clinical phenomena post operatively, and after a rapid course ended fatally, was ascribed to the operation. By the lumbar puncture, we are now informed about the condition of the meninges at the time of the operation. The result of the lumbar, puncture, however, cannot provide any contraindication against the operation. We have fortunately overcome the standpoint that a cloudy lumbar puncture contraindicates an operation. We certainly, thereby, do not mean to say that we should operate also every far advanced case of purulent meningitis. An unfavorable prognosis of an operation can, however, only be foretold by the clinical symptoms of the patient (deep coma, paralysis, Cheyne-Stokes), and never by the result of the lumbar puncture. Again, we must always remember that even a very marked purulent, cloudy liquor may occur in cases of brain abscess, labyrinth suppuration or sinus thrombosis (Körner, Voss).

We now proceed to the discussion of the operation. The first demand is to remove the suppurative focus from the ear as completely as possible. We accomplish this in acute cases by antrotomy and in chronic cases by the radical operation. With simultaneous suppuration of the labyrinth a wide opening of the labyrinth spaces starting from the vestibule and the promontorium is indicated, at the same time removing the petrous bone, until we obtain an unhindered flow of the liquor; so in some cases, it becomes necessary to expose the inner auditory canal.

In operating purulent meningitis, the object is the free drainage of the middle and posterior cranial fossae. which chiefly are involved in otitic meningitis. We accomplish this purpose by first removing the lower part of the squama, and the tegmen tympani. Then the sinus and the dura of the posterior cranial fossa in front and behind the sinus are exposed and by the removal of the upper edge of the petrous bone, both openings to the size of a dollar are connected at the level of the tentorium. In cases of labyrinth suppuration the exposure of the dura of both cranial fossae precedes the labyrinth operation.

. Finally we must see to the drainage of the intradural spaces. This drainage is obtained by an extensive incision of the dura. According to our present experience, we should recommend four incisions, two on the middle cranial fossa, one between the sinus and the labyrinth, and one behind the sinus. Every incision should be ½ cm. long; large blood vessels should be avoided in order to prevent hemorrhage.

By a simultaneous ventricle puncture the drainage of the cerebrospinal spaces is accomplished (Boenninghaus). Preysing's knives serve for the incision of the dura and the brain.

For a long time I have used knives 4 cm. long, sharp on both sides and provided with marks (5 mm.).* One of these knives is straight; the other is curved 45° on the angle, and the third 45° or the flat.

Of course, it is not necessary to make multiple incisions in all cases. The more we are convinced from the clinical symptoms and the operation findings on the ear that the meningitis is limited to a region easily accessible for surgical treatment, the greater will be the chances for the efficiency of a single incision in the region. Thus, for example, it is recommended to make the incision between the sinus and the labyrinth in sinus phlebitis and meningitis; with purulent labyrinthitis and clinical phenomena of a meningitis limited to the posterior cranial fossa (marked rigidity of the neck, abducens paresis, etc.) after the removal of the posterior wall of the petrous bone, one incision into the dura of the posterior cranial fossa will do. With localized disease of the tegmen tympani, accompanied by meningitis, the incisions should be above the tegmen. If at the same time we meet with extradural ichorous suppurative foci, we will have to avoid the ichorous parts of the dura and give preference to the more intact regions for the purpose of making the incision, provided we do justice to the chief requirement; i. e., that the incision should be made at that place where the meninges were first attacked by the otitic disease. If the bone and the dura seem unaltered and the latter is not under increased tension, we are sometimes (case 1) able to refrain from incising it.

In all cases the meningitis is combined with acute brain edema, which causes the brain surface to immediately bulge forward into the incision opening of the dura. If the edema is of a slight degree and the dura substance itself still intact, the gaping incision opening will hereby be closed. If the brain is mascerated, it will jut forward and sometimes in only a few seconds large prolapse will develop. With edema of slight degree the drainage may be made by introducing short sterile strips of gauze into the intradural spaces (Manasse).

The drainage of the intradural spaces is maintained by frequent changes of dressing. The first change may take place on the day the operation is made; however, during the first week we will, of course, have to limit ourselves to the renewal of the peripheral layers of the dressing; the strips of gauze

*To be had at Reiner's, Vienna, 1., Franzensring.

covering the wound-cavity are only shortened, and, as to the rest, it is left in situ. A repetition of the lumbar puncture after two or three days is also recommended. Each time a quantity of 20 ccm. can be withdrawn without running any risk.

As to the prognosis, we can at this time hardly give any general information. It is certain, however, that two main factors are to be considered: (1) Whether any microorganisms are present, their kind, their virulence, and (2) whether by the meningeal changes at the time of operation we may recognize a topical relation with the auditory organ.

In regard to the first point as to the proof of microorganisms, reference is made to the material discussed herein. It is certain that every pathologic admixture of the liquor cerebrospinalis has to be considered as indicative of meningitis, and the mere presence of polynuclear leucocytes proves meningeal changes. If microorganisms are present at the same time, we have to deal with an infectious purulent meningitis, provided that we succeed in making the positive culture test. If the nutrient culture medium remains sterile, the finding of microorganisms in the stained specimen is not free from objections, for, in addition to contaminations and mistakes in examination, or bacteria in the reagent, non-viable microorganisms that accept strong stains may lead us to the microscopic diagnosis of an infectious meningitis, whereas an attempt to make a culture proves negative. It is also important to know that in some instances (especially in the initial stages) with infectious purulent or tubercular meningitis the lumbar puncture is found to be free of microorganisms. Only in later stages (after repeated lumbar punctures) we may succeed in such cases in demonstrating microorganisms. Testing the virulence is best made by experiments on animals after a positive culture test. The experiment on animals alone allows us to value and judge the case properly. Accordingly, the cases without microorganisms, or those with degenerated forms, are prognostically far more favorable than the infectious kind and especially those of great virulence. As regards the second point, i. e., the topical relation between the ear suppuration and the meningeal changes, frequently we can speak definitely at the operation. Those cases in which the purulent inflammatory changes extend from the ear to the intradural spaces prove to be the most favorable. In these cases we not only have the certainty of the close pathogenic connection between the ear disease and the meningitis, but from a technical standpoint we are able to begin the operation at the correct location of the suppurative focus on the brain and to expose it sufficiently; i. e., over the limits of the pathologic changes. In such cases we are, of course, not certain whether there are no other seats of the disease on the dura, but it always means a good sign when we are able to establish during operation a localization of the meningeal changes in the region of the ear. If we cannot find such localization, the causes may be that it never existed, that we had to deal with a metastatic meningitis from the very beginning; i. e., with a diffuse meningitis. But even in cases where the meningitis developed by continuity through the extension of the purulent ear inflammation, we cannot expect that the contiguous tissues of the inflammatory region remain unaltered during the whole length of the disease. Pathologic changes of the bone, especially in the regions extending to the dura, will certainly furnish us a valuable indicator, but quite frequently we will find in an advanced stage of the disease only a trace or absolutely no pus in the ear itself and on the portions of the brain near the ear; the pathologic changes of the bone then give us the impression that pus must have been everywhere, but ruptured into the brain. It is clear that these latter cases prognostically are very unfavorable.

Also, those cases are not promising in which during operation the dural regions of the temporal bone are entirely unaltered and only slight changes are met with in the middle ear. In these cases when operating we frequently form the opinion that we have not to deal with an otitic meningitis at all, and it is certain that in some instances the differentiation of an otitic meningitis from a meningitis probably originating from the pharynx or the nose is exceedingly difficult if the examination of the ear shows the existence of a purulent, especially a chronic purulent, middle ear inflammation.

Finally, that form of purulent meningitis in which the intradural infection starts from multiple inflammatory plaques on the pachymeninges are unfavorable. This is a form of meningitis which is best illustrated by tubercular meningitis with caries of the base of the skull. In such cases we find within the ear region circumscribed or diffuse bone suppuration reaching to the dura. The removal of these suppurative foci, however, appears to afford no relief, because, as we learn from the autopsy, on other places of the base of the skull (orbital roof, lamina cribrosa of the ethmoid bone, wing of sphenoid) corresponding bone changes have led to meningitis.

In this respect the middle ear is best to be compared with the vermiform process (Wicart). Wicart arrives at the conclusion that the fulminating course of so many cases of otitic meningitis depends on anatomic variations of the temporal bone consisting in circumscribed attenuation or atrophy of bone and must be taken into consideration in so far as the plates of bone by means of which the middle ear is normally isolated from the skull cavity, are attenuated or dehiscent. As to this view, which has been taken in regard not only to meningitis, but frequently also to other intracranial otitic diseases, my cases furnish little evidence. It may even be that a thick sclerosed bone plate furnishes a better protecting wall than a normal bone. As far as normal bone is concerned, we cannot judge a thin bone plate differently from a thick one, the thickness of which has chiefly been increased by diploetic of pneumatic spaces. A thin bone plate is always strengthened by the periosteum, and the spaces appear only as permeable spaces on the macerated specimen, while on the living body they are filled by connective tissues which in substance, i. e., as regards the lymph and blood vessels (upon which the extension of an inflammation chiefly depends) are the same as the bone. If, on the other hand, the bone is thick and contains much diploe, in consequence of the strong increase of the blood contents, the possibility of infection is increased. In case there are many pneumatic spaces, the danger of an inflammation resembling empyema will again arise and the great possibility of retention. We, however, must admit that every inflammatory process having its origin in the bone greatly endangers the dura on the bone, and we therefore can not simply speak of "dangerous, normal anatomic varieties of the temporal bone." On the other hand, we agree with Wicart, especially in regard to meningitis having a severe course, that the power of resistance of the patient and his state of nutrition are of greatest importance, and that in these cases chronic alcoholism blood and constitutional diseases (diabetes) will, of course, still more diminish the chances of recovery.

REFERENCES.

Full references are given to the works of Boenninghaus and Voss. The later articles of Körner following my contribution can be referred to only by reviewing same.

Alexander. Ueber die chirurgische Behandlung der otogener Meningitis. Deutsche med. Wochensch., 1905, No. 39.

Bertelsmann. Ueber einen geheilten Fall von otogener Meningitis. Deutsche med. Wochenschr., 1901.

Billroth. Ueber akute Meningitis serosa and akutes Hirnödem nach chirurgischen Operationen. Wiener med. Wochenschr., 1869, No. 1 u. 2.

Boenninghaus. Die Meningitis serosa acuta. Wiesbaden, 1897.

Breuer. Bemerkungen zur Diagnose der tuberkulösen Meningitis durch die Lumbalpunktion. Wiener klin. Rundschau, 1901.

Brieger. Verhandlgen d. Deutschen otolog. Ges., 1899, S. 78, Gradenigo. Arch. f. Ohrenheilk., Bd. 47, 62.

Grossmann. Arch. f. Ohrenh. Bd. 64.

Gruning. Abst. Zentralbl. f. Ohrenheilk., Bd. III, 1904.

V. Haberer. Wiener klin. Wochenschrift, 1906.

v. Haberer. Wiener klin. Wochenschrift, 1906.

Hinsberg. Verhdlgen d. Ges. deut. Naturf. u. Aerzte. Breslau, 1905.

Ibid. Z. f. O., Bd. 36.

Körner. Die otitischen Erkrankungen des Hirns usw. Nachträge zur 3. Aufl. 1908.

Körner-Kühne. Z. f. O., Bd. 54. Ibid, Münchener med. Wochenschrift, 1897, Nr. 8 u. 9.

Lemoyez and Bellin. Zur chirurgischen Behandlung der akuten otogenen Meningitis. 7 int. otol. congress, Bordeaux.

Leutert. A. f. O. Bd. 54.

Ibid. Münch. med. Wochensch., 1897, No. 8 and 9.

Leutert-Schencke. Geheilter Fall von Meningitis. A. f. O., Bd. 53.

MacEwen. Die infestiös-eitrige Erkrankungen des Gehirns u. Rückenmarks. Wiesbaden, 1908.

Maljean. Meningitis cerebrospinalis acuta nach Influenza-Otitis. Annal. des. Mal. de l'oreille, Oct., 1903.

Neumann. M. f. O., 1904, S. 330, No. 7.

Oppenheim. Zur Encephalitis acuta non purulenta. Berlin. klin. Wochenschrift, 1900.

Ibid. Encephalitis und Hirnabszess. Nothnagels Handbuch der spez. Path. u. Ther. Bd. IX., 2.

Politzer. Lehrbuch der Ohrenheilkunde. 4 Aufl.

Ruprecht. A. f. O. Bd. 50.

Schenke.

Schulze. A. f. O. Bd. 57.

Siebenmann-Oppikofer. Ztschr. f. Ohrenh. Bd. 40.

Sokolowsky. Zur Diognose und zur Frage der Operabilität. d. otogenen diffusen eitrigen Meningitis. A. f. O. Bd. 63.

Urbantschitsch. Demonstration in d. österr, otolog. Ges. Sitzung vom November, 1907.

Voss. Bericht über die Ohrenklinik Passow, 1902-1903. Charité-Annalen, Bd. XXVIII.

Ibid. Die Heilbarkeit der otogenen eitrigen Meningitis. Charité-Annalen, Bd. XXIX.

Wicart. Ueber foudroyante Meningitis in Gefolge von Ohraffektionen. Progres med. 1907. No. 23.

Witte und Sturm. Z. f. O. Bd. 39.

Wolff. Beitrage zur Lehre vom otitischen Hirnabszess. Dissert. Strassburg, 1897.

Zeroni. Postoperative Meningitis. Arch. f. O., Bd. 66.

ABSTRACTS FROM CURRENT OTOLOGIC, RHINO-LOGIC AND LARYNGOLOGIC LITERATURE.

I.—EAR.

Preventive and Abortive Treatment of Mastoiditis.

W. Sohier Bryant, New York (*New York Medical Journal*, January 30, 1909), calls attention to the close relation anatomically of the ear and nasopharynx and the important role that the latter plays in causing infection of the ear and mastoid. His conclusions are as follows:

"The preventive treatment of mastoiditis should be directed to the nasopharynx and its preservation in normal condition. Preoperative treatment is a question of: (1) General systemic treatment with saline laxative and rest in bed; (2) the application of heat for the pain; (3) drainage of the middle ear: and (4) treatment of the nasopharynx. What he wishes especially to emphasize is that nasopharyngeal treatment is the treatment for prevention and abortion of mastoiditis."

Harris.

Thiosinamin in the Treatment of Deafness.

Maupetit and Colat (*Revue Hebdomadaire de Laryngologie, D'Otologie et de Rhinologie*. May 1, 1909) have conducted a series of investigations regarding the efficacy of thiosinamin in deafness along the lines conducted by Lermoyez and Mahu. They have confined its use to two classes of chronic deafness—to those cases of cicatricial otitis following suppuration of the ear where fibrous tissue has been thrown out, and, second, to cases of chronic adhesive otitis media of the dry variety. usually dependent upon affections of the nose and throat. They have employed thiosinamin in such case only after the use of inflation and massage of the drum have failed to give any further improvement to the hearing. They apply it locally and have endeavored to check their results by using iodid of potassium (one to one hundred) with sterile water in the other ear. where both ears were affected. As a result of such investigations carried on in some thirteen cases, they are convinced that the drug has no therapeutic value in ear disease and in consequence its use has been abandoned in the clinic of Moure at Bordeaux.

Harris.

Deafness Following Febrile Diseases, and Its Prevention.

J. A. PRATT, Aurora, Ill. (*New York Medical Journal*, May 15, 1909). There seems to be little doubt that adenoids and enlarged tonsils are responsible for the majority of ear diseases. It is the mechanical obstruction to the Eustachian tube and the interference with the ventilation and drainage of the middle ear which causes the trouble. Where adenoids and tonsils are present, there are usually ear complications even in slight nasal congestion and practically always in febrile diseases, while in those free from these growths the ears are not affected in severe colds. Authorities disagree as to the presence of germs in the normal middle ear, but the author, from the common sense point of view, believes that they are, although the infection may spread from the nose and throat. He believes that germs forcing their way into the internal ear are often the cause of sudden internal ear deafness which has been attributed to toxins. Through ignorance and carelessness, the proper prevention of these troubles, the early and complete removal of all hypertrophied lymphatic tissue, is being neglected and, since so large a proportion of children have adenoids and enlarged tonsils, the time is coming when the State will take the matter into its own hands.

Harris.

Voluntary Rhythmic Nystagmus in Its Relation to Infections of the Vestibular Labyrinth.

PIETRI and MAUPETIT (*Revue Hebdomadaire de Laryngologie, D'Otologie et de Rhinologie*, January 23, 1909) have studied the symptom of voluntary nystagmus in a series of labyrinthine cases; first, where the diagnosis has already been made, and secondly, in cases of middle ear suppuration where a question of labyrinthine involvement was under consideration. They also carefully studied it in a series of deaf mutes. The results of their examination prove, on the whole, the importance of the symptom, and yet, in their opinion, it is not impossible to put too precise and absolute value-upon reflex nystagmus. Certain sources of error càn occur. Among these are: First, that the nystagmus varies in certain professions to such an extent that one cannot, in these cases, make a positive diagnosis. Second, it varies also in certain individuals, particularly in those who are nervous and alcoholic, and these variations are very irregular and inconstant. In their opinion this is due to a lowering of the reflexes. Third, it varies with the age of the patient also in an irregular way. Finally it varies in individuals, and at times in the same individual in successive examinations made at intervals of several days.

Harris.

Hemorrhage of the Cavernous Sinus.

MOLINIE. Marseilles (*Revue Hebdomadaire de Laryngologie, D'Otologie et de Rhinologie*, June 26, 1909). A man of forty-three had suffered from suppuration of the right ear since infancy. When seen by Molinie, persistence of discharge and pain necessitated a radical operation, which revealed a small sequestrum in the roof of the attic. The patient was a man of bad habits. The convalescence was faulty, granulations soon followed and intense pain returned to the head. One night there was a hemorrhage. This phenomenon repeated itself every two or three days. The hemorrhage stopped spontaneously. The estimated loss of blood each time, according to the patient, was from one to two litres. Six weeks later a second operation was performed when the roof of the attic was found extensively necrosed, the osteitis extending to the roof and in part to the cerebellar wall of the antrum. There was no exposure of the lateral sinus or cerebellum. Much pain followed the operation in the region of the zone of the trigeminal nerve. Six days later a severe hemorrhage took place followed by another one in two days and death.

The autopsy showed a necrosis of the entire upper portion of the pyramid which had caused ulceration of the wall of the cavernous sinus, accounting for the repeated attacks of severe hemorrhage. Blood had burrowed underneath the dura and upper wall of the pyramid and thus escaped through the roof of the attic.

Harris.

The Modified Blood Clot After Mastoid Surgery.

SAMUEL McCULLAGH, New York (*New York Medical Journal*, June 13, 1908), is a strong believer in the modified blood clot method of inducing healing after the mastoid operation. He quotes Reik's well known views explaining how healing takes place in this method. The author employs only silk worm gut for suturing. A running subcutaneous suture is introduced and rubber tissue, properly folded, for drainage is placed between the last two stitches. This is allowed to remain from twenty-four to forty-eight hours. Care is necessary to avoid including any layers of skin in the suture. McCullagh believes that in this way infection is liable to occur. A certain rise of temperature after the operation is not, in itself, a sufficient cause for immediate removal of the suture. He does not regard any constitutional disease, with the exception of diabetes, as a contraindication. Only where an intracranial involvement exists should the method be avoided. He lays much stress upon the time saved in healing as well as the lessened discomfort to the patient. He believes that prompt healing will succeed, under proper diagnosis and in well selected cases, in seventy-five per cent of cases so treated. In spite of a number of complications, such as sinus thrombosis, that have occurred, he does not apprehend any evil consequences in cases where the clot breaks down.

Harris.

Sinus Thrombosis of Otitic Origin and Its Relation to Streptococchemia.

EMIL GRUENING, New York (*New York Medical Journal*, June 5, 1909), in a paper read before the New York Academy of Medicine, calls attention to the value of the examination of the blood in complications of middle ear suppuration. "In the last ten cases of thrombosis of the lateral sinus occurring in the otologic service of Mt. Sinai Hospital, blood cultures were made. In seven of these the result was positive and in three negative. The microorganisms causing the infection were, in five cases the streptococcus pyogenes, in one case streptococcus mucosus, in the other bacillus proteus. The same organisms had been previously found in the purulent discharge of the ear. The blood used in these cultures was taken from the median vein before and after ligation of the internal jugular vein. Of the ten cases here grouped together. eight patients recovered and two died. One death occurred from meningitis in a case of the blood of which was reported negative, and the second death took place in the case infected by the bacillus proteus. These observations go to prove that blood taken from the veins of the arm will demonstrate the presence of the microorganisms in the general circulation more convincingly than the blood taken directly from the sinus." Furthermore the presence of the streptococcus in the blood does not necessarily lead to a fatal result but permits of a favorable prognosis. Gruening finally refers to the fact that a positive culture from the blood will aid in the diagnosis of sinus thrombosis where the objective evidences are lacking.

Harris.

Report of a Case of Cerebral Abscess With Masked Symptoms.

ROBERT EMMET COUGHLIN, Brooklyn (*New York Medical Journal*. April 11, 1908). The report of a fatal case of brain abscess illustrating the difficulty at times met with in arriving at a correct diagnosis. The patient was a woman of twenty-five who, when seen, had been complaining of headache in the right occipital and parietal region for two months. Once or twice there had been attacks of vomiting and vertigo. There was a history of pain in the right ear two years before. The eyes were found to be normal. The ears were examined and only a congestion of the right drum was found. A lumbar puncture was made but a dry tap resulted. There was a polynuclear count of eighty-six per cent. The temperature ranged from $99\frac{1}{2}$ to 101; for most of the time it was normal. The pulse rate ran from 82 on admission to 145 before death. In the presence of no localizing symptoms an operation was decided against and the patient died about two weeks after first being seen. The necropsy showed an abscess in the left side of the brain just external to the lateral ventricle. A connection existed with the right ear.

The author calls attention to the impossibility in this case of having discovered the abscess if the brain had been exposed in the locality of the pain complained of.

(The case is a most unusual one and. so far as we know. unique in that the abscess was located on the side oppo-

site the affected ear. Except for this not easily to be explained fact, there would seem to have been sufficient indication to trephine the skull in the region of the temporo-
sphenoidal lobe.—Abstractor.)

Harris.

Indications for Operation in Acute Mastoiditis.

ERNST DANZIGER, New York (*New York Medical Journal,*
June 26, 1909), is of the opinion that there is such a thing
as sound conservatism in deciding when to operate for acute
mastoiditis. He points out that in inflammation of the
middle ear, the inflammatory process is not limited to the
middle ear, but the mucoperiosteum of the antrum and
mastoid cells participate to a greater or less degree and
that it is only later that a true pathologic change takes
place here, which is in the nature of an osteitis followed later
by a thrombophlebitis of the smaller veins of the mastoid.
He argues that inasmuch as the midle ear disease is usually
secondary to an affection of the nose and throat, we should
expect to find the temperature typical of the original disease. When the middle ear is involved the temperature
should become higher and assume a septic aspect. After
the performance of paracentesis of the drum, the temperature will asume the typical picture of the original disease.
Reasoning from this and the fact that the physiologic
edema and the mucoperiosteum of the drum will cause retention and resorption, we should regard the continuation
of the fever as no indication in itself for operation. Only
when fluctuation occurs with chills and sweats is there a
distinct indicaton for operation. The presence or absence
of a rise in temperature is not an absolute indication for
surgical interference. Pain over the mastoid antrum and
tip of the process is characteristic of all acute affections of
the middle ear and usually disappears after proper drainage
of the tympanum. Only when it persists or becomes more
severe and boring, especially at night, are we to assume that
necrosis has taken place. An increase in the amount of the
discharge from the middle ear with a change in its character and the sink'ng of the upper posterior wall of the canal
are also important indications for operation.

Harris.

A Contribution to the Pathology of the So-Called Circumscribed Otogenous Meningitis.

ENGELHARDT (*Deutsch medicinische Wochenschrift,* February 25, 1909). Körner's recent investigations would seem to show that a circumscribed purulent meningitis is not as common as was formerly believed.

It is a question whether anatomically a circumscribed meningitis occurs as frequently as the clinical diagnoses appear to prove.

Even the cases of Gradenigo, in which clinically the symptom complex, acute inflammation of the middle ear, persistent pain in the temporal and parietal regions and paralysis of one or both abducens nerves—as a rule without involvement of other cranial nerves—was present, were not proved anatomically.

The inspection of the exposed dura, without an incision through it, is not sufficient to make a diagnosis of a suppurative meningitis.

Manasse in his work "The operative treatment of otitic meningitis," states that when symptoms of meningitis are present, the suppurative process in the mastoid should be cleaned out and the dura exposed, and unless extradural abscess, sinus thrombosis or brain abscess are complications, a waiting policy should be followed out.

In a case reported by Grossman, however, in which the bone was healthy, the exposure of the dura was followed by a secondary infection of the sinus, a complication that could have been avoided.

He also reports another case with fully developed symptoms of meningitis: vomiting, rigidity of the neck, facial paralysis and cloudiness of the fluid obtained by puncture, which entirely cleared up after the mastoid operation, without exposure of the dura or lateral sinus.

The author reports the following interesting case: A young man aged 25 years, was operated upon five years before coming under his observation, for mastoiditis, and had been apparently in good health up to March 10, 1908. Then he developed pain and discharge in the same ear with inflammation of the old cicatrix and tenderness on pressure. There was a right-sided abducens paralysis. At the operation a large cholesteatoma, which had destroyed part of the labyrinth, was found.

The dura of the middle fossa was not exposed. On the

following day there was some rigidity of the neck, retracted abdomen and headache. Pupils were contracted, and there was double vision and a right-sided abducens paralysis. Kernig symptom absent.

The patient made an uninterrupted recovery without exploration of the brain. The author comes to the following conclusions:

1. In purulent circumscribed meningitis there is anatomically perhaps first a diffuse leptomeningitis.

2. Even when intracranial complications are suspected an exposure of the dura is not always advisable in performing the mastoid operation, in fact in some cases it is contraindicated.

Theisen.

Clinical Investigations on Disturbances of Equilibrium of Labyrinthine Origin With Especial Reference to the General Methods of Examination and That by Means of the Goniometer.

GEORGE W. McKENZIE (*Archiv. f. Ohrenheilkunde*, Vol. 78, Nos. 3 and 4). The relation of disturbances of equilibrium to disease of the labyrinth has been somewhat in doubt. Certain observers have been of the opinion that such irregularities went hand-in-hand with the cardinal symptoms of vertigo and nystagmus, disappearing when the latter disappear; others have regarded them as dependent upon meningitis or general weakness; still others that they were of meningeal origin; while certain careful observations have pointed to their labyrinthine origin. With the aim of arriving at some definite conclusion, McKenzie has carried out a series of careful investigations covering a number of months and representing the repeated examination of over thirty cases of labyrinthine disease by means of the various functional and caloric methods and by the goniometer. He has, for this purpose, made use of the apparatus modified by Alexander, the patient being carefully instructed in the proper position of holding the knees and standing erect. The feet are bared for the test and covered with powder. As a result of his investigations he has found that disturbances of equilibrium bear no relation to the degree of vertigo and nystagmus and persist after the latter have disappeared. His results in the examination of normal ears are quite in line with those of von Stein. The normal case shows, after the first or second examination, no equilibrium disturbance by Romberg, or the forward or backward bending, or by hopping, nor on the goniometer, up to an angle of about thirty degrees, except in about five per cent of cases where hysteria or excessive nervousness was shown, and even in these cases after a time the usual results were obtained. McKenzie made his tests on cases from six to eighteen months after the onset of the disease. As just stated, in all these cases nystagmus and vertigo were not present, yet disturbances of equilibrium persisted. This was especially noticeable where both labyrinths had been involved. From this the author concludes that incoordination cannot proceed from the semicircular canals but that disturbances of incoordination must depend upon the end organs of the vestibule, namely the macula utriculi and the macula sacculi. Among the conclusions which he draws from the use of the goniometer are: First, that disturbances of equilibrium can be exactly shown: second, that in cases of acute disturbances of equilibrium the angle of inclination corresponds to the grade of disturbance; that is to say, in cases of pronounced acute disturbance only a small degree of inclination can be arrived at; third, that the examination by means of the goniometer allows us only to determine in regard to the disturbance of incoordination as such; whether it is of labyrinthine origin or not can only be determined by other methods of examination.

Harris.

Clinical Studies on the Functional Examination of Labyrinthine Disease by Means of the Galvanic Current.

GEORGE W. MACKENZIE (*Archiv. f. Ohrenheilkunde,* Vols. 77 and 78). These studies covered a period of eleven months. The galvanic current in the examination of the inner ear has, in the past, been of scientific rather than general value. It is necessary for it to be used for each ear by itself. The author has employed it by a method of his own in a large number of cases both with normal and diseased labyrinths. He makes use of a ball electrode which he places upon the temporal bone of the ear to be examined. The other electrode, a flat plate, four to five centimetres in length, is held in the patient's hands. An assistant to take charge of the motor is desirable. The patient is instructed to fix his glance on some object upon the wall a short distance over the head of the examiner, who wears a head light for the purpose of detecting the nystagmus. The current is gradually increased until a positive reaction is obtained. It is then gradually diminished and the electrodes are changed. This procedure is followed for both ears. In certain cases the opening of the current produces nystagmus and vertigo. The nystagmus produced in this way is compared with that obtained by the closing of the current. This fact has lead Mackenzie to compare the nystagmus in all cases of the current opening and the current closing.

He gives in detail the result of the functional examination of thirty cases of unilateral labyrinthine disease occurring in patients seen in the Allgemeine Polyclinic in Vienna. From the analysis of these testings he draws certain important conclusions in regard to its availability for detecting disease of the labyrinth.

In the healthy ear the galvanic reaction of the kathode and anode ranges from one and a half to seven milliamperes or an average of four milliamperes. In the same individual there was never more than a difference of one milliampere between the two ears. Cases of unilateral labyrinthine destruction had the following points of differentiation in common: (1) The history gave at least one attack of typical, violent vertigo. (2) All cases showed more or less violent nystagmus of greater intensity towards the sound side. (3) All cases showed inactive caloric excitability of the diseased labyrinth. (4) All cases showed a higher grade of diminution of the nystagmus toward the diseased side when placed on the turning stool as compared with the labyrinth of the other side. (5) All cases showed an equal degree of diminution of the galvanic nystagmus towards the diseased side, the galvanic excitability of the diseased side being diminished compared with the normal or healthy side In a few cases it was not possible to use a sufficiently strong current for the kathodal test on the diseased side or the anodal test on the healthy side, since the patients became restless when seven or eight milliamperes were employed. In the remaining cases 't was necessary to use from fourteen to sixteen milliamperes in order to get a positive reaction.

The result of the examination of the cases of unilateral labyrinthine destruction gave the following conclusion:

(1) From the fact that unilateral destruction gives a positive reaction on this side it follows that the vestibular nerve is not attacked, or at least its conducting power is preserved. (2) In cases in which, in order to obtain a kathodal reaction, it is necessary to employ a current two or three times stronger than on the diseased side, we must assume that the static nerve ends are not functionating. (3) From the evident diminution of the kathodal reaction upon the diseased side, we must conclude that the galvanic reaction in the normal ear is given by the nerve end organs and by the nerve ends themselves. It is clear, therefore, in cases of destruction of the labyrinth, that to bring about a distinct kathodal reaction a much stronger current must be used than if the organ be intact. As regards cases of unilateral labyrinthine disease with pathologically increased excitability, the following common symptoms were obtained: (1) History in all cases of subjective noises and attacks of vertigo. (2) All cases give evidence of positive reaction upon the diseased side. (3) In all cases diminution of nystagmus in being placed upon the turning stool as compared with the normal and healthy ear. (4) In all cases cardinal labyrinthine symptoms were present—difficulty of hearing with shortened bone connection; lowering of the upper tone limits. (5) Disturbance of the equilibrium as shown especially by the goniometer. (6) All cases were alike in that upon the normal side anodal reaction was produced by a weaker stream than by the kathodel. The author concludes from these findings that the galvanic reaction represents a very valuable quantitative reaction for the static labyrinth and is especially important in unilateral disease with pathologically increased excitability; better, indeed, than upon the turning stool when the differential diagnosis between the normal condition and that of the increased excitability produced by disease is so small that it cannot be made out.

Harris.

Etiology of Acute Otitis.

NEUMANN and RUTTIN, Vienna (*Archiv. f. Ohrenheilkunde,* (Vol 79, parts 1 and 2), have examined ninety-one cases of acute otitis with reference: First, to whether the epi- or mesotympanic situation of the suppuration has an influence upon the course of the disease, and especially whether one of these localities leads constantly, or in the great majority of cases, to purulent otitis, or whether this is due to other causes; second, whether one particular excitant oftener than others gives rise to acute mastoiditis, or whether this also is dependent on other causes. The bacteriologic examinations have been carried out with the utmost care to get pure cultures, and the methods employed by them are carefully described. In cases where the drum membrane has not spontaneously burst, the paracentesis was made with a small glass rod. In only a few cases was it necessary, on account of the thickness of drum, to use a paracentesis needle.

In the table, mixed cultures are regarded only as such from a pure bacteriologic standpoint. They represent seven cases. Of the cases which were examined, representing ninety-seven ears, forty-three came to operation, of which seven had an epi- and thirty-six mesotympanic perforation. Fifty-four healed spontaneously; of these eleven were epi- and forty-three mesotympanic suppurations. The answer, then, to their first question is that the occurrence of an acute suppuration of the mastoid is not dependent upon the locality of the suppuration in the middle ear. In regard to the second inquiry—whether the character of the pus has an influence in causing acute purulent mastoiditis—they found fifty-four cases healed without operation; three were "kapsulkokki otitides" and fifty-one were cocci otitides produced by an excitant without capsule. Of the forty-three cases which came to operation, fourteen showed "kapsulkokki otitides" and twenty-nine capsule free microorganisms. We see, therefore, that otitides caused by capsulated cocci have a higher percentage and, therefore, more frequently lead to mastoid and cranial complications than capsule free microorganisms.

These agree with the previous investigations by them of ninety cases. The smaller number of "kapsulkokki otitides" is to be noted. This is at variance with Supfle, who, however, included a number of children in his studies. The authors call attention to the fact that on account of the difficulty in making pure cultures in children, they have excluded all children under four years of age, who, it appears, are more liable to "kokki otitides" and, because of the still present bone fissure mast, periosteal abscess is more likely to form. Of the "kapsulkokki otitides," the streptococcus mucosus in pure culture in eighteen cases examined by them out of which sixteen came to operation; only two healed spontaneously. These findings are at variance with the common opinion of the malignity of the streptococcus pyogenes aureus. As regards its power for producing mastoid complications, of the thirty-four cases of streptococcus infection, twenty healed spontaneously, and only fourteen came to operation. In the authors' opinion the anatomic form of the mastoid is of more importance than the character of the infection in the production of acute mastoiditis. In most of the cases where severe bone complications resulted, they were able to demonstrate the existence of the pneumatic form of mastoid. Every acute otitis is an inflammation of all the pneumatic cells of the temporal bone and gives rise in these cells to an exudate which is an excellent breeding place for bacteria. It can easily be seen that a sclerotic mastoid would be less liable to cause an extension of the disease.

They admit regretfully that our present methods of examination fail to detect the pneumatic mastoid, but the presence of spontaneous pain over the mastoid in acute otitis in the course of the first few days they feel should make one suspicious of such a condition. This pain soon disappears when the inflammatory process in the mastoid disappears, but returns when the simple inflammation of the mastoid changes into an empyema.

While the character of the infection is of less importance than the anatomic formation of the mastoid in producing an acute mastoiditis, it has an influence on the course of the disease. While they found it impossible to indicate particular cocci, they were able to determine, with reasonable satisfaction, that the "kapsulkokki" have a much more virulent effect than the capsule free cocci.

In comparing these two groups they found that the course of an acute otitis as regards the development of the mastoid complication forms, in the case of the capsule free cocci, a crescendo curve, while in that of the "kapsulkokki" the curve was a descending one, and after a long interval again rose. With the streptococcus mucosus there was an entirely characteristic picture. Such an otitis can spontaneously heal, but there was little tendency for a permanent healing, and it appears that cases formerly regarded as primary mastoiditis were in reality due to an otitis of streptococcus origin. Characteristic of such an otitis is the receding of the inflammation in the middle ear in the first or second week, the continuance of considerable difficulty with the hearing, for the most part associated with subjective noises and appearance of the drum membrane which suggests a secretory catarrh. The general contour is still recognizable but the details and the sharpness of the light reflex are not sharply defined; there is no pain, only a minimum amount of tenderness. Of their cases, two had extradural abscess, one meningitis, one brain abscess and five Bezold abscess. The symptoms can be extraordinarily light so that the patient does not go to the physician. The histories of fourteen cases are given illustrating the peculiar character of this infection.

Of the capsule. free cases, the streptococcus pyogenes aurens produces a fairly characteristic otitis. There is a sudden painful onset followed by symptoms of redness, bulging of the drum, pain on pressure over the mastoid and fever which is soon succeeded by a spontaneous rupture of the drum, giving rise to a sero-bloody secretion. From this stage the otitis goes on without any complication to prompt healing, or in some cases acute mastoiditis develops. Their opinion that the streptococcus pyogenes aureus has no particular malignity in producing mastoiditis is confirmed by the fact that five of the cases of streptococcus infection examined by them had double sided otitis where the condition did not vary. These cases were all dependent on influenza. All five cases had a central perforation and healed spontaneously without operation.

Harris.

II.—NOSE.

A Case of Accessory Sinus Disease With the Symptoms of an Osseous Tumor of the Orbit.

BURTON CHANCE, Philadelphia (*New York Medical Journal*, March 14, 1908). The patient was a lad of fourteen who showed a hard bulging mass in the right orbit pushing the eye outward and downward. The tumor was not sensitive to deep pressure. There was no obstruction or discharge from the nose or throat. The accessory sinuses were not examined. A diagnosis was made of an exostosis of the orbit. The operation revealed a closed cyst of the ethmoid filled with thick mucus. The cavity extended back to the sphenoid and up to the frontal sinus. An opening was made into the nose. A prompt recovery followed the operation.

Harris.

Pathogenesis and Treatment of Ozena.

LAVRAND (*Revue Hebdomadaire de Laryngologie, D'Otologie et de Rhinologie,* July 17, 1909) calls attention to the widely varying views regarding the etiology of ozena and also to the unsatisfactory methods of treatment generally employed. Of these the use of paraffin locally has seemed to give the best result. In his opinion, however, this is an illogical form of treatment, and in his hands it has failed to give as good results as others have obtained. In a study of cases of ozena where no treatment has been instituted, he has always been impressed that the secretions have proceeded from the region of the middle meatus. Acting upon this suggestion, he has carefully probed the middle meatus and has always found signs of an osteitis of the ethmoid shown by a sensation of denuded bone. The extent of the osteitis is in proportion to the abnudance of the discharge and the intensity of the odor. An exception to this observation he has yet failed to meet. Where there is a unilateral osteitis, the ethmoid upon the healthy side has always been normal. The histories of a number of cases are given where an ethmoiditis has been discovered and, after operation, the ozena symptoms have been relieved. In the author's opinion, then, in all cases of true ozena we have to do with necrosing ethmoidal osteitis demanding surgical intervention.

Harris.

The Treatment of Suppuration of the Accessory Sinuses of the Nose.

HAJEK (*Archives Internationales de Laryngologie, D'Otologie et de Rhinologie* January-February, 1909) places a great deal of importance on the general treatment of the acute affections of the accessory sinuses. In all cases of sinusitis depending upon acute colds or influenza, he is wont to obtain speedy cures by means of sweating through the use of aspirin in fifteen to thirty grains. He continues this for three or four nights in connection with dry friction twice a day of the whole body. He also is a firm believer in the value of a change of climate in effecting a speedy cure. The particular climate does not seem of as much importance as a change from the climate in which the disease developed. In the treatment of chronic cases of frontal sinus, Hajek is able to effect a cure in many instances by intranasal measures. He practices resection of the middle turbinate, removing it at its extreme anterior portion from the agger nasi with curved scissors, in this way laying open the infundibulum. Where this does not succeed in effecting a cure in a reasonable time, which means in some cases months or even years, he practices the external opening according to the Killian method. He does not favor the primary closure of the external wound, regarding it as the cause of the frequent failures in this operation. He condemns the osteoplastic operation because of the many cases of recurrence.

Diseases of the ethmoidal labyrinth demand exenteration intranasally. Only in cases where the extreme anterior cells are involved is it necessary to do the external operation. He urges the importance of careful cocainization of the operative field before beginning the operation, removing only such portions of the disease at a single seance as the patient can endure and the application after the final operation to the granulations which spring up of three to ten per cent of nitrate of silver.

As regards the treatment of the sphenoid, he does not attach a great deal of importance to the lavage nor to enlarging the osteum because of its tendency to close. He believes that the greatest relief will be had in the thorough removal of the middle turbinate and ethmoid and the anterior wall. To do this, he uses either his hook or one of the several models of cutting forceps or the electric trephine.

Harris.

III.—LARYNX.

A Plea for Systematic Use of Bronchoscopy in Our Routine Work.

WOLFF FREUDENTHAL, New York (*New York Medical Journal*, May 23, 1908) gives a description of a bronchoscope jointed two and one-half inches from the end. In the author's opinion, the use of such a form of instrument greatly facilitates the ease of introduction and overcomes the difficulties encountered with Jackson's solid tube. For purposes of illumination, he uses a light carrier similar to that used in the Jackson instrument.

Harris.

New Contributions to Laryngotracheostomy.

MELZI and CAGNOLA (*Archives Internationales de Laryngologie, D'Otologie et de Rhinologie*, March and April, 1909) report three additional cases operated upon successfully by laryngotracheostomy. They all occurred in children of eleven years or under and were, in each instance, the result of diphtheria.

The stenosis in the first case took the form of a general atrophy in the size of the larynx, due to the prolonged intubation. There was a general narrowing of the passage, but no spot of cicatricial deformity.

The second case showed a thick cartilaginous growth, which was removed by the Hartmann conchotome, which they recommend as especially indicated for this purpose. The result in this and previous cases reported by them render them very enthusiastic for this form of treatment for stenosis of the larynx. In place of the gutta percha recommended by Killian, Prof. Ferreri uses compressed cotton, known in this country as a Bernay's sponge, and the authors employ a tampon of hard wood covered with iodoform gauze, which is cubically shaped above and grooved below to conform to the tracheal cannula to which it is attached. They urge never to lose sight of the operative field and never to leave any portion unpacked.

Harris.

Some Experiences in the Direct Examination of the Larynx, Trachea and Esophagus.

A. BROWN KELLY (*Journal of Laryngology*, June, 1909) states his object in this paper to be "to indicate the possibilities of endoscopy of the lower air passages and esophagus and the desirability of making a routine use of the method."

He has used the Rosenheim tube for esophagoscopy and the Killian for bronchoscopy, but of late has found the Bruening telescopic tubes available for both. He has tried various methods for lighting.

Most of his examinations and operations have been conducted with the patient recumbent and under chloroform. He describes certain of his examinations, showing how the direct method has facilitated correct diagnosis in many cases. In children and unduly sensitive adults, the direct method renders certain operative procedures much easier.

In the past tracheoscopy and bronchoscopy have been chiefly employed for the removal of foreign bodies, but Dr. Kelly has found them of much assistance in discovering the cause in stenosis of the trachea and bronchi.

He believes that the routine use of the direct method may lead to the detection of malignant diseases at a stage before they become inoperable. He, himself, has investigated a number of growths at various depths in the esophagus and in some instances has removed fragments.

By the employment of esophagoscopy he has been able to discover the cause of the dysphagia in several cases which undoubtedly would otherwise have been classed as hysterical.

Harris.

Fulguration and Laryngotomy in Cancer of the Larynx.

LAURENS (*Archives Internationales de Laryngologie, D'Otologie et de Rhinologie,* January-February, 1909) reports two cases of laryngeal cancer treated by the method of Keating-Hart. The report is confessedly of little importance as regards the permanent value of the operation, inasmuch as they were performed only a month before the report was made. The author gives a detailed account of the operation and the laryngoscopic appearance afterward.

In both cases the disease was a limited one. The author describes the various steps of the laryngotomy, calling attention to the necessity of employing, as far as possible, only instruments made of glass. He then enumerates the different post operative phenomena seen in the larynx, which were: First, a moderate edema of both arytenoids lasting for thirty-six hours, more pronounced on the fulgurated side; second, intense erythema; third, a fibrinous eschar which was spontaneously thrown out on the fourth to the sixth day without any hemorrhage through the tracheal orifice; fourth, hypersecretions from the larynx, first mucous and then muco-purulent; fifth, ecchymosis of the lateral wall of the larynx; sixth, a laryngeal picture suggesting the destruction of the healthy vocal cord. The convalescence was rapid in both cases and Laurens is enthusiastic for the method, not only in cases of limited disease, but also in cases where the neoplasm has extended widely into the neighboring tissues. He concludes by giving a careful account of the technic employed in the fulguration, as described by Keating-Hart, and which is now practiced by himself representing two steps: First, the macroscopic removal of the growth without any attempt at its entire obliteration and of the surrounding glandular tissue; second, the fulguration practiced from five to ten minutes under chloroform anesthesia reinforced by applications of cocain to prevent undue movement of the larynx.

Harris.

Treatment of Four Infants Suffering from Papilloma.

VAN DEN WILDENBERG (*Archives Internationales de Laryngologie. D'Otologie, et de Rhinologie,* March and April, 1909). For removal in these cases the author has successfully employed the intralaryngeal method by means of the Killian tube spatula. The ages of the first three children weie seventeen and eighteen months, and of the fourth child eight years. General anesthesia was employed. The greatest difficulty presenting itself was the form of the epiglottis, which at that age is very small and not easily controlled. Local anesthesia is not recommended on account of the great fatality wont to follow its use in children of such a tender age. The author does not use adrenalin, checking the hemorrhage entirely by compression.

In the second case, where the larynx was found completely filled with the papilloma, cyanosis occurred during the removal of the growth and a tracheotomy was necessary. The operation was continued the following day, when the larynx was found free. Two days later masses were seen below the cords. which were removed.

In the third case, no anesthesia was employed at the first three operations, when papilloma were removed, but a general anesthetic was given for the removal of the papilloma situated in the angle of the cricoid. Soon after roughness of the voice returned. Two months later intense dyspnea showed a pronounced recurrence and tracheotomy was then performed. For six months the papilloma were removed from time to time intralaryngeally. The child died later of convulsions. The autopsy showed the respiratory tract below the cannula perfectly normal. It demonstrates the uselessness of our interference as regards the cure of papilloma in this case. The larynx was covered with a profuse mass of papilloma extending to the tracheal opening. He does not recommend the method employed here except in cases of very young children who can be easily held, and only for the removal of papilloma

situated in the upper larynx. He advises the removal of only
a few at a time and keeping the field well in view. The introduction of the tube spatula is wont to cause a fit of crying
with a spasmodic closing of the larynx, which will be followed
by a deep inspiration opening wide the larynx. The sitting
position favors the avoidance of wounding the mucous membrane. There is usually no reaction and the procedure can
be repeated two days later.

The fourth case was that of a child of eight, who had for
over four years worn a tracheotomy tube because of papilloma
in the larynx, which had been removed at the time of the
tracheotomy. Here laryngotomy was performed.

Harris.

IV.—PHARYNX.

Acute Unilateral and Recurring Hypertrophy of the Tonsils.

MUNCH, Paris (*Revue Hebdomadaire de Laryngologie,
D'Otologie et de Rhinologie*, February 13, 1909), reports a
case of a child operated on by morcellement at four years of
age for adenoids and enlarged tonsils and twice afterwards at
intervals of two and three years for acute and unilateral hypertrophy of the left tonsil. A careful histologic examination
was made of the tissue removed and, in spite of suspicion of
malignacy, the findings showed nothing but the ordinary picture of hypertrophied tonsil tissue. The author comments
upon the rarity of the occurrence and quotes a similar case
reported by Lavrand.

Harris.

Two Cases of Syphilis of the Nasopharynx.

TRAPENARD, Menton (*Revue Hebdomadaire de Laryngologic, D'Otologie et de Rhinologic*, January 30, 1909). The report of two cases occurring in children of eight and ten years
respectively where the nasal obstruction was of recent date.
The soft palate showed marked engorgement, one case with
a tendency to perforation. Hutchinson teeth were present in
the younger child. The growth in the nasopharynx was soft
to the touch. Both cases recovered promptly under specific
treatment.

The author is of the opinion that syphilis of the nasopharynx in children is not as uncommon as is usually thought.
The difficulty of diagnosis leads him to advise that where the

respiratory trouble is of short duration, we should always bear in mind the possibility of syphilis, even where it resembles the ordinary adenoid growth.

Harris.

Neurasthenia in Its Etiologic Relation to Nasopharyngitis.

ROYET, Lyons (*Archives Internationales de Laryngologie, D'Otologie et de Rhinologie,* January-February, 1909), is of the opinion that many symptoms usually ascribed to neurasthenia are dependent upon disease of the nasopharynx localized in the fossa of Rosenmueller. He calls attention to the anatomy of this fossa and its liability to inflammation and thus becoming a closed cavity retaining secretions. He also refers to the structures lying in close proximity as capable of causing many of the symptoms which he enumerates, such as headache, mental asthenia, nasal hydrorrhea, nervous coughs; referable to the ear: subjective noises, deafness, hyperacousis, vertigo and inco-ordination of gait, muscle anesthenia and sensation of "casque." This latter symptom is often associated with headache and is met with in ear diseases which have their origin in the nasopharynx. Of general symptoms depending on nasopharyngitis, he names insomnia, tachycardia, digestive troubles, neuralgia and motor and sensory affections of the throat.

Harris.

Ulcer of the Palate of Strepticocci Origin.

JACQUES (*Revue Hebdomadaire de Laryngologie, D'Otologie et de Rhinologie,* July 10, 1909). The ulcer occurred in an adult laboring man of thirty-eight and, when seen, was of about a month's duration. There was a complaint of constant pain in the throat, not benefited by gargles. The ulcer was situated at the base of the epiglottis. It had rounded borders and a diameter of about a franc piece. It was not covered with detritus, showed considerable vasculation, had a vermilion tint and presented a loss of substance of from ten to fifteen millimeters, but blended gradually with the healthy mucosa of periphery. There was no other lesion in the neighborhood, neither of the tonsils nor gums, no enlargement of the glands. The application of iodid of glycerine and potassium iodid internally, on the supposition that it was of mycotic origin, gave satisfactory results, and in the course of a month the ulcer was healed.

An extensive bacteriologic examination was made, which showed a microbe reported by Klava some years ago and described by him as leuconostoc hominis resembling in many ways the streptococcus pyogenes.

Harris.

Three Cases of Primary Gangrene of the Pharynx. Cure in One Case by Injection of Anti-Streptococcus Serum.

CITELLI (*Archives Internationales de Laryngologie, D'Otologie et de Rhinologie,* January-February, 1909). The first case was that of a young woman, twenty-five years old, of excellent health. Eight days before seen by Citelli, she noticed two small white spots on the tonsils, which gradualy extended, giving rise to only a little difficulty in swallowing. When seen by him, the patient was clearly septic—breath very offensive, pronounced glandular enlargement. On examination of the throat, the two tonsils could no longer be recognized; in their place one saw a lardaceous colored mass, which gave rise to an unbearable odor. In spite of the use of anti-diphtheretic serum and of local and general treatment, the disease gradually extended and the patient died fifteen days after the onset of the disease.

The second case was a child of eight years, where the picture of the disease was similar to that in the first case. Here local disinfectants seemed to have the happy effect of limiting the necrosis to the affected tonsil, but twenty days later the same phenomenon broke out in the other tonsil and the child died.

In the third case, a man of thirty, Citelli was able to effect a cure with one injection of antistreptococcus serum.

He emphasizes the well-known gravity of this disease and urges the discovery, if possible, of the particular germ which is the cause and combating it by the use of a suitably prepared serum.

Harris.

Digital Enucleation of the Faucial Tonsil. The Otitic Significance of Tonsillectomy With Reference to Digital Enucleation.

A. MORGAN MACWHINNIE, Seattle, and H. P. BLACKWELL, New York (*New York Medical Journal,* May 29, 1909). The interest which at present is being shown in the procedure for the removal of the faucial tonsils is seen in two papers on digital enucleation by men living at widely removed distances. Dr. MacWhinñie advocates the employment of the index finger for the complete removal of the tonsil without the aid of any instruments. He works under general anesthesia and claims for the method "simplicity, rapidity, safety and thoroughness." The essential point in his method is carrying the finger "outside the capsule in the posterior inferior portion of the sinus, working up to the supratonsillar fossa." The same procedure is carried out posterior to the anterior pillar. He states that the bleeding is very slight and the reaction insignificant.

Blackwell, instead of depending upon the finger entirely, first separates the attachment of the tonsils to the anterior and posterior pillars by means of a Leland knife. The left index finger is then introduced into the supratonsillar fossa and each tonsil is gently shelled out of its bed. He stops short of complete removal in this way, leaving the tonsil attached at its inferior pole. The operation is then completed by means of the cold wire snare.

Harris.

V.—MISCELLANEOUS.

Positive Proof of Adrenalin Reaction of Meltzer and Loevi in a Case of Accidental Section of the Sympathetic and Pneumogastric Nerve.

BRINDEL, Bordeaux (*Revue Hebdomodaire de Laryngologie, D'Otologie et de Rhinologie,* April 24, 1909) has demonstrated that the pneumogastric is the regulating and the sympathetic the accelerating nerve of the heart. Injury to the pneumogastric and section of the sympathetic produces a slowing of the pulse, diminution of the pupil and a shrinking of the eyeball. Meltzer and Loevi have found that adrenalin introduced into the healthy eye has no effect, but put into the eye of an animal where the superior cervical sympathetic has been removed, a mydriasis was at once produced and myosis resulted after section of the nerve. Brindel has recently seen a case of a man who had received a wound of the neck. When seen by him thirty-three days after the accident, a complete paralysis of the left vocal cord was noted. The characteristic diminution of the size of the left eyeball was to be detected, and the left pupil was much smaller than the right. There was no tachycardia. In the presence of such symptoms, a diagnosis was made of a section of the pneumogastric and sympathetic nerves, and it was possible to confirm the experiments of Meltzer and Loevi of the effect of adrenalin in such cases.

The author concludes by commenting upon the rarity of the simultaneous section of the pneumogastric and sympathetic nerves, having been able to find but three probable cases in the literature.

Harris.

The Physiologic Action of Strong Cocain-Adrenalin Solutions.

John Leshure, New York (*New York Medical Journal,* February 6, 1909), in a carefully prepared article, takes up the relative absorption of the common solutions of cocain and adrenalin used in nasal surgery. "Both cocain and adrenalin have the power of contracting superficial and deep vessels, but the degree and rapidity of this contraction seems to be proportionate to the strength of the drug solution used." Strong solutions are seen to do it promptly, as any solution is rapidly diluted by the copious mucous exudate. By a strong solution, the author means one made by dissolving a gram of cocain hydrochlorid in a cubic centimetre of a one to one thousand solution of adrenalin chlorid. This solution represents fifty-five per cent by volume and has a specific gravity of 1110. As he rightly says, we should seek to bring the solution to the vessel walls and anesthetize the vasomotor fibers, but not allow it to pass through them. He shows that with the ordinary solution (from four to twenty per cent), we have a specific gravity of only a little over a thousand. He also calls attention to the law of fluids, that absorption is in inverse proportion to the density of the fluid. From this, he logically reasons that the light solutions of common use are much more liable to become absorbed into the system than the heavy solution employed by himself. Such a clear physiologic explanation of the toxic effects of cocain and adrenalin, in view of the accidents occurring from their use, is most timely. The solution is applied upon a cotton applicator to the part of the nose to be operated upon. A few wipings at intervals for ten to fifteen minutes will produce complete anesthesia.

Harris.

ANNALS

OF

OTOLOGY, RHINOLOGY

AND

LARYNGOLOGY.

VOL. XVIII.   DECEMBER, 1909.   No. 4.

XLVII.

THE TOPOGRAPHIC ANATOMY OF THE THYROID GLAND.*

By Peter Potter, A. M., M. D.,

Butte, Mont.

The problem was suggested by Prof. Waldeyer, of the Anatomical Institute of Berlin, and the work was begun in his laboratory in the summer semester of 1904.

It was recognized that many observations had been made upon the topography of the gland, but since they were made before the present methods of preservation of material were in use it seemed advisable to undertake this work. Accordingly most of the material used was formalin hardened, the remainder being hardened by arterial injections of alcohol 2 parts, carbolic acid 1 part, and glycerin 1 part. The material consisted of 23 fetuses, ranging in age from five months

*From the Anatomical Laboratory of St. Louis University.

to term—all formalin hardened[1]; 19 children from 1 to 7 months of age, formalin hardened[2]; 55 adults from 20 to 70 years of age, 30 formalin hardened, 25, alcohol-carbolic acid-glycerin hardened.

Two methods of making the measurements were used, (1) from sagittal and transverse sections, and (2) from dissections.

The sagittal sections show at once the position of the isthmus of the gland with reference to the vertebral column and the trachea. The transverse sections were reconstructed on profile paper, so as to show the relations of the gland to the vertebral column and surrounding organs. (The reconstructions were made according to the method described in the Topography of the Thorax and Abdomen, University of Missouri Studies, Science Series, Vol. I, No. 1.)

When the neck region was dissected in the ordinary way, the measurements were made by driving a steel pin vertically through the isthmus of the gland into the vertebral column and using it as a point from which to measure in all directions. A point on the profile paper was taken to represent the position of the pin, and all of the structures were located on the paper in accordance with the measurements on the body. The measurements were taken in a horizontal plane and not over the convex surface of the gland. When the gland and other soft parts had been removed, the vertebral column was mapped out in the same way as the gland by using the point where the pin entered the column as the starting point for the measurements. In some cases the soft parts only were measured, thus giving the relations of the gland to the trachea.

In the following description the gland will be considered as composed of an isthmus and two lateral lobes. The gland as a whole is roughly U-shaped.

Each lateral lobe is more or less cone shaped, with its apex extending considerably above and its base only a little below

---

1. Most of these were material belonging to Dr. Jackson, University of Missouri, upon which he worked out the topography of the pancreas. This part of the work was done in Prof. Waldeyer's laboratory.

2. The neck organs were removed at autopsy by Dr. Thompson, Dept. of Pathology, St. Louis University, and placed in formalin.

the plane of the isthmus. The external surface of the gland is markedly convex from side to side, and slightly so from above downward. The internal surface is concave from before backward, fitting accurately over the sides of the larynx, trachea, pharynx and esophagus. The isthmus is the thin plate of gland substance molded over the anterior surface of the trachea, uniting the contiguous surfaces (margins) of the lower part of the lateral lobes.

The relationship which the gland bears to the other structures in the region is well shown in Figures 1 and 3.

The anterior surface of each lateral lobe is covered by the sternothyroid muscle and separated from it by a thin layer of fascia. The inner margin of the sternohyoid muscle overlaps the inner margin of the sternohyoid a few millimeters, so that the uncovered (intermuscular) portion of the gland is reduced to a small area. This interspace becomes smaller from above downward, since the muscles of the two sides almost meet in the midline at the lower margin of the isthmus, thus leaving only a small V-shaped portion of the gland not covered with muscle. This medial portion of the isthmus is covered with superficial fascia and skin containing small veins of the inferior thyroid and anterior jugular systems. The anterior margin of the sternomastoid crosses the region of the lateral lobes obliquely from below upward and outward.

Each lateral lobe lies between the carotid sheath externally, the trachea internally, and the above named muscles anteriorly. The upper part of the lobes usually extend as far back as the sides of esophagus and pharynx. In the child and fetus the lobes protrude, in many cases, into the post-pharyngeal space, and while they seldom meet behind the pharynx the two lobes hold it in a firm grasp.

While the thyroid is a true cervical organ, it comes into close relationship with such thoracic organs as the lungs and thymus gland. The lower pole of each lobe is separated from the apex of the corresponding lung in the adult by a small interspace containing the vertebral and ascending cervical vessels and the arch of the thoracic duct (on the left side).

In Figure 1 the apices of the lungs, which lie only about 2 mm. below the surface of the section, are indicated by the dotted lines in the quadrilateral spaces bounded by the first ribs and the scaleni and longus colli muscles.

Figure 2 shows the relative levels of the lung and gland in the adult, while Figure 4 shows the relation in the fetus at term where the gland is much higher in the neck, and consequently not in close relation with the lungs.

By comparing Figures 1 and 2 with 3 and 4 it will be seen that the superior division of the mediastinum is much larger proportionately in the fetus than in the adult and is filled, in its anterior portion, by the thymus gland, which comes into close relationship with the lower part of the thyroid. In many of the dissections of the fetus these glands were in direct contact.

The parts of the gland will be located with reference to the vertebral column and then with reference to the trachea and larynx; first as determined by projections from dissections and then by projections from cross sections.

THE ADULT GLAND.

1. *As Measured from Dissection.* The isthmus lies over the seventh cervical and first thoracic vertebrae. In every case the upper border of the isthmus was below the disk between the sixth and seventh cervical vertebrae. In more than 50% of the cases the upper border of the isthmus is below the disk between the seventh cervical and first thoracic vertebrae, but in only two cases is it below the first thoracic vertebra.

It lies upon the three first rings of the trachea. In 66% of cases it completely covers the first ring, but in no case does it overlap the cricoid cartilage to any considerable extent. In every case its upper border is above the middle of the second ring. The isthmus is so variable in size and width that its lower border may be found anywhere from the third to the sixth ring. In the few cases, three in the series, in which it reaches the fifth or sixth ring it extends below the lateral lobes. More than half of all the cases cover rings two and three.

The apex of the right lobe varies from the upper part of the fifth to the lower part of the sixth cervical vertebra, with the greater number opposite the fifth vertebra and fifth disk. The apex of the left lobe is never higher but often a little lower than the right, the difference being only a few milli-meters in any case.   However, a much larger number of the left than of the right were below the fifth intervertebral disk.

The lower poles do not show so much variation as do the apices, nor do they differ as much from each other. The ordi-nary variation in position is from the middle of the first to the lower part of the second thoracic vertebra, with the larger proportion of the cases above the second vertebra.

Each lateral lobe extends upward and backward along the sides of the larynx and pharynx into a conical space bounded internally by the larynx and pharynx, anteriorly by the sterno-thyroid and omohyoid muscles, and posteriorly by the carotid sheath and the prevertebral fascia.   The upper part of the anterior border follows more or less closely the attachment of the sternothyroid muscle to the oblique line of the thyroid cartilage.

In 27 cases the thyroid cartilage was projected along with the gland to show the relative position of the apex of each lateral lobe to this cartilage. The united portion of the ante-rior portion of the alae is used as the basis of comparison.   In 13 of the 27 cases the apex on the right was as high as the upper end, while only six of the left lobes reached this level. Of the other 14 right lobes, 9 reached the middle and 5 only the lower end of the anterior border. On the left side six were on a level with the upper end, 13 the middle, and 8 the lower end of this border.

2. *As Measured from Cross Sections.* The projections made from cross sections show the relation of the glands to the vertebral column only, since these projections were made for a different purpose and the larynx and trachea were not included in them.

The average position of the isthmus is over the first and second thoracic vertebrae.   Its upper border may be as high as the middle of the seventh cervical, and its lower border as low as the third thoracic disk, but since it is usually about as broad as a vertebra and disk, when the upper border is high, the lower border is correspondingly high, and vice versa.

The apices of the two lateral lobes are at about the same level in most cases.   They vary from the fourth to the sixth cervical disk, a majority being opposite the fifth and sixth vertebrae.   The lower poles of the two lobes are usually at about the level of the first thoracic vertebra. In nearly every case the lower lobes were above the second thoracic vertebra.

THE GLAND IN THE CHILD.

From the material at hand it was only possible to locate the gland with reference to the larynx and trachea, because all the material at this stage had been removed at autopsy. The upper border of the isthmus touches the cricoid cartilage in a majority of cases. The cricoid is completely covered in 7 of the 19 cases. In every case except one the first ring of the trachea is covered. In this one case the isthmus is very narrow and might be said to be absent, for it is difficult to distinguish any thyroid tissue in it macroscopically. The isthmus covers rings 2 and 3; one-half ending below ring 3, and the other half passing over ring 4.

The lateral lobes appear to be proportionately larger and less conical than those of the adult. In nearly every case the apex is at the level of the base of the superior cornu of the thyroid cartilage. They cover most of the cricoid cartilage and that part of the thyroid cartilage below and behind the oblique line, so that the sternothyroid muscle is displaced upward and forward at its attachment to the thyroid cartilage and is made to hook over the anterior border of the gland instead of passing to its attachment in the plane of the body of the muscle, as it does in the adult.

THE GLAND OF THE FETUS.

Most of the specimens were full term fetuses hardened in the dorsal position by injection with formalin.

The gland is very much like that of the young child in size and position. The isthmus corresponds to the fifth and sixth cervical vertebrae (Figs. 2 and 4), usually not extending below the middle of the sixth. It lies over the first four rings of the trachea. In about 30% of the cases it was high enough to lie over the cricoid, but in these cases it usually did not reach below the third ring of the trachea.

The lateral lobes extend high up into the space between the thyroid cartilage, sternothyroid and omohyoid muscles and carotid sheath. In many cases they extend beyond the outer border of the omohyoid muscles into the superior carotid triangles. These lobes are so thick anteroposteriorly that they displace the sternothyroid muscle at its attachment to the thyroid cartilage, as in the child. The apex of the lateral lobe is usually high upon the posterior part of the thyroid cartilage, being as high as in the child and almost constantly higher than in the adult.

VARIATIONS AND ANOMALIES.

The middle lobe or pyramid varies more than any other part of the gland, both in size and position. It may be entirely absent, or vary from a small tubercle on the upper margin of the isthmus, or one of the lateral lobes, to a well developed band of gland tissue extending upward to the hyoid bone. It is more often connected with the left lobe at its union with the isthmus than with any other portion. of the gland, though it not infrequently connects with the right lobe. Nearly every gland has a more or less well developed band connected with its upper border, though only about three-fifths of these bands contain any gland tissue. This band can be traced to the hyoid bone, to the posterior inferior margin of which it is attached. The usual structure of this band is connective tissue, containing gland substance below and muscle fibers above—the muscle fibers may or may not fill in all of the remaining portion of the band. Occasionally two or more separate nodules of gland tissue are imbedded in the band and connected to each other by muscle fibers. When the muscle fibers are well developed and the gland substance reduced to a small nodule on the upper part of the isthmus it is called the levator glandulae thyroideae, but all of these conditions should be classed together as being persistence of the thyroglossal duct.

The isthmus is rarely absent. though many times it is only a very thin band of gland substance. In this series it was entirely absent in one fetus and one adult, and practically absent in two other cases.

Among the glands which were dissected there were several with one or more accessory slips of muscle. When there was but one slip it was considered as the levator glandulae thyroideae. even though it was not connected with the isthmus of the gland. In a few cases this middle slip was found along with an extra slip to each lateral lobe. Figures 5 and 6 show this condition. In these cases the muscle fibers arise from the fascia covering the anterior surface of the gland and end by blending with the inner margins of the thyrohyoid muscles. In Figure 5 the fibers end near the lower part of the thyroid cartilage, while in Figure 6 they remain more or less separate up to the hyoid, where they insert along with the inner fibers of the thyrohyoid. In Figure 5 the middle slip (f) does not contain many muscle fibers, but from its position and appearance it may be taken to represent the thyroglossal duct. In Figure 6 this middle slip (i) is muscular and well developed and arises from both surfaces of a small pyramidal lobe

Figure 7 has two well developed slips symmetrically placed, but without any well defined remains of a median portion. These fibers arise from the fascia along the upper margin of each lateral lobe and may be traced to the hyoid bone as the inner portion of the thyrohyoid.

Figure 8 is from a child seven months old. It shows a condition different from those described above. Here the three slips are found, but the right one arises from the fascia on the posterior surface of the gland, while the left one arises from the anterior surface. Otherwise this case does not differ from the others.

These muscle slips do not correspond to the extra muscles of this region, as described in Porier and Charpy, in that they do not connect with the constrictors of the pharynx.

CONCLUSIONS.

1. That the thyroid gland is smaller, proportionately, in the adult than in the fetus and young child.

2. That the thyroid gland descends upon the vertebral column with the assumption of the erect position.

3. That there is an apparent descent of the thyroid gland upon the neck organs. The gland is lower on the thyroid and cricoid cartilages of the adult, but it is attached to the same rings of the trachea. This apparent descent may be due to the fact that the hyoid, thyroid and cricoid are telescoped upon each other in the fetus and young child and thus brought closer to the fixed part of the thyroid gland.

4. That some remains of the thyroglossal duct can be

found in almost every case, and that a pyramid is present in over three-fifths of all cases.

5.   That the isthmus may be very small, but that it is rarely entirely absent.

6.   That accessory muscle slips are to be found, which seem to be aberrant slips of the thyrohyoid or possibly of the sternothyroid. They do not appear to have any special function, but act in conjunction with the fascia to hold the gland in position.

EXPLANATION OF FIGURES.

Figure 1. Section through lower portion of first thoracic vertebra. Adult.

sp. c. spinal cord.
d. m. dura mater.
c. centrum of first thoracic vertebra.
r. first rib.
l. c. longus colli.
v. v. vertebral vessels.
n. eighth cervical nerve with its junction with first thoracic nerve.
th. d. arch of thoracic duct.
sc. a. scalenus anticus.
c. s. carotid art., jugular vein and vagus nerve in carotid sheath.

p. platysma.
a. j. v. anterior jugular vein.
st. hy. sternohyoid.
st. th. sternothyroid.
th. gl. thyroid gland.
tr. trachea.
i. th. v. thyroid vessels (inferior).
oe. esophagus.
s. g. inferior cervical sympathetic ganglion.
tr. p. transverse process of vertebra.

Figure 2. Reconstruction of thyroid gland and surrounding structures from set of sections to which Figure 1 belongs.

m. manubrium sterni.
cl. clavicle.
l. lung.
r. rib.
v.-vii. cervical vertebra.
i.-iv. thoracic vertebra.

Figure 3. *Section through sixth cervical vertebra. Fetus at term.

o. h. omohyoid. Other labeling same as Figure 1.

Figure 4. *Reconstruction of region of thyroid of fetus, of which the section shown in Figure 3 is part.

thym. thymus gland. Other labeling same as Figure 2.

Figure 5. Thyroid gland with accessory muscles.

5a. front view.
5b. right lateral view.
5c. left lateral view.
a. thyroid cartilage.
b. cricoid cartilage.
c. thyroid gland.
d. extra muscle of right lobe.
e. extra muscle of left lobe.

f. fascia, etc., representing remains of thyroglossal duct.
l. hyoid.
m. thyrohoid.
n. sternothyroid.
o. oblique line of thyroid cartilage.
p. sternohyoid.

Figure 6. Thyroid gland with accessory muscles.

6a. front view.
6b. right lateral view.
6c. left lateral view.
h. extra muscles of right lobe.

g. extra muscles of left lobe.
i. levator glandulae thyroideae.
Other labeling same as in Figure 5.

Figure 7. Thyroid gland with accessory muscles.

7a. front view.
7b. right lateral view.
7c. left lateral view.
k. extra muscle of right lobe.

j. extra musle of left lobe.
Other labeling same as in Figure 5.

Figure 8. Thyroid gland of child with accessory muscles.

*Figures 3 and 4 are from a reconstruction by Dr. H. D. Kistler, awarded a gold medal by the International Jury of Awards, L. P. E., St. Louis, 1904.

XLVIII

THE X-RAY EXAMINATION OF THE MASTOID REGION.*

By Samuel Iglauer, B. S., M. D.,

ASSOCIATE PROFESSOR OF OTOLOGY, LARYNGOLOGY AND RHINOL-
OGY, OHIO-MIAMI MEDICAL COLLEGE, UNIVERSITY
OF CINCINNATI,

CINCINNATI.

In many branches of medicine and surgery the Roentgen rays have become almost indispensable as an aid to diagnosis, and frequently the nature of some obscure condition is absolutely determined by the radiogram. The value of radiography has become well established in the field of rhinology, especially in the examination of the accessory cavities of the nose, so that sinusitis, or tumors of the antrum of Highmore, of the ethmoids, and the frontal sinus, can be definitely outlined. Radiography in rhinology not only lays bare pathologic conditions, but also gives valuable aid in outlining anatomic relations, so that the surgeon may proceed with greater assurance in opening these cavities when they are diseased. Thus Beck[1], after obtaining an exact outline of the frontal sinus in the skiagram, turns down the anterior wall of the sinus and subsequently replaces it by a plastic operation. Ingalls[2] does not hesitate to drill into this cavity by the nasal route, after he has determined its anatomic position in the radiogram. To Caldwell[3] belongs the credit of having established the proper angle for the delineation of both frontal sinuses upon the same plate.

In exposing the temporal bone to radiographic examination, greater obstacles are to be met with than in examining the sinuses and bones of the face, because it is difficult to obtain a profile of one temporal bone without superimposing upon it

*Thesis presented to the American Laryngological, Rhinological and Otological Society, January 1st, 1909.

the shadow of the other. In fact, the chief difficulty in radiography of the cranium is to establish the proper angle at which the picture is to be taken, in order to avoid the shadows of the thicker portion of the skull.

Thus Voss[4] and Winckler[5], by taking pictures in the transverse diameter of the skull, report excellent results in outlining the mastoid region as well as determining its condition of health or disease.

Kuhne[6] and Plagemann[7] prefer taking pictures in the occipito-frontal direction, since thereby an image of both mastoid processes is obtained at one time and upon the same plate. Judging from the illustrations accompanying their article this method is open to objection, since the temporal bone is too far removed from the plate to give a sharp image, and only a portion of the mastoid process appears in the Roentgen picture.

Considering the difficulties frequently encountered in diagnosticating diseases of the mastoid process, it has for some time past seemed advisable to me to obtain radiograms of the mastoid region; and I was fortunate in having an expert radiologist, Dr. S. Lange, kind enough to undertake this work. To him I am indebted not only for his untiring efforts, but also for valuable suggestions.

The greatest obstacle to be overcome was in establishing the proper angle from which uniform results might be expected. At my suggestion the oblique profile of the temporal region was employed. Subsequently Dr. Lange suggested taking measurements of the angle of inclination of the X-ray diaphragm, so that greater precision might be had. These points will be further elucidated in describing the technic.

We have taken radiograms of the dry skull, of the cadaver and of a considerable number of patients. In all we have collected about fifty plates.

TECHNIC.

The technic is as follows:.

A small piece of lead foil is plastered to the tip of the mastoid process in order to fix this point in the Roentgen picture. For the same reason a coil of wire is introduced into the auditory meatus. The auricle is then drawn forward and fastened by adhesive plaster to the cheek of the patient in order to hold it away from the mastoid region. The patient then lies on his side on the table, or sits upon a chair, with the ear to be examined in contact with the photographic plate. The diaphragm of the X-ray tube is then adjusted immediately below the parietal eminence on the opposite side of the patient's head, and is given a slant, so that the rays will be directed through the cranium toward the sigmoid sinus and mastoid process of the ear which is being radiographed. (See Figs. 1 and 3.) In this position, the temporal bone on the upper side of the skull is left almost entirely out of the radiographic field. Dr. Lange has measured the angle of inclination of the axis of the diaphragm and finds it to be as follows:

First, it is inclined 25 degrees to the basal plane of the skull, and secondly, it is tilted backward 20 degrees from the coronal plane of the skull. (See Fig. 1.) This step of the technic is very important because it assures uniform results.

The time of exposure varies from 20 to 50 seconds with an electrolytic interrupter, to 4 minutes with a mercury turbine interrupter. For comparison it is advisable to radiograph both temporal bones at the same sitting.

Figure 2 shows a quarter section of the dry skull, in which some of the landmarks are brought out by filling them with lead foil. This experiment enables the observer to fix the anatomic relations in subsequent pictures. This radiogram shows very well the internal structure and relations of the temporal bone and requires no further description.

The next illustration (Fig. 3) shows the mastoid region traced from a radiogram taken through the entire skull. The anatomic structures are here very distinct, and it will be observed that the one mastoid is entirely out of the field

Figures 4 and 5 are tracings from radiograms of normal mastoid regions in different patients. It is impossible to reproduce some of these plates except by tracings. These illustrations show the relative position of the middle fossa of the skull, the outline and cellular arrangement of the mastoid process, the position of the external auditory canal and frequently of the sigmoid sinus.

As may be judged from the illustrations, practically all of the skiagrams delineate very accurately the anatomic relations of the mastoid process. Considering the great variability in the structure of the temporal bone, it is apparent how valuable this knowledge obtained prior to an operation may become. Indeed, should radiography give no further information than this, it would still repay the otologist to obtain those Roentgen pictures. As a matter of fact, however, the skiagrams reveal not only anatomic relations, but also, in some cases, pathologic processes in the interior of the mastoid process.

In certain cases of chronic suppurative otitis media the radiograms showed practically an absence of mastoid cells, the sclerosed bone throwing a dense shadow. Such pictures were obtained in five cases. (See Fig. 6 and 7.) In four instances the Roentgen pictures were confirmed by operation.

In one case, that of a man 21 years, with chronic otorrhea, osteosclerosis was diagnosticated in the right ear, with the probable absence of mastoid cells. (Fig. 7.) The left ear taken at the same time for comparison, showed a massively developed pneumatic process. Operation revealed a dense mastoid process with a very small antrum, which was only uncovered after working according to the method of Stacke.

A second operative case was that of a boy of twelve, with chronic suppuration in the left ear. The sinus, the tegmen tympani and the mastoid process were found exactly in the condition indicated by the picture. (Fig. 8.)

The third case was one of tuberculosis of the middle ear in a man of forty-five. The two radiograms, taken at intervals before the operation, showed a very large mastoid process of penumatic type with hazy outlines of its cells. Operation revealed a large mastoid process with numerous large cells, most of which were filled with a clear serous fluid. The middle ear and antrum contained granulations. (Fig. 9.)

The fourth case was operated upon too recently for description.

From the experience gained by this investigation, the following conclusions may be drawn:

First. It is quite feasible to radiograph the mastoid region.

Second. The best skiagrams are obtained by directing the rays so as to give a slightly oblique profile of the temporal region.

Third. The radiogram distinctly outlines the anatomic relations of the external anditory meatus, the limits of the mastoid process and of the mastoid cells. The floor of the middle fossa of the skull is shown, as well as the thickness of the tegmen tympani. The sigmoid sinus is frequently delineated and its position indicated.

Fourth. Osteosclerosis of the mastoid bone, following prolonged otorrhea, may in some cases be determined by the X-ray examination.

Fifth. It is possible that pus and granulations (Voss), as well as sequestra (Winckler), in the mastoid process can be diagnosticated by means of the X-ray. It must be stated, however, that acute inflammataion of the mucosa is difficult to differentiate from softening of the bone (Plagemann).

Sixth. In general it may be stated that radiography should prove of great value in the determination of both the anatomic and pathologic conditions within the temporal bone.

BIBLIOGRAPHY.

1. Jos. Beck. Jour. Am. Med. Assoc., August 8, 1908.

2. E. Fletcher Ingals. Jour. Amer. Med. Assoc., May 9, 1908.

3. E. W. Caldwell. Amer. Quar. of Roentgenology, January, 1907.

4. O. Vos. Verhand. der Deutsch. Otologischen Gesellschaft, May, 1907. Reprint pub. by Gustav Fischer in Jena. Also Ref. Zeitschrift f. Orenheilkunde. Bd. LIV. Heft 2, p. 208, July, 1907.

5. Winckler. Zeitschrift f. Ohrenheilkunde. Bd. LIV. Heft 2, p. 209, July 1, 1907.

6. Kuhne and Plagemann. Fortschritte auf dem Gebiete der Roentgenstrahlen. Bd. XII. Heft 5, September 1, 1908.

7. Plagemann. Verhand. der Deutsch. Roentgen-Gesellschaft. Bd. IV. September, 1908.

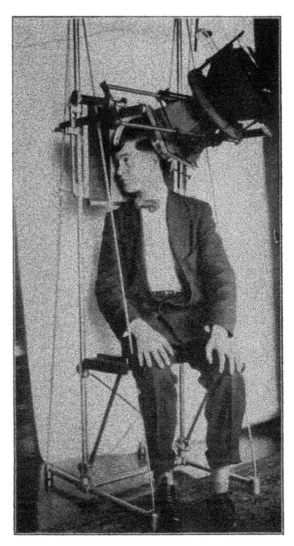

FIGURE I.

Radiography of Mastoid Region, showing relative positions of plate, X-ray diaphragm and patient's head. Note the inclination of the X-ray diaphragm. (The radiograms may be taken to advantage with the patient lying on his side, but with the diaphragm in the same relative position as in Fig. I.)

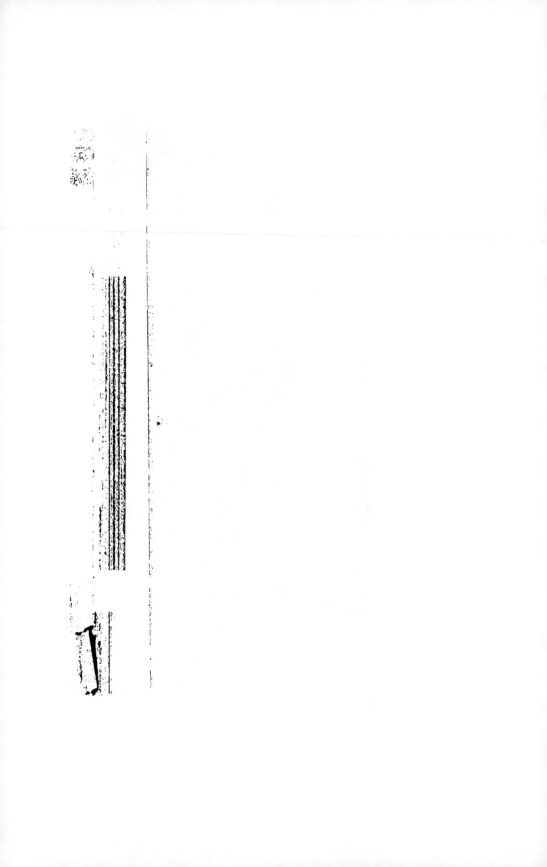

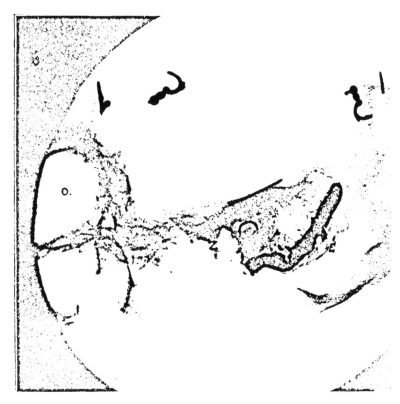

FIGURE II.

Quarter section of a skull with lead foil in the sinus, and a
in the auditory meatus and in the middle fossa. (P F) Post
fossa. (E) Foramen for emissary vein. (Arrow) Indicates des⸱
ing portion of facial canal. (O) Orbit. (Z) Zygoma.

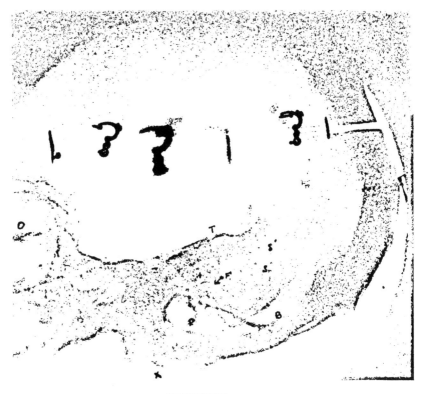

FIGURE III.

Radiogram of a dry skull, showing left mastoid region taken in an oblique profile. The lower shadow (X) is the right mastoid thrown out of the field by the oblique direction of the X-rays. (M) Meatus. (T) Tegmen. (SS) Sinus. (P) Styloid process. (Arrow) Facial canal, in the mastoid. (Z) Zygoma. (O) Orbit. (B) Floor of post-fossa.

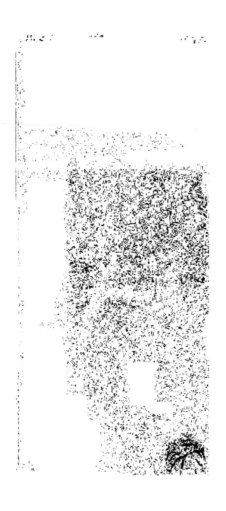

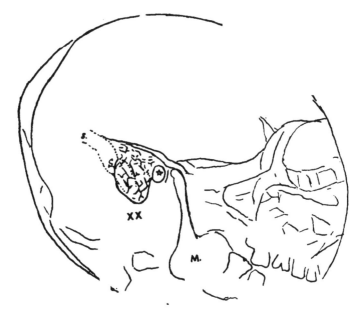

FIGURE IV.

Print and tracing from plate of a normal mastoid region in a young woman. (*) Meatus. (X) Mastoid cells. (SS) Sinus. (M) Mandible. (E) Middle fossa.

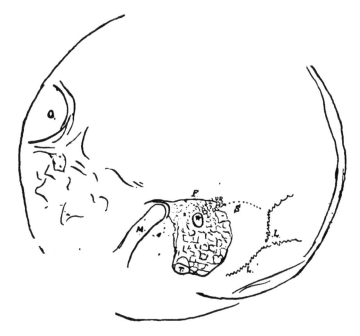

FIGURE V.

Tracing from a radiogram of a normal, left mastoid in a man of
37. (*) Meatus. (T) Large cell in the mastoid tip. (F) Middle
fossa. (S) Sinus (?). (LL) Suture lines. (M) Mandible. (O)
Orbit.

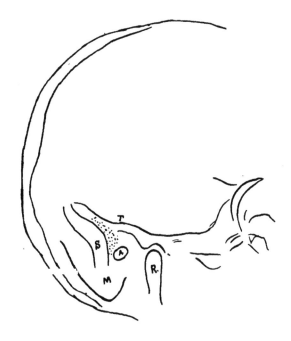

FIGURE VI

Tracing from a radiogram. Right mastoid region in a case of chronic otorrhea of many years' standing. Note absence of mastoid cells, i. e., osteosclerosis. (S) Forward-lying sinus. (M) Mastoid. (A) Meatus. (T) Tegmen. (R) Ascending ramus of mandible. (Patient of Dr. William Mithoefer.)

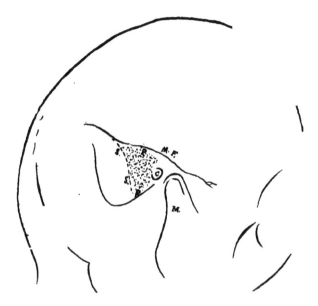

FIGURE VII.

(Case I.) L. K. Right mastoid region, showing: (PP) Osteosclerosis of mastoid. (SS) Sigmoid sinus. (M) Mandible. (MF) Middle fossa. (C) Meatus. (Confirmed by operation.)

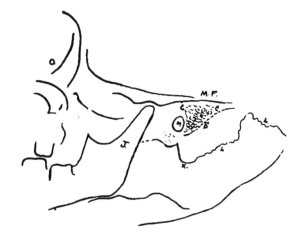

FIGURE VIII.

(Case II.) Tracing from a radiogram. Left mastoid region. (M)
Meatus. (MF) Middle fossa. (CC) Mastoid cells. (S) Anterior
border of sinus. (J) Mandible. (LL) Suture lines. (O) Orbit.
(X) Top of mastoid.

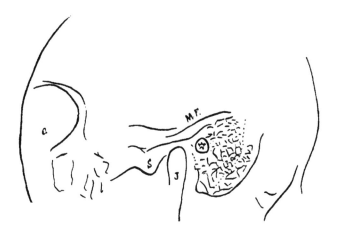

FIGURE IX.

(Case III.) Radiogram tracing tuberculosis of middle ear and mastoid. Large mastoid of pneumatic type. Cells appear hazy in the radiogram. (Confirmed by operation.) (*) Meatus. (S) Zygoma. (O) Orbit. (MF) Middle fossa. (J) Mandible.

XLIX.

REMARKS ON THE PHYSIOLOGY AND DEVELOPMENT OF THE NOSE AND ACCESSORY SINUSES AND NASAL REFLEXES, WITH SPECIAL REFERENCE TO THE FUNCTION AND IMPORTANCE OF THE TURBINATED BODIES.

By Henry J. Hartz, M. D.,

Detroit.

The nose constitutes a protective mechanism important for the economy of the body. Its physiologic significance is underestimated, especially during infancy and childhood, when the nasal organ is more or less predisposed to inflammatory obstruction.

Disse, the embryologist, and others have demonstrated that the nasal passages of the child differ in relative size and form from those of the adult; for while in the infant at birth the ethmoidal portion of the nasal space is twice as high as that of the maxillary portion, in the adult they are of equal height. Somewhere near the eighth year the nasal space assumes relative adult proportions, the maxillary portion equals in height that of the ethmoidal portion, and with this growth and the descent of the hard palate, the nostrils develop slowly.

Figure 1 shows a section of a fetus eight months old, by Mihalkovics, to represent the difference in height of the ethmoidal and maxillary part of the nasal chamber. The ethmoidal is twice the height of the maxillary portion of the nares.

During the first three years respiration is confined chiefly to the upper ethmoidal portion, the lower portion being very narrow and the inferior turbinated bone touching the floor of the nose. (See Figure 1.)

In this manner we may account for the dangers of acute inflammation of the nares in the infant, which become distressing and dangerous on account of interference with proper feeding and oxygenation.

Figure 2 shows a frontal section of the facial structure of a child four years old, by Mihalkovics, showing an undeveloped lower nasal chamber; the ethmoidal part of the nasal fossae is still larger than the maxillary part.

Figure 3 is Mihalkovics' frontal section of the facial structure of an adult, showing the development of both the maxillary and ethmoidal part of the nose, they being equal in height.

Figure 4 is Chiari's section of a newly born infant, showing the predominence of the cranium over that of the face, and the ethmoidal nasal space over the maxillary. The face, while helping to form the orbit and nasal cavity, is essential for the jaws and teeth. The greatest change is the downward growth of the face. In the infant the face is to the cranium as one to eight; at two years as one to six; at five years, as one to four; at ten years, as one to three; and in the adult, as one to two.

DEVELOPMENT OF HEAD AND FACE.

The head and face grow more rapidly in two periods. The first is from birth to the eighth year. The second begins at puberty, or at the fifteenth year, when the head and face develop in all directions alike, and are completed in the female about the nineteenth year; and in the male at about the age of twenty-one. During the intervening period, from the seventh to the fifteenth year, much less growth takes place. The development of the child's face may be divided into three stages. During the first year the development of the head and face is general, but the face gains distinctively on the cranium, more especially in the lower nasal cavity. The second stage is ushered in at the second year, to continue to the fifth year, when the face grows more in breadth. From the fifth to the seventh year the face grows more in length, while the nose develops chiefly in the lower region. The hard palate, forming the floor of the nose, descends to increase the dimensions of the space above. At birth, the hard palate, if prolonged back, would strike near the junction of the basillar process and sphenoid. At the age of three it has grown downward to strike near the middle of the basillar process, and at the age of six it may be seen on the plane with the edge of the foramen magnum, which is nearly the relationship of the adult palate. The choanae, likewise, exhibit changes indicative of palate descent. At birth the height of their cavities is about six mm., and the breadth a little more. At the first year it has doubled, at the second year its height has increased more rapidly and has changed from a circular to an oblong channel; at the seventh year its perpendicular axis is twice the length of the horizontal and has assumed at this early time the relative adult form.

DEVELOPMENT OF THE NARES.

We have said the nasal spaces increase in size by the downward growth of the hard palate.

Figure 5 shows section of a child's nasal space at the age of three years, having developed so that the maxillary portion represents one-third and the ethmoidal portion two-thirds of the nasal cavity. The mouth of the eustachian tube is on an even plane with the hard palate.

Figure 6 is a section of a child's nasal space at the age of three years, having developed so that the maxillary portion of the nares represents little more than one-third, while the ethmoidal portion occupies the remainder. The mouth of the eustachian tube is on an even plane with the hard palate

Figure 7 is a section of child's nasal space at the age of eight years, showing that the nasal chamber has developed so that the maxillary part equals that of the ethmoidal. The palate has grown downward and the eustachian tube is above the plane of the palate

In proof of this it may be seen that in the embryo the hard palate is above the level of the mouths of the eustachian tubes, while in the newborn it lies on an even plane, and later, about the eighth year, considerably below it. (See Figs. 5, 6 and 7.) The nasal space is lengthened by the growth of the pa'ate in the anteroposterior direction, and by the development of the alveolar process, which affords space for three molar teeth, and which has its beginning near the seventh year, to be comp'eted at the time of full dentition. This development of the nasal space in the anteroposterior direction pushes the maxillary bone forward and causes the orthognathous face of the child to assume the more prognathous form. A notable development of the nares takes place with the eruption of the milk teeth, when the superior maxillary bone, which is very vascular, increases in its dimensions and gives rise to the formation óf the maxillary sinus.

Unlike other bones, those of the face are not developed from cartilage, þut are produced within sheets of connective tissue, and are, therefore, spoken of as arising by intramembranous development. At birth the body of the superior maxillary bone consists almost entirely of the alveolar process, the'sockets of the teeth being in contact with the orbital p!ate. However, the growth of the face takes place simultaneously with that of the maxilla by the formation of spongy bone between the alveolar process and the orbital plate of the maxilla, and in this way the alveolar process, along with the teeth, becomes separated from the orbital plate. Coincident with the increase in the cancellous tissue upon the facial and dental aspects of the bone, a process of absorption apparently takes place upon its nasal and orbital surfaces, which causes the formation of the sinus and the broadening of the nasal chambers. This simultaneous process of growth and absorption continues until the eruption of the wisdom'teeth, at about the twenty-fifth year of life, when the antrum reaches its complete adult form.

THE TURBINATED BODIES AND NASAL MUCOSA.

These soft structures are under control of the vasomotor and cerebrospinal system of nerves, and are, therefore, capable of assuming (through the action of dilator and constrictor nerves) different degrees of turgescense in response to local stimulation of whatever nature. The membranes respond physiologically to meet variations of climate, and supply humidity, warmth and filtration to the air.

Figure 8 is Spalteholz's lateral section of the nasal chambers, showing the sphenopalatine ganglion nerve distribution to the turbinals, the anterior ethmoidal nerve to the mucosa, and the distribution of the nerve of smell.

In winter time the blood vessels of the membranes enlarge and supply heat sufficient to raise the temperature of cold air 12 degrees C., during the transit from nose to pharynx. Conversely, in summer time, during the hot weather, or by strong light, the nasal mucosa contracts to a thin membrane, while the erectile tissue maintains its normal state of partial venous congestion. During dry weather or in heated houses the mucous membrane furnishes sufficient moisture to nearly saturate the air.

Figure 9 is a section of nasal mucosa from the floor of the nose, by Schiefferdecker, exhibiting the plasma channels, through which numerous leucocytes are passing. The first layer is of the columnar type, and below is represented the basement membrane, and the numerous canals which furnish lymphlike moisture in abundance, and few of which are seen perforating the basement membrane

The moisture is derived from the plasma channels that connect directly with the lymph system. While its source is probably the lymphatic system, and also the product of some special cells, its specific gravity is less than that of lymph fluid. The perforating canaliculi carry the fluid to the surface of the membranes in such liberal quantities that the structure is literally held in suspension. Especially is this true of the ciliary layer of the epithelium, which carries on its highly specialized activity under the same fluid, which possesses, besides a nutritive, also a bactericidal property.

The surfaces of the nasal membranes are constantly covered by a layer of mucus supplied from the mucous cells and the becherzellen and leucocytes. This layer of mucus entangles foreign bodies that are not arrested by the vibrissae at the entrance of the nose, and the dust and germs thus held by the sticky mucus are transported by the cilia·waves towards the choanae. The cilia activity, aided by phagocytosis and the bactericidal plasma fluid, is important to nasal integrity—nearly sterile conditions being maintained within the nasal cavity. In 80% the nasal contents have been found sterile and only a few organisms were found in the remainder. When the cilia cells are destroyed by suppurative processes or by operative procedure, they do not replace themselves, but the squamous cell without cilia action is substituted.

The erectile tissue of the turbinated bodies is found on the anterior end of the lower and middle, and the posterior end of all three bones. Its circulation is contrary to that of the tubercle of the septum, composed of veins of thick coat, stronger than arteries, deriving its vasomotor control from the sphenopalatine ganglion. The glandular structure of the erectile tissue is so scarce that its function for supplying moisture is nil, but the mucous membrane supplying the remainder of the nasal region has abundant glands for that purpose. The erectile bodies contain numerous large vascular spaces, forming a cavernous plexus, formed by the arterioles breaking up into capillaries. The venous sinuses thus formed have thick walls and contain much muscular tissue, which upon contraction empties these vascular spaces of their contents. The bone and membrane of the inferior turbinate are intimately connected, the nutrient blood vessels perforate the bone, so that in event of hypertrophy or atrophy both structures are affected alike.

Figure 10 is a histologic section of the mucosa of the middle turbinated body, by Schiefferdecker, showing the ciliated epithelium with the basement membrane. Leucocytes are seen traversing the intracellular spaces. The perforating canaliculi, carrying fluid to the epithelium, are represented by the clear channels passing through the basement membrane. The becherzellen, furnishing mucus, are seen between the long spaces in the region of the cilia layer. The leucocytes, represented by the dark cells, seem for a normal membrane to be in excess. The cellular activity of the cilia is carried on under fluid supplied by the plasma canals.

Figure 11 is transverse section of the lower turbinated body from the posterior end, by Schiefferdecker, showing the erectile tissue composed of arteries dividing into capillaries, and these in turn into veins, which form the large vascular spaces, also termed venous sinuses. The lowest line points where a vein is in communication with a sinus. The vascular spaces are veins, with coats stronger than arteries, and supplied with muscular fibers. The mucous membrane of the middle turbinated body is thinner and blends with the periosteum, while in the inferior region it is separated from it by a thick vascular layer.

The turbinated bodies, more especially their erectile tissue, and the tubercle of the septum have the function of regulating the inspiration by offering physiologic resistance, by their normally swollen and spongelike state, to each inspiration, thus affording sufficient time for moistening, warming and filtering the air. It seems probable that the lower and middle by their resistance retard expiration, and thus assist in maintaining a positive air pressure in the hypopharynx during expiration and aid in regulating the supply of residual air within the bronchial tree.

PROTECTIVE MECHANISM.

The architecture of the nose, its tortuous passages, with its moist mucous membrane and the erectile tissue of the turbinated bodies, together with the tubercle of the septum, are designed as a protective mechanism and favor the deposit of impurities of the atmosphere, such as dust and bacteria. The respiratory portion of the nose is provided with ciliated epithelium, which transports impurities towards the choanae. Nasal respiration modifies the air by moisture, warmth, and filtration, so as to render it practically sterile within the bronchial tubes and alveolar region.

The nerves of smell and taste combine to serve in the gratification of the sense of taste, the volatile substances of the food and drink reaching the olfactory region by diffusion during expiration. Zwaardemaker has well termed this the act of gustatory smelling. The olfactory and glossopharyngeal nerves in association constitute also a protection, acting as they do the part of a sentinel placed at the entrance of the alimentary and respiratory tract, giving warning of the approach of unwholesome food or unsanitary air. The sensory branches of the trifacial nerve aid in the protection against the ingress of dangerous gases or irritating air, by the involuntary closure of the nostrils, which is partly accomplished by the tubercle of the septum. an arterial erectile tissue, situated opposite to the anterior portion of the middle turbinate bone. Its situation is favorable for aiding the dilator nares in regulating the space for inspiration and by its engorgement to exclude irritating air from the nose. For that reason it has been referred to as a rheostat for the inlet of air.

THE NOSE AS A PATHWAY FOR AIR.

Atmospheric pressure acts on the body equally from all sides, and also in those internal air spaces which are in direct connection with the outer air, such as the respiratory tract, the sinuses of the frontal, superior maxillary and ethmoid bones. If such air filled space be closed off from the outer air for some time, rarefaction of the gases in the space occurs —it is followed by congestion of its membrane, as a result of the absorption of oxygen, and its replacement by a smaller volume of carbon dioxid. The air pressure in the nasal cavity during inspiration is negative, and contrarily, during expiration it is positive. In slight deformities of the septum and other structures of the nose, the air currents, creating alternating states of rarefaction and condensation of the atmosphere within the nose, easily become factors in begetting and maintaining acute and chronic states of inflammation, by partial or complete closure of the nasal lumen and the orifices of the sinuses or that of the lacrimal duct. The inspired air takes an upward curved direction into the middle and superior meatus, it traverses the olfactory region to descend toward the choanae.

Figure 12 shows Paulson's schematic representation of the pathway of air during inspiration. Partial vacuum having been created within the lungs, the zone of rarefaction extends to the upper air tract, hence inspiration takes place under negative pressure. Thus the main air current influences the inspired air to take an upward curved direction toward the middle and upper meatus, traversing the olfactory region to descend to the choanae.

In its passage the air meets resistance offered by the tubercle of the septum, the erectile tissues of the turbinates and the mucous membranes of the nose, the resistance of which is sufficient to keep the air within the nasal cavity long enough to be modified.

The investigations of Kayser and Schutter reveal that there is but little difference, as far as heat and moisture are concerned, between the air inspired through the nose and that inspired through the mouth. Schutter found the air of the nose has a temperature of 33 C., and that of the mouth 32 C., and that the air of both shows a humidity of 7-9. Saturation and blood temperature of the inspired air is attained only when it reaches the bronchial tubes, this being accomplished by the glandular and vascular tissue of the oropharynx, pharynx and trachea. Thus the usually accepted theory that the nose alone serves to heat and moisten the inspired air is not borne out by experiment. While in mouth breathing, or through a tracheal canula, the air may be sufficiently moistened and warmed, it must be clear that it cannot be purified as in nasal breathing. Normally the expired air is under positive pressure and is completely saturated with moisture of blood temperature and contains CO' gas, and is 11% more voluminous than the inspired air. Unlike the negative air currents of inspiration, it does not rise, but chooses the path along the floor of the nose, there being no rarefied air currents to deflect it.

Experiments appear to corroborate the pathway. A particle of wool placed in the middle and inferior meatus yielded readily by a forceful expiration from the lower, but with difficulty from the middle meatus. The expiratory current thus meets the inferior turbinated body, which in its swollen state offers resistance to its free escape, aiding in air storage in the nasopharynx. Normally the inspiration is initiated by the descent of the diaphragm and the contraction of the chest muscles creating a partial vacuum in the lungs. By its proximity, the air nearest the zone of rarefaction is first to move, hence the air in the bronchi, the trachea, the nasopharynx, and from the middle of the nose descends before the atmospheric air gains access to the nose.

The inspiratory current, normally, is of negative pressure, which induces suction upon the accessory sinuses, and they partially empty themselves of air, producing rarefaction in all the sinuses, which, however, is equalized at the end of each inspiration to atmospheric pressure. The full inspiration being completed, expiration ensues under positive air pressure, practically in the entire air tract. The fluctuations of air pressure differ considerably.

According to Mink, of Holland, the normal during quiet inspiration is 10 mm., water negative, in the trachea; 8 mm. in the nasopharynx; 6 mm. in the middle nose and sinuses; 4 mm. in the prechoncal space and 2 mm. in the vestibule. Normal expiration is carried on under positive pressure, and the manometer registered 10 mm. water below the glottic region; 8 mm. water in the nasopharynx; 6 in the turbinal region; 4 in the preconchal space and 3 in the vestibule of the nose. If the mouth be open, then the pressure, either negative or positive, is equalized in the trachea or pharynx. Careful experiments by Mink reveal the interesting fact that when turbinates are contracted by cocain, the air pressure is reduced from 8 mm. to 4 mm. water.

Figure 13 is a diagrammatic illustration of the pathway of

the air through the nose, during expiration, after Mink, of Holland. The chamber represents the nasal cavity, b, its outlet, while c, and a, constitute an imaginary inlet and forced expiration. When tobacco smoke is gently forced into the tube, a, it is seen to move in a direct line to b, along the floor to the outlet. When, however, greater force is employed in blowing, various sizes of whirls of smoke are formed, proportional to the force. Expiratory currents of air under positive air pressure descend to the floor of the nose, while inspiration under negative pressure ascends proportional to the suction.

The same relation of air pressure exists in atrophic catarrh. This observation seems to indicate a physiologic function of the turbinated bodies, especially the inferior, namely, that by the swelling of the erectile tissue, a resistance is offered to expiration, which aids in maintaining a storage of residual air under positive pressure in the nasopharynx.

Figure 14 is a graphic illustration of the air pressure within the nose during expiration, by Mink, of Holland. When the turbinated bodies are contracted by cocain, the air pressure is reduced from 8 mm. water to 4 mm. water, revealing the physiologic significance of the swollen turbinates of maintaining a positive air pressure equal to 4 mm. water in the nasopharynx.

The spongy tissue thus assists in equalizing the amount of expired air in a unit of time, irrespective of the depth of the preceding inspiration. It may be said that the turbinates are an auxiliary to the function of the glottic constrictors, that of protecting the lower air passages, as well as maintaining automatically at all times the required amount of air in the respiratory tract for the purpose of oxygenation. The adaptability of the turbinates thus appears to have an influence in regulating the lumen of the nose, keeping up a reciprocal relation with the automatic center, which presides over the demand for oxygen for the body as a whole.

ACCESSORY SINUSES.

The accessory sinuses act in an esthetic sense as subsidiary resonators. Together with the nasal fossae they impart quality (timber) and resonance to the singing and speaking voice. The vocal effects of sopranos and contraltos differ in timber. The soprano is found to possess more often the narrow and contracted facial structure,—the dolychocephalic head with small sinuses, while the contralto has the broader face with larger accessory sinuses—the brachycephalic structure. The proximity of the cavities to the olfactory region gives rise to the theory that they aid the olfactory nerves in perception of odors. Paulson experimented to this end, and concluded that in the process of smelling, the forced inspiration sends branches of the main current of air into these various sinuses, and by diffusion aids in the perception of volatile odors.

Luschka looked upon the accessory sinuses as the reservoirs for the heated and moistened air. Actual measurement by Braune and Clasen showed that the capacity of all the sinuses was only 45 ccm. It is evident that this small amount of air as a carrier of warmth and moisture would have no effect on a current of air of at least 500 ccm. It was also thought that the cavities might have some effect on the direction of the air current during inspiration, but Paulson held that the cavities had no influence and showed that the rarefied air current within the upper part of the nasal chamber had some influence in drawing the air to the middle and superior meatus.

Figure 15 is an apparatus devised by Vohsen, of Munich, to demonstrate the ventilation process of the accessory sinuses by the nasal air currents. The apparatus is made of glass, with a soft rubber tube attachment, and a glass globe-shaped bottle, hermetically sealed, with an outlet into the glass chamber, d. By slight suction upon the soft tube at a, the niveau 6c is seen to slowly descend, simultaneously a few drops of the liquid escape at the funnel d. When the tube is released, the atmosphere at once rushes in at a, and finds its way through the funnel a, and passing through the liquid ascends to the space above the liquid 6c, which again causes a few drops of water to escape through the funnel d. The glass chamber represents the nasal space, the glass bottle represents the sinus and its orifice, the suction through the tube may be imagined to take the place of the negative air current, which causes a slight syphonage of either air or fluid.

The ventilation of the sinuses is influenced by the inspiratory currents of the nose, which being negative in pressure, causes syphonage through the orifices. At the end of each inspiration, however, the negative pressure of air in the sinuses is equalized by a sudden inrush of air to atmospheric pressure. Thus the sinuses, like the entire tract, undergo fluctuations of air pressure, changing with each inspiration and expiration from partial negative to atmospheric and then to partial positive. Their mucous membrane is continuous with that of the nose, but considerably thinner in the maxillary and frontal, and thinner still and less adherent in ethmoidal and sphenoidal regions. Their resistance to disease is less than that of other tissues, but being supplied with periosteal nutritive layers on both sides of their bony walls, rapid necrosis and formation of fistulous tracts are prevented. The mucous membranes are lined with cilia, whose activities sweep secretion toward the orifice into the nasal fossa. The membranes around the orifices are loosely adherent and tend to form folds which easily become obstructing by inflammation.

OLFACTION.

We live in a world of light and sound, but also in one of odors, says the renowned investigator Zwaardemaker, in his book on the Physiology of Olfaction. The truth of this statement is evident when our attention is called to the fact that nearly every organic body of the animal and plant kingdom has its characteristic odor. The human olfactory organ is said to be in a state of retrogression and has lost some of its original power of perception. It is related by M. Fee that some of the lower human races have retained some of their acuteness of smell that is possessed by the lower animals, and are able to anticipate the approach of and to classify their enemies by the sense of smell.

With the diminished sense of smell, the human being is still marvelously influenced by the pleasurable and the disagreeable odors conveyed by the air. The one imparts a sense of pleasure and of well being; while the other produces disgust and even illness. The pleasurable effects are accomplished reflexly through the stimulus being conveyed by the olfactory nerves alone, or in association with the sensory branches of the trigeminus to the vagus, which responds by increased function of respiration and circulation. Unpleasant odors, irritating substances, or strong electrical currents exhibit the reverse effect and produce either decreased or transient arrest of the functions of the heart and lungs.

NASAL REFLEXES.

The nose is endowed with nerve ends which have the capacity of setting in motion and of receiving a variety of reflex stimuli. Its intimate association with the sympathetic and central nervous system permits of the establishment of vasomotor reflex paths, which link the nasal organ with remote parts of the body.

A most intimate relation exists between the nasal nervous mechanism and the nerves regulating the action of the heart and lungs. The earliest investigator, Johannes Muller, announced that the respiratory apparatus, through its nerves, could be reflexly affected by a stimulus applied to the surface of the mucous membrane of any part of the body to such an extent as to cause not only convulsive movements, but also pathologic processes.

Modern physiologists have narrowed Muller's very wide interpretation of reflex action of the nose and the respiratory apparatus. A normal reflex effect demands, as its name "Reflexion" implies, a return or bending, hence a true reflex action consists of a peripheral stimulus traveling towards the centre (centripetally) along a nerve end, returning centrifugally towards the periphery. A reflex may be initiated from any part of the nasal membrane, but most effectively through the erectile tissue of the turbinated bodies. The sensory nerves of the nose are derived from the trifacial, and they are responsible for the physiological reflexes of the nose that are positively established, such as sneezing, coughing, spasm of the glottis, expiratory spasm, vasomotor, dilatation and constriction of blood vessels.

Nasal reflexes consist of three varieties and effects.

I. A peripheral stimulus of the sensory nasal nerve most frequently produces a dilatation of the vessels of the nose, seldom contraction.

2. Peripheral stimulus of a sensory nerve of the nose will be followed by a dilatation of the blood vessels of the head, while the reverse, a contraction, takes place in all other parts of the body.

3. Stimulus applied to sensory nerves of remote organs may either dilate or contract the blood vessels within the nose.

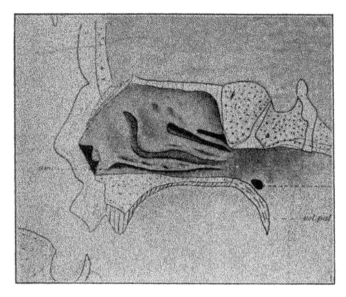

FIGURE 5.

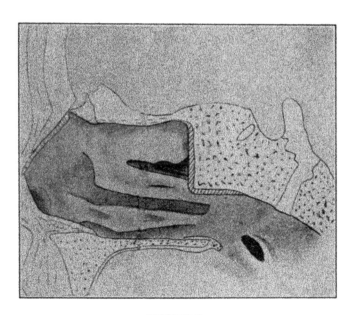

FIGURE 6.

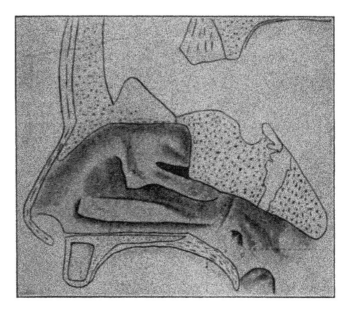

FIGURE 7.

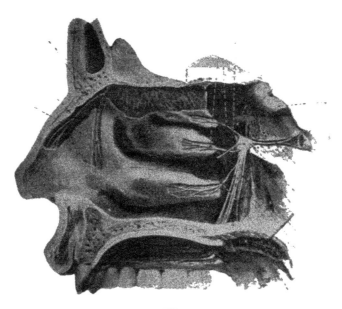

FIGURE 8.

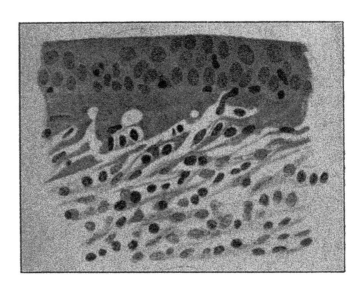

FIGURE 9.

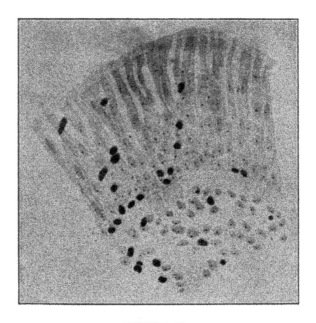

FIGURE 10.

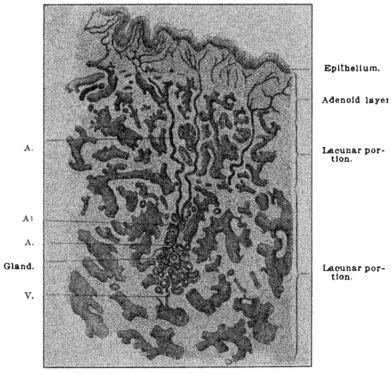

Epithelium.

Adenoid layer

Lacunar portion.

Lacunar portion.

FIGURE 11.

A represents branches of artery, perforating at A¹, which break up into capillaries in the adenoid and epithelial layer of the mucous membrane. V shows an artery communicating with one of the vascular spaces.

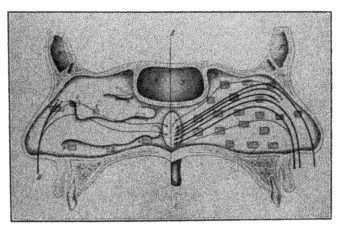

FIGURE 12.

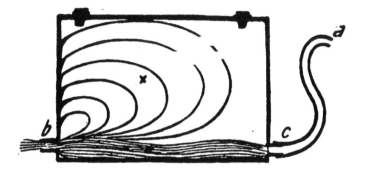

FIGURE 13.

a. Soft rubber tube atachment.
c. Opening into chamber.
b. Outlet of chamber.

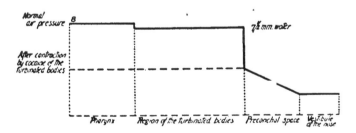

FIGURE 14.

d

m

x

FIGURE 15.

a. Soft rubber tube.
b.c. Niveau.

d. Opening into.
m. Glass chamber.

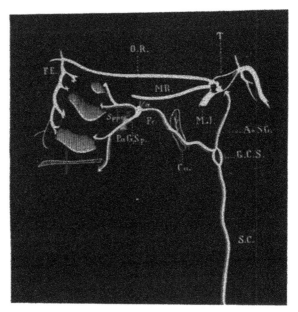

FIGURE 16.

Diagrammatic representation of the communication of the three divisions of the 'fifth or trifacial nerve and branches, with the sympathetic nerve and the gasserian, the sphenopalatine and superior cervical ganglion. These nerves serve to establish a vasomotor reflex path between the nasal organ and remote paths. (By François Franck.)

T. Trigeminus or trifacial nerve.
O. R. Ophthalmic division.
F. E. Ethmoidal nerve supplying the mucosa.
M. R. Superior maxillary division.
G. S. P. Ganglion sphenopalatinum.

S. C. Sympathetic nerve.
G. C. S. Ganglion cervical superior.
An. S. G. Connecting the sympathetic nerve with the Gasserian ganglion.
M. T. Inferior maxillary division.

THE PRESENT STATUS OF THE TONSIL OPERA-
TION: A COLLECTIVE INVESTIGATION.*

By George L. Richards, M. D.,

OTOLOGIST AND LARYNGOLOGIST TO THE FALL RIVER, UNION
AND ST. ANNE'S HOSPITALS,

FALL RIVER, MASS.

This paper is based on 130 replies to a series of questions
addressed to prominent laryngologists in this country and
Europe, and on such of the recent literature as covers certain
of the same points concerning which information was
requested.

The questions to be considered are: the physiologic function of the tonsil, the use of chemical caustics in its treatment,
its relation to tuberculosis and the cervical glands, its relation
to rheumatism, indications for its removal, the choice of
operation, the necessity of re-operation, present technic, and
the question of hemorrhage connected with the operation.

I wish to express my thanks to all those who so carefully
and conscientiously replied to my questions. I regret that
the length of the paper precludes the possibility of giving them
all individual credit. Certain of them will be referred to by
name, and the results of the work of all will be found incorporated in the body of the paper.

I have commented somewhat on the various opinions and
stated my own views, which I wish to qualify in advance by
the statement that as the arc of the circle which any one man's
experience subtends is necessarily small, too much weight
must not be given to any one person's opinion until experience
has proved or disproved its value.

*Presented before the American Laryngological, Rhinological
and Otological Society at its annual meeting held in Atlantic City,
N. J., May 31, June 1-2, 1909.

PHYSIOLOGY.

Only 77 attempted to answer the question "What is the function of the tonsil?" in any way whatsoever. The general tenor of these answers seems to show that few laryngologists have troubled themselves very much about the physiology of the tonsil or its value as an organ in the throat, being mostly concerned with its removal or treatment when manifestly abnormal. Having discovered that apparently its removal in no sense prejudices or endangers the life of the individual, but, on the contrary, that most cases of removal have been to the decided advantage of the individual, they have assumed that its value in the normal physiologic economy is practically very slight, whatever it may be theoretically.

Thirty-four considered the tonsil of value when normal, as an arrestor of the entrance of pathogenic organisms. In early life it assists leucocytosis and gives off phagocytes, but when diseased it loses its function and serves to spread disease. Seven considered it as a lymphatic gland of no special function, and nine as a producer of white cells when in a state of health. Ten considered that it has no further function or any physiologic value; four that it secretes an antitoxin and furnishes moisture to assist deglutition in the throat, and five considered its function unknown.

Goodale considers the function of the tonsil to be identical with that of the cervical lymph nodes, of which it is the distal unit. He regards the tonsils as constituting protective organs, not in the sense of themselves producing phagocytic leucocytes, but rather as representing unusually open channels of communication between the interior of the organism and its exterior, along which polynuclear leucocytes make their way from the blood vessels to the surface of the mucous membrane[1]. In normal tonsils, both of men and also animals, large mononuclear phagocytes are present, which appear to be derived from a proliferation of the endothelial cells of the reticulum[2].

Price Brown, of Toronto, considers that the tonsil is probably of the same nature, though not the same, as the thyroid and thymus glands, effecting some change in metabolism.

Dr. Jonathan Wright very kindly replied somewhat in detail to my question as to the physiologic function of the tonsil, and as he has given considerable attention to the subject, I present in very nearly his own language his views, quoting from recent papers as well as from his personal communication:'·'

"It is a very definite organ, and in the human race is the most highly developed of all the lymph glands, having an extent and a complexity, considering the whole faucial and laryngeal ring, entirely in excess of any other local aggregate of lymphoid tissue, except the spleen.

"If its normal state is one of comparatively little obstruction to the passage of food and air, such a condition varies between wide limits of volume, and it is impossible to draw any line between the minute structure of the normal and that of the abnormal in size.

"The enlargement becomes pathogenic, or less accurately pathologic, only when it injures the system more by its presence than it assists in whatever physiologic acts of assimilation or defense it may have to perform.

"Many large tonsils exist from childhood to old age without in the least being either a source of danger or even of inconvenience. Their existence, even when originating in temporary disturbance of the organism (inflammation?) may not subsequently be a menace to health.

"Of course, they may and frequently do reach such a size as to injure the patient's health. From their size they may really cut off the proper air supply; the irritation of their presence in the fauces may excite constant hyperemia and paresthesia, etc., but all these classical symptoms by constant iteration have been much exaggerated. There are a large number of children, especially in the country, who are never inconvenienced in the slightest by moderately projecting discrete faucial and pharyngeal and lymphoid hypertrophies.

"The pits of the tonsils are retorts in which the germs are either destroyed or modified so that they may live at peace with their host, or they are allowed to pass through only in such numbers as can be dealt with by internal processes without the destruction of the host.

"From various clinical facts, it seems likely it is the small, sunken, ragged tonsil, and not the large tonsil, which lets through the dangerous germs.

"Whatever may be the conclusions as to their marked enlargement, the knowledge derived from all these sources and the experimental evidence unite in pointing to the function of the tonsil as one of defense against infection. The tendency to enlargement seems a persistence of the process by which the function was evolved.

"It has been shown that dust or inanimate matter passes through the tonsillar epithelium. It has been shown that oil globules, at once saponified when applied, also readily pass. It has been shown that bacteria of the same size as the dust and oil globules do not readily pass, though constantly in contact with the epithelium of the tonsillar crypts It has been noted that dust (carmin) particles when applied, pass through the layer of bacteria on the surface and on into the tonsillar structure without carrying in any of the bacteria. Yet we know that under certain conditions bacteria, especially the pathogenic bacteria, do pass through the epithelium of the tonsils and of the intestines. I have attempted to show from collateral evidence that this action probably arises from the difference between the potentials of surface tension of the epithelial cell on the one hand, and that of the bacterium and the dust particle on the other. Since one is a living colloid state of matter and the other is so-called inert matter, we could hardly expect any other experimental result than has been obtained. How has this distinction arisen in the animal organism? I have attempted to show that the one kind of matter being often harmful and the other kind of matter usually harmless, evolution, by natural selection or otherwise, has stepped in, and in the phenomena exhibited by the tonsil we find evidence of its influence.

"The experiments of Loeb furnish a possible physical explanation of just how the difference of potential comes about, whereby at one time the streptococcus or the staphylococcus pyogenes, for instance, is excluded and at other times (cold taking, infection, etc.) is allowed to enter. For, knowing as we do that these germs and perhaps others are more or less constantly found on the surface of the tonsil when in health, and beneath the surface in disease, we must have some sort of an explanation of how this surface tension may be made to vary."

In Dr. Wright's personal communication he states that he does not think we can speak of the function or the physiology of the tonsil in the usual acceptation of the meaning of these terms. He attempts to discuss not the function or the physiology of the tonsil, but rather the part it plays in the process of infection and immunity. He says, "It seems hardly possible to explain the selective action of the tonsillar epithelium upon dust and upon bacteria, at times preventing the latter from passing and at times allowing them to pass into the lymph channels, from laws revealed by the usual work on immunity. This is almost exclusively concerned with what happens to the bacteria after they come in contact with internal body fluids. The problems belong chiefly to biophysics. Consequently, it seemed necessary that the dynamic phenomena exhibited in the process of absorption of bacteria from the surface of the tonsil should be studied in the same way as we study other phenomena of osmosis, but evidently we have here to do with living matter which obeys the laws of heredity and evolution, and if these are left out of account, the solution of our problem is hopeless.

"For instance, a bacteriolysin might perhaps destroy bacteria after they pass the epithelium, though the microscopic evidences are not suggestive of this; but no bacteriolysin can explain why they pass in or why they are kept out. This, which is at the very beginning of all we want to know, has been all but completely neglected in the work on immunity.

"Adaptation by natural selection or otherwise must eventually occur to one as the explanation why the protoplasm of the cells of the epithelium of the tonsillar crypts acts in the way it does. The colloid of cells is in the colloid state by virtue of the surface tension on the molar or molecular masses of protoplasm of which they are made up. The same is true of the bacterial cells lying in contact with the cryptal cells."

George B. Wood has published several papers on the histology and physiology of the faucial tonsil. In his latest paper he states that the faucial tonsil is covered by stratified squamous cells, the structure of the tonsil resembling somewhat that of a lymph gland, differing, however, in that it possesses no afferent lymph vessels and no periglandular sinuses, and does possess those peculiar structures, the crypts or lacunae. The crypt of the tonsil is its most peculiar and characteristic structure, and consists of an invagination of the surface of the epithelium, which has undergone a very interesting anatomic change The subepithelial connective tissue which exists beneath the surface epithelium, disappears as soon as the epithelium starts to form the crypts. This permits the epithelium to come into direct contact with the lymphatic structure of the tonsil, and very frequently it is impossible to distinguish a dividing line between the epithelium of the crypt and the interfollicular tissue. This epithelium does not form a compact, unbroken barrier of protection. For the greater part of its extent it presents an intact line, possibly three cells in thickness, and there are occasional spaces between these cells.

In the crypt, then, we have a loose disintegrated epithelium which, so far as any mechanical barrier is concerned, presents an open door to microbic infection, and it has been shown that minute inert foreign bodies readily pass between the cells. In the faucial tonsils the gross arrangement of the crypts is such that frequently they form pockets and recesses capable of retaining large numbers of bacteria which find plenty of nourishment in the desquamating epithelium.

Hence, it would seem that unless the vital resistance is considerably greater in the tonsil than in the surrounding structures, the tonsillar tissue ought to be the vulnerable spot in the throat. This being the case, it was thought possible that there might be developed in the tonsil certain antibodies which would make this structure especially resistant to germ invasion. Experiments to determine this were carried out, but they resulted in failure to find immune bodies in the tonsil, due either, Dr. Wood states, to a lack of sensitiveness in the technic, or to the simple fact that the reasoning concerning this subject has been false, or it may be that soluble substances are so easily removed by both the blood vessels and lymph channels that immune bodies as well as the toxins and antitoxins cannot accumulate in the tonsil. The blood supply of the tonsil is fairly rich, and the efferent lymph stream is a decided entity, so that a soluble substance could probably not remain long in the tonsillar structure. The rapid and marked systemic intoxication seen in cases of simple tonsillitis shows that some toxins, at least, are readily absorbed from the tonsil into the general circulation, and it is more than probable that the first general symptoms are due to toxic absorption through the blood vessels. The slowness of the lymphatic method of infection is shown by the fact that enlargement and tenderness of the tonsillar lymph gland at the angle of the jaw is not always present in simple tonsillitis, and is almost never present at the- very beginning of the attack. This failure to find any considerable amount of immune bodies in the tonsillar tissue as has been indicated, leaves us still uncertain as to the degree of vital resistance of the tonsillar structure.

As the lymph chain of the neck presents a rather formidable barrier against the invasion of microorganisms, the large majority of patients suffering from microbic infection of the tonsil pass through the disease without any true bacteremia'.

F. H. Bosworth has contended for many years that the tonsil is not a physiologic organ but a diseased process which practically constitutes a morbid growth or tumor, and should be thoroughly removed in the same manner as any other tumor, whether it be fibroid, malignant or any other'. In his answer to me he adds: "Incalculable miscief has resulted from the early anatomists describing it as a normal organ of the body."

In accord with this is the observation of Spohn that in the throat of the healthy child there are practically no tonsils. He examined one hundred infants soon after birth, and not one had a tonsil that was perceptible. There was no elevation, not even a roughness between the pillars of the fauces'. This observation, being made by the sense of touch only, can not be considered as definite, as the tonsil may be so small in the infant as not to be evident to the sense of touch or sight.

On the other hand, the anatomic work of Mosher, based on the examination of embryos of four, five, six and seven months and full term infants effactually disproves the statement that the tonsil is absent at birth. The reason that it is overlooked in the newborn child may be due to its position, since at birth the tonsillar opening and the tonsil are practically horizontal, and at such time the tonsil is more a part of the palate than of the wall of the pharynx. As the face grows downward, the tonsil also grows downward, forward and inward'.

DIRECT OR APPARENTLY DIRECT RELATION BETWEEN ENLARGED CERVICAL GLANDS AND THE TONSIL.

One hundred and seventeen personal reports were positive as to this point; namely, that there is a direct relation between the two, the tonsil being apparently the gland through which the infecting agent comes, as evidenced by the cessation of the adenitis after removal of the tonsils.

Five observers did not know of any relation between the two. This statement is the more remarkable, considering the fact that two of the observers, Professor Chiari and Seth Scott Bishop, are men of large experience, and it would seem that the import of the question must have been misunderstood by them, as it would seem hardly possible that they have never seen cases of cervical adenitis which were apparently of tonsillar origin.

The anatomic investigations of Poirier and Wood have shown that the lymphatic drainage of the faucial tonsil runs directly to the upper deep cervical glands, which glands by a rich system of anastomosis are connected by efferents and afferents with practically all the lymph glands of the neck and head. The tonsillar lymph gland is generally situated just below the posterior belly of the digastric where it crosses the anterior border of the sternomastoid. This spot is located just behind and below the angle of the jaw, and in tuberculous adenitis of the neck it is this gland which is almost invariably the first one to become enlarged, the others being involved subsequently'.

It would seem, therefore, as though this question had been sufficiently determined to admit of this relation being stated as a positive fact. That following the removal of the tonsil there may be in some instances—as was stated by two or three reporters—at first an enlargement of the immediate glands, followed later by their subsidence, is an undoubted fact, and has been observed by me on several occasions. This is easily accounted for by the traumatism from the operation, with the resulting direct absorption for a short time of more or less material from the throat and consequent gland enlargement. The observation made by Chambers, that infected cervical glands are always accompanied by large tonsils, is hardly warranted. On the contrary, the investigations of Jonathan Wright and Lee M. Hurd have shown that in some cases of cervical adenitis the tonsil itself may be quite small and belong to the submerged type.

Goodale has treated cervical lymphadenitis by the introduction of medicinal substances into the tonsils, and has proved the ability to reach the angular lymph glands in this manner. In one of his cases there was a steady diminution in the size of the gland, which had previously been increasing in size, while the tonsils. themselves appeared to be essentially normal[16].

R. B. Canfield says that enlargement of the cervical glands is one of the general indications for the removal of the tonsils, and this has been my experience; so much so that in all cases of this kind where possible I have the tonsils removed as a part of the treatment for the enlarged glands.

Albert E. Rogers says that the surgeon should first extirpate the tonsil before resorting to an incision through the skin in all cases of cervical adenitis which have not already broken down[17].

Griffin states that the person who has a tonsil at birth will always have enlarged cervical glands or enlarged glands elsewhere. The truth of this statement would seem to be doubtful, as, in spite of various statements to the contrary, it is probable, from the testimony of the best observers, that the tonsil is always present at birth. It is also equally true that there are a great many persons who have enlarged tonsils who do not have enlarged cervical glands. Enlarged cervical glands are probably caused by or are the result of infection from or though diseased tonsils, but not all persons who have diseased tonsils have enlarged cervical glands, since the gland not infrequently has sufficient resisting power to ward off the infecting process from the tonsil.

CONNECTION BETWEEN THE TONSIL AND TUBERCULOSIS.

Fifty-seven had no knowledge of any connection between the two, while 39 had. The others did not answer the question. Goodale has seen several such cases, already reported. Hurd reports seven cases out of nine in which the clinical diagnosis of tubercular tonsillitis was made, mainly from the condition of the cervical glands, and in which Jonathan Wright found evidence of tubercle bacilli in the tonsils. In one case out of ten in which the clinical diagnosis was simple chronic inflammation of the tonsil, Dr. Wright found tuberculosis evident in the tonsil. He thinks the tubercular cervical glands at the angle of the jaw are almost always secondary to primary tuberculosis of the tonsil.

Dr. Hurd and Dr. Wright have recently made further investigations which show that the larger and freer the tonsil the more it resists the invasion of harmful organisms; also that it is exceptional to find associated with such a tonsil much enlargement of the lymphatic glands The small submerged tonsil is much more likely to be the soil for invasion of the tonsil with tuberculosis. Dr. Wright examined the tonsils in sixty cases where the protruding portion only was removed, and did not find tuberculosis in any of them.

The tubercular tonsil is usually pale, the crypts contain cheesy debris, and the edge of the anterior pillar shows passive hyperemia, and the associated lymph glands are enlarged. The stump of the partially removed tonsil is quite as liable to tubercular infection as if originally submerged.

The examination of the tonsil is difficult as to the diagnosis of tuberculosis, since spots of granular protoplasm representing tonsillar regression are accompanied by a grade of fibrous tissue such as is found in old healed tubercular areas at the apex of the lung.

George B. Wood found that tubercle bacilli passed through the tonsil to the lymph glands five days after inoculation of living tubercle bacilli in the guinea pig, showing that even while in an apparently normal state the tonsil is unable to filter out living tubercle bacilli[1].

Koplik regards the tonsil as the source of infection when the lymph nodes are found to be the seat of isolated tubercular infection of a primary nature. Isolated tuberculosis of the tonsil is very rare. The infection may occur during the act of swallowing[1].

Swain voices a somewhat different opinion, in the statement in answer to this question, that the lateral column of the pharynx, all of its postnasal surface, and the pharynx, can and do contribute lymph in inflammation of the neck, and says that if he were to have any deleterious matter absorbed, he would rather have it go through the tonsils, where a host of phagocytes live, than any other less protected place.

Theisen has had cases in which examination of the removed tonsils showed the presence of giant and tubercular cells in the tonsillar tissue. The children from whom the tonsils were removed had enlarged cervical glands, yet the examination of the lungs was negative.

Lermoyez regards chronic lesions of the tonsils as an open door to tuberculosis.

Thompson advised the removal of diseased tonsils in an

adult woman, which was refused. She returned two years later for the removal of the tonsils and a large mass of tubercular glands in the neck. Recovery took place. There was no tuberculosis anywhere else in the body.

E. L. Shurley reports, on the other hand, that according to his observations there are very few cases of tonsillar tuberculosis, and he has seen but few cases where any causal relation could be even suspected.

Professor Chiari says that primary tuberculosis of the tonsil originates either through the air passages or through the ingestion of tubercular milk. It is possible for the tuberculosis to extend from the tonsil to the entire body. He has not had the opportunity, however, for direct observation of this.

Moure, of Bordeaux, does not believe that the tonsils are very often the starting point of tuberculosis.

Solenberger says that in Colorado there as so many cases of reinfection, not a few after an attack of acute tonsillitis, that he is forced to think there is a causal relation between the two. In several hundred cases of tubercular patients, 62 per cent have had tonsillitis at intervals from childhood and severe attacks of swollen cervical glands.

From all of which somewhat conflicting testimony, it would seem that the question of the entrance of tuberculosis germs through the tonsil has been definitely determined by a sufficient number of careful observations to render the fact an undisputed one, even though only a minority of observers have reported thereon. This, taken in connection with the results in cervical adenitis, would seem to give a sufficient reason for excising the tonsil whenever there are any symptoms suggestive of possible incipient tuberculosis or cervical adenitis. I have to admit that I have myself no direct knowledge of general tuberculosis where examination of the tonsil has proved the presence of either giant cells or tubercle bacilli, but I am firmly convinced that such relation does exist.

THE RELATION OF THE TONSIL TO RHEUMATISM.

The relation of the tonsil to rheumatism is one of the as yet unsolved problems to which considerable attention is being given. At the outset of such an inquiry one is confronted with the question as to what rheumatism is, and on this question there is as yet no unanimity of opinion. The older theories as to dependence on cold or wet and the uric acid theory seem about to be superseded by the theory of direct infection. Sufficient proof is perhaps not yet at hand to make this a certainty, but the tendency is all in this direction.

Since the investigations of Birch Hirschfield in 1888, the bacterial origin of rheumatism has been suspected and studied. Sahli, von Leyden, Achalme, Triboulet, Coyon, and Apert isolated in rheumatism bacilli of the diplococcus type, which caused the death of guinea pigs from pericarditis, valvular lesions and the like, but in no case produced arthritis. At about the same time Wasserman isolated from a case of rheumatism, with complications, a diplococcus which when injected into animals developed after an incubation period of three to ten days a periarthritis without pus formation. Alkaline media were essential to the best growth of this diplococcus. Meyer followed by isolating a diplococcus from twenty-five cases of rheumatic tonsillitis, which he injected into the ear veins of rabbits, and then obtained from the joints a pure culture not differing essentially from that obtained by previous investigators. In one hundred rabbits inoculated, a polyarthritis developed, and in twenty-one endocarditis was produced.

Passing over the individual work of the other various investigators, I come to that of Frissell. His first efforts to obtain from joints or nodes an organism having a causal relation to rheumatism being failures, he next made cultures from three cases of tonsillitis occurring during an attack of acute articular rheumatism. He obtained a streptococcus in nearly pure culture, but when this was injected into rabbits, the results were negative so far as arthritis was concerned. In March, 1904, he isolated from the throat of a patient suffering from acute articular rheumatism, with diffuse reddening of the tonsils and faucial pillars, but without exudate, an organism in mixed culture which after injection into the joints of a rabbit produced a polyarthritis. This organism, while culturally not readily distinguished from other diplo- or streptococci, yet had a special affinity for joints. This was shown by the fact that ten out of eleven rabbits injected had a polyarthritis, the other dying of pericarditis and pleurisy. It sometimes produced pus in the joints with disintegration of the joint itself, while no pus was found elsewhere in the body. The course of the disease was towards spontaneous recovery. The pus formation he regards as probably due to the large amount of serum injected. He does not claim with certainty to have isolated a coccus which is specific in the sense that it will cause the disease known as acute articular rheumatism, but one that has an affinity for joints. Rheumatism may be due, not to a specific coccus, but to a coccus group intimately-allied, though perhaps indistinguishable from each other by present cultural methods, the individual strains of which would vary greatly in virulence. He says, "Such a group might well contain the ordinary harmless streptococcus, a common habitant of the tonsil, so many of which were injected in our experiments into the animal circulation without producing symptoms. It might also include a variety causing an arthritis which tends to spontaneous cure unless the number of the invading host be too great, and range up to the malignant streptococci, causing septic joints, septic endocarditis and pyemia. Exposure to cold and wet, so long held as potent factors in the causation of rheumatism, may be considered as lowering body resistance, thus giving the bacterium a chance to attack the temporarily unprotected organism. The angina of tonsillitis often precedes and is frequently a symptom of acute rheumatism. What more natural supposition than that here the invading organism gains its access to the body, or is here overwhelmed by the resistance of the phagocytes, such an abortive attack constituting the ordinary tonsillitis. One is forced to look beyond the common joint affection to gain a clear idea of such a protean disease attacking, to be sure, oftenest the joints, but too frequently skin, pleura, and heart. Granted a point of entry, probably the tonsil, as the frequency of tonsillitis would suggest, the various conditions vaguely called rheumatic, as well as the out and out attack of acute articular rheumatism, seem best explained by considering the essential condition to be a blood infection[4]."

Rosenheim reports the careful study of eight cases in which there was an apparent relation between tonsillitis and rheumatism. In four, streptococci were found in pure culture; in two, streptococci and staphylococci; and in two, streptococci and other organisms were found in the tonsils. Two cases had serious endocarditis, in both of which the streptococcus was found in pure culure. All were improved after removal of the tonsil, from which he concludes that bacteria penetrate deeply into the substance of the tonsil, and the organisms found in the tonsil are probably the causal agents of the attack of acute rheumatism[15].

The replies to my question have in the main clinically substantiated the foregoing relation between the tonsil and rheumatism, more than two-thirds of the reporters believing in such relation. Eighty-three replied in the affirmative as to rheumatism in general; two qualified by applying it to muscular rheumatism only; six thought it occurred, but only occasionally; three thought so, but had no proof; four had observed endocarditis and one pericarditis after tonsillitis. Thirty-five were doubtful as to any relation or did not believe there was any.

As to the question of whether the tonsil showed any partieular lesion which would be suggestive of its being the cause of the rheumatism, the answers were as follows:

The characteristic rheumatic tonsil may be hypertrophied, fibroid, and have crypts filled with detritus. It may have stringy, white fibrous deposits and a peculiar soft, velvety red color. There may be moderate swelling with edema in the adjacent region. In other cases the tonsil may not be at all characteristic in appearance. Pain is an early manifestation. While usually enlarged the tonsil is not always so, but is congested, tense, and tender. Ingals, who has studied the matter considerably, says there is nothing in the appearance of the tonsil to indicate any relation between the two, but an analysis of cases seems to prove the relation[16].

Phillips had a case in which severe rheumatism followed an attack of acute tonsillitis in a subject who had never previously had rheumatism.

A. R. Elliott cites one case of rheumatism showing very marked improvement after tonsillectomy, and two other cases in which marked improvement of septic conditions, one of them being rheumatic, occurred after local treatment of the tonsil. He thinks it is not unreasonable to assume that the tonsils may originate the toxins causing chorea[17].

Levy thinks the opinion in regard to the apparent relation between the tonsil and rheumatism arises from the ease with which the infection causing rheumatism can or does enter through the tonsil. One causes the other. The specific infection which produces rheumatism is the same that may produce tonsillitis. This is a reasonable and probably correct opinion.

Ross has seen many cases where the inflammatory rheumatism asserted itself concurrently or almost immediately after the subsidence of the throat condition.

Lee Cohen, of Baltimore, reports a case in a male of forty, who had suffered for a number of years with chronic subacute articular rheumatism, for which he was treated six weeks medicinally with no results. Then as an experiment he had the tonsils removed. The tonsils were found to be more like membranes than glands. Medicinal treatment was stopped, and the patient left the hospital fourteen days after the operation without the assistance of crutch or cane, and since then has had no return of the rheumatism.

Welty reports twelve cases of rheumatism cured by the removal of the tonsil. Diagnosis was based on the fact of the association of rheumatism and tonsillar disease in adults. The tonsils were all partially or almost completely submerged and had concretions in the crypts.

C. M. Robertson is certain that the tonsil is the offending factor in as high a percentage of cases as thirty in acute and ninety in chronic rheumatism.

In regard to the important question as to whether the rheumatism disappears after the removal of the tonsil, the replies indicate that while this does not always occur, the attacks are milder and occur less often where they do not altogether disappear. Twenty-nine reported "no" or "not always"; twelve said, "in some cases," while thirty-seven reported cessation or diminution in severity of the rheumatic attacks after the removal of the tonsil. One reported that the rheumatism was worse after the partial removal of the tonsil; another that the pharyngeal wall can perform some of the functions of the tonsil after removal, which observation accords with the history of one of my own cases. The patient was a woman of 45 years, who had suffered from severe rheumatic attacks for many years, located largely in the throat, and with considerable pain running to the ear, always coincident with tonsillar trouble. The tonsils were of the submerged type, small, but showing the results of frequent inflammation. They were removed by thorough enucleation and for an entire year there·was no sign of rheumatic trouble in the throat or elsewhere. Then she had an attack somewhat suggestive of the old tonsillar rheumatism, but much less severe. Examination of the throat showed no sign of tonsil, but some granular tissue which had filled in the space formerly occupied by the tonsils. This may be a case in which the infection entered through the granular tissue.

Griffin thinks that quinsy is a rheumatic disease and the rheumatic tonsil very common, but has not found that the rheumatism disappears after removal. As he does not perform a thorough enucleation, but only tonsillotomy, this may account for the lack of good results after removal. It seems to me that good results or the lack of them will depend on the type of the operation done, as it is not logical to expect the best results unless entire removal of the gland has been effected.

Isaac Taylor says that acute articular rheumatism is due to some species of streptococcus; muscular rheumatism to some bacterial infection, perhaps of a highly attenuated streptococcus. In many cases of tonsillar origin the muscles of the neck and shoulder are especially affected[1].

I have had several cases where removal of the tonsils has been done solely for rheumatism and with good results. Sufficient time has not elapsed to enable me to say whether or not permanent relief from the rheumatic attack has been attained, but I think it has. I have recently removed some tonsils with diseased crypts in a woman of forty-two, who had rheumatism of the neck and shoulders for many years. This ceased after thorough enucleation of the tonsils, and has not recurred.

Aneurism, appendicitis, erysipelas, meningitis, iritis, pleuritis, pericarditis, endocarditis, pneumonia, paraplegia, strabismus, nephritis, osteomyelitis, phlegmon, oophoritis, orchitis and general septic infection are all found in the literature as of tonsillar origin or occurring with or as a result of tonsillar inflammation. Investigation of all these would lead me beyond my present field. They all show the possibility and probability of the tonsil as a portal of infection, and prove that whatever of protective value to the organism the tonsil may theoretically have, practically it is of little value; on the contrary, it is not infrequently a decided menace to the organism.

ON THE USE OF CHEMICAL CAUSTICS.

Of 126 replies, 65 did not use any form of chemical caustic in the treatment of tonsillar troubles. By chemical caustics, I mean those commonly used to reduce inflammatory growths, to lessen the size of the tonsil or to destroy diseased crypts, and, in general, any chemical which applied directly is used to get the tonsil into a more healthy condition, leaving out of consideration the treatment of acute tonsillar inflammation. The chemical caustics which seem to be principally used are: nitrate of silver in varying strengths and the fused salt on the probe, trichloracetic acid, chromic acid, carbolic acid with glycerin and silver nitrate, London and Vienna paste, suhlimate in alcohol, lactic acid and zinc chlorid. Forty-two out of 125, or about 33 1-3%, still employ these to a greater or less extent, while 18 have abondoned their use.

Many formulae for the use of these measures have been given me, with various combinations of these materials, the essential thing being to carry the substance as deeply into the crypts as possible, with the result of destroying or making the crypts smaller and bringing about a healthier state of the crypt wall, thus lessening the amount of secretion which exudes therefrom, shrinking the tonsil and getting it into a healthy condition.

While the advocates in favor of these measures are decidedly in the minority, I cannot agree with Dr. Freer, who regards chemical caustics as the resort of the timid manipulator who shuns surgery because he is afraid to do it, as many of the users of chemical caustics are good surgeons and cannot be said to use these because of fear of more radical measures. Certainly this is not true of Leland, Professor Chiari, Beck, D. C. Greene, Jr., Thomas Hubbard, Anderson, Roy, Clarke, Gleason and others.

There occur in the practice of most laryngologists a certain number of cases of diseased or hypertrophied tonsils in which for one reason or another radical surgery seems contraindicated, or, if indicated from the standpoint of the operator, is not accepted by the patient. In these cases I am satisfied from a considerable personal experience that fused nitrate of silver on the probe, chromic acid or trichloracetic acid carried deeply into the crypts reduces the size of the tonsil very materially, and adds to the comfort of the patient, and will often be accepted when more radical measures will be refused. Other substances, no doubt, act equally as well. That these measures take the place of complete removal of the tonsil when this is indicated is not claimed, but that they have a place far more important than would seem to be indicated by the opinions I am quoting is, I am sure, the case.

Beck has recently been using the new bismuth paste—bismuth subnitrate 30, vaselin 70—injected while in a warm liquid state, by means of a glass syringe, into the crypts in cases of chronic lacunar tonsillitis, and reports good results from its use. As to the ultimate value of this, it is too soon to state.

Goodale has used a five to ten per cent nitrate of silver injected interstitially in hemophilia.

In mycosis, chromic acid and trichloracetic acid are used by several operators after removing the leptothrix masses. The chemical caustics are also used after slitting up the crypts.

Lermoyez, on the other hand, regards all chemical caustics as useless and bad for the voice. I cannot see how, properly used, they injure the voice at all or are likely to do so.

Beatle's fluid (iodin gr. 160, phenol gr. 320, glycerin 6 oz.) is used by E. B. Gleason in the diseased crypts of chronic inflammation.

C. M. Harris uses iodin glycerin, tincture of iodin and silver nitrate applied directly to the crypts, especially in early acute troubles.

INDICATIONS FOR THE REMOVAL OF THE TONSIL.

For many generations surgeons have recommended the removal of large hypertrophied tonsils; that is, those tonsils which appear to be obstructive in the throat, the so-called hypertrophied or large tonsil. It was formerly taught that only those tonsils which project beyond the anterior pillars are hypertrophied and to be removed. The common type of guillotine or tonsillotome was invented and adapted for this purpose, the forks being afterwards added so as to pull the tonsil out a little beyond the pillar, in order to make sure that a sufficient amount would be removed. From some 125 answers to the question as to the indications for the removal of the tonsil, I received the following:

Recurrent tonsillar abscess, or quinsy.—This would seem to be a sufficient indication, since in these cases there is a pocket at the superior and outer portion of the tonsil, which fills rapidly, and the history is that the patients who have had one attack are quite likely to have another. Thorough enucleation, and not tonsillotomy, is the only operation that will fulfill the indications and prevent subsequent attacks of quinsy.

Recurrent simple tonsillitis.

Benign tumors and new growths of any kind when their removal is not prejudicial to life.

Diseased crypts, with or without hypertrophy.—The tonsil in these cases is sometimes submerged or imbedded and sometimes not. Among the diseased crypt cases are also included those of mycosis. Many of the tonsils with diseased crypts are small and are visible only on retracting the anterior pillar. On grasping the tonsil with a hook it is found to lie rather deeply to the outer side and usually to be much larger than would be supposed from a superficial examination of the throat.

The coexistence of rheumatism and tonsillitis.—This has occurred so often that many operators regard recurring attacks of rheumatism associated with diseased tonsils as a distinct indication for their removal. Along with the studies in regard to rheumatism has come the growing conviction, based on a study of the lymphatic drainage of the tonsil, that enlarged cervical glands owe their origin in a large majority of cases to hypertrophied or diseased tonsils. Certain it is, that after the removal of such tonsils we have improvement.

Middle ear involvement, such as deafness and tinnitus, especially the progressive type, seems to be influenced unfavorably and even to be caused by enlarged tonsils as well as adenoids, and when so caused, the tonsils should be removed.

Mouth breathing, accompanied by hypertrophied tonsils, is sufficient cause for their removal, if for no other reason than to improve the facial aspect and the breathing.

General toxemia, impaired nutrition and systemic dyspnea, are perhaps more often evident with the tonsil as a cause than is recognized. A recent case of my own illustrates this: A policeman, who was in the habit of going to sleep and snoring

whenever he sat down, very large and continually putting on
flesh, was referred to me for examination of the throat. The
faucial tonsils were so large that they met in the middle line.
On their enucleation the symptoms of dyspnea and general carbonic acid intoxication, as evidenced by the tendency to
sleep, entirely disappeared, and the individual's entire character changed.

Remote reflexes, such as vomiting, cough, chorea, irritable
and granular pharynx and enlarged glands, when the tonsils are the probable cause, should have for treatment the
removal of the tonsils.

With reference to tuberculosis, there seems to be a difference
of opinion. If tuberculosis is evident or suspected, it may do
to remove the tonsil when the case is seen very early; but so
competent an observer as Freudenthal advises against the
removal of the tonsil in advanced cases of tuberculosis, since
he has found it not only of no advantage to the individual,
but a distinct disadvantage. Chambers cites a case of tuberculosis where the tonsils were thoroughly removed, following
which there was increasing pain and rapid involvement of the
entire operated area.

With reference to children, if one accepts the dictum of
Bosworth that the tonsil is not a normal gland at all,
hypertrophied tonsils in children should always be removed,
even though there are no symptoms. It is probably the custom of many operators at the present time when operating
for adenoids to remove the tonsils at the same time, even
though there are no particular symptoms which lead one to
do this, since we are uncertain, as to their function and we
know that they often cause trouble. Since apparently no
one ever misses them when they are out, it seems better to
give the child the benefit of the doubt and when the adenoid
operation is done to remove the tonsils at the same time.
This is my own practice if there is any suspicion of hypertrophied or diseased tonsils.

As opposed to this view, G. H. Wright has recently shown
that there are four periods of molar tooth eruptions, with
some variations in time, when the tonsils may enlarge without infection; viz., at two, six, twelve and seventeen years
of age. Even if slightly enlarged, if not infected, the tonsils
return to a normal condition with complete eruption of the

teeth. Diseased teeth are prolific sources of enlargement of the glands, directly by infection or by toxins. He advises that operations on the tonsils be deferred during these periods until the molars erupt. In a series of cases he found that the tonsil, while showing inflammation and enlargement during the period of eruption, returned to normal as soon as the tooth came through the gum. He regards the tonsil as having some value as a protector of the organism from the products of dental infection. Tonsillar enlargement without infection is a normal expression of the active function of the tonsillar gland, and when the tonsil becomes infected, it does so because of its lack of power of resistance to the invasion of micro-organisms".

In general, some of the statements seem to me too sweeping and others too conservative. For instance, Gildea and some others would remove every tonsil that shows any tendency to disease, whereas I think that many diseased tonsils are curable by local measures without removal. On the other hand, Gleitsman would remove only those tonsils that protrude beyond the palatine pillars. As many of the most troublesome tonsils, so far as the general economy is concerned, are those which do not protrude at all, this is necessarily too conservative.

Welty, of San Francisco, regards all tonsils in persons over twenty years of age as diseased, and says that the tonsil, when once diseased, predisposes the individual to any kind of infection, more especially the whole group of infectious diseases.

Professor Chiari, of Vienna, would limit the removal of the tonsils to individuals under forty, in the absence of further inflammatory symptoms and when there is no suggestion of hemophilia.

Several writers in speaking of the indications for the removal of the tonsils use the phrase "adherent pillars," "bad adhesions to the pillars," and the like. These terms seem to be misnomers, and I am quite of the opinion of Dr. Robert C. Myles, who has been claiming for years, in various papers written by him on the tonsils, that there is no such thing as adhesions to the pillars in the sense in which that term is ordinarily used. All tonsils are adherent to the pillars, anatomically so, the tonsil being a gland covered with mucous membrane on its free surface with a capsule on its external

side, set in between the anterior and posterior pillars and
necessarily attached to them on the anterior, posterior and
superior aspects, and to the mucous membrane adjoining the
side of the root of the tongue on its inferior aspect. That
the anterior pillar frequently forms folds known as the plica
supratonsillaris and the plica infratonsillaris is well known,
and this is what may be meant by the adhesions of some
writers. As a matter of fact, these plicas are merely redupli-
cations or folds of the free surface of the anterior pillar. In
cases in which this does not exist, the mucous membrane of
the edge of the pillar divides into two parts, one becoming
continuous with the capsule of the tonsil and the other continuous with the mucous membrane covering the tonsil, the
two together forming the attachment of the pillar to the
tonsil which is invariably present. This line of attachment is
the first thing to be severed in complete removal, in whatever manner it may be done. This gives access to the edge
of the capsule, which is adjacent to the superior constrictor
muscles of the pharynx, some of the fibers of which frequently
penetrate it. I cannot see, anatomically, any reason for
speaking of "adherent tonsils," or "bad adhesions to the pillar," except as one refers to the complete operation of tonsillectomy, in which, owing to the character of the areolar
tissue, it may be more difficult sometimes than others to perform complete dissection. Also, the two folds going from the
anterior pillars are sometimes thicker than at others, but they
are true anatomic structures and always present.

The size and position of the tonsil with reference to the
pillars, sometimes projecting, again submerged, varies
greatly according as it projects into the cavity of the throat
or is partially or completely submerged.

Finally tonsillar tissue should be removed when its pathological condition cannot be cured with treatment, when it obstructs
the nares or oral cavities or interferes with their physiologic
functions. This has no reference to the size, as a small
diseased tonsil often causes more trouble than a large mass.

TONSILLOTOMY OR TONSILLECTOMY.

Twenty-eight favored tonsillotomy; 57, tonsillectomy; 32 do
tonsillotomy in young children for simple hypertrophy, tonsillectomy in older children or at any age where there are dis-

tinct pathologic changes; two do tonsillotomy in adults and tonsillectomy in children.

The opinions given in answer to the question as to the preference for tonsillotomy or tonsillectomy show a gradual perceptible change towards the more thorough operation; since only 28 out of the entire number still range themselves as absolutely on the side of tonsillotomy, although the answers in the way of technic would seem to show that some of the operators who use the term tonsillectomy are content with rather less than the absolute removal of the entire tonsil gland. The tendency, however, is in that direction, and it is probably only a matter of a few years when the others—the 32 who use tonsillotomy for young children or in cases of simple hypertrophy and tonsillectomy in older children or when the tonsil is manifestly diseased—will use tonsillectomy in all their cases, since it is certainly not rational to remove a gland at all unless one removes it as thoroughly as possible, with a view to the prevention of any future possible complication.

To take some answers a little more in detail, Gleason, of Philadelphia, advocates tonsillotomy in simple hypertrophy, because it requires no general anesthesia and there is no risk. In recurrent tonsillitis and quinsy, with retention of cheesy matter, he uses more or less complete tonsillectomy, but with reluctance and a feeling that the remedy may be worse than the disease; he says it is theoretically comparable to the rough surgery of the Civil War. To which I would reply that a clean tonsillectomy is not rough surgery, but quite the proper operation for the purpose for which it is done.

Dr. Farlow uses tonsillotomy generally, because it has less risk, and thinks tonsillectomy has a risk out of proportion to its advantages.

Dr. Frank Miller says that tonsillotomy correctly done never causes hemorrhage, but there is bleeding if all the tonsil comes out, leaving the capsule, while tonsillectomy is very often dangerous, with sudden hemorrhage five to eight hours after when not expected.

Ross, of Montreal, finds tonsillotomy always satisfactory.

Professor Chiari uses tonsillotomy only, as the remaining portion of the gland atrophies, and in tonsillectomy there is danger of injury to the tonsillar artery in the capsule. Personal observation in Professor Chiari's clinic corroborates this statement as to practice, for I have never seen any operation done there except tonsillotomy.

Professor Gerber, of Koenigsberg, believes tonsillotomy sufficient, and thinks tonsillectomy more likely to cause hemorrhage than tonsillotomy, an opinion which seems to be of slight value, since he does not do tonsillectomy.

Pooley says tonsillotomy is the safest and the easiest, reasons which hardly carry much weight.

Luc does tonsillotomy with the cold snare

Sir Felix Semon has found tonsillotomy sufficient with very few exceptions.

As showing that the leaven of completeness in tonsillar surgery has not leavened the whole lump, so experienced an observer as Dr. Gleitsmann says he uses tonsillotomy and does not see any reason why the whole organ must be removed.

Dr. G. Hudson Makuen advises tonsillectomy, since the remnants of the tonsil after tonsillotomy do not easily drain their crypts into the pharynx, and secretions are more readily absorbed into the system.

Randall and Gradle do tonsillectomy by choice, but have had good results from less complete operations. This last remark, that is in accordance with everybody's experieuce, as it is an undoubted fact that many of the cases of tonsillotomy done by all of us have apparently served the purpose for which they were intended. As, however, a number of them have not, and as the trend of all working medicine should be towards improvement, and we have learned that tonsillectomy is apparently always a success, why should we in the future do any operation but the best one?

Kyle thinks the essential thing in all operations is to thoroughly free the upper and lower parts of the tonsil, and that in many instances, if this were carefully and thoroughly done, it would make very little difference whether the tonsil were removed or not.

Ellis has found that secondary hemorrhage is much less likely to take place if the tonsillar tissue has been completely removed, and for ragged, submerged and irritable tonsils he always uses tonsillectomy, particularly in adults.

T. R. French thinks that other things being equal it is desirable to leave the base of the tonsil in infancy.

Ballenger performs tonsillectomy, removing the tonsil with the capsule intact. The crypts of the tonsil extend to the capsule, and it is the crypts that usually form the atrium of infection. If the capsule is not removed, the surgeon is not sure that all the diseased tissue is removed. If tonsillotomy is practiced, a careless and imperfect operation is too often passed as a sufficient operation. A partial operation is frequently followed by recurrent tonsillitis and by the regrowth of the tonsil tissue. He has never seen recurrence after removing the tonsils with the capsule intact.

Bryant thinks both operations indicated in special cases. He uses tonsillotomy when the symptoms are only local; tonsillectomy when extended, such as cases of enlarged lymphatic glands.

A large number of others have abandoned tonsillotomy for tonsillectomy, since they have found recurring trouble after tonsillotomy.

Ward reports 800 cases of tonsillectomy, of which 129 had been previously operated on by tonsillotomy, having been brought back for reoperation on account of the remains of septic tonsillar tissue. It is not the size of the tonsil but its septic condition which is of importance[20].

Contrary to the oft expressed opinion as regards the difference in procedure between children and adults, Theisen, of Albany, always does tonsillectomy in childhood, since incomplete removal is frequently followed by recurrence of lymphatic tissue. In adults he finds tonsillotomy is often sufficient.

If one is to differentiate at all between the two, I should regard this opinion as more nearly correct than that of tonsillotomy in children and tonsillectomy in adults.

REOPERATIONS: AFTER ONE'S SELF OR AFTER OTHERS.

One hundred and six reported in the affirmative as to both; that is, they had operated on the same individual more than once and also after a previous operation performed by someone else. Ten replied in the negative, and five said they had reoperated after others, but not after themselves. This statement is easily explainable, as it not infrequently happens that a second operation is done by another operator. Nearly every operator who now does tonsillectomy reported that all of those secondary operations had been done after tonsillotomies and that no occasion had been found to reoperate after tonsillectomies. That the tonsillar tissue seems in a measure to reform when the basal portion is left, is evidenced by the testimony of several good observers, such as Emil Mayer, Gleitsmann, and others. Packard states that he has operated at least a dozen times on cases that had been previously operated on by men who operate thoroughly. He has come to the conclusion that the tonsils may recur even when apparently a thorough operation has been performed. He truly states that as of course most cases go to another operator for a second operation, the statistics are necessarily misleading.

Joachim, of New Orleans, has not noticed the necessity of re-operation since tonsillectomy has been performed. Percy Fridenberg has never seen regeneration. He has reoperated, however, when for some reason or other removal of the tonsils was not complete.

As to the question of regeneration, Berens, who has reoperated in several instances, cites one case where a very large tonsil was removed from each side. Observation of the throat nine months later showed a very large tonsil had returned on one side, the removal of which was not followed by its regrowth. Here it was possible that the tonsil was not removed in toto in the first instance, and that either the action of the muscles of the neck forced the tonsil into prominence, or else there was a certain amount of true regeneration.

Hajek says that he has reoperated, and that in the case of small children, after amputation of the tonsil, the remainder of the tonsil can again become hypertrophic. Lermoyez says there is no need for the return of the tonsil if it is properly removed in the first instance. Gradle thinks the remnants can enlarge. Professor S. S. Bishop says he has always removed the whole tonsil; hence there was never any need to operate subsequently. As, however, in the description, of his technic in detail he merely does an amputation, as completely as possible, with the Mackenzie tonsillotome, the statement as to his having always removed the whole tonsil may admit of honest doubt. Professor Luc says that since doing complete removal he has never had occasion to reoperate. Logan Turner thinks that in some cases there is distinct regrowth.

The practical unanimity of opinion as to occasional need for reoperation after tonsillotomy, not to quote individuals further, would seem to show that tonsillotomy is certainly an incomplete operation and that it does not fulfill, as so many of its advocates aver, all the indications.

ANESTHESIA.

There is quite a difference in usage in regard to the question of anesthesia. In operations on children several operators use no anesthesia whatever, and it is well known that it is not the custom on the continent of Europe to anesthetize children for adenoid and tonsil operations. In America, most parents prefer that the child shall be spared the shock and pain of the operation, even though it be not so very great. Anesthesia also has the advantage that it allows time enough to do a better operation, especially in the dissection of the tonsil, and with few exceptions all of the persons reporting to me are in the habit of using anesthesia in operations on children. For local anesthesia, cocain in some form or other is mostly in vogue, either by injection or painted on in varying strengths. The reports on this question were as follows:

Sixty-three use ether as the anesthetic for children; 10, gas and ether; 10, chloroform; 1 uses chloroform up to twelve years of age, ether after this age; 7, ethylchlorid; 5, somnoform; 2, nitrous oxid; 3, ethyl·bromid; 2, ethyl-chlorid and chloroform.

Packard thinks mixed anesthesia is no more dangerous than any any other. Care should be taken that no food is taken beforehand; twice he has nearly lost a patient on account of food having been taken beforehand. He has not found the use of atropin satisfactory. Pierce, on the other hand, advises its use to lessen the amount of mucus during the operation.

Yankauer has obtained satisfactory local anesthesia by injecting with a long needle 15 minims of a 1% solution of cocain into the sheath of the middle and posterior palatin nerves as they leave the bony opening in the posterior part of the hard palate at the junction of the alveolar process with the horizontal part of the bone.

Ether seems to be the anesthetic of choice. I invariably use it, and have had no serious accident from its use. On one occasion during etherization and before the operation was commenced, a child with very huge tonsils became asphyxiated, stopped breathing, and artificial respiration was required for a few moments. The result was all right and the operation was performed as usual, although for a few moments things looked rather bad. I was on another occasion badly scared with chloroform. The child blanched out, the pulse stopped, and the outlook seemed dubious. Recovery, however, took place, and the operation was performed. The difference between ether and chloroform is, that ether gives a warning usually sufficient to enable one to remedy the condition, while chloroform acts so quickly that it may be too late. Of 29 fatal cases reported, 26 were due to chloroform. Chloroform does not seem to be indicated in the lymphatic diathesis. I have had no personal experience with the other .anesthetics, but assume they have been satisfactory to the persons using them. Ether would seem, according to all the testimony, both as here given and as found in literature, to be the safest of the anesthetics, although, of course, not without a certain danger itself.

As to the method of giving ether, the drop method, the cone, and some form of bulb and pipe apparatus, are all used. Up to the present I have relied on the closed cone. For deep narcosis, in an operation which may be at all prolonged, the bulb and pipe apparatus is doubtless preferable.

Operation under general anesthesia should be done in the hospital or home, and not in the physician's office.

POSITION.

In operating upon children under anesthesia, the dorsal position is preferred by 25, the prone on one side or the other by 40, the semi-recumbent by 2, the Rose or Trendelenberg by 7, and the upright by 27, the various recumbent positions being still further modified in accordance with individual preference. It is somewhat remarkable that the upright position is used almost exclusively by operators in the New England States and by several scattered over the West and South, who were former house pupils in Boston hospitals.

Phillips believes the upright position to be unnecessary from the standpoint of skill, and to be fraught with danger of syncope, suffocation, flooding of the larynx, and puermonia. Packard thinks this position adds greatly to the danger of ether and chloroform and to the risk of detached tissue entering the larynx and causing dangerous obstruction.

On comparing the reports of accidents, hemorrhages and the like, I do not find that they have been any more common in those who operate in the upright position than in those who operate in the dorsal or recumbent. The operating room nurse in our own hospital has told me that all the unpleasant experiences coming under her observation in the past four years were in cases operated upon in the prone position. Without exception, everyone who operates on adults under local anesthesia does so in the upright position, and as all those who use no anesthetic whatever operate in the upright position, it would seem, from anatomic reasons of position and comfort of vision, that the upright position was preferable to the recumbent or dorsal, unless there are manifest reasons why one is much safer than the other. I almost invariably operate in the upright position, in most cases in adults, as well as in children. I usually give general anesthesia, and, when completely anesthetized, the patient is put in a chair facing the light, or else I use a head mirror and artificial light. The patient is not so profoundly anesthetized as to abolish the reflexes, and I have not had, so far as I know, any accident due to position. It is true that at a demonstration at a meeting of this society I had an unfortunate experience in an operation done in the upright position, tracheotomy having been required. That, however, as I stated at the time, was due entirely to a fault in the matter of technic in the introduction of the gauze pressure sponge too heavily soaked in peroxid of hydrogen, and was not at all dependent on the position which was used. The same thing was just as likely to have occurred in the three following cases, done at the same time in the same position and without accident. As never before nor in the year that has elapsed have I had any trouble incident to the question of position, I defend the upright position as perfectly proper, and to be used by those operators who prefer it, without in the least condemning the prone or horizontal position, since, so far as thoroughness is concerned, it is possible to do the operation as well in one position as in the other. In the case of severe hemorrhage, where there is danger of swallowing considerable blood, and where a large pad of pressure material may have to be introduced, the Trendelenberg or Rose position is probably more advantageous as interfering less with respiration. I occasionally operate on adults in some of the recumbent positions. Even then I prefer the head and shoulders somewhat elevated. The advantage of the upright position is that the anatomic relations are normal and one has a good view of the entire area. In my operations the amount of blood vomited afterwards is comparatively slight, and I have found no discomfort in any way from it.

<h3 style="text-align:center">INSTRUMENTS.</h3>

The armamentarium is a matter depending entirely upon the type of operation to be done. For simple tonsillotomy, a mouth gag, tongue depressor, tonsillotome, and perhaps a pair of grasping forceps, seem to be all that is necessary; whereas when one sets out to do a complete enucleation his armamentarium depends entirely upon the particular type of operation he intends to do and the instruments which he individually prefers to attain that end.

For tonsillectomy all of the following instruments have been mentioned; mouth gag, tongue depressor; grasping forceps of the following varieties—rat-toothed, Ballenger's, Richards', type special to reporter, tenaculum, and vulsellum; separators —blunt, right-angled and saw-edged, Yankauer's, Sajous', Leland's, Ingall's, Freer's and Freeman's knives, spud and finger nail; cutting instruments—scissors curved on the flat, Robertson's scissors, Farlow's and Peter's snares, various types of Mathieu's and Mackenzie's tonsillotomes, Casselberry's knife, galvanocautery, curved and straight knives, and ecraseur; punches—Myles', Farlow's, and Rhodes'.

<h3 style="text-align:center">TECHNIC.</h3>

The technic of tonsillotomy seems to be unchanged over the years, with the exception that the punch is used by many in the attempt to remove what may be left after the tonsillotomy, the tonsil forceps are employed to get more of the tonsil into the ring, and pressure on the outside of the throat is made by many. The technic, as given by the operator citing the largest number of tonsillotomies, is extremely simple; his technic for children and adults being given as follows: "Patient seated in a chair—cocain—Mathieu's tonsillotome—cut." ..

As to the results in tonsillotomy, it cannot be denied that a good tonsillotome, followed by the punch forceps, removes the greater portion of the offending gland. I have examined a good many of my earlier cases of tonsillotomy, some after the lapse of many years, and have found, in the main, that the results have been satisfactory. In several of them, however, there has been quite too much of the gland remaining for me to consider that the operation had done all that it might have done for the individual had the tonsils been completely enucleated, and there have been a few peritonsillar abscesses.

The replies to the question as to the technic of tonsillectomy show that each operator starts out to remove the entire gland, but evidently with varying conceptions as to how this is best accomplished. There is a difference of opinion as to the capsule, some saying that they leave the capsule, or punch out everything to the capsule. Thorough enucleation of the gland requires the removal of the tonsil with its capsule, and this is evidenced by the reports of the technic of all those who really do a thorough enucleation. To enucleate requires, first, the separation of the attachments (to my mind the miscalled adhesion) of the outer and inner surface of the tonsil to the mucous membrane and edge of the anterior pillar, which edge at this point divides into two layers, one continuous with the capsule, and the other continuous with the mucous membrane of the tonsil surface, the free mucous portion of this, with probably a few muscle fibers, sometimes folding over the front of the tonsil and sometimes above and below, forming the so-called plica. The tonsil is attached to the posterior pillar as well, and to the superior border where the two pillars meet. When this separation is made, the tonsil is detached with its entire capsule from its attachment by fibrous fascia to the inner border of the superior constrictor muscle, some of the fibers of which seem to run into the capsule at times, so that occasionally this detachment is impossible without the removal of an occasional muscle fiber. In other cases the capsule can be separated without apparently removing a single muscle fiber. To accomplish this requires some form of dissecting instrument, sharp or blunt. These are various, consisting of the knives, scissors and blunt spuds already mentioned, which are used while traction is being made on the tonsil, in this way everting it from its bed. Many operators, including myself, find that this separation is made very readily with the finger, which gives one control of the sense of touch, and with a sharp, clean finger nail it is in most instances easy to make the first line of cleavage with the nail, and then follow it up until the tonsil is pretty thoroughly shelled out, when any detaching instrument can be thrown over the portion that remains, which is the portion at the base of the tongue. Several types of grasping forceps, over which the detaching instrument can be placed, have been recently devised. Other operators, grasping the tonsil, take knife or scissors, cut along the edge of the pillar until the white edge of the capsule is reached, and then follow the dissection with knife, scissors or blunt instrument. Quite a variety of instrumental methods can be used to accomplish exactly the same result; namely, the shelling out of the tonsil from its bed and the cutting off of its attachment at its lower border near the base of the tongue. One can also do this entirely with the finger, as is proved by Dr. Charles W. Richardson and others. I was under the impression that I was one of the first to use the finger nail as a dissector of the tonsil, and I was certainly one of the first in American literature to describe a finger-nail dissection.[22] I am not, however, the earliest in the description of this, as the following quotation from Lambert Lack shows:

"In enucleation an incision is made through the mucous membrane between the anterior pillar of the fauces and the anterior border of the tonsil, through which the finger or blunt instrument is introduced and the tonsil shelled out of its bed. This little operation is not at all difficult to perform if care be taken to keep outside the tonsil capsule, this being but loosely attached to the surrounding areolar tissue. It takes a few minutes to complete, however, and a general anesthetic is advisable. Its advantages are:

(1) There is no risk of hemorrhage, the vessels being torn across outside the tonsil, where they are healthy.

(2) Complete removal, a point of importance in case of frequently recurring tonsillitis. When a tonsil is removed with a guillotine or snare, the tonsil crypts will be found open on the cut surface; that is, some of them have been left behind.

(3) In some cases of flat tonsils there is no other practicable method."

One of the advantages in using a finger·nail is that in buried tonsils, where it is sometimes hard to get good traction with the forceps, without tearing, and where there may be danger of cutting·the pillar with sharp instruments, it is possible by the sense of touch alone to do nearly the entire dissection. It is my own habit not to apply any form of traction forceps until after the dissection is partly made and the tonsil somewhat pedunculated. The forceps, whatever their type, are then less likely to tear through. In my first operations of this kind, I seized the tonsil with the grasping forceps, having the tonsillotome swinging on the blades. Later I devised one of the many types of ringless forceps, with the idea that after once getting a good hold it would be possible to throw the detaching instrument over the forceps and the tonsil. As to the type of cutting instrument, these vary with individual usage. Personally, I prefer a ring tonsillotome of the old Mathieu type, without the forks. (I think it is known in the instrument catalogues as Casselberry's.) Before getting these I had removed the forks from my old instruments, and they work equally well. I also use the snare, which is efficient and is preferred by some, but I do not feel certain that there is less hemorrhage after its use, as is often claimed. When well applied it follows the natural inequalities of the tonsil perfectly. Norval Pierce uses a separate snare for each tonsil, looping and tightening the first, applying the second, and then detaching them in the same order. He claims this method lessens hemorrhage. A thorough operation can be done with the Robertson scissors, and Robertson, who demonstrated his method at the meeting of the American Medical Association at New Orleans, is entitled to very much of the credit for the operation of thorough enucleation, being one of the first to describe that method. His operation consisted of detaching the tonsil from the pillars with a double-edged sickle knife, grasping the tonsil with the vulsellum, and going in behind it with specially constructed scissors. He made the statement, which has been borne out in some instances in my own expericuce, that if bleeding occurred afterwards, some portion of the tonsil had been left. I have found that sometimes, in the final cutting or in the necessary dissection, a piece of the tonsil

is left either above or below, and after detachment of the
tonsil I invariably feel with my fingers between the pillars and
above where they meet, to see if any portion of the tonsil can
possibly be left; if so, it is again grasped with the forceps.
Care should be taken not to have too much traction when the
final detachment is made, on account of the danger of making
too deep a wound at the base of the tonsil.

Yankauer divides the plica triangularis at its junction with
the anterior pillar, after freeing the upper part of the tonsil,
using an ordinary pair of surgical scissors curved on the flat.
This is done because after dissection of the plica the tonsil becomes freely movable, so that if downward traction is made upon
it the entire organ can be pulled down from its place of conceal-
ment in the velum of the soft palate, even when the velar lobe is
quite large[23].

J. L. Goodale's method is to pull the tonsil toward the
median line by forceps passed through the loop of the snare,
make a semilunar incision with a sharp knife from just outside the base of the uvula toward the mucous membrane covering the anterior aspect of the tonsil, downward to the base.
With the same knife the tonsil is freed from its attachment
until the main fibrous trabeculum is reached, this being cut
through slowly with snare. This operation affords minimum
subsequent discomfort, the muscular parts being cut out with
a sharp instrument.

Thomas Chew Worthington, of Baltimore, whose method
was referred to by several, uses vulsellum forceps and knife;
otherwise he employs the usual methods of enucleation[24].

West dissects the tonsils from the posterior pillar with a
right-angled knife, makes a circular cut around the tonsil
through the mucous membrane, using traction while cutting
through the loose tissue connecting the capsule to the fascia
of the superior constrictor muscle with a knife, thus completing the enucleation. He begins posteriorly, as he finds
the hemorrhage is less this way[25].

F. E. Miller, who has done over eleven thousand tonsil and
adenoid operations, says that the beveled knife and beveled
fenestrum Mackenzie form ideal instruments. He operates
under gas anesthesia, which he considers relaxes the muscular
fibers more than any other anesthetic. One whiff often relaxes
the pillars, and the tonsil falls almost out of the capsule, at

which moment it is cut. He says these instruments are equally effective for submerged tonsils.

It would seem, from the reports given, that adult tonsils are removed less thoroughly than in operations upon children, many contenting themselves with pinching out the adult tonsil, or with less thorough dissection. If, however, the adult tonsil is to be removed for rheumatism, it would seem necessary to do it as thoroughly. The whole trend of thought seems to be in favor of complete enucleation, with the capsule, and the accidents so far seem to be few.

The throat is sorer after tonsillectomy than after the old tonsillotomy, but the result justifies the discomfort. In the adult a week elapses before the soreness disappears.

HEMORRHAGE.

In reply to the question, "How often and in what class of cases have you had hemorrhage; how many within a few hours, delayed primary; how often secondary?" I received a variety of answers, showing great variation in individual experience. One hundred and seventy-nine cases of primary hemorrhage and 54 of secondary hemorrhage were reported. Individually, they vary from none at all, reported by several, to as high as 10%, bleeding sharply at the time. There is evidently great variation in what is understood by primary hemorrhage. Secondary hemorrhage has occurred all the way from one to seven days after operation, several of them being serious, and not all of them in hemophiliacs by any means. Two of my own had secondary hemorrhage, one, somewhat alarming, six days after, and another five days after. As to primary hemorrhage, we are wont to think that if this is at all serious we have to do with a hemophiliac, and that is sometimes the case; nevertheless, the possibility of bleeding in every tonsil operation should be considered. For this reason I have ceased to do the tonsil operation in my office. Nor do I consider it wise to operate when the tonsil is inflamed, and would prefer not to operate on females during the menses. On one occasion when I did a tonsillotomy in my office on an adult, under local anesthesia with cocain and adrenalin, there was no bleeding at the time of operation, but four hours after there was most alarming hemorrhage, controlled with difficulty. Since that time I have abandoned the use of any adrenalin preparation in the removal of tonsils under local anesthesia, preferring to have my bleeding at the time of operation, rather than several hours later.

Comparing tonsillotomy with tonsillectomy, I have found, contrary to some observers, that there is less bleeding after tonsillectomy than after tonsillotomy. Nevertheless, I have seen one case of most severe bleeding in a child a few hours after tonsillectomy.

Griffin reports that he has done over thirty thousand cases of tonsillotomy and has had only one hemorrhage, and that one a bleeder.

E. M. Holmes, of Boston, has had twenty delayed primary and three secondary hemorrhages in twelve thousand operations.

Francis R. Packard has had to pass a ligature, by means of a curved needle, to stop the hemorrhage; and Sprague, of Providence, has had the same experience.

F. E. Miller observed many hemorrhages from various causes, several five days after the use of the galvanocautery snare.

Wilson now avoids hemorrhage by dissecting, for the most part, with the finger, after which he finds the bleeding is less.

One reporter gives two cases of severe bleeding in children, one fatal. The other required transfusion, after which recovery took place. He also had one adult who bled to faintness.

Stout has seen in adults many cases of profuse, though not dangerous, bleeding.

Ballenger says he does not find that hemorrhage depends to any extent upon the class of cases, but upon whether the muscles forming the sinus tonsillaris are injured. In all classes of cases hemorrhage may follow the decapitation of the tonsil, perhaps more often in the fibrous or sclerotic tonsils. Otherwise the hemorrhage depends largely upon the injury of the muscles of the anterior and posterior pillars and the superior constrictor of the pharynx. As the arteries are either buried in or are external to these muscles, they will not be injured if the muscles are not injured. The tonsillar artery, while external to the superior constrictor muscle of the pharynx, is one large stem. In passing through, it subdivides into three or four branches. If, therefore, this muscle is injured, the main trunk may be divided and the hemorrhage be great, whereas, if the tonsil is removed without injury to this muscle, only the branches are divided and the hemorrhage is correspondingly less.

Barnhill has found-primary hemorrhage frequent, 10% bleeding sharply at the time. He has had two cases that bled to the point of alarm several days after the operation, but no fatalities.

Kenefick has previously reported a case of death in a hemophiliac, and ever since then has been afraid of hemorrhage, although he has had none since.

Hajek has seen troublesome hemorrhage only after tonsillectomy, an opinion not in accord with that of most American operators who do tonsillectomy.

Levy says he should estimate roughly that delayed primary hemorrhage has occurred in about 10% of his cases, and that it often comes when the form and appearance of the tonsil least lead one to expect it.

Matthews, who has done many operations on children, has seen troublesome bleeding in the first twenty-four hours, once after complete enucleation with the finger; several after tonsillotomy.

Munger has had to use the tonsillar clamp.

Beck says that one in twenty bleed freely after the local anesthetic passes off. One of his cases oozed for a week.

Cohen found after a careful analysis of 111 cases that four tonsillotomies bled, two severely, and of the tonsillectomies three bled primarily and three secondarily; all but one easily controlled.

Getchell finds hemorrhage infrequent; but often enough to give him some anxiety in every case. He thinks a patient ought to remain in bed in the same building in which the operation is done for at least six hours.

Professor Chiari reports one case of bleeding after four hours, one after 24 hours, in two adults over forty, one of whom had to have compression applied for half a day, and in the other the pillar had to be sutured. He does not think tonsillotomy should be performed in adults with very large tonsils, on account of the danger of hemorrhage.

Thrasher, of Cincinnati, says that when the operation is done with the head far below the body, there is always free hemorrhage immediately, and then probably no more. He has had secondary hemorrhage on the following day twice in 3,000 cases.

Luc reports two cases of severe hemorrhage, one to syncope.

Sir Felix Semon has had very serious hemorrhage three times, twice immediately after the operation, and once several hours later.

Welty has seen only one case of hemorrhage after 300 cases of tonsillectomy, and thinks that all hemorrhage after tonsil operations is dependent upon the amount of tonsillar tissue remaining. In the one case that bled there was some tonsillar tissue remaining, as he discovered later. After other methods he has had severe hemorrhages several times.

Todd has had no hemorrhage not controlled at the time of operation since ceasing to use sharp instruments.

Moure, of Bordeaux, reports a case of severe hemorrhage occurring twelve days after a galvanocautery operation.

Brainard, of Boston, has had two secondary hemorrhages in adults, neither fatal, but both alarming.

Pynchon gives his patients a most elaborate paper with minute directions as to what to do in case of hemorrhage, so that he must consider that bleeding occurs sufficiently often to render this necessary. There are four pages of closely printed directions and two pictures in this circular. He gives chlorid of calcium by the mouth or rectum in 10 grain doses in 2 ounces of water, repeated hourly for three doses. After the three days it is discontinued for a few hours before being used again. Forty to 60 grains in 24 hours is the maximum dose. He also mentions lactate of calcium in single doses of 30 grains.

Turning now to the recent literature, one finds a good many cases of hemorrhage, although Haymann thinks a great many more occur than are ever reported, since the tendency to relate unpleasant experiences is not great.

Damianos and Herman report 50 cases of severe bleeding after tonsillotomy, in only five of which there was any definite etiology suggesting hemophilia. There were eight deaths, only two of which occurred in hemophiliacs[10].

There is only one case in literature where the internal carotid was injured. This operation was done by a quack, and is related by Biclard and referred to by Bardeleben. There is a second case which is said to have been an injury of the carotid, but careful reading would seem to show that this was not the case.

Heuking reports. six cases of severe hemorrhage occurring in his practice, in all of which the operation was done with the tonsillotome, and the injury was at the junction of the anterior and posterior pillars, or else at the beginning of the posterior pillar. In none was the hemorrhage from the stump of the injured tonsil. They were all stopped by digital compression with a gauze sponge, and might have been stopped by compression forceps, as in all the cases the hemorrhage ceased without torsion. The ages varied from fifteen to sixty years. Death occurred in several of the cases. The free border of the posterior pillar was caught in the ring of the tonsillotome, thus leaving an open vessel without good opportunity for retraction, and not particularly visible. Owing to the action of the muscle, coagulation was hindered by coughing, vomiting, and gagging".

In 1904, Harmon Smith reported six fatal cases of tonsillar hemorrhage and 48 cases of severe hemorrhage, three of them being his own, in which the bleeding was controlled only by the tonsillar pad hemostat. The special causes of hemorrhage are given as hemorrhagic diathesis; fibroid tonsils; age (adults rather than children) ; sex (males rather than females) ; acute inflammation; anemia; malignancy; abnormalities in the distribution of the blood vessels, such as the ascending pharyngeal artery; abnormally large tonsillar artery; abnormal internal carotid; large vessels in the anterior pillar of the fauces; wounding of large venous plexus at the lower and outer border of the tonsil; arterial sclerosis. The exciting causes are traumatism and local anesthesia, combined with an astringent".

I find the following reports in recent literature, mostly since Smith's article, and not included in those reported by him:

Lamb has reported a case of very severe hemorrhage, requiring the suturing of the pillars".

Stewart removed the tonsils and adenoids under ether in a boy of seven; there was free hemorrhage, which soon stopped. but two hours later blood extravasation took place in the neck and subcutaneously. Death occurred 32 hours after the operation".

Murray has reported three alarming cases of hemorrhage, one six days after operation, requiring etherization and the sewing up of pillars. The second case bled for six hours after the operation and required the suturing of the wound[11].

Brown reports three cases of serious hemorrhage, the first primary, the second two days later, controlled with difficulty; the third 15 days later, persisting for several hours[12].

Roberts had one patient who nearly died from hemorrhage after using the tonsillotome. Operation was done in the upright position[13].

Jarecky reports two cases of secondary hemorrhage, due to injury of the plexus of veins at the tonsil base[14].

Bulson, ten hours after an operation on a boy of six, had hemorrhage so severe as to exsanguinate the child. Saline injection and hypodermics of strychnin and whisky were given. The temperature went to 106, and at one time the child was supposed to be dying. The hemorrhage seemed to cease of its own accord, but it left the child in such a collapsed state that life was maintained with difficulty a sufficient length of time to recover somewhat from the loss of blood[15].

Hayman reports one of his own cases, in which death occurred after operation on adenoids and tonsils. The child was fourteen years of age, operated on at 11 o'clock in the morning in the usual way. There was no unusual amount of bleeding, and what there was apparently stopped completely. Two hours after the operation slight, but continuous, bleeding came from the nasopharynx, soon followed by considerable vomiting of blood and hemorrhage from both tonsil stumps. Peroxid of hydrogen was used, as well as powders and tamponing. These stopped the bleeding from the adenoid region, but not from the tonsils. Cauterizing remedies were then used. The bleeding stopped, but a few hours later began again, so that the entire pharynx wall showed the presence of blood, the exact origin of which was difficult to find. Adrenalin was used hypodermically to no purpose. Gelatin was then injected subcutaneously. The bleeding became more profuse from the tonsils, the two pillars were sewed together over a gauze tampon, and the nasopharynx plugged absolutely tight. Later collapse came on, pulse 140. Digital compression against the stumps of the tonsils was next made and then the Mikulicz tonsil clamp was used. The bleeding stopped for about half an hour, then began again. The tampon came away under the stitching, and the two tonsil pillars were again sewed up over a heavy gauze tampon, but all to no purpose, as the patient collapsed again. Respiration became bad, and two hours later death occurred. At the autopsy the organs were found completely normal. All the portions of the throat were taken out and carefully examined, but the autopsy was made so late that it was impossible to have any microscopic examination. The only history suggesting hemophilia was that the child bled rather easily after injury to the finger, but earlier in her youth she had been operated on for enlarged glands without any special bleeding having been noticed".

There is a tendency to call all such cases as the foregoing cases of hemophilia, even though other signs of hemophilia are absent. Leukemia can give us a dangerous bleeding. A wax-like pallor of the tonsil is characteristic of this condition. Zarniko and Berger have each reported a death after tonsil operations on leukemic cases. The sharpness or dullness of the instruments used does not make any material difference. Haymann reports twenty-one cases of severe bleeding in three thousand, which is less than one per cent. Of these, two thousand were operated on during the first ten years of life, and eight hundred in the next ten years of life.

Lack, of London, has seen most alarming hemorrhage after tonsillotomy, persisting for hours and ending only on faintness. He thinks severe hemorrhage will occur in three out of four cases in fibrous tonsils of adults if cutting instruments are used".

Without carrying these statistics further, we can see that with rare exceptions every operator doing any amount of work has had hemorrhage at some time or other. It seems to me that this is less likely to occur after the operation of tonsillectomy, but I do not deny that it may and does occur after this operation.

Chevalier Jackson says that oozing after tonsillectomy is exceedingly rare, and that it is bleeding from a vessel concealed back of the anterior pillar that is usually mistaken for oozing.

The hemorrhage seems most likely to come from the vessels around the base of the tonsil or from injury to the pillars, since when no portion of the tonsil is left, the vessels of the muscular tissue of the superior constrictor usually contract to such an extent as to completely close the mouths of the vessels.

As to the best methods of handling hemorrhage, simple pressure with a good-sized cotton or gauze tampon carried into the tonsil cavity and maintained for a short time, will usually be sufficient. If it is not, the tampon may be soaked in a weak solution of nitrate of silver or in peroxid of hydrogen. In this case one must be careful that there is no free fluid or excess on the sponge. Should this be the case when peroxid of hydrogen is used, there may be too great formation of gas, with the danger of inhaling some of it into the trachea with resultant difficulty in breathing. If the simple pressure is insufficient, the bleeding point can be grasped with the tonsil hemostat and the vessel twisted or tied. Tying the vessel is very difficult and will seldom be necessary. Suturing the pillars over a pad of gauze is efficient and much easier than tying the tonsil. This suture is removed in twenty-four to forty-eight hours. For continuous oozing, lactate or chlorid of calcium may be used. Monsell's solution should be avoided as dirty, not very effective, and as having danger of secondary hemorrhage when the slough comes away. The large tonsil pad hemostat may be needed, but is very uncomfortable for the patient, and should be avoided if possible. There is also danger of slough from its use.

Dr. Chevalier Jackson, of Pittsburgh, has reported six cases of ligature of the external carotid for hemorrhage. Dr. Jackson's cases were seen by him as consultant after everything else had been tried and the patients were moribund. In one case caustics had previously been used, and when the slough began to separate there was oozing again, and had the carotid not been tied the patient would have bled to death. Dr. Jackson's experienec is somewhat unique. In most cases it is probably possible to stop the hemorrhage, even where the bleeding is severe, without resorting to so formidable an operation.

From the reported cases there is no particular proof that dangerous bleeding occurs more often in adults than in children. There seems to be sufficient testimony in favor of the use of calcium chlorid and calcium lactate as preventives of hemorrhage to warrant their future use. Pierce gives the chlorid for a week before operation, while most operators advise its use for three days.

Bryant gives the calcium salts two or three days before operating, and has no annoying hemorrhage.

Lermoyez always gives his patients three grams a day of calcium chlorid for three days preceding the operation. He says there is hemorrhage when the pillar is injured and when the whole tonsil is removed at once in an adult.

OTHER ACCIDENTS.

Exclusive of hemorrhage, the following accidents were reported:

Sixteen have seen injury to the uvula, the pillars or the palate, even to the point of temporary paresis of the soft palate. 'I have seen one such case as a result of twisting the artery in the soft palate after troublesome hemorrhage. The condition lasted about a week, followed by perfect recovery. While the paralysis lasted the voice was much altered. Three others report alteration of speech from injury to the pillars.

Quinsy from incomplete operation, and as a result of injury with the snare, double otitis media with double mastoid, and acute otitis media were reported. Four observers had mild cellulitis follow, once claimed to be due to unclean instruments used by students. Severe surgical shock with deep sloughing in the tonsillar region was twice seen by Berens after the use of the snare. Simple infection is reported four times. Jackson reports a case of cervical cellulitis from operation; three cases of respiratory arrest, one of cardiac arrest, all requiring tracheotomy and with recovery in all cases. Torticollis was observed in one case; and one reporter nearly lost two cases from chloroform anesthesia.

The following deaths were reported:

E. M. Holmes, a case of general staphylococcus infection, death on the tenth day, with staphylococcus aureus in all the organs. He states there was no other known way of entrance, as everything was as aseptic as possible at the time of operation. As, however, a submucous operation on the septum was done at the same time as the tonsil and adenoid operation, it is hard to say to which operation, if any, death was due. The operation was done on the back. After the boy was returned to the ward he turned blue, the heart became rapid and weak, and death ensued.

Hubbard cites two deaths, one from pneumonia, chloroform anesthesia, erect position. The other was in the practice of a colleague, where a mixture of chloroform and ether was given, with a local injection of ten to fifteen minims. Death occurred with the symptoms of adrenalin poisoning in about one minute.

MacBride reports one death from chloroform and one from sepsis or malignant scarlet fever on the second day.

Cohen has knowledge of a death from spasm of the glottis during etherization, and now fears to operate unless he has facilities for intubation and tracheotomy at hand.

Thompson had a death from chloroform from respiratory failure after the operation was completed.

Gradle had a patient who was said to have died from an abscess in the throat one and a half weeks after a perfectly smooth tonsillotomy done with the tonsillotome, but does not know the details.

I have had one case where after removal of the tonsil a pledget of gauze wet with too much peroxid of hydrogen was placed in the tonsil cavity to stop the bleeding. There was so much gas formation that some of it was inhaled, interfering with respiration and requiring tracheotomy. Recovery took place. This is the same case referred to under the section on position:

EFFECTS ON THE VOICE.

The question of injury to the voice is one that merits discussion, inasmuch as the laity have considerable fear that the tonsil operation will injure the voice. By far the great majority of the reporters have seen only improvement and not injury to the voice. Those physicians having most to do with professional singers, however, give somewhat guarded replies, and admit that for the time at least there is an alteration in the voice, followed later, as a rule, by improvement, most of them having found that higher tones were obtainable than before, an exception being DeBolis, who finds the voice generally lowered.

E. L. Shurley has seen many cases where the tone or quality and the sustaining power of the voice are impaired by the removal of part of the tonsil.

Gleason reports that an actress told him that her singing voice had been ruined and her stage course ended after a tonsil operation, and he has also had numerous complaints from adults that the voice was injured by an operation done years before.

F. E. Miller says incomplete removal injures; thorough removal raises the pitch and increases the amplitude of the voice.

Price Brown has had singing masters say that the voice was injured, but has never had that experience. He never removes the entire gland and is careful not to injure the pillars.

Professor Chiari says the power and range of the voice is changed in adults, so that he does not entirely remove the tonsil in adults, but only makes it smaller.

D. Crosby Greene, Jr., says that in two professional singers the voice improved in every way, but one month elapsed before effective singing could be done. If the uvula or soft palate is injured, there may be permanent change.

Coolidge says that professional singers have the voice thrown out of adjustment for some time.

George B. Rice, who treats a great many singers, says the voice is frequently changed somewhat, but is soon adjusted to the new conditions. In children a nasal twang may come on after the complete operation, but this disappears later.

Lack has found that singers sometimes entirely lose their singing voice, and public speakers, teachers, etc., find that they are unable to speak so well or so long as before the operation, and the use of the voice causes them a hitherto unknown aching feeling in the throat. This consequence of tonsillotomy in adults he has repeatedly met with, and does not think it is generally sufficiently considered. The greater the enlargement, the longer it has persisted, the greater the risk. A medical friend of his had his tonsils removed a few years ago, and not only did he have most alarming hemorrhage lasting nearly twelve hours and ending only on faintness, but at the same time he entirely lost his singing voice.

Levy reports stiffness of articulation for a time, soon disappearing.

Makuen finds the final results satisfactory, but singers may have to make changes in the use of the muscles.

T. P. Berens reduces the tonsils very slowly in singers, while Smyth refrains from the operation in trained singers.

Hajek says the quality of the voice is changed somewhat.

Luc, Lermoyez and Sir Felix Semon have never seen any bad results.

Ballenger finds the voice impaired for about six weeks, but the ultimate effect good.

I believe that the range and power of the voice should be increased, provided the pillars are uninjured, after complete tonsillectomy, as in many cases the tonsil, by its firm attachment to the pillars, especially if it is enlarged, hinders the mobility of the muscles. I have always believed that the reported cases of injury to the voice were due to the fact that the tonsil stumps were still present, hindering the mobility of muscular action, or else that the pillars themselves were injured by the operation.

CONCLUSIONS.

Further study of the physiology of the tonsil seems desirable, as it is still a question how important the tonsil may be at certain periods of life. If of value to the economy, the tonsils ought not to be removed to as great an extent as at present.

Under diseased conditions the tonsil is one of the avenues of entrance for the tubercle bacillus and for the specific organism of rheumatism, whatever that may be. There is sufficient amount of undoubted clinical evidence to show that it is also the avenue through which the infection enters in many other constitutional disorders.

The small submerged tonsil is quite as apt to be deleterious to the economy as the large one.

Local measures in the treatment of tonsillar troubles have their place.

Any condition in which it is evident that the tonsil is exerting a deleterious action upon the entire organism, and which cannot be averted by local treatment, is an indication for removal.

Ether is the safest general anesthetic.

According to the testimony of most observers, some form of horizontal position is the safest for general anesthesia, though the writer believes that the upright position, properly safeguarded, is equally safe.

Tonsillectomy should always be done in preference to tonsillotomy. Any method that completely removes the tonsil with its capsule, and with the least traumatism, is satisfactory.

The voice is improved rather than injured, provided the pillars are uninjured in the operation.

BIBLIOGRAPHY.

1. Goodale. Boston Med. and .Surg. Jour., September 25, 1902.
2. Goodale. Jour. of Med. Research, May, 1902.
3. Wright, Jonathan. New York Med. Jour., August 8, 1908.
4. Wright, Jonathan. New York Med. Jour., October 10 and November 7, 1908.
5. Wood. Transactions of the Henry Phipps Institute, 1906.
6. Bosworth. Medical Record, January 11, 1902.
7. Spohn. Laryngoscope, January, 1905, p. 73.
8. Mosher. Laryngoscope, November, 1903, p. 817.
9. Wood. Transactions A. L. R. & O. Society, p. 376.
10. Goodale. Boston Med. and Surg. Jour., May 19, 1898.
11. Rogers. Medical Record, November 28, 1903.
12. Wood. Laryngoscope, May, 1906.
13. Koplik. American Jour. of the Med. Sciences, November, 1903.
14. Frissell. Medical Record, May 12, 1906.
15. Rosenheim. Johns Hopkins Hospital Bulletin, November, 1908, p. 338.
16. Ingals. Laryngoscope, September, 1907, p. 712.
17. Elliott, A. R., Chicago. New York Medical Journal, May 1, 1909.
18. Taylor. New York Med. Jour., March 31, 1906.
19. Wright, G. H. Boston Medical and Surgical Journal, May 20, 1909.
20. Ward. Surgery, Gynecology and Obstetrics, April, 1909.
21. Richards, Geo. L. Boston Med. and Surg. Jour., September 24, 1908, p. 411, and Am. Jour. Clinical Medicine, February and March, 1908.
22. Lack. Journal of Laryngology, October, 1901, p. 599.
23. Yankauer. Laryngoscope, May, 1909.
24. Goodale. Jour. of A. M. A., May 25, 1907.
25. West. Johns Hopkins Hospital Bulletin, November, 1908.
26. Damianos and Herman. Wiener klin. Wochenschrift, 1902.
27. Heuking. Archiv fuer Laryngolgie. Vol 17, 1905, p. 64.
28. Smith, Harmon. Laryngoscope, February, 1904, p. 121.
29. Lamb. British Medical Journal, November 15, 1902.
30. Stewart. London Lancet, November 15, 1902.
31. Murray. Laryngoscope, December, 1903.
32. Brown, Edw. J. Laryngoscope, February, 1905, p. 106.
33. Roberts. Transactions A. L. R. & O. Soc., 1904, p. 397.
34. Jarecky. Medical Record, April 30, 1904.
35. Bulson. Laryngoscope, March, 1903, p. 219.
36. Haymann. Archiv fuer Laryngologie, Vol. 21, p. 15.
37. Lack. Journal of Laryngology, October, 1901, p. 599.

LI

CASE REPORTS.

By Lewis A. Coffin, M. D.,

SURGEON, THROAT DEP'T, MANHATTAN EYE, EAR AND THROAT
HOSPITAL; LARYNGOLOGIST AND OTOLÒGIST TO THE
CITY HOME AND WORKHOUSE,

New York.

(A) CAVERNOUS SINUS THROMBOSIS.

While still at her country place, on the morning of October 4, 1908, Miss J. G., 59 years of age, was seized with a sharp and violent pain in the right anterior aspect of her head. For four or five days following, beside the severe pain located about and in the right eye, there was nausea and vomiting, and patient complained of a blowing or rushing noise. The nurse said she could hear the same noise with her ear at the patient's temple. About the fifth day after the onset of pain some bulging of the right eye was noticed and diplopia developed.

The temperature during this time was never over 99½ degrees F., nor did it rise higher during the subsequent history of the case.

On October 12th patient was moved to the city, and I being asked over the phone to call, was told of the severe pain over, and bulging of the right eye. Wrong as it may seem, my diagnosis of disease of the nasal accessory sinuses was made, and I hastened to make the call, prepared to confirm the long-distance diagnosis. I found patient in condition described, but history was not gone into as minutely as should have been done. The right frontal sinus was darker on transillumination than the left, and very tender on percussion and pressure. No discharge was seen in the nose. Drainage I believed to be blocked, and the eye condition due to pressure. Septum was markedly deviated to the right, and there was a broad ecchondroma on that side of the nose. Owing to this intranasal condition and the temperament of the patient, who declared she would consent to no operation except under general anesthesia, I decided to do a radical Killian operation. I asked Dr. C. G. Coakley to see the case with me. He confirmed the diagnosis and agreed that a radical operation offered the best solution of the case; suggesting, however, that we delay operation to obtain a radiograph of patient's head. Dr. Caldwell made the exposure on the afternoon of October 13th, and on the morning of the 14th delivered an excellent negative, which showed cloudiness of both frontal and ethmoidal regions; greater cloudiness showing on the right side. A complete Killian operation was done in the afternoon. I was much surprised to find in the frontal sinus no pus, polypi or granulations. The lining membrane was, however, very thick from congestion as was the membrane lining the ethmoidal and sphenoidal cavities. Bleeding was very profuse, and although there may have been at some point a diseased cell or pus, I was not able to recognize it. Recovery from operation was uneventful, except for condition about the eye. Immediately the pain disappeared, and the exophthalmus was reduced and continued steadily to improve; but there developed a marked chemosis of the lower lid. Sixteen days after the operation, the chemosis persisting, I asked Dr. Egbart LeFevre to see the case. He gave as his opinion that we had been dealing with a thrombosis of the cavernous sinus, and said, further, that he believed that the operation had been of the greatest benefit, as by reducing the edema about the tissues of the eye by the extensive bleeding we had probably saved the sight of the eye if not the life of the patient. To reduce the coagulability of the blood as well as to break up any existing thrombus or clot, large doses of lemonade were ordered. A slightly astringent wash and light pressure were applied to the eye. Improvement in the chemosis was immediate and steady, and patient was considered well on November 12th. Her nurse left her on November 14th, and I find this entrance on her chart, "Patient in A No. 1 condition."

Thrombophlebitis is of traumatic or septic origin. In the region under discussion thrombophlebitis from traumatism may be ruled out. Herbert Parsons[1] says: "Thrombosis of the cavernous sinus may arise from extension from the ophthalmic vein, the source of infection being wounds or septic infection of the skin, etc., or from the ear, nose, and accessory sinuses, pharynx, tonsils, etc., or as a metastasis in infectious diseases or septic conditions."

Thrombophlebitis is a progressive and cumulative disease, as long as the source of infection persists; but the source removed, the disease is marked by retrogression and self-limitation. The last holds good, of course, only when the source of infection has been removed before the disease has progressed to a point beyond repair.

H. Siguard[2] says the prognosis of thrombophlebitis is very gloomy, and he is inclined to believe with Parker that thrombophlebitis of the cavernous sinus is equivalent to a death warrant. He cites seven cases, however, in which recovery from a condition diagnosed as thrombosis of the cavernous sinus followed operation on and about the mastoid.

In my own case it is probable that the source of infection was in some one of the accessory sinuses of the nose, that by the operation the source of infection was removed. Much of the edema and pressure were removed immediately by the local blood-letting. Liquefaction of the clot and a re-establishment of circulation through the sinus was probably hastened by the administration of the lemon juice. This question then presents itself: given a case of thrombosis of the cavernous sinus in which no trouble can be found about the ear or elsewhere, which may be considered as the septic focus, would we be justified in doing a radical Killian operation in the hopes that the septic origin might be in some of the accessory sinuses of the nose? I believe we would.

(B) TERATOMA OF THE SOFT PALATE.

In the latter part of October, 1908, Mrs. H. R. consulted me on account of a tickling in her throat and a constant desire to cough on lying down.

Mrs. R. is a lady 66 years of age, very large, of a nervous temperament, and has very large varicose veins about the sides and at the base of the tongue. For years she has had what she calls strangling spells, the tendency to which has been well controlled by cathartics and nitroglycerin. When told of the tickling and cough I, not being in a condition at the time to examine the throat thoroughly, thought probably it was caused by the varicose condition at the base of the tongue and prescribed accordingly. About ten days later, on the phone, I was told her condition was no better. The patient was asked to come to my office. With a small mirror, in the back of the throat I discovered what seemed a small tumor lying just behind and above the uvula, and of the shape of the uvula. Hooking the velum forward and up with the mirror, a tumor as large as my thumb hung free in the pharynx. I asked Dr. Jonathan Wright to see the growth in situ. Dr. Wright and myself both thought it to be a simple papillomatous growth. I snared off what I could of the growth through the mouth and gave it to Dr. Wright for microscopic study. His report was as follows: "This specimen is apparently primarily a teratoma; cells included in the tissue probably from embryonic life. They are apparently branchiogenetic cells. Unfortunately there are areas where the endothelium of the blood vessels is so infiltrating the tissue as to leave little doubt in my mind that we have here an endotheliomatous growth of serious import. The surface epithelium is hyperplastic, assuming the form of papilloma. Dr. Wright asked me to submit the slides to others for an opinion. Dr. Hodenpyl, of Columbia University, reports as follows:

"At your request, I have carefully examined two microscopic slides of a growth taken from the soft palate of Mrs. H. F. R., and have the following report to make:

The tissue consists partly of a new growth and partly of the underlying normal tissue. This latter consists of mucous glands, a loose stroma with blood vessels, etc. The growth itself consists of two parts. The major portion is composed of intercommunicating strands of squamous epithelium arranged in such a manner as to resemble a papilloma. On either border the growth is of different character. Here and originating in the columnar epithelium the growth is distinctly glandular in type. It gradually becomes atypical (i. e., bordering on carcinoma), and finally becomes merged into the papilloma.

The growth is infiltrated with a moderate number of leucocytes, and careful research reveals but a very few leucocytes.

I should regard the growth as a papillary adenocarcinoma,

and I think it took its origin just at the junction of squamous and columnar epithelium. From the specimen I gain the impression that the growth is not very malignant, at least, some of the signs denoting malignancy are wanting. Not knowing the history of the patient, I am unable to speak definitely upon this point. However, I would suggest the advisability of removing any remaining traces of the growth if there be such. Yours sincerely,   EUGENE HODENPYL."

In accordance with the advice of Drs. Wright and Hodenpyl, I operated for the removal of the base of this tumor, which was situated in the median line just posterior to the septum, in the following manner:

Under cocain anesthesia a transverse incision from molar to molar was made through the tissues of the hard palate in a line parallel to and just anterior to its junction with the soft palate. The posterior flap thus made was dissected back until free of the hard palate, when the incision was carried through the soft palate into the nasal pharynx. The soft palate was then separated into two layers; the posterior containing the growth was cut out as near the Eustachian tubes as possible. The transverse incision was stitched up and healed by primary union, except for a small slough in the center. The opening thus caused was completely filled by granulation and contraction in about one month. Bleeding during the operation was practically nil. Dr. Wright has given much study to this growth and has made it subject of many consultations, and sends me the following report for this paper:

"In going over the reports of the case of Mrs. R.—which we made you from the laboratory without a view to their being incorporated in a report for publication—in looking over the sections and in considering the various expressions of opinion as to the tumor by competent histologists to whom the sections were submitted, there is so much conflicting evidence that I am unable to say more than that it was regarded as an epithelial growth of a malignant nature. I was inclined at first sight of the piece removed for microscopic examination to think it a teratoma of branchiogenetic origin, with evidences of malignant potentialities of a feeble character in certain cells, some of which were of endothelial appearance and some of an epithelial nature. On examining the whole tumor, there can be no doubt 'that the fimbriated extremity from which we on inspection in the mirror made the diagnosis of a benign papilloma presented the structure microscopically which warranted it, but deeper down, closer to the base, were various appearances of graver import which, when revealed by the microscope, justified the operative course pursued.

Frankly, I do not know what name to give the growth, and a minute and exhaustive description of the objective appearances would extend this report beyond the limits suitable for your purpose.   JONATHAN WRIGHT."

· The soft palate seems to be a favorite field for the development of trouble-making tumors—trouble for the pathologist as well as the possessor.

They are often diagnosed as mixed tumors, but in several instances have been classed as teratoma. Serapin[3], in discussing these tumors, says:

1. The mixed tumors of the palate form a group by themselves from the pathologic, anatomic, and chemic point of view.

2. They have a common origin with teratomata and teratoid tumors.

3. From a clinical point of view they are benign in character, easy to enucleate, and not inclined to recurrence.

4. Garel[4] has reported a teratoma of the soft palate. Fullerton, R.[5] has reported a teratoma arising from the right tonsillar region.

So far as I have been able to look the matter up, mixed tumors of this region have been reported by the following men:

REFERENCES.

1. Herbert Parson. Path. of the Eye, Vol. IV., p. 1226.

2. Siguard, H. Thrombo-Phlebitis des Sinus Caverneux d'Origin Otitique. These de Paris, 1904.

3. Serapin. Mixed tumors of the palate. Russ. Archiv. f. Chirurg., February 2, 1903.

4. Garel. Tumeur rare du voile du palais (Teratoma of Soft Palate). Bulletin de la Soc. Med. des Hopitaux de Lyon II. 1903. Seance du 24 Fev., 1903.

5. Fullerton, Robert. Teratoma arising from the right tonsillar region. Brit. Med. Journal, Oct. 12, 1907.

Gevaert. Les tumeurs du voile du palais. Belg. Med. V, 1898, p. 385.

Cordes. Ein Fall von Endothelioma myxomatodes palati mollis. Deutsche méd. Wochenschrift, 35, 1900.

Halstead. Mixed tumor of the soft palate. The Laryngoscope, September, 1906.

Leto (Luigi). Tumore misto del palato. Archiv. Ital. di Laringologia III, 1906.

Chaput. Tumeur glandulaire (adeno-myxome) de la voute palatine. Bull. et Mem. de la Soc. Anat., No. 9, 1900.

Gross, G.

Floche, G. Tumeur mixte du voile du palais. Societe de Medecine de Nancy, Seance du 23 Juillet, 1902.

Hoche. Revue Medicale de l'Est, 1 Novembre, 1902.

LII

SOME RECENT CASES OF NASAL SARCOMA. SUBMITTED AS A COROLLARY TO A FORMER PAPER UPON THE SAME SUBJECT.*

By J. Price-Brown, M. D.,

Toronto.

It is acknowledged that in our professional life we should hold no secrets in the treatment of disease. Every method should be as open as the day. And if after long experience we have found faith in one method above all others, by which valuable lives have been saved, no matter how long and tedious may have been the path of the finding, it becomes our duty to proclaim it to others; and to continue to proclaim it until our confreres not only give us a patient hearing but also grant to the method a reasonable examination.

Six years ago I reported to this Association three cases of nasal sarcoma. All of them had exhibited the usual classical symptoms; continued obstructive growth, repeated hemorrhages, etc. All had been previously operated upon. All had been of long standing; and pathologic examinations of sections taken from each individual case verified each diagnosis. Two were reported at that time to be cured; one was still under treatment.

Four years ago I submitted a further report upon the last of the three. At that time it still required, occasionally. operative treatment at the basic spot, at the juncture of the posterior naris with the vault.

This necessity is now over, and two and a quarter years have elapsed since the last cauterization was made.

To-day all three men are perfectly well, following their usual vocations as bread winners for themselves and families. It is fourteen years since the first was last operated on; seven years the second, and over two years the third.

*Read at the annual meeting of the American Laryngological Association in Boston, June, 1909.

CASE 4. In the December issue of the ANNALS OF OTOLOGY for 1906 I reported my next case, of which I offer a brief note. The patient was a butcher, aged 58. His father had died of cancer of the stomach at the age of 72. On examination 1 found the left nasal passage from the anterior to the posterior naris filled with a dark, dense growth, which bled on being touched. After removing a section with a knife, microscopic examination by a pathologist proved it to be round-celled sarcoma. The treatment was on similar lines to that reported in the previous cases. In two weeks the growth was, seemingly, entirely removed, and the nasal passage cleared of obstruction. The growth in this case was from the outer wall, the middle and inferior turbinals being involved and softened. The electrocautery operations numbered seven or eight, being done at intervals of one or two days. At the expiration of the time mentioned there was complete restoration of normal breathing through that nostril. His temperature when he first presented himself was 99 2-5, and it continned more or less elevated throughout the treatment, running between 99 and 102 degrees. As the operative treatment drew to a close septic symptoms developed. He lingered about two months and then succumbed to them. He died, I believe, from the absorption of toxins from the site of the original tumor. There was, however, no return of the sarcoma, nor of inflammatory vegetations; and both the patient and his friends were spared the horrible and unsightly disfigurement and distress which usually attends death from this disease.

Taking this as one fatal case out of four, 75% of recoveries have been the result of the electrocautery method of treatment, which was adopted in all of these cases—a fairly good showing, when we consider the far smaller percentage of recoveries which have followed the usual surgical methods of operation.

More than two years elapsed. Then, on April 1st, 1909, Dr. Kerr, of Toronto, referred:

CASE 5. Mr. C. C., age 35. His general health had been good, also his family history. He was a bachelor, and a weaver by trade. For several months there had been gradually increasing stenosis of the left nasal passage, and for the past few weeks complete occlusion, affecting even the right side. Taste and smell were both gone and the voice had a thick, nasal twang.

Examination.—Left nasal passage packed with a red, fleshy growth, which bled on being touched. On applying cocain and adrenalin, the tumor was found to be widely sessile and attached chiefly to the triangular cartilage of the septum. It extended to, but not into, the nasopharynx. A segment was at once removed by knife and submitted for pathologic examination. Drs. Carveth and Davis gave the following report:

"The specimen is for the most part composed of small, round cells with deeply staining, round nuclei and but little cytoplasm. There is a small amount of interstitial reticulum. There are many blood vessels with undeveloped walls, some showing only the endothelial lining, and in some cases they seem to be blood spaces rather than vessels. The microscopic examination, together with the clinical history, incline us to believe that the growth is a small, round-celled sarcoma."

Electrocautery operations were repeated almost daily for a period of two weeks, the sloughs presented being a portion of what was taken away during that period. By the time that the growth was fully removed the nasal passage was quite free and breathing had become normal again. For the six succeedings weeks he has been under observation. The sense of smell has returned, and for more than a month he has been doing his regular work. There is no indication of the redevelopment of the sarcoma.

CASE 6. April 9th, Mr. W. S., age 20, was referred by Dr. Nicol, of Cookstown. For more than two years he had suffered from a constantly increasing growth in the right nasal passage. For the whole of this period he had lost the sense of taste and smell. Nine months ago the stenosis had become very severe, and, being referred to a surgeon, segments had been removed. by one means or another. from then until now —each one being attended by excessive hemorrhage. As the tumor continued to increase in size, he was finally brought by his family physician to the city and placed in the Toronto Western Hospital under my care.

I found complete occlusion of the right nasal passage by a red, inflamed mass, which extended from the anterior naris backward into the postnasal space. There it assumed a globular form and seemed to be attached to the right summit of the septum. It bore no resemblance either in attachment or appearance to adenoid tissue. The slightest touch caused bleeding; yet, notwithstanding this fact, the hardness within the nasal cavity was so dense that, on first examination, I considered the obstruction to be partly due to a cartilaginous and bony ridge of the septum; which, after a free application of cocain and adrenalin, I attempted to remove with a saw. But the instrument met with neither bony nor cartilaginous resistance. It simply removed a mass of tissue which, upon pathologic examination, proved to be a portion of an angiosarcoma, as verified by Drs. Davis and Carveth, as follows:

"Examination of specimen from nostril. We find that this is an angiosarcoma, composed of small, round cells in a fibrous reticulum, having in it large and numerous blood vessels with thin walls. Myoxmatous degeneration is found in places."

The bleeding was excessive and nasal packing had to be resorted to.

On the 11th the tampons were removed, and electro-cautery operations were done on the 12th, 13th, 14th and 15th of April.

On the afternoon of the 15th he had a severe rigor, and in the evening, when sleeping, had a large, involuntary movement of the bowels. Nasal operations were consequently suspended.

On the 18th the patient awoke in the morning with agonizing pain around the left ankle, on the side opposite to that of the sarcoma. This was followed by swelling. The treatment at first was by fomentations and subsequently by poultices; but the leg was not opened until May 3rd, when a large amount of streptococcal pus was evacuated. Several days later a smaller abscess was operated on on the opposite side of the foot. Since then the leg has completely healed.

To return to the sarcoma. On the 19th, the day after the chill, the nose was cauterized, but not again until the 29th, after which the cautery operations were repeated almost daily until May 17th, the rule being to cleanse the nasal cavity and anesthetize it with cocain and adrenalin, and then to cauterize as much of the growth as was deemed advisable each morning, and to follow this by an evening dressing.

By this time the nasal cavity was tolerably free from the growth all the way back to the nasopharynx. So, on May

18th, chloroform was administered, and a large portion of the nasopharyngeal portion of the tumor removed by means of a modified Lowenburg's forceps, and as the growth had been fissured in several places by the intranasal operations, this lessened the hemorrhage. The attachment was to the anterior part of the roof of the nasopharynx, to the septum, and also to the outer wall and the upper side of the soft palate.

Subsequently I operated almost daily with the electrocautery upon the fragments of the growth still remaining and upon the base of the nasopharyngeal pedicle. This could all be done by means of a strong light through the nasal cavity. These operations were continued until last Saturday, when the treatment was almost complete.

The nose is free, and practically all that remains of the tumor are a few disintegrating sloughs, which will soon cease to form. In this case, too, the sense of smell has returned. Still when I return I may find a few minor cauterizations necessary.

CASE 6. On April 12th, 1909, Mr. S. W., age 18, was referred to me by Dr. W. M. Brown, of Neustadt. The history in some respects was more severe than in the last mentioned case. For several years the left nasal cavity had been filled with a similar growth, extending into the nasopharynx, where it assumed a much larger size than in the case of Mr. S. During the last two years he had undergone very many operations by snare and forceps and cautery, each being attended by abundant hemorrhage.

On examination, I found nasal breathing on either side impossible. The left passage was filled by the growth swelling out in a roundish form to within half an inch of the nostril. The right side, while narrowed by the pressure from the opposite chamber, was filled with pus. In the postpharynx was a large, globular mass, completely filling it. He was at once placed in the Western Hospital.

I need not detail the treatment in this case, as it was on similar lines to the preceding one, which resembled the method practiced in all the cases I have reported.

In this, however, there was no preliminary operation of any kind to secure a section for pathologic examination. That was deferred until later, the daily cautery operations being commenced at once. As the main object was to reduce the size

of the tumor as speedily and as safely as possible, the attacks
were made on the central part, leaving the shrinkage shell
as a protector to the normal tissues. Consequently, although
the sittings were long and tedious to the operator, they produced little pain to the patient. Little by little the heart was
eaten out of the nasal portion of the tumor and the nasopharynx was reached. In the meantime I had discovered that
the attachment was to the middle turbinal and upper posterior
end of the septum and nasopharynx; and, like the former
case, there was also an adhesion to the soft palate. Many
sloughs were taken away during the first month of treatment,
and the nasal cavity became quite free. Still, breathing
through the nose was quite impossible, owing to the presence
of the postnasal section of the growth, although several
cautery cuts into it through the nasal passage had been made.

On the thirty-first day of treatment chloroform was administered, and the body of the tumor removed, post-nasally, with
cutting forceps. The bleeding was severe, much more so than
in the previous case just reported, and post-nasal packing had
to be done. Two days later this was removed, when I discovered one piece of tumor still attached to the post-pharyngeal wall, low down and immediately behind the left posterior
pillar. It presented the appearance of a hard, misplaced
uvula. Another segment occupied the posterior part of the
nasal cavity and was attached to the middle turbinal and the
summit of the septum. These were both removed by electrocautery. Since then many other spots have required to be
burned in the nose and post-nasal space, but all were done
directly through the nasal cavity.

During the last week the improvement in every way has
been very marked. There are now no vegetations of the
growth to be seen anywhere, only sloughing spots from recent
burnings, which are removed daily. Nasal respiration is perfectly free. The vault is open to the fullest examination. The
affected nostril is much wider than the other one all the way
through, and the posterior chaona at least three times the
size of its corresponding fellow. The sense of smell, entirely
absent for more than a year, has likewise returned. A noticeable feature, particularly marked in this case, is the ease with
which any recrudescence of the disease could be attacked
again *per vias naturales*.

In one respect the pathologic examination in this case differed from the preceding two. The section taken was from the center of the mass removed in the major operation from the nasopharynx. The report is here appended:

"I have examined the specimen of tissue from the nasopharynx, and consider the condition to be one of myxosarcoma. The myxomatous tissue, forming a greater part of the growth, is exceedingly vascular, the vessels as a rule having poorly developed walls, and in different areas of the growth there are masses of small, round cells, the individual cells being separated by very scanty stroma, which in places contains thin-walled blood vessels. The condition I believe is one of sarcomatous transformation of a myxomatous tissue.

Yours faithfully,
(Signed)   H. B. ANDERSON,
Assoc. Prof. Clin. Med., Univ. of Toronto."

In reviewing these cases, it may be noted that the whole seven cases occurred in males; that the ages were, respectively, 18, 20, 21, 21, 35, 50, 58; and that two of them occurred in the right nasal passage, and five in the left. Three out of the seven have permanently recovered, one died, the fifth had no return six weeks after healing; and in the last two the growths have been removed, the patients being still under treatment. They were all private patients.

In view of these facts, I think I am entitled to present this subject in the light of research work, not in pathology, but in operative treatment; and, in doing so, there are several points I would like to touch upon, basing them upon the history of these cases, with the fourteen years' experience which they have afforded, and the fact that the process and results have made me a stronger advocate of the treatment here outlined than ever.

1.   In sarcoma of the nose the usual site of origin is in the soft tissues, and not in the bony framework which supports them.

2.   That the origin is usually in the form of a pedicle, which rapidly becomes sessile.

3.   That as the sarcomatous mass enlarges and presses upon the surrounding mucosa, abrasions take place that **are** quickly transformed into adhesions. These in time may become almost coextensive with the disease itself.

4. These adhesions never attain the vitality and virile power possessed by the pedicle. Hence, when once destroyed, they are not likely to reform again.

5. Recrudescence, however; may take place in the region of the pedicle; and, in view of this contingency, this region should be kept under regular observation and control.

6. Owing to the fact that in many cases of nasal sarcoma the affected cavity becomes entirely filled by the hemorrhagic growth, that its adhesions are extensive and that it is impossible at the time of examination to locate them, attempts at intranasal removal by the ordinary knife are inadvisable; but that gradual and systematic dissection out by the cautery knife, in suitable cases, is a method which is always available and should be encouraged.

LIII

PURULENT OTITIS MEDIA OF INFANCY AND CHILDHOOD.*

By H. O. Reik, M. D.,

ASSOCIATE IN OPHTHALMOLOGY JOHNS HOPKINS UNIVERSITY,
SURGEON IN THE BALTIMORE EYE, EAR AND
THROAT HOSPITAL,

BALTIMORE.

In selecting this topic for my paper I was influenced more by a desire for information than the hope of presenting to you anything new in relation to the subject. From both reading and observation I have conceived the idea that some members of the profession seem to look upon suppurative otitis media occurring in children as a different disease from that bearing the same name in adults. Certainly a different line of treatment is often recommended, and there appears to be some question as to whether the affection does not pursue a different course in the two classes of patients. I am led, therefore, to ask a question—does suppurative otitis media occurring in infancy or early childhood differ at all from that disease as observed in adult life, and, if so, in what respects? As forming a basis for discussion, I shall avail myself of the privilege of suggesting a few points wherein there may be grounds for supposing that the disease varies in some way, either as to its course of procedure or the response to treatment, and I trust you will not only discuss these, but add to the list any that have a practical bearing upon the question.

Purulent otitis media is an infectious disease, dependent, in the main, upon the action of the pyogenic microorganisms. We cannot suppose, therefore, that there is any difference in the etiology of the affection in the two classes of patients, at least in so far as the active agent is concerned.

*Read at the meeting of the Southern Section Amer. Laryngological, Rhinological and Otological Society, Richmond, Va., February 14, 1909.

It has been said that there are differences in the tissues upon which the germs have to work, that the younger, more nearly embryonic, tissue of the middle ear of the infant is more susceptible to inflammation and possesses less resistant power to the action of the pathogenic bacteria. I am by no means sure this is true; clinical experience does not furnish very strong support to the theory. That children are more susceptible than adults to middle ear inflammation is probably quite true, but the reason for this more likely lies in the factors that predispose to infection than in any peculiarity of histologic development of the tissues. The great prevalence of otitis media in young children has seemed to me to be largely due to the coexisting very great prevalence of adenoids and diseased tonsils at that period of life. The family physician is beginning to recognize the predisposing relationship of these affections to middle ear inflammation, but I sometimes wonder if even the otologist fully comprehends the intimate relationship often existing between nasopharyngitis, adenoids and tonsils and the progress and persistence of the middle ear disease. This point, bearing upon both etiology and pathology, may be considered one of the most pronounced differences in the disease, as viewed in childhood or in adult life. The etiologic influence we all teach, but do we always pay the proper amount of attention to the predisposing factor as a part of the aural treatment? Once the middle ear disease has started we are possibly too prone to devote attention principally or wholly to the ear, perhaps entirely ignoring the continued existence of such an important element in the original cause of the disease. It may be possible—in many instances it certainly is—to heal the aural affection by local treatment, but how frequently do we find that the otitis resists all treatment until the offending tonsils or adenoids have been removed? If these abnormal pharyngeal growths can occasion persistence of the otitis media, and if chronicity of the tympanic suppuration favors the development of more serious complications, how often might the latter conditions be prevented in children by an early recognition and treatment of the causative factor. The greater prevalence of adenoids, especially in early life than among adults, is an important difference in the etiology of otitis media in these two periods, and that adenoids and diseased tonsils may play an important part in the pathologic course of the ear disease there can be little doubt.

This fact has brought about a discussion as to whether surgical treatment of the nasopharyngeal disease should be instituted immediately, as an essential part of treatment for the aural disease. or whether it should be delayed until the acute evidence, at least, of the otitis has passed away. So many possibilities enter into a consideration of a problem of this sort that it is exceedingly difficult to give an answer applicable to all conditions, but, as a general proposition, I believe it a wise rule to remove adenoids and tonsils, whenever they are found in connection with suppurative otitis media, at the earliest possible moment. Furthermore, I believe the operation should be a most thorough and complete one, for anything less than perfect ablation of the hypertrophied lymphoid tissue is fairly sure to be followed by a recurrence of the growth and a continuance or recurrence of the otitis. The day for tonsillotomies and partial adenoidectomies has passed, and only a skilled, trained operator can properly perform the modern operation of tonsillectomy, and as the adenoid operation is usually required and can be performed at the same time, it seems to me this organization should sound a note of protest against the attempted performance of these operations by the family physician unless he has adequately prepared himself for the task.

While considering possible differences in the pathology of otitis media at different stages of life. we might well ask whether the disease is more destructive in early than in adult life and whether complications are of more frequent occurrence.

My own answer to this query would unhesitatingly be in the affirmative. I do not mean that we see more cases of meningitis, sinus thrombosis, or brain abscess among children than in adults, but are there not other important complications occurring to children that are not so well recognized? It is a matter of common observation that spontaneous perforation does not occur so early nor so readily in children as in adults. Some have supposed that the tympanic membrane is thicker or more resistant in the young. I am not aware of any anatomic proof of that idea, but it is not a point of great practical importance. A more probable explanation of the non-rupture of the drumhead is that it is not subjected to the same strain as in the case of the adult; owing to the greater patency of the tympanopharyngeal tube, an accumulating secretion in the tympanum will force an exit in that direction before it reaches a degree of tension sufficient to effect a break in the membrane. In infants and young children, therefore, we probably have in cases of suppurative otitis media a more or less constant escape of infective secretions from the tympanum into the nasopharynx, and this material is swallowed, into the gastrointestinal tract, or by way of the larynx and trachea reaches the pulmonary structures. Aural examinations are not a common procedure in the day's work of the average physician, and the diagnosis of otitis media purulenta is not made by inspection of the tympanic membrane, but, as a rule, by the flowing of pus from the external auditory meatus. Now, if the membrane does not rupture and pus does not appear in the canal the child passes through a period of obscure febrile disease until, after a lapse of a week or ten days, the condition is diagnosed as enteritis or bronchopneumonia. Not a small number of these unfortunate children die of the secondary disease, or a general septicemia, without the primary affection having ever been suspected; autopsy records show a surprisingly large number of such cases. Of the greater (facility with which purulent otitis media may invade the cerebral cavity in the young, because of the unclosed petrosquamosal suture or other dehiscences in the bone, we need hardly speak. It is an obvious fact that complications of suppurative otitis media occur with greater frequency than in adults, and that, therefore, it is extremely important that the primary ear disease should be recognized at the earliest possible moment and proper treatment instituted to cure the local disorder or prevent its spread.

Are there any differences in the symptomatology dependent upon age? I have already mentioned the possible delay in the appearance of otorrhea due to the tardiness of spontaneous rupture of the tympanic membrane. The fever accompanying otitis media in children is apt to be of a higher degree than that of adults, but as this is true of all children's disorders it is not a matter of special clinical value. The only differing symptom that has particularly impressed me refers to the onset of complications, really to the onset of mastoiditis.

I have frequently found it rather difficult to determine whether a child was developing mastoiditis, or, having shown some evidence of this involvement, whether the mastoid·disease was increasing. Variations in the subjective symptoms of pain and tenderness cannot be accurately gauged in children; indeed, it is often difficult to determine whether tenderness actually exists. · Blood examinations are of service, of course, in such cases, but there is one objective symptom—enlargement of the posterior cervical glands,˙either superficial or deep—that has seemed to me a reliable indication of mastoidal involvement. I am inclined to the opinion that these glands are usually enlarged in young children suffering with mastoiditis, and that their palpable presence in any case of purulent otitis media of infancy demands most careful consideration. If the glandular swelling persists for several days, and the other evidences of an infection are not abating, a mastoidectomy had better be performed.

This brings us to the consideration of treatment; is there any difference here to be based upon the age of the patient? I think not, except that, from what I have said regarding the gravity of the disease in young children, as compared to adults, there is greater necessity for the prompt application of the generally recognized therapeutic laws. We should endeavor to teach the family physician the necessity for making aural examinations in every case of obscure febrile disease occurring in young children, and that he errs on the safe side, if at all, when he has the tympanum opened early. A clean incision of the healthy tympanic membrane does no harm, and it is far better to open an infected tympanum one day too soon than one hour too late. It is not safe to wait for spontaneous rupture of the membrane in a case of acute otitis media. Again, when there are symptoms indicating a spread of the middle ear disease to the mastoid or neighboring structures an operation should follow with the slightest delay. We are all familiar with the marvelous recuperative powers of children, and have observed the rapidity with which they respond to proper treatment; here is a marked difference in their favor that should be taken advantage of, for, if given half a chance, they make record recoveries.

In conclusion, reverting to the question which formed the basis of this paper—does suppurative otitis media occurring in infancy or early childhood differ at all from that disease as observed in adult life, and, if so, in what respect?—I would say: .

1.   There are no fundamental differences in the disease as seen at different periods of life. Suppurative otitis media is a distinctive clinical entity, is caused by any one of a certain group of pyogenic microorganisms and progresses according to a definite pathologic- course.

2.   Owing to the prevalence of abnormally developed lymphoid tissue in the nasopharynx of young children, they are more susceptible than adults to aural infections.

3.   Because of certain well recognized anatomic differences the opportunity for extension of the infection to other organs and structures is much greater in children than in adults, and the disease, therefore, becomes one of more serious consequence.

4.   The greater gravity of the affection requires that the physician should be more alert in diagnosing it in children during the earliest stage and most prompt in applying the treatment appropriate to the stage at which the diagnosis is made.

LIV.

OTOSCLEROSIS: TREATMENT.

By W. Sohier Bryant, A. M., M. D.,

New York.

In 1892, while the author was connected with the Massachusetts Charitable Eye and Ear Infirmary, Dr. E. D. Spear demonstrated to him the relation between what was then called otitis media catarrhalis insidiosa—now called otosclerosis—and the nasopharynx, and showed how the otosclerosis could be controlled by applications made to this part of the upper air tract. The object in view in these cases of otosclerosis is to bring the mucosa of the upper air tract into as normal a condition as possible, and, also, by iritating the mucous membrane, to cause a counterirritating effect on the ear.

For the counterirritant the author uses a solution of nitrate of silver of from 5 to 10 per cent strength, or a saturated aqueous solution of ammonio-ferric sulphate, taking the precaution not to push the effect to much local reaction. The applications are made through the inferior nasal fossae to the back and side walls of the nasopharynx. At first the treatment is repeated every day, for three to seven days, then at gradually lengthening intervals, and is discontinued when the mucosa and ear seem to have ceased improving. Should the exigencies of the case demand it, general constitutional treatment, and local ear treatment, such as inflation, etc., should be instituted, in addition to this counterirritating measure. The beneficial effects of the treatment are soon apparent in the improvement in the hearing, which improvement generally lasts for a long time.

A continuous series of 31 cases, treated according to the method outlined above, gave the following results: All of these cases had shortened time of bone conduction, while they had relatively increased bone conduction. The hearing tests given are for air conduction. No case had any history of middle ear suppuration. The following five cases are sufficient as examples of the entire series:

CASE 1. Woman, 38 years old. Mother, father and grandfather deaf. Loud various tinnitus and deafness commenced at 23 years of age. Normal tympanic membranes and tubes; manubria malleorum pink, movable. Watch not heard; Politzer acoumeter—right ear, 6 inches; left ear, 1 inch; high tone limit—both ears—21,000 S. V.; low tone limit—both ears—156 S. V. The patient received two treatments each week for five weeks. These treatments consisted of general tonics and hygiene, nasal insufflations of powdered suprarenal gland, applications of solutions of $AgNO_3$ gr. 40 to dr. 1 of water to the nasopharynx, and vibratory massage about the ear.

Results.—Hearing much improved, tinnitus relieved. No congestion of manubria malleorum. Watch not heard. Politzer acoumeter—right ear, 48 inches; left ear, 5½ inches; high tone limit—both ears—26,000 S. V.; low tone limit, 26 S. V. Improvement maintained while under observation for four years.

CASE 2. Man, 42 years of age. Family history of deafness—great-uncle, two uncles, and one aunt out of seven, four cousins, deaf, two of the latter deaf only when old. Deafness commenced at 17 years of age; occasional tinnitus and vertigo. Normal tympanic membranes and tubes; mallei pink and movable; promontories appear pink through the membranes. Watch not heard; Politzer acoumeter—right ear, 5½ inches; left ear, 12 inches; high tone limit—right ear, 30,000 S. V.; left ear, 21,000 S. V.; low tone limit considerably raised. The treatment was chiefly directed to the maintenance of hygiene, and to the insistence upon more regular habits and less stimulants. Two or three times a year applications were made to the nasopharynx of a 10 per cent solution of nitrate of silver or saturated solution of ferric alum. This treatment covered a period of four years.

Results.—Slightly improved hearing. Relief from tinnitus and vertigo. No congestion of mallei and promontories. P. acoumeter—right ear, 9 inches; left ear, 24 inches; high tone limit—right ear, 31,000 S. V.; left ear, 28,000 S. V.; low tone limit—right ear, 128 S. V.; left ear, 113 S. V. Improvement maintained while under observation during seven years.

CASE 3. Man, 43 years old. Paternal grandfather deaf. Deafness began at 25 years of age; various tinnitus. Tympanic membranes and tubes normal. Watch—right ear, 4 inches; left ear, 2 inches. Treatment consisted in nasal insufflation of suprarenal glands twice a week. Once or twice a month applications of saturated solution of ammonio-ferric sulphate were made to the nasopharynx. This treatment was continued for three years.

Results.—Hearing much improved and tinnitus relieved. No change on inspection. Watch—right ear, 36-inch watch heard 10 feet; left ear, 7 feet; high tone limit—left ear, 49,000 S. V.; right, ear, 53,000 S. V.; low tone limit, 28 S. V., both ears. Improvement maintained while under observation for nine months.

CASE 4. Woman, 45 years old. Family history of deafness. Deafness commenced at 33 years of age, following childbirth; tinnitus. Normal tympanic membranes and tubes; membranes show promontorial blush; manubria malleorum pink; mallei movable. Watch not heard; Politzer acoumeter—right ear, 1 inch; left ear, 1½ inches; high tone limit—right ear, 15,650 S. V.; left ear, 21,000 S. V.; low limit raised; Gelle test negative. No change in bone conduction on compression of air in external meati. Treatment consisted in nasal insufflations of adrenal gland powder twice a week at first. Later the treatment was given every two or three weeks. Applications of supersaturated solution of persulphate of iron above the lower turbinates were made at first twice a week. Treatments were later given every two weeks, and were continued for 16 months.

Results.—Hearing and tinnitus improved. No congestion of mallei and promontories. Watch not heard; Politzer acoumeter—right ear, 8 inches; left ear, 6 inches; high tone limit—right ear, 16,500 S. V.; left ear, 22,400 S. V.; Gelle test still negative. Improvement maintained while under observation 15 months.

CASE 5. Man, 24 years old. Mother and brother deaf. Deafness one year with tinnitus. Normal tympanic membranes and tubes. Treatment consisted of nasal insufflation of suprarenal gland powder. Applications were made to the nasopharynx with nitrol of silver solution 40 gr. to the ounce. The treatments were given about every six days and were continued

for two months. Watch not heard. Politzer acoumeter—
right ear, 12 inches; left ear, not heard.

Results.—Hearing much improved and tinnitus stopped.
No change in appearances. Watch—right ear, 6 inches; left
ear, 48 inches; Politzer acoumeter—right ear, 8 feet. Improvement maintained while under observation for four years.

Conclusion.—Otosclerosis is amenable to treatment, with
the expectation that in most cases the process of otosclerosis
will be arrested and the hearing improved. The more advanced
the case, the less benefit will be derived from treatment. Very
advanced cases, however, can be benefited to a degree.

LV

CHRONIC PURULENT OTITIS MEDIA IN ADULTS.*

By S. MacCuen Smith, M. D.,

Philadelphia.

In discussing the pathology of suppurative otitis media, we have two processes to consider, especially in relation to its subsequent invasion of the mastoid cavity, through which it passes, and the changes incident thereto. The first produces a condition of malnutrition, in which the intercellular structure is destroyed, finally converting the several spaces into one large cavity. A continuation of this process of absorption by a persistent invasion of the greedy leukocytes and osteoclasts renders the cortex exceedingly thin, resulting in erosive perforation. On the other hand, the osteitis may terminate in resolution, or, as is more frequent, in osteosclerosis, the exudate being converted first into fibrous tissue, which gradually undergoes ossification and becomes dense bone.

The second form presents the characteristics incident to hypernutrition, which, after passing through various abnormal histologic changes, produces the condition known as sclerosis of the mastoid cells, condensing osteitis, or hyperostosis of the same process. A chronic inflammation of the mucosa lining the tympanic cavity and antrum produces a secondary hyperemia of these structures, enveloping the pneumatic cells, which in turn becomes chronic, and this in time, owing to an increase of cellular structure, entirely obliterates the pneumatic spaces, eventually producing a solid, eburnated mastoid process.

This condition, having its origin during a suppurative otitis media, may continue after all tympanic discharge has ceased. Furthermore, it is during the course of such pathologic changes that the sinus is frequently pushed so far for-

---

*Read before the Southern Section of the American Laryngological, Rhinological and Otological Society, at Richmond, Va., February 13, 1909.

ward that the posterior osseous canal becomes the anterior-wall of the sinus, the antrum is partly or completely obliterated, and we are apt to-find the tympanic branch of the facial nerve in an abnormal position, the changed relations rendering the performance of a mastoid operation most difficult. Pain or neuralgia in the vicinity of the mastoid may also be attributed to the same process, and should make us more mindful of such conditions, even though the ear is dry and has not been the site of a suppurative lesion for some time.

I wish to reiterate the fact that in my experience a chronic recurrent suppurative otitis media is relatively productive of more complications, intracranial and otherwise, than the continuous variety. The danger point appears to be during the period of the acute exacerbation, which seems to be productive of lighting up an old abscess formation or a chronic labyrinthine disease, both of which nature may have walled off by protective coats, thereby causing them to remain latent until aroused to action as the result of an acute exacerbation.

Gruber defines cholesteatoma as small, degenerated epithelial cells, between which lie cholesterin crystals and other fatty deposits. If we are to adhere strictly to the composition thus defined, we must conclude that true cholesteatomatous masses are not so common as some would have us believe. In any event, we are all familiar with the great frequency with which we find larger or smaller masses of desquamated epithelium within both the tympanic cavity and the mastoid process, and furthermore, we have learned from experience, and probably sad experience, that this formation of what we are pleased to call cholesteatoma is the result of a chronic suppurative otitis media, and, moreover, is frequently the chief etiologic factor in the development of a majority of the serious intracranial complications that we are called upon to treat. In other words, as aurists we are confronted with a disease of the osseous structure, the etiology of which, in consequence of this peculiar formation, is unique and serves to distinguish it from diseases of bone in any other part of the human economy.

Some authors properly regard this subject as of sufficient importance to be treated as a separate disease, and yet from the fact that it is dependent upon an otorrhea for its existence, as well as clincally inseparable from the same, it must remain an important development of chronic suppurative otitis media.

Without warning, and in the absence of symptoms, this formation slowly develops and advances until accumulating coats, one upon another, assume such proportions that finally the patient, from pressure necrosis, is warned that the temporal bone is the site of a grave lesion.

An immediate radical operation at this time will, in all probability, eradicate the disease, while delay will favor the rapid development of some serious endocranial complication, the exact nature of which is governed by the location of the mass and the direction of its pressure erosion. The symptoms resulting therefrom will determine the route which surgical measures for relief should take.

The pathologic changes caused by a chronic suppurative otitis media necessarily differ from those resulting from the acute disease, and usually develop from heedless neglect of the primary lesion.

During the acute disease the mucosa becomes macerated and peels off, exposing the unprotected and defenseless osseous structure to the ravages of the various microorganisms present. By this process is ushered in the grosser pathologic changes, which mark the beginning of bone erosion and all the serious intracranial and general complications incident thereto. Eventually, granulation tissue replaces the normal mucous lining, and the consequent proliferation may be sufficient to fill the entire middle-ear cavity and extend into the antrum and cells. The outward extension of granulation tissue through this process of proliferation may fill the external osseous canal, and finally, after passing through various histologic changes, result in a polypoid growth sufficiently large to reach the coucha.

Coincident with the above, the ossicles and tympanic walls become necrosed and exfoliation takes place, which finally results in the middle ear becoming emptied. In the meantime the labyrinth may have become implicated. and the mastoid process will almost assuredly have suffered from disintegration. If, however. the fenestrae escape injury and the stapes remain fairly movable, the hearing power will continue good. On the other hand, should the ossicles remain in situ and become ankylosed or firmly fixed by fibrous bands, or the membrane covering the fenestrae become opaque or calcified. great loss of hearing must result. Masses of epithelial scales from the external canal may pass through the perforation in the membrana tympani, coat the walls of the tympanic cavity, reach the attic and antrum and there form cholesteatomatous masses.

The presence of cholesteatoma and the character of the discharge are valuable aids in determining the advisability of operative interference. The generally accepted rule today is that we should advise immediate operation when convinced that cholesteatoma is present in the tympanic cavity, especially the superior part, and the mastoid antrum or cells. Indeed, this rule holds good if there is even a strong probability that the same exists. We must not, however, confuse the diagnosis on account of the presence of desquamated epithelium in the external auditory canal, as cases do undoubtedly exist where laminae of epidermis in considerable quantity are present in the canal, but have not entered the tympanic cavity through a perforation. Cases of this character will yield to non-operative treatment, and should be carefully differentiated.

We should recognize three distinct types of otorrhea; the first and most common is that having its origin in the nasopharynx and the Eustachian tube, which is ropy and mucoid in character; that arising from the tympanic cavity alone, which is less abundant and yellowish in character; while a discharge brownish-yellow or greenish-yellow in character, and having a decidedly offensive odor, indicates extensive bone erosion, occurring more frequently in the tympanic attic and mastoid antrum. All these regions may be involved at the same time, and in long-standing cases this is frequently true. A further diagnostic sign in these cases is the appearance of blood, indicating the presence of granulation tissue, which in turn is usually an outgrowth of carious bone.

We must not lose sight of the fact, however, that non-fetid pus frequently contains large quantities of pathogenic cocci, which are highly infectious and just as dangerous to life as the more offensive type of discharge.

The question as to the particular line of treatment to be instituted in the chronic suppurative disease of the ear is still agitating the professional mind. While all of us may have operated unnecessarily on some of these chronic cases, yet on the whole I venture to say we are probably too conservative, as shown by an unfortunate occurrence in some particular case where ultra-conservatism dictated the treatment.

The great difficulty heretofore, as at present, has been our inability to appreciate the destruction that is slowly but surely taking place through carious erosion within the temporal bone. Certainly a fair proportion of patients presenting graunlation tissue and polypoid growths will yield to properly directed non-operative treatment, except in so far as surgical means are necessary for their removal. Those of us who conduct large clinics are continually being impressed by this fact, and it is a daily occurrence for us to examine cases with marginal cicatrices and perforations, the results of middle-ear suppurations which have healed without operation, in which state they have remained for years. It would seem, therefore, that notwithstanding granulation tissue may be the outward expression of circumscribed carious destruction, the latter will frequently yield to non-operative treatment of the major type. It is generally conceded that in the absence of urgent symptoms we should not recommend radical operative interference until the more simple lines of medication have been exhausted, and furthermore, the radical operation should not be performed in the average case until minor surgical measures have failed. It is probable that a limited amount of caries and even cholesteatoma are not of themselves absolute indications for the radical operation, but if to these are added the symptoms of an acute exacerbation, or some intracranial, sinus, or labyrinthine complications, the surgeon should immediately operate. If the case fails to yield to the removal of granulation tissue and polypoid growths, if such are present, as well as to properly directed medication, and still presents no special indications for more radical measures, it would become our duty to first resort to ossiculectomy and removal of all pathologic products that can be reached through the external auditory canal. As to choice between this measure, however, and a modified operation known as the Heath, I have reason to express some preference in favor of the latter. In a paper on the subject, read before the Eastern Section of the American Laryngological, Rhinological and Otological Society, at Philadelphia, on January 9th of this year, I exhibted some patients, who showed in a striking manner the benefits of the modified procedure. Heath's contention is that the mastoid antrum is usually the site of the continued suppuration, rather than the cavity of the middle ear. Such being the case, we can readily appreciate why the removal of the ossicles and membrana tympani does not correct a discharge the origin of which is in the mastoid antrum or cells, as these cavities cannot possibly be reached through the external auditory canal.

Then, again, the preservation or improvement of hearing, especially if both ears are involved in childhood, is a matter of the greatest importance. Ossiculectomy will undoubtedly improve temporarily the hearing power in the majority of cases. This, however, will almost assuredly decrease gradually in the course of time; whereas, in the Heath operation, we preserve the membrana tympani and ossicles, or any fragment of the same that remains, the natural tendency being, therefore, toward a betterment of the hearing power as well as the correction of the discharge.

From a purely surgical viewpoint, it does not seem sound operative technic to deliberately retain pathologic products, however minute, within the organ of hearing, and yet a goodly number of the cases seem to justify the procedure, from the fact that it not only preserves the hearing power present at the time of operation, but actually improves it to an appreciable degree in the majority of cases. Then, again, it is suitable in both the advanced acute and chronic variety of cases and will probably supplant the operation known as ossiculectomy for the cure of an otorrhea,

If the Heath operation is advised, this should be done under the same conditions as would an ossiculectomy; in other words, the operation should be continued to a radical at some future date, in case the patient is not relieved by the simpler procedure.

LVI.

SPOON ENUCLEATION OF THE TONSIL.

By A. Morgan MacWhinnie, M. D.,

Seattle, Wash.

The value of any tonsillar operation consists in the thoroughness of the enucleation. Consequently no tonsil operation should be considered thorough unless the capsule be included in the enucleation. The question of hemorrhage is usually what alarms most operators, but if the tonsil is removed with the capsule intact, regardless of the teaching that may exist from previous operators, it is my experience that bleeding instantly stops. That we occasionally have a stubborn hemorrhage of the oozing variety is probably due to the fact that the tonsil capsule is composed of fibrous tissue. Fibrous tissue, as we well know, does not possess a great deal of contractility. Existing between the carotid side of the capsule and the superior constrictor muscle there is a varying amount of connective tissue, this possessing a greater amount of contractility than the capsule itself. Consequently, when a tonsil has been enucleated and a part of the capsule remains, we lose this contractile power which is necessary for the closure of the blood vessels, thereby preventing hemorrage, when no injury has been inflicted upon either the anterior or the posterior pillars. When bleeding continues it is fair to assume that some portion of the tonsillar capsule remains, for these arteries pierce this capsule and ramify through the tonsil. Hemorrhage might also takes place if in the enucleation some fibers of the supraconstrictor muscle may have been brought up as well. This can be readily obviated by the use of the instrument which I have devised. Secondary hemorrhage is practically unknown if the details as above have been carried out. I believe if the anatomy was better understood we would not have any amputations or punching of this tonsillar tissue. At its best, part of the capsule still remains, and the added danger of injury to the superior constrictor ensues. Using the various punches, it is

almost impossible to empty the supratonsillar fossa, where
90 per cent of our abscesses occur. While it is generally conceded that a clean-cut surface will heal more quickly and is
less liable to infection, it has not been my experience to have
had any infection or to have the healing process delayed
beyond a period of about ten days after using the tonsil spoon,
when healing is complete. I do not deem it necessary to
massage this fossa during the period of healing, as suggested
by Pynchon, because a certain amount of irritation is thereby
caused, and exuberant granulations are liable to spring up,
necessitating their removal. Careful cleansing with an alkaline wash, followed by a 50 per cent argyrol solution, constitutes the only treatment that is necessary after enucleation
of the tonsil in the intact capsule. True it is there are some
cases in which this fossa does not fill with connective tissue
under four or five weeks, but this is the exception and not the
rule.

The methods by which enucleation may be done are numerous and vary with each operator, and he may have some special device of his own which seems to suit his method. The
danger of using a knife in the separation of the pillars and
the extirpation of a tonsil is such, that only when we have an
extremely tranquil patient and are exceedingly dextrous in
its use, are we justified in using it in the separation of the
tonsil from the connective tissue. While the advocates of the
knife use the blunt end to separate the tonsil from the connective tissue, using the sharp portion only to separate the
pillars, by means of my spoon the pillars are separated as well
as the tonsil. Obviously the knife can only be used by a very
few.

The method of removing with the finger is undoubtedly the
best, causing the least trauma, as well as possible injury to
the surrounding parts, and undoubtedly as quick as any.
Ether is generally necessary for such cases, but there are
some patients who object to a general anesthetic for this purpose. While I have enucleated a number of cases under cocain
by my finger, in 15 to 20 seconds usually, the patient gags and
retches to such an extent that the time of removal is lengthened and possible injury to surrounding parts increased. With
the idea of overcoming this I have devised the spoon shown in
the cut, by which the tonsil is removed, with the capsule intact,

with a minimum amount of loss of blood, and leaving a fossa which readily heals in a period of a week to 10 days. A 10% cocain and adrenalin solution is injected at two points between the anterior pillars and the tonsillar capsule, and at two points between the posterior pillars and the tonsillar capsule, corresponding with that made anteriorly. An ordinary hypodermic, or, preferably, a Luer glass, syringe is used, but a special gold needle four inches long is attached, which allows a deep penetration. A lapse of five minutes is allowed, so that anesthesia becomes complete. The tonsil is then grasped well into the supratonsillar fossa and the infratonsillar fossa, so as to engage the capsule as well as the tonsil. Otherwise we might grasp the tonsillar tissue, which is soft and readily tears out. I believe this is the point where failures are often made in enucleation. A tongue depressor is not necessary,

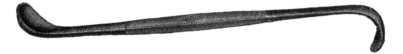

the handle of the volsellum taking its place. The spoon is then entered between the posterior pillars and the tonsillar capsule, rapidly separating from below, upward to the supratonsillar fossa. The spoon is then moved rapidly forward, separating the tonsil as it comes forward from the connective tissue beneath. The same process is carried out inferiorly and anteriorly. This spoon has semi-sharp edges, which act better as a separator on the connective tissue than a sharp instrument would do, without the added risk of leaving some of the capsule. The spoon fits so accurately over the tonsil that injury to the pillars should not be considered. The extreme traction by means of the volsellum brings the tonsils so well forward into the pharynx that it leaves very little separation necessary. many changes that were necessary to make this spoon of practical value.

LVII

CHRONIC EPIPHARYNGEAL PERIADENITIS IN ADULTS.

By Jas. E. Logan, M. D.,

Kansas City.

As its name implies, this is a disease of the tissues in the vault of the pharynx. The writer is not content with the term periadenitis—as interpreted literally it would indicate that the structures surrounding the glands are alone involved, while it is intended to comprehend a pathologic process extending throughout the glandular, muscular, vascular and connective tissues.

In 1903 I read before this association a paper entitled "Adenoid Growths with Special Reference to Adult Condition," in which I recited my experience in operating upon sixty-five cases of adults over twenty-five years of age. I shall attempt to give further proof of the importance of recognizing this as a distinct disease deserving a separate classification along with other inflammatory processes of the upper respiratory tract. Writers upon this subject have generally considered this condition as an extension of inflammatory processes either from the nose or from the pharynx into the epipharynx, making this a secondary and not a primary affection. In the light of our experience, we are convinced that in these structures are developed the etiology and pathology of many diseases which have baffled the efforts of our greatest men in the sphere of investigative research. We have been taught to believe that after the age of puberty has passed, the lymphatic glands undergo atrophy and ultimately disappear, and clinical facts bear out the fact of this statement within certain limitations. Whenever the age of childhood has passed without establishing pathologic processes of a chronic nature within these structures, then atrophic changes take place that very soon obliterate their existence. But whenever chronic inflammations once become installed, they seldom, if ever, disappear. In entering upon the discussion of the pathology of this disease we shall not attempt to go into the details of the acute forms of this affection, leaving that to some future time.

In 1868 Luschka described indefinitely a chronic disease of the nasopharyngeal bursa, to which he gave the name "Chronic Nasopharyngeal Bursitis." Later, in 1885, Thornwaldt gave a more detailed account of this affection, to which our textbooks have ascribed the name "Thornwaldt's Disease." D. Braden Kyle refers to it in the last edition of his work as a suppuration of rare occurrence in the pharyngeal bursa presenting symptoms very similar to those of empyema of the sphenoidal sinus—the latter condition he regards the more frequent. Ballenger mentions it as a disease of the recessus medius due to inflammatory adhesions of the median borders of the adenoid mass. Schwabach regarded it as a disease of congenital origin, situated in the remnant of the middle cleft.

In determining the actual pathology of this disease I have submitted a number of these growths to Dr. Frank J. Hall, of Kansas City, who has spent much time investigating the characteristics, and I am indebted to him for valuable aid. I give his report at length: "The tissue removed from the epipharyngeal region of Mr. D. by you and sent to me for microscopic examination and description presents the following: The gross specimen is roughly circular, one inch in diameter and three-eighths of an inch thick. Sections made at right angles to the surface present the following: The covering is squamous epithelium, which is broken at one point by an ulcer whose floor is composed of polymorphonuclear leucocytes held in a reticulum of fibrin. At one other point the surface epithelium is being invaded by leucocytes and round cells. This area lies directly over a lymphoid deposit resembling tonsillar tissue.

"Beneath the epithelium at all points the submucosa is liberally infiltrated with round and polymorphonuclear cell exudate. Here and there is a deposit of lymphoid tissue whose lymph sinuses are choked with inflammatory products. Deeper down, groups of mucous glands are encountered. The lumina of these glands are wide and filled with a liberal amount of secretion. About the glands just mentioned are liberal deposits of inflammatory round cells of the plasma of the small leucocyte type. In the planes of connective tissue at the level of the mucous glands is a noticeable amount of fibrin, almost sufficient to constitute a severance of the overlying submucosa from the gland-bearing area. Still deeper, planes of voluntary muscles are encountered. Between the individual fibers of the muscles is a great quantity of inflammatory material, both cellular and fibrinous, constituting a real interstitial myostitis.

"Throughout all the section and particularly marked in the upper layer of the submucosa are many degenerated nuclei of the proper connective tissue. These degenerated nuclei are drawn out in the most bizarre fashion into clubs, strings, etc. No giant cells or other specific histologic cell elements or arrangement of same is noticeable. Blood vessels are all the seat of thickening of the intima and media."

You will observe from Professor Hall's report that this disease does not alone involve the glandular structure, but extends to the muscular, vascular and connective tissues as well. We believe this to be of especial importance with reference to the muscles concerned in the function of hearing. The tensor tympani, tensor palati and the levator palati are to be mostly considered in this connection because of their attachments into and around the orifice of the tube, influencing as they do the action of the drum membrane, together with the effect upon the lumen of the tube, by the opening and closing functions of the levator and tensor palati. These muscles originate in and around the orifice, and any inflammatory process in adjacent tissue undoubtedly involves these fibers and must of necessity interfere with their physiologic action. This might serve to explain the yet unsettled theories of sclerosis of the middle ear. Chronic catarrhal inflammation of the middle ear has been the bugbear of every pathologist. He has never been able to establish its identity. We know that these cases progressively increase in deafness, even when they are given the very best attention. In the light of these facts, it is already evident that either these conditions are irremediable or the etiology, pathology and its elimination are yet unknown. Buck, in his third revised edition, p. 41, says: "As yet we are unable to form any very accurate idea of the extent to which the impaired hearing in this class of cases (referring to chronic catarrhal deafness) is to be attributed to the abrogation of the functions of the tensor tympani and stapedius muscles. The sclerosing process undoubtedly invades both of them, and to a greater or less extent paralyzes their action; and it is also conceivable that in certain cases a state of permanent contracture may be produced whereby the membrana tympani on the one hand and the stapedio-vestibular-annular ligament on the other are kept by these muscles permanently in an abnormal state of tension."

Retraction of the membrana tympani is more often dependent upon the lack of resiliency of the tensor tympani than upon any perceptible encroachment upon the lumen of the tube. This fact can be proven in a large proportion of cases by catheterization. It can also be proven by the unimpeded introduction of the bougie through the tube. If the tube permits of the entrance of air and also of the introduction of the bougie, then why does the membrana tympani remain retracted? The answer to this question seems to me to be found in the foregoing statement, viz., the lack of the resiliency of the tensor tympani. Admitting that sclerosis (a process hard to define) does become established within the drum, then it must have a cause, and that cause in a great majority of cases is to be found in a diseased condition of the epipharynx. This disease may exist indefinitely without producing any disturbance in the function of the ear, though this is the most frequent complication.

Whenever the tissues in the vault have been the seat of repeated attacks of acute inflammation, supervening upon the chronic process, we have found these patients frequent victims of acute rhinitis and of epidemic influenza. The reason for this lies in the productiveness of this soil for the cultivation of all forms of pathogenic bacteria. In forty-two cases of acute epidemic influenza in adults, in which were found the catarrhalis, every one exhibited a greater or less amount of lymphoid and connective tissue hypertrophy in the vault. I desire to lay special stress upon the question of the amount of this hypertrophied tissue. In my experience the smallest amount of it is sufficient to furnish a field for the cultivation of infectious material.

We must realize that in adults the process of deterioration of this lymphoid structure can leave but a little of the growth in all but exceptionable cases, but the point we wish to bring out is that even the slightest amount may be the origin of widespread invasion. In the cases of No. 1 and No. 2, there existed the smallest possible amount of hypertrophied tissue, yet the removal of it brought about good results. In the cases of No. 3 and No. 5, it is our purpose to show the presence of this periadenitis was the determining pathologic process of the chronic suppurative otitis media. The case of No. 4 is of especial interest, showing the effect of bacterial invasion into the right ear during measles in childhood and the development of a chronic progressive deafness in the left ear at the age of twenty-eight.

DIAGNOSIS.

Diagnosis of this disease is a matter of little difficulty. In the routine of all nasal, aural and pharyngeal examinations we carefully inspect the vault in every instance. With the rhinoscopic mirror we can in most cases determine fairly well the condition of the epipharynx; but we should always go farther and introduce the finger behind the soft palate. By this means every evidence of adventitious tissue in this space cannot fail to be discovered. This upholstered mass may exist in considerable thickness without destroying the symmetry of the cavity.

The obtuseness of the angle made at the juncture of the basillar process with the spinal column varies greatly in different skulls, consequently the mirror alone may lead to mistaken idea of the amount, while the keen sensibility of a clean finger is a never-failing indicator.

PROGNOSIS.

The prognosis in these cases is usually favorable so far as the vault condition is concerned. As to the disappearance of complications, this depends upon what organs and functions are involved, the age of the patient, and the amount and character of the impairment. Within the last six years I have operated upon 652 cases of adenoids, both young and old, in my private practice. Of this number 368 were below the age of 25 years and 284 were from 25 to 59 years. Of the 284 adults, 162 were males and 122 were females; 167 between the ages of 25 and 35; 106 between 35 and 45 and 11 between the ages of 45 and 59.

I have seen one case 64 years of age, with large epipharyngeal growth, but was not allowed to operate. Of the 284 adults, 210 suffered from chronic progressive deafness in varying degrees of severity; 24 were victims of recurrent attacks of acute and subacute catarrhal otitis media; 17 had chronic suppurative otitis and 33 exhibited no ear complications of any moment. Of the 210 cases of progressive deafness 182 showed noticeable improvement after operation. This number represents those who faithfully persisted in the after-treatment and whose conditions were not so disastrous as to preclude the possibility of some benefit. Twenty cases were of such long standing and of such a character that the after-treatment failed to bring about any appreciable improvement. These patients gave marked evidence of internal ear complications; the remaining eight cases were operated upon and little or no after-treatment was given.

Of the 24 cases of recurrent acute and subacute otitis operated upon, 16 have had no recurrence of the discharge, and the hearing has been improved; 5 have had recurrent attacks —in 3 of these I have recently done the preliminary stripping and secondary removal, as in the first operation I failed to get rid of the hypertrophies about the orifice of the tubes; 3 cases were operated upon and I have lost sight of them.

Of the 17 cases of chronic suppuration of the middle ear occurring in adults over 25 years of age, five have had no recurrence after the removal of the growth in the vault; eight required subsequent curettage of the necrosed tissue of the middle ear, and four demanded the radical operation. Of the 33 cases operated upon showing no ear complications, all of them exhibited symptoms of nasal and epipharyngeal diseases of various kinds. Four were in-patients who had recurrent hemorrhagic expectoration without evidences of lung complication, and so far have had no return of the trouble. Five cases had active suppurative inflammation in the epipharynx accompanying atrophic rhinitis. Twenty-four were cases of various nasal and pharyngeal conditions where the periadenitis seemed to be the predominant etiologic factor. In more than 75 per cent of these cases turbinal hypertrophies were present. Deflections of the septum existed in the usual proportion. Sinus complications were present in 22—a little less than 10 per cent.

In summing up the question of prognosis, my experience leads me to say that whenever a case presents itself exhibiting any disease whatsoever of the nasal or accessory sinuses, the middle ear, the pharynx or larynx, and at the same time there is evidence of the smallest amount of adventitious tissue in the epipharynx, the prompt removal of this mass adds greatly to the chances of permanent relief. If I may be pardoned for appearing extreme and overzealous, I will go still farther and say that permanent good is practically impossible if this fertile field of infection is not destroyed.

SYMPTOMATOLOGY.

It is hardly necessary to dwell at length upon the symptoms of this disease, as to go into detail would involve the question of complications which are so varied that your patience would cease to be a virtue. Just a few points I desire to bring to your attention. First—The general symptoms are those complained of by patients suffering from the ordinary phases of nasal inflammations, viz., repeated attacks of acute coryza, especially of the infectious influenza type; sensations of fullness in the vault and pharynx and a more or less desire to hawk and expectorate, especially upon arising. Each morning the patient may remove a large mass of inspissated muco-pus; during the day a large amount of mucus and muco-pus is secreted.

As heretofore stated, a very large majority of my cases were coexistent with hypertrophies of the nasal mucosa, and in many deflections of the septum were present. Consequent symptoms of these conditions were present. The same may be said of those showing sinus complications. Secondly—The invaluable aid given us by the mirror, enabling us to see the actual conditions, and lastly, and by all means the most important, information revealed by the introduction of the thoroughly sterile finger behind the soft palate—all conspire to render plain the symptoms of this disease.

TREATMENT.

The treatment of this condition can be nothing less than a total extirpation of the diseased tissue. If allowed to remain it will suffer repeated invasions of acute inflammations and render ultimate relief, even to the remotest complication, impossible.

Situated as it is, high up in the vault and in the fossae on either side, it has been almost impossible to devise an instrument that will serve the purpose of total extirpation. Failing in so many instances to remove the tissue in the fossae and about the orifices of the tubes, I have resorted to the following **method**:

Thoroughly cleanse the epipharynx and the nose with a warm sterile normal salt solution by means of the postnasal syringe. Through the nose, by means of long, curved applicators wrapped with cotton, apply an 8 or 10 per cent. solution of cocain several times for ten or fifteen minutes. In the intervals of this application I also apply a solution of suprarenal extract about twice through each nostril. Within this time the vault is well anesthetized. With thoroughly sterile hands the right index finger with long, sharp nail, is introduced behind the palate. Beginning at the lower border of the left eustachian orifice, proceed to break up all the adhesions and upholstered mass within the vault. In other words, strip the growth away from its bed, wherever it can be felt. The result of this preliminary operation is to free the tubes and the fossae of the resisting mass. which is almost impossible to remove by forceps or curette. An active inflammation follows this procedure, which renders the tissue brittle and susceptible of easy separation from the underlying structures. After an interval of forty-eight hours the secondary operation is performed. This is done by the us of the curette in a large proportion of cases. In well-trained throats the Brandagee forceps may serve good purpose. In the selection of the curette I prefer the Beckmann pattern. After the operation the finger should be introduced behind the palate to make sure that none of the growth remains. The size of the curette depends upon the width of the space between the tubal orifices —the No. 4 Beckmann is the size I usually employ. Another important point is that the curette should be pushed high into the vault, following closely the posterior border of the septum, so as to engage the mass. Then changing the grasp of the instrument so that the dorsum of the hand is upward, firmly and quickly with a wrist movement. cut backward and downward, following the under surface of the basillar and the anterior surface of the spinal column. This procedure, if done with a sharp instrument, will deliver the growth into the mouth —sometimes out into the lap of the patient or upon the gown of the operator.   I have performed this operation in this manner more than 200 times and have not had occasion to use a general anesthetic.   In fact, I would hesitate a long time before giving ether or chloroform to an adult, first, because the operator is at a great disadvantage by reason of the lying-down position of the patient, and secondly, there is much greater danger of hemorrhage.

The advantages of the primary and secondary operations are: First—The operator can break up all adhesions easily and strip the mass from its bed in the fossae of Rosenmuller, where it exists in greatest abundance. Second—This mass cannot be removed in its entirety in these fossae without the greatest difficulty by the use of forceps or curette. Third—The finger will detect hypertrophies where the mirror will fail to reveal them. Fourth—The danger of severe hemorrhage is practically eliminated by the preliminary stripping of the mass. This procedure breaks up the continuity of the blood vessels, which undergo degeneration within forty-eight hours, at which time the growth is removed.   In all of my experience with this method so far have had but three cases of hemorrhage which required plugging.

CASE No. 1.—Miss W., aged 28; light eyes, brown hair; applied to me for treatment July 9, 1908. During the winter of 1904 she sufferd an attack of double acute catarrhal otitis media, which lasted some two or three months. Previous to that time had noticed that her hearing was becoming impaired, especially during attacks of "colds."   Since the attack of double otitis she realized that she was fast losing ground. Being a music teacher she became greatly alarmed at this condition. Upon testing her ears found watch hearing, right ear 3 inches and left ear 4 inches. During attacks of acute rhinitis hearing in both ears reduced to bare contact of watch. Bone conduction increased; drum membranes of both markedly retracted. Schrapnell's membrane showed signs of previous acute inflammations. Catheterization showed both tubes open and the bougie passed readily into the middle ear.

Examination of nose revaled slight hypertrophies of both turbinals. The epipharynx was the seat of some thickening in and about the orifices of both tubes. The left posterior lip bound down with three bands of adhesions to the posterior border of the fossa of Rosenmuller—only one small adhesion on right. As represented in the plate, you will observe that there showed but little evidence of thickening except in the two fossae. With the finger I detected great depth to the fossae, which was filled to almost a level of the grooves with a mass of tissue. This mass not observable through the mirror and would have been overlooked but for the use of the finger.

Diagnosis.—Chronic epipharyngeal periadenitis with progressive catarrhal deafness.

During the after-treatment she complained of great discomfort from what she termed her ears "clicking." This symptom has partially disappeared. This "clicking" sensation I regard as an interference with the free action of the tensor tympani, levator and tensor palati muscles, rather than the interrupted entrance and exit of air.

I am reporting this case to illustrate the facts: 1. The mirror alone did not reveal the true condition of the epipharynx. 2. Air passed readily into the middle ear, yet the drum membrane remained constantly retracted. The bougie passed both tubes unobstructed.

CASE No. 2.—Mrs. W. H., age 54; married; one grown daughter. Applied for treatment February 27, 1906. Gave history of progressive deafness of more than thirty years' standing. Right ear the seat of recurrent acute otitis in childhood. Left ear had never been involved in any acute inflammations. Hearing tests: Watch at contact in right ear; at bare contact in left. Bone conduction increased in left: tuning fork on vertex, forehead or teeth intensified in left: indefinite in right. Whisper heard in left at two inches; not at all in right. Drum membrane in right showed many scars and was deeply retracted; ossicles displaced high up in attic and bound by adhesions. Left drum membrane slightly thickened; above firmly retracted; lower portion normal in color.

Examination of the nose revealed turbinal hypertrophies of both inferior bodies. The epipharynx exhibited but a slight ridge on left side extending from the basilar, down the posterior wall blending with some hypertrophied tissue, which began with the upper portion of the fossa of Rosenmuller and disappeared under the posterior eustachian lip of that tube. The right fossa of Rosenmuller was more nearly filled with a mass of larger size—one small adhesion on left side. The finger confirmed the presence of a mass greater than the mirror showed. This patient complained of much annoyance from the "clicking" sensation in left ear; she complained of very occasional tinnitus.

Diagnosis.—Chronic epipharyngeal periadenitis—fixation of tensor tympani and probable ossicular anchylosis in right ear. Partial fixation of tensor tympani and palati muscles in left ear and vault.

This was a most unpromising case. The patient talked in such low voice as to be almost inaudible. She observed the movement of the lips in those conversing with her very closely.

Prognosis.—Very unfavorable so far as the hearing was concerned. I removed a mass of considerable size from the vault on March 25, 1906. She remained under my charge constantly for more than a year, during which time I catheterized both tubes and introduced bougies twice each week. She persistently complained of the "clicking" in left ear, which even now occasionally troubles her. She called on me May 27, 1909, at which time I found the following conditions: Hearing—Right ear, ½ inch; left ear, 2 inches; whisper test, 6 feet; no tinnitus; hears ordinary conversation at 8 feet distinctly.

CASE No. 3.—Mrs. B., age 34; German parentage; married; one child; light blue eyes, brown hair; strong, robust. Applied to me for treatment November 15, 1905. Had measles at seventeen years of age, followed by a suppurative otitis media in left ear that had never ceased discharging in seventeen years. At the time of my examination found left ear excreting a very foul pus in great quantity. A large perforation, including almost the entire Schrapnell's membrane; the tip of the handle of the malleus was yet intact below the margin of the opening. Incus was destroyed, large granulations protruding through opening. Mastoid had been involved, according to the patient's statement; but no evidence of trouble at the time of her visit to me. Patient heard watch—left ear at bare contact when first examined. Right ear normal.

Examination of nose and epipharynx showed the presence of extensive inflammations. The vault was upholstered with a mass of hypertrophied tissue which under the microscope proved to be an inflammation of the muscular, vascular and lymphoid structures.

This seemed a fit case for radical operation, though I felt warranted in postponing such action until the growth in the vault was removed and the granulations in the ear destroyed. I operated upon her November 20, 1905, removing the growth. Ten days later curetted out the granulations through the perforation in drum membrane; packed the canal with iodoform gauze. This treatment continued for three weeks, after which time the discharge ceased and has not again recurred.

This case with that of No. 5 are exhibited here for the purpose of showing some of the different phases into which this periadenitis enters as determining etiologic factor.

CASE No. 4.—A. J. D., aged 28; single; clerk in dry goods store; dark eyes and hair; not robust; pale and anemic. Applied to me for treatment January 27, 1909, threatened with attack of acute otitis in left ear; severe pains in ear; some temperature, etc. This condition lasted but a few days, then subsided.

Examination of this case showed right ear had been seat of suppurative otitis in childhood following measles; almost total destruction of drum membrane and contents of middle ear. At present only slight discharge. Hearing, right ear, nil. Left ear soon regained its normal condition, so far as any inflammatory process was concerned. The function, however, had been long since impaired. This loss of hearing became noticeable at about eighteen years of age. Following this acute attack, for which he visited me, left ear showed watch at bare contact, which improved to three inches when all acute symptoms subsided. Membrana tympani firmly retracted; some evidence of thickening.

Examination of nose showed prominent inferior turbinals; septal deflection to left side. This patient was operated upon March 29th, after a preliminary stripping done on the 27th. The growth removed was typical of periadenitis and is the last one examined by Dr. Hall, whose report I have submitted to you.

CASE No. 5.—Mrs. G., age 28; light hair, blue eyes; anemic; weight 105 pounds; family history good. At 12 years of age patient suffered an attack of scarlet fever. Right ear became seat of a destructive suppurative otitis media, which continued uninterruptedly for 15 years. Received treatment of various kinds, with no permanent results up to the time of coming to me. Upon examination of the right ear found hearing completely destroyed; a very offensive discharge of pus, not great in quantity; discharge consisting of pus with much desquamation; epithelial cells becoming inspissated about the walls of external canal. The drum membrane exhibited a large perforation, including the entire posterior superior quadrant; Schrapnell's membrane, the seat of great inflammation, extending high into the attic; the incus had been destroyed, but the malleus and the stapes remained; granulation tissue protruded through the perforation in the drum membrane. During acute attacks some tenderness and swelling appeared over mastoid; but none was present at the time of her visit to me.

Upon examination of her throat I found an inflammatory thickening of the lining of the vault. In the fossa of Rosenmuller on both sides could be seen a considerable mass of hypertrophied tissue, enough to almost obliterate the folds surrounding the tubes, the right mass being much more distinct. Thick adhesive bands extending from the pharyngeal wall to the posterior eustachian lips. The lip of the right tube was very much enlarged; there was little or no hypertrophy in the middle of the vault. The entire surface was covered with a thick mucopurulent secretion and could be seen from the crevices between the folds of hypertrophied tissue. The nasal mucous membrane was greatly thickened, especially over both inferior turbinates and a cartilaginous deflection of the septum to the right side of slight degree.

This seemed to me a very unfavorable case and so informed the patient, telling her that I regarded a radical operation necessary to a complete recovery. To this she demurred. On July 9, 1908, I did the preliminary operation of stripping the vault tissue, and on the 11th removed the mass exhibited to you. This patient made a rapid recovery. The discharge ceased in twenty-one days after the operation, and up to the present time there has been no recurrence.

LVIII.

THE INCISION FOR THE SUBMUCOUS RESECTION.*

By Sidney Yankauer, M. D.,

New York.

The clinical results which have been obtained in the treatment of deflected nasal septa by the submucous removal of all the deviated cartilage and bone, as well as the universal applicability of the operation to all varieties of this condition, have placed this operation upon such a secure footing as the operation of choice, that further discussion of its clinical advisability would be superfluous. But on account of the large variety of pathologic conditions which present themselves, and the consequent varying clinical experience of different operators, a consideration of some of the details of technic may be of some value and interest.

The entire character of the operative procedures, many details of technic, the choice of instruments, and the after-treatment are dependent upon the manner of making the incision in the mucous membrane. From this point of view, two classes of operations may be distinguished—operations through a linear incision, and flap operations.

In Killian's method a curved vertical incision is made in front of the deviation with its convexity forward. The anterior end of the deviation is embraced in the hollow of the curve. When the deviation is very pronounced the lower end of the incision is extended backwards in a horizontal direction along the lowest part of the septum near the floor of the nose, thus converting the operation into a flap operation.

Hajek makes an incision further forward, corresponding to the anterior border of the cartilage, and its removal is begun from this point. As the hyaline cartilage of the septum proper becomes gradually changed into fibrocartilage along this anterior border there is sometimes difficulty in separating the

---

*Read before the American Laryngological, Rhinological and Otological Society, June, 1909.

mucous membrane at the beginning of the operation. This incision makes it necessary at times to perform the whole operation from the side of the concavity, a decided technical error. It also leaves the tip of the nose supported by a strip of cartilage which has only one attachment to the bony framework of the face, namely, at its connection with the nasal bones. The support of the columna is taken away entirely, and I have seen one case in which a considerable drawing up of the columna took place, resulting in a hook-shaped nose, a very noticeable deformity.

Both the Hajek and Killian incisions are open to the objection that the entire incision is made upon the septum itself; hence it is mechanically impossible to separate the mucous membrane from the cartilage without stretching it. As the mucous membrane is often very thin along the bony crest, this becomes a dangerous procedure. It becomes particularly objectionable after the removal of the cartilage, when access to the bony portions of the septum can only be obtained by forcibly stretching the mucous membrane open with long-bladed specula. These incisions, which have been aptly termed "button-hole cuts," are altogether too small to permit of access to the deeper part of the septum. They are entirely too small to give a sufficient view of the parts when the deviation is complicated by fractures or dehiscences in the cartilage, or by unusual deviation or exostoses of the bony parts.

A better exposure of the septum may be obtained by making a flap of the mucous membrane, the so-called open operations. Two incisions, meeting at an acute or obtuse angle in the form of a V or an L, or three incisions, in the shape of a U, may be made in various directions, so that the resulting flap may be turned upwards, forwards or backwards. Of these the reverse L incision of Freer is the most popular.

While these incisions permit of better access to the deeper parts of the septum than the smaller incisions of Killian and Hajek, they present, in the opinion of the writer, a number of disadvantages. The flap is free in the nose and becomes unmanageable, and is apt to be caught in the forceps and injured, unless it is held back by means of a retractor; this requires the undivided attention of an assistant. As one assistant is always required to sponge the wound, etc., two assistants become necessary. This is a disadvantage, not only in private practice, but also in clinical practice, where many such operations must be performed; for it delays the clinic and retards other work of equal importance.

One of the incisions which bound the flap is always a horizontal incision. Every incision means a scar, and every scar is covered with squamous epithelium. A horizontal band of squamous epithelium on the septum is a particularly undesirable condition. For the one function of the septum is to afford a large unbroken surface of· ciliated epithelium, which by its capillary proximity to the turbinates constitutes the long arm of the nasal syphon, by means of which the entire nose, including the accessory cavities, is drained. A horizontal band of squamous epithelium constitutes a break in the syphonage. The normal secretion of the nose is held up by this form of epithelium, upon which it dries and forms crusts..

Another objection to the flap operations is the increased danger of perforation.· Whatever method of making the flap is employed, the incision is so designed as to include, within the area of the flap, the most prominent part. the apex. of the deviation. On the concave side of the septum. the deepest part of the concavity corresponds to the apex of the deviation on the convexity. The mucous membrane of the deep part of the concavity is very thin; it is often so sharply folded upon itself that the bend consists of little more than a layer of epithelium. Moreover, the mucoperiosteum is here closely bound down to the bone; it is continuous with the layer of dense fibrous tissue which lies on top of the bone: sharp serrations from the ends of the bony crest are embedded within it in this situation; its separation, therefore. presents many difficulties. and it is occasionally torn during the necessary manipulations. This possibility is increased by the fact that we are working upon the distant side of the septum. and that it is not infrequently necessary to separate the periosteum over the edge of exostoses which may project prominently into the other nostril. When a tear of any magnitude occurs in the mucous membrane of the concavity. within the area corresponding to the flap. a permanent perforation is sure to result.

These several objections to the flap methods may be overcome by providing sufficient facilities for the work. and by care and skill in operating: on the other hand. a difficulty which is inherent to the method itself is the delayed convalescence. Every plastic flap has a tendency to retract. When the flap retracts, as it does after this operation, an open space is left, which must heal by granulation, followed by epithelialization. An open wound in the nose, exposed as it is to every breath of air which the patient breathes, invariably becomes infected, even though the infection may be, and usually is, of a mild type. Such an infected wound secretes a considerable amount of fluid, which dries and forms crusts. When bone has been exposed and cut, the healing of the wound may be delayed for several weeks, until the slow-forming bone-granulations are built up. In proof of these assertions permit me to quote from a recent article by one of the ablest exponents of the flap operation:

"Up to the tenth day of the operation the patient is directed to keep the naris closed with a pledget placed in the nasal vestibule and changed when it becomes filled with secretion. In this manner dust is excluded and the interior of the nostril kept moist, so that no scabs can form. After this period the patient may use the nostril for breathing, is told to spray it out with normal salt solution and to insert a little plug of wet cotton into it for a few hours at a time, whenever it becomes necessary to soften dried secretion. In addition an ointment is swabbed into the nasal vestibule by the patient to prevent hardened mucus from adhering.

"In most cases it is necessary to continue this cleansing treatment for a period of from four to twelve weeks, for during this time, if the nose be neglected, scabs will form upon the septum."

Now, in Dr. Emil Mayer's clinic at the Mount Sinai Hospital, where most of my operations are performed, such a long period of convalescence from septum operations is quite unknown. Our cases return on the second day for the removal of the packing, and on the fourth day nearly all of the cases can be discharged with the wound healed and the nose free from crusts or secretion. Moreover, in nearly 300 successive cases of deviation of pronounced or extreme degree, there has not been a single perforation resulting from the operation. Nor have such results been limited to the cases operated upon by me personally, for my colleagues at the clinic, as well as others whom I have taught my method of operating, have had similar experience; they may, therefore, be attributed to the technic, employed, which is dependent, as previously stated, upon the method of making the incision in the mucous membrane.

The mucous membrane incision which I have devised for this operation has been previously described as follows: Beginning behind the attachment of the lower lateral cartilage, and about 1 cm. from the dorsum of the nose, the incision is made vertically downwards to the lower border of the nostril, to the point where the mucous membrane of the nasal floor meets the skin of the vestibule. It is then carried outwards along the mucocutaneous junction, half way to the outer nasal wall. This incision permits the mucous membrane of the septum to be reflected upon the outer wall of the nose, that of the inner half of the floor being laid upon the outer half. The opening into the septum is just behind the nostril, and when the tip of the nose is raised, is nearly parallel to it. It is as large as the nostril itself, without stretching the mucous membrane, and any instrumentation that can be done through the nostril can be done through this opening.

When the deviation is not pronounced, the incision is begun several millimeters behind the reflection of mucous membrane which marks the posterior border of the attachment of the lower lateral cartilage to the septum; when the deviation extends far forwards, the incision may be begun at this reflection. When the septum is so twisted that the cartilage of the anterior slope of the deviation crosses the median plane and projects from the other nostril, it will usually be found that the bone of the anterior nasal spine (intermaxillary crest) is correspondingly twisted; the incision is then made along the line of crossing, which always brings the lower part of the incision in the desired place.

As the mucous membrane of the convexity remains anchored to the nasal floor, the flap can be readily controlled from the nostril without the use of deep retractors or long-bladed specula. When it has been properly freed it is ballooned outwards by the act of inspiration, and often sticks to the outer nasal wall through the tenacity of the normal nasal secretions. In the beginning of the operation, until the mucous membrane has been properly separated, it may be necessary to retract the membrane, but this can be done by the operator himself with a spatula or with one of the blunt separators; when the deeper parts of the septum are reached, the shank of the instrument that is being used serves as a retractor. It thus becomes possible' to operate without an assistant, and many of my operations were so performed.

The incision permits of an excellent exposure of the lower anterior corner of the septum and of the angle between this part of the septum and the nasal floor, just underneath the deviation. This part of the septum has not received as much notice in the literature as its importance demands. For, on account of the mobility of the organ in this region, its liability to traumatism, the frequent occurrence of ulcerations, the dislocation of the cartilage from the bony connections, and dehiscences in the cartilage itself, an increased amount of fibrous tissue develops between the cartilage and bone, as well as under the mucous membrane and in the periosteum. This fibrous tissue is very dense and resistant, and has more the nature of cicatricial tissue than of ordinary connective tissue. For these reasons the thorough exposure or opening of the septum in this region is of the utmost importance, especially in difficult cases, in which the uncovering of the anatomical arrangements in this region constitutes the key to the entire situation.

As a result of these considerations we may conclude as follows: A sufficient exposure of the septum to permit of good access to the cartilaginous part of the deviation is essential in all cases, but the incision should be so planned as to permit a sufficient exposure of the bony deflection as well. This is particularly important in extreme and difficult cases, for in these the removal of the bony part is usually indispensable for the correction of the deformity. Just as the anterior portion of the bent cartilage shuts out from view its deeper parts, so the anterior part of the bony deflection, the deviated intermaxillary crest, closes the bend in the bony parts and shuts from view the deeper parts of the deviated vomer. The proper exposure of the bony part of the deviation is, therefore, an essential part of an open operation, and in the experience of the writer can not be obtained by any of the incisions that have heretofore been suggested or practiced so well as by the method herein advocated.

LIX

AMPUTATION OF THE EPIGLOTTIS IN LARYN-GEAL TUBERCULOSIS.

By Lorenzo B. Lockard, M. D.,

Denver.

By far the most fatal, as well as the most painful, localization of tuberculosis in the larynx is the epiglottidean; a type always resistant to treatment, rapid in development and extension, and deplorable in the subjective symptoms evoked.

The picture presented by the unfortunate subject of such a process is well known to all, and no other condition, with the possible exception of a malignant growth, induces a feeling of such utter helplessness as to either cure or effective pallia-tion.

That it is possible, however, through radical extirpation of the involved organ, to effectually relieve the pain in practically all of these cases and to permanently cure the larynx in a small proportion, has, I believe, been conclusively demonstrated.

Extensive studies upon the living and dead have shown that approximately one-third of all consumptives have, in greater or lesser degree, coincident involvement of the throat, and sta-tistics prove that in over twenty per cent of the laryngeal cases the epiglottis is involved. That this estimate is conservative is shown by the following table:

Author.	Cases of laryngeal tuberculosis.	Lesions of epiglottis.
Mackenzie	500	175
Mackenzie	100 (Postmortems)	81
Lake	329	68
Carmody	155	58
Stein	100	65 (Est.)
T. J. Harris	125	35 (Est.)
Author	961	136
	2,270	618—27.22%

In the above table the number of cases of epiglottidean involvement has been compared with the total number having laryngeal tuberculosis. In the following table the number of epiglottidean cases is compared with the total of laryngeal lesions, a method that gives a much smaller percentage, as each individual usually has several distinct foci:

Author	Lesions of the larynx.	Lesions of the epiglottis.
Gaul	140	27
Mackenzie	1,174	186
Lake	859	82
Phipps Institute	150	14
Author	1,671	127
	3,994	436—10.91%

These statistics show that this form of the disease, instead of being a rare manifestation, as is commonly believed, is a relatively frequent complication.

A tuberculous lesion of the epiglottis, while occasionally the sole localization of the disease in the throat, occurs, as a rule, in patients with older and well-developed foci of other segments of the larynx, notably of the arytenoid cartilages and aryteno-epiglottidean folds. Isolated epiglottidean disease, in individuals having pulmonary tuberculosis, has been observed in only a few instances, of which the following may be cited:

Author.	Laryngeal disease limited to epiglottis.
Stein	2
Barwell	1
T. J. Harris	1
H. Bert Ellis	5
Lake	4
Carmody	1
Besold and Gidionsen	8
Author	4
	26

On theoretical grounds the possibility of an epiglottidean focus being the first and only lesion in the body must be admitted, but from a practical standpoint the question scarcely deserves serious considertaion. B. L. Shurly, in a personal communication, reports one case of apparently primary infee- tion, and one to which considerable doubt attaches is recorded by Lake, the only ones found in a close review of 4,991 cases.

As already shown, epiglottidean tuberculosis is practically always associated with advanced disease of other segments of the larynx and of the lungs, and to this fact, in large meas- ure, can be accredited its appalling mortality, for even if the epiglottidean disease were capable of arrest or cure, the patient would usually succumb to these concurrent processes. Even when the pulmonary and other laryngeal foci are incipient or quiescent, their advancement is rapid after breaking down of the epiglottis, for the severe dysphagia and resultant cachexia soon destroy what little vitality the tissues have retained, and these conditions have generally supervened by the time the case comes under observation.

Even in the incipient cases little is to be anticipated from medicinal treatment, for, as a rule, they progress rapidly from bad to worse, while in those with advanced lesions we are even powerless to control the terrible dysphagia.

From such statistics as are available it would seem that the general mortality of these cases, including both the incipient and advanced, is in the neighborhood of ninety per cent. If one took into account the advanced cases only. those associated with severe dysphagia, it would be found 'that not more than one to two per cent result in local healing. Many eminent laryngologists place the death rate, in this class of patients, at 100 per cent.

These statistics, moreover, do not show the full extent of our helplessness, for. in addition to the failure to cure or even temporarily arrest the process, we achieve but little in the way of relief; success in conquering or markedly lessening the dysphagia would palliate, in large degree. our lack of success in overcoming the disease.

Any method of treatment, therefore, that offers some hope of local cure in favorable cases, and promise of euthanasia in the incurable. deserves serious consideration, and such a method we unquestionably possess in complete amputation.

Although the number of enduring cures of the patient, as a result of the operation, is small and must ever remain so, because of associated conditions in other organs, the procedure does undoubtedly save an occasional case, and I feel that the statement is justifiable that no palliative operation, in the whole domain of surgery, gives more brilliant immediate results.

That eventual cures are not more frequently attained is no valid objection to its performance, for the vast majority are already irrevocably doomed when they come under the laryngologist's observation, and we are confronted by a single problem: the relief of pain. In a not inconsiderable proportion of these cases, however, a complete arrest of the laryngeal process is attained, and in a small number the removal of this complication enables the body to conquer the basic disease.

Of the twenty-seven cases operated by the author, twenty-six were completely relieved of pain; in eight the larynx was cured, and in five the pulmonary process eventually became quiescent. Three cases are still under treatment. In one case the palate was also involved, but even in this instance deglutition was greatly facilitated.

Of the cured cases one has endured five years and a half, and one four years and eight months.

When it is recognized that these cases, if operated early, before the vitality is hopelessly impaired and the accompanying conditions advanced to an incurable stage, are susceptible of cure, the operation will take its place as a curative as well as a palliative procedure.

The average length of life after operation, the usual way of estimating the utility of such a procedure, is of absolutely no importance in this connection, for it is no way an index of its effectiveness; the amputation, nine times out of ten, is made with the sole idea of relieving pain, with the knowledge that life cannot be prolonged more than a few months at most; hence statistics are certain to be misleading and disappointing.

Thus Lake, in summarizing his results according to this method, says: "By these methods I have removed the epiglottis some fifteen times. Speaking from this experience, I consider the average duration of life after operation in bad cases, to be not less than three months, and seldom more than nine months; and in a certain number, in which the epiglottis is attacked earlier than usual in the course of the laryngeal and pulmonary disease, a complete cure may result."

Since the results are very favorable when the operation is performed before the concurrent processes are far advanced, a triple classification in tabulating the cases will be attempted.

(a) Results in patients who, were it not for the epiglottidean involvement, might be classed as favorable.

(b) Results in patients suffering from dysphagia due to involvement of the epiglottis, in whom the pulmonary or other laryngeal lesions would warrant an unfavorable prognosis, even if the epiglottis were not affected.

(c) Because of the impossibility of getting definite data regarding the general condition of a large number of cases operated, a separate table, including these cases, must be made.

In cases of the first class a large percentage of enduring cures may be anticipated; in the second class, comprising the great majority, an occasional cure only may be attained, but these would undoubtedly succumb under other methods of treatment, and in those that do not recover the dysphagia will usually completely disappear.

NUMBER OF CASES, 240.

Heryng	100
Barwell	30
Lake	15
Freudenthal	10
Harris	2
Carmody	9
Schmidt	9
Hajek	1
Moeller	20
Beck	1
Gleitsman	3
Flatau	1
Sollenberger	2
Gruenwald	1
Gerber	*3
Sokolowski	*3
Potter	†1
Bennett	1
Newman	1
Author	27
	240

The operation has also been done, a number of times, by Besold and Gidionsen.

*Some additional cases. Number not specified.
†Cancer.

ANALYSIS OF 134 CASES.

CLASS "A."

Cases.	Pain relieved.	Epiglottis healed.	Larynx healed.	Patient cured.
11	11	11	8	5
			3 under treatment.	3 no report. 3 under treatment.

CLASS "B."

Cases.	Pain relieved.	Epiglottis healed.	Larynx healed.	Patient cured.
83	79	70	3	0

CLASS "C."

Cases.	Pain relieved.	Epiglottis healed.	Larynx healed.	Patient cured.
40	25	25	8	7

TOTALS.

Cases.	Pain relieved.	Epiglottis healed.	Larynx healed.	Patient cured.
134	115	106	19	12

	Class A.	Class B.	Class C.
Pain relieved	100.00%	95.18%	62.5%
Epiglottis healed	100.00%	84.33%	62.0%
Larynx healed	72.72%	3.61%	20.0%
Patient cured	45.45%	0.00%	17.5%

TOTALS.

Pain relieved.	Epiglottis healed.	Larynx healed.	Patient cured.
85.82%	79.1%	14.17%	8.95%

An additional 100 cases, reported by Heryng in a personal communication, are not included in this report, since general conclusions only were given. He says: "I have operated about 100 times, 70 times with the double curette and perhaps 25 times with the galvanocautery snare. The cautery seemed, in a number of instances, to provoke severe and prolonged reaction. When possible, I remove either the entire epiglottis, or one-half, with the double curette or cold snare, because after their use there is only the slightest reaction, and the dysphagia disappears more promptly. Evil consequences, such as severe bleeding, I have never experienced."

Of the six other cases not included in the report, five could not be analyzed; the sixth was a case of cancer, involving the epiglottis, in which amputation gave wonderful relief.

In considering these figures, allowance must be made for two sources of error: in the first place, in a small number of cases, after varying periods of complete relief, some pain recurred, owing to progression of complicating laryngeal lesions, and, on the other hand, some cases benefited to a considerable degree were not classed as successful, for I have attemped to tabulate as relieved only those in whom no dysphagia persisted.

Many cases pass from observation after relief of the subjective symptoms, hence the statistics regarding the eventual outcome of the disease in the lungs and larynx are very incomplete.

Of all the authorities consulted, who have performed the operation, only one believes it to be unwarranted: Sokolowski, of Warsaw.

He writes: "Gradually, from year to year, I have departed from the surgical treatment of laryngeal tuberculosis, because by general treatment, combined with local treatment (carbolic, menthol, lactic acid, etc.), I achieve improvement and healing without the bad results of the surgical procedures. For the same reason we have given up complete and partial amputations of the epiglottis, which I previously performed in some cases without any striking results. Recently my long-time assistant, Dr. Erbrich, operated, in our hospital, three cases of advanced laryngeal tuberculosis with severe dysphagia, after ineffectual local treatment, by excision of the epiglottis, but the results were not satisfactory, as the dysphagia was not relieved."

A considerable number opposed the procedure on theoretical grounds, and a yet larger number, who had not done the complete operation, favored, in certain cases of limited involvement, the excision of small areas. As this paper deals only with the complete operation, their valuable work cannot be quoted.

The general opinion of those who have had considerable experience with the operation is well reflected by Jorgen Moeller, of Copenhagen, who wrote to me as follows: "As you see, I have this time. (10 unreported cases) no brilliant results to record. The cases, however, were all very bad, and in which the indications for operation, as previously adhered to, were extended to embrace all cases of severe dysphagia due to the epiglottis, even when the lungs were hopelessly diseased. (In his previous ten cases, in which the line was more strictly drawn, he had three cures: two of these are still well, and one has had a recurrence.) It appears to me, however, that the history of these cases supports the correctness of this extension of the indications for amputation, because almost without exception there was wonderful relief that lasted for a longer or shorter time, frequently until death."

INDICATIONS.

There need be no confusion regarding the types of cases in which amputation is indicated.

1. The operation is imperatively demanded in every case of involvement accompanied by severe dysphagia, regardless of the state of the lungs.

2. Immediate removal is indicated even when dysphagia has not supervened, provided the lesion is extensive and there is still hope of arresting the pulmonic disease. The existence of such a focus is a constant menace, because it may at any moment give rise to severe pain and in a brief period cause irreparable injury.

3. Any lesion that resists treatment should be excised.

4. If the condition of the epiglottis is such as to hinder correct treatment of underlying lesions, it may be removed to render these parts more accessible.

METHODS OF AMPUTATION.

The methods employed are unimportant, provided they permit of complete excision and leave a smooth stump. If the lesions are sharply circumscribed, only the affected parts need be removed, but when there is considerable involvement, or if doubt exists as to the true limits of the disease, the entire organ should be amputated.

The preference of the individual may decide in favor of the cutting forceps, the cold snare, or the electric snare.

In my earlier cases I used the galvanocautery snare, but early abandoned it, owing to the severe reaction experienced in nearly every instance. In one of my last cases I used the cold wire, as advocated by Gerber, of Koenigsberg, who has operated three times in this way. In its favor he claims (1) slight reaction in the neighboring tissues, (2) slight pain and little bleeding, (3) rapid performance.

In my case the first two indications were fulfilled, but owing to a slight slipping of the loop it was necessary to remove the central base with the forceps.

Gerber says: "I have frequently removed the epiglottis, formerly with the cutting forceps and cautery. Of late, however, with especially good results, by means of the cold snare. I have undertaken this for the relief of severe dysphagia, and have had very good results.

"An influence upon the general disease in cases of extensive tuberculosis has not been experienced or expected."

With perfect adaptation of the snare much time may be saved, as it is rarely possible, with the cutting instruments, to thoroughly remove the organ with less than three distinct sections—one for the central portion and one each for the lateral thirds.

Of the cutting forceps there are two of almost equal utility; the Lake-Barwell and the Spiess. The great fault with the Spiess instrument, as commonly made, is that it has the same length of shaft and curve as the instruments designed for endolaryngeal work, so that, in many instances, when the cutting blades are in position, the shaft impinges against the palate to such an extent that free manipulation is impossible. In one instance, when no other instrument was available, nearly three hours were consumed in the operation, as the irritation produced in the attempts to introduce the instrument caused uncontrollable gagging. With the correction of this defect it would be a very valuable instrument. In the Lake-Barwell forceps this fault does not exist. The operation is likewise simplified by the possession of several instruments of various sizes, with the blades placed at different angles to the shaft, for in no two instances is the epiglottis of the same size and shape.

In several instances I have successfully used a modified lingual tonsillotome.

The parts can be so completely anesthetized with 20 per cent cocain as to make the operation practically painless; never have I seen even the most sensitive and nervous patient rebel.

Hemorrhage is seldom severe and it is not necessary to make preliminary applications of adrenalin; after each section there is free bleeding for a few seconds, necessitating a brief period of waiting before the following cut can be made. In only one case, of which I have record, has the bleeding been even profuse; this occurred in the practice of Harold Barwell, but no especial procedures were necessary for its control.

The report of an interesting case of hemorrhage was sent me by Moeller, of Copenhagen. He writes: "Immediately (after the amputation) severe bleeding occurred, which, despite the local use of ice, persisted, unabated, for an hour, when I was able to get a good view of the larynx, and found the wound covered with a firm coagulum and no bleeding point; the patient also declared that his sensations were the same as during a previous pulmonary hemorrhage. He was, therefore, sent to the hospital. After six weeks he was discharged feeling very good; there was, however, no demonstrable improvement of the pulmonary process. The amputation wound was almost completely cicatrized; the disease in the interior of the larynx needs further treatment."

In nearly all of my cases the organ was removed as near as possible to the base, but never was there any bleeding of moment. The last vestige of blood in the sputum has usually disappeared within a quarter of an hour.

In its exposed condition, subject to constant insult by the pulmonary secretions, it would seem probable that postoperative infection would be a danger of considerable magnitude, but this contingency has only rarely materialized. Lake reports one case of infection of the stump that responded to treatment, and I have seen two cases in which superficial ulceration occurred; in both instances the ulcers disappeared under the use of antiseptic sprays and cauterizing pigments. In one case the stump became infiltrated, but did not produce any particular discomfort. In several additional cases, in which the dysphagia was completely relieved, the stump was not entirely healed at the time of death, but including these, it leaves, in my series, twenty-three cases of perfect healing in a total of twenty-seven.

Barwell, in thirty amputations, has not met with one where there was postoperative ulceration or inflammation; Gleitsmann has removed the organ three times without subsequent local infection; T. J. Harris did not have it in either of his two cases, and Dr. Carmody, of nine cases which he operated, had two in which the wound was not completely cicatrized at the time of death; in the remaining seven local healing was perfect.

Aggravation of the pulmonary process must be an accident of extreme rarity. Barwell, in a personal communication, says: "In nearly all of my cases the excision has been performed merely for the relief of dysphagia, for in my experience infiltration of the epiglottis seldom occurs until the disease in the lungs and other parts of the larynx is so far advanced that cure is out of the question. I have never seen any shock; hemorrhage has never been dangerous, and only profuse in one case. I have never found the general condition made worse by the operation. The wound never becomes inflamed nor acts as the starting point of ulceration; in most cases where the general condition is fairly good it tends to heal rapidly and often becomes completely healed in about fourteen days. In every case the severe dysphagia has been much improved and frequently quite abolished, but in some removal of the arytenoid swelling has become necessary as well."

Dr. Freudenthal, in summarizing the results of his ten operations, says: "A reinfection was stirred up that caused death in some cases within a week."

In one of my cases, a man of twenty-three years, there occurred, ten days after operation, a miliary outbreak in the pharynx and nasopharynx that soon produced wide destruction of tissue. The patient had large cavities in both lungs, universal laryngeal involvement, and a large tuberculous ulcer of the right cheek, above and posterior to the last molar, forming a necrotic pouch as large as a hickory nut. At the time of operation this ulcer was extending to the anterior pillar, and the temperature was ranging around 103 degrees. Two weeks before the epiglottis was removed he was operated for appendicitis. The miliary outbreak could hardly be accredited to the operation, which was performed because deglutition had become impossible and he was starving to death. The pain was greatly lessened by the operation and thereafter could be largely controlled by cocain and morphin.

In very exceptional cases the cough is temporarily aggravated and the sputum increased, but these symptoms rapidly subside. In the great majority of instances the exact opposite obtains, and the cough is almost at once diminished in frequency and severity, sometimes to an extent that seems almost incredible. Occasionally the temperature is slightly elevated for one or two days, but usually there is a decided and almost immediate fall from the average maintained during the preceding weeks, the declension, in several cases, amounting to three and four degrees within the first few days.

AFTER-TREATMENT.

Because of theoretical considerations it was long the author's practice to have the patients fed by nutrient enemata during the first week; today he permits the taking of non-irritant liquid food within a few hours of the time of operation. As a rule little pain is experienced, but as paroxysms of coughing are occasionally, though rarely, provoked, it is advisable that solid food be withheld for a couple of days. In a number of instances a full meal has been eaten at the end of forty-eight hours. If difficulty in swallowing is experienced within the first days the food should be taken through a tube, while the patient lies prone with the head well below the level of the body. In the short interval during which solid foods are withheld the strength is maintained by raw eggs in milk, custards, beef-juice, Biftick a la Tartare, raw oysters, gelatines, etc.

During the first twenty-four or thirty-six hours comfort is promoted by keeping the air of the room impregnated with steam, and there is nothing more soothing than the following mixture, one teaspoonful to the pint of boiling water:

> Ol. pinus pumilionus ....dram i.
> Menthol ....gr. xxv.
> Milk of magnesia ....oz. ij.

Until healing is complete the cough is controlled, if excessive and irritating, by sedatives and expectorants; the larynx is cleansed several times a day by a one-half per cent formalin solution, followed by a daily application of 20 per cent argyrol, and if pain persists, the injection of orthoform emulsion, according to the formula of Freudenthal.

Immediately after the operation, as soon as bleeding has stopped, the stump is thoroughly rubbed with lactic acid. Heryng advises the use, at this time, of a two per cent alcoholic solution of malachite green.

To one who has not previously performed this operation two things are a decided revelation; the wonderful and almost immediate relief of pain and the insignificant amount of postoperative inflammation and discomfort, unless there are accompanying conditions themselves provocative of pain. Even in these cases the suffering is greatly diminished. One naturally presupposes a prolonged period of odynophagia and dysphagia, but in practice it is found that the odynophagia almost immediately disappears, that there is little subsequent soreness, and that deglutition, previously difficult or entirely impossible, becomes at once almost normal.

I believe it can justly be claimed that by this operation we save a certain number of lives that otherwise would most certainly be sacrificed; that in the vast majority, when a cure is not to be thought of, we effectually conquer the pain, and that we succeed, even in those in whom the suffering is not entirely controlled, owing to the presence of complicating lesions, in diminishing it to a notable degree.

LX.

A NEW METHOD FOR INFLATING THE EUSTA-CHIAN TUBE AND MIDDLE EAR.*

By Edmund Prince Fowler, M. D.,

New York.

For forty-five years Politzer's method of inflating the middle ear has had no rival for simplicity and but few for efficiency and safety. The reason for its pre-eminence in otologic practice is that it makes use of the act of swallowing to open the pharyngeal mouth of the Eustachian tube, and this is the method by which nature mainly and best maintains the normal pneumatic balance in the air channels of the middle ear. Politzer's method is, however, sometimes impotent to effect an entrance into the closed tube, and we are driven to modifications or other methods of inflation.

Although you are all fully cognizant of these modifications of Politzerization, I will briefly state the most important.

Instead of swallowing water at the moment of air compression in the nasopharynx, the simple act of swallowing may be performed, or a lump of sugar or other substance may be held in the mouth to increase the secretion of saliva and so facilitate deglutition. Simply lifting the soft palate will occasionally open the mouth of the tube; so also acts phonation, especially of words containing the syllables "hic," "hac" and "huk," etc., and the letter "k." Blowing into and puffing out of the cheeks, or inspiring through the nearly closed lips, or through a small tube inserted between the lips, all tend to elevate the palate and shut off the nasopharynx from the aural cavity, and so enable the air pressure to be increased in the former during the air insufflation. Whereas at times one of these methods may succeed in aiding Politzerization, it is rare to have it so happen, and we are usually forced to catheterize

*Read before the Section on Otology, New York Academy of Medicine, January 8, 1909.

the tube to obtain the desired increase in the intratympanic pressure in different cases.

In children, we are frequently dependent on their cries for closure of the soft palate, and in adults and children it is not an uncommon occurrence to fail miserably, because we cannot with sufficient accuracy time the air-bag pressure so that it will coincide with the shutting off of the patient's nasopharynx.

Stenosis of the pharyngeal orifice of the Eustachian tube from edema or tenacious mucus frequntly blocks the entrance of air by Politzer's method, and even cleansing or shrinking the tissues with adrenalin or cocain fails to permit entrance of the air. Likewise, narrowing or closing of any portion of the tube will often effectually block all attempts at inflation.

Now, although we have in catheterization of the tube a most efficient and dependable means for inflation of the middle ear, there are many reasons why we should prefer Politzerization, if the latter is feasible. Briefly, these reasons are—its simplicity of application, which enables not only the general practitioner to successfully treat many ear affections, but also adapts it for use by the patient himself; its possibility of use in many cases in children and adults where catheterization is impossible because of deformities or pathologic conditions in the nose or nasopharynx, or because of the pain, discomfort or irritation caused by the introduction of the catheter into the nose or tubal mouth.

I will not go more fully into the advantages and disadvantages or dangers of Politzerization and catheterization in this paper, as they are well known to all otologists, and space will not permit. I have briefly summarized the matter as above, to better lead up to the consideration of the method with which I desire to acquaint you. as it was partly through the contemplation of facts such as I have noted that I was led to devise it.

During the experiments incident to the testing of my instrument for diagnosing and differentiating ossicular anchyloses, I was struck with the fact that after Valsalva's experiment, or inflation of the middle ear by other means, the normal pressure in the tympanic cavity was reestablished with much more facility on swallowing than was the case after swallowing following Toynbee's experiments or deflations by other methods. It was clearly apparent that the Eustachian tube would permit of air transit towards its pharyngeal end with more

facility than in the opposite direction. It was also to my mind
quite clear why this should be the case, aside from the action of
the cilia, or the form or patency of the Eustachian tube. I rea-
soned that although the tube could not be exactly compared
to a soft tube outside of the body, its membranous portion, and
especially the pharyngeal end, could be so thought of, and
that a partial vacuum or condensation of the air, distal to its
pharyngeal mouth, would act similarly to a partial vacuum or a
condensation of air distal to a closed section of very soft rubber
tubing. In both cases it needs no elaborate argument to prove
that a diminished air pressure distal to the stricture would tend
to hold in approximation the stenosed segment, or that an increased pressure would tend to make it more readily patent.

These results would likewise hold in kind, if pressure was
brought to bear from the proximal ends of the tubes, and they
would open much more readily under this air pressure if the
air contained in the distal portions was in a state of condensation than if it was below normal atmospheric pressure. These
facts throw light on the subject of Eustachian tube permeability, and the vicious condition which tends to perpetuate itself
once the normal air pressure in the tympanic cavity is lowered
by tubal strictures. They also suggested to me a method of
effecting the permeability of the Eustachian tube, of relieving
conditions of diminished air pressure within the middle ear,
and of treating middle ear diseases concomitant with these
lowered tensions.

The method consists of bringing an increased air pressure
to bear on both extremities of the closed portion of the tubal
lining by simultaneously condensing the air in the middle ear
and in the nose and nasopharynx. To accomplish this end we
may construct apparatus in several ways, and I will describe
two.

The simplest form consists of an air bag connected by means
of a Y tube to a nose-piece and an ear-piece. The former is
preferably a large, olive-shaped nozzle, and the latter one of my
ear massage cups—as both of these devices are more agreeable
to the patient, easy of application, painless, sufficiently tight,
and cleanly. I regularly substitute a magnifying Siegle's
speculum for the ear cup, during the first few inflations, and
obtain a magnified view of the tympanic membrane, to be sure
that the air has entered the tube, as many people cannot recog-

nize its entrance, owing to the meatal air compression preventing the drum from violently distending, as is the case in Politzerization. The patient holds the nose-piece with one hand tightly in either nostril, and closes the other nostril with the fingers of the same hand. The surgeon adjusts the ear-piece tightly into or about the ear, depending upon which contrivance he is using, and holds the air bag with his right hand. The patient is told to swallow, and ás he does so the surgeon quickly compresses the air bag, thus bringing to bear on the tympanic membrane, middle ear contents and outer extremity of the Eustachian tube, an increased air pressure, and simultaneously an increased nasopharyngeal pressure on account of the closure of the soft palate, and if the act of swallowing has opened the tubal mouth the air pressure extends through the tube toward the middle ear.

If for any reason the pharynx was not properly shut off from the nose, the force of the air expends itself against the posterior pharyngeal wall, and in the nose and oral cavity, and a slight wave reaches the ear drum through the branch going to the ear-piece. This latter cannot be of much consequence unless the air pressure in the tubing is increased by the closure of the nares and soft palate.

If it is desired to bring suction to bear on the nose and middle ear, it is necessary to at once release the air bag after the inflation, keeping the apparatus in place and the nostrils tightly closed. In stenosed or blocked tubes suction does not often act through the pharyngeal mouth of the tube, as the moment it is exerted the inner portion of the tube collapses and the suction affects the tympanic cavity only through the partial vacuum in the external meatus.

In cases with patent tubes it is often possible to bring alternately suction and compression to bear on both sides of the drum if the tubes are maintained open by elevating the palate by forced inspiration or expiration through the lips.

The above described method is sometimes annoying, for the same reason as is Politzerization, namely, failure to correctly time the compression.

To obviate this difficulty and to more perfectly regulate the amount of pressure exerted, and to almost wholly eliminate any pressure on the external surface of the drum membrane, except there be a successful condensation of air in the nose and nasopharynx, I constructed the following apparatus:

The tube from the ear-piece is joined to the nose-piece, or enters the latter's tubing very close to the nose nozzle. The tube to the air bag is constricted just before it gives off the branches to the nose and ear, and an elastic reservoir bag is placed between this constricted portion and the air compression bag. The latter is provided with a valve, as in double bulb atomizers, so that although the supply of air to the second bulb is intermittent, the latter through its elasticity maintains a continuous current of air through the distal constricted portion

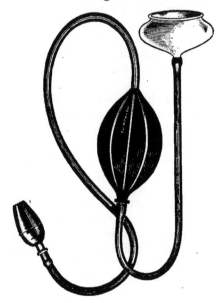

Aural Inflater.

of the tubing. This constricted portion must be of such a lumen as to retard the escape of air sufficiently to permit of its accumulation in the storage bulb.

By the above arrangement we are relieved from the necessity of noting the exact instant of our patient's swallowing, for no matter when he accomplishes the act, or in other ways opens his Eustachian tubes and closes his nasopharynx, the air from the apparatus is pouring into his nose and will increase the pressure in the nasopharynx the instant its escape into the oral cavity is cut off. Moreover, at this instant and not before, the pressure in the ear portion will be increased by the same means which bring about an increased air pressure in the nasal cavity.

By continuing to supply air to the reservoir bag as long as it is desired to continue the treatment, and every time the patient swallows or in other ways opens his tubes and approximates his soft palate to the posterior pharyngeal wall, so often will we accomplish an inflation of the Eustachian tube.

If it is undesirable to inflate both ears, one may be closed with a moistened finger to prevent its tympanic membrane from bulging during the treatment, but I find that this is seldom necessary, for as a rule the ear under treatment alone is inflated. Two ear cups are used if double inflation is desired.

After a little practice one can demonstrate on himself and learn that the ear under simultaneous compression requires less pressure to open its tube than does its fellow.

The possibilities of simplifying tubal inflation by this method are numerous; for instance, we can substitute for the hand bag a foot pump, or a compressed air reservoir, or the electric air pump, and easily arrange that just so much pressure is exerted during the treatment.

The indications and contraindications for using the method are not as yet fully worked out, but I believe it is indicated in preference to Politzerization or catheterization in many cases, especially in children: if the drum ear is atrophic; during tubal or middle-ear congestions or inflammations; in the after-treatment of suppurative otitis.

Unless the drum membrane is movable or permeable the method is not applicable.

To prove its usefulness, I hope some of you will give the method a trial, and report pro or con at some future meeting of the Section.

LXI

A SIMPLE ACUMETRIC FORMULA ADOPTED BY THE EIGHTH INTERNATIONAL OTOLOGIC CONGRESS AT BUDAPEST, 1909.*

By Jörgen Möller, M. D.,

Copenhagen.

For many years otologists have felt the need of a simple method of indicating the results of the functional tests for hearing. Nearly everybody who tests the hearing has his individual formula, which fails more or less to be understood by his colleagues, especially those from other countries, unless it is explained anew in every publication. If the acoustic functional tests were everywhere made in the same way it would indeed be most acceptable. This, however, is not the case, nor is it necessary. What can be done, however, and what should be done, is that the chief tests ,which are everywhere used, should be noted in the same way and with the same international signs, so that everybody may know at once what they mean.

As early as the Congress at Bordeaux the question of a simple acumetrie formula was discussed, and Drs. Politzer, Gradenigo and Delsaux proposed a formula which was praetical and easily understood. However, the subject was given over to an international commission by the Congress for further study. The majority of the members of this commission agreed upon a proposition, which was laid before the recent VIII Otological Congress, held at Budapest, and which was accepted by it. The formula agrees in its main points with the Bordeaux formula, but has been modified in many points. The commission has considered only the so-called qualitative functional tests, while the quantitative tests, testing of the hearing, etc., was left to each one's taste. Moreover, the commission did not desire to establish a collection of tests which

---

*Translated by Clarence Loeb, M. D.

should be exclusively and invariably used. They desired, rather, to make the formula so comprehensive that each man could find therein just what he needed, and could omit whatever seemed to him superfluous. However, the commission thought that a certain number of tests were necessary if it was desired to carry out a functional test which would be exact and of diagnostic value. Above all, however, the commission was intent upon devising an international notation, a system of abbreviations, which would be understood everywhere, no matter in what language the author wrote.

PROPOSAL OF THE COMMISSION.

In order to be able to write down the results of the functional tests in a manner as simple as possible and one understood by everybody, it is necessary that the fundamental formula established by the commission be used and that, furthermore, if abbreviations are employed only those established by the commission should be used. The abbreviations of each test are the initials of a corresponding Latin name, but the pitch is always designated according to the German musical method. The formula adopted by the commission has the following appearance (in order to assist its understanding the figures of an imaginary functional test are given, such as might be found in a right-sided middle ear affection):

A. D. and A. S. mean *Auris Dextra* and *Auris Sinistra*.

W means *Weber's* test. The lateralization is shown by an arrow pointing in the proper direction. If there is no lateralization after the W an = sign is placed. If the tuning fork is not heard by bone conduction a 0 is placed. Tuning fork a^1 (435 v. d.) is used. S means *Schwabach's* test. The difference in time from the normal perception time is indicated with a $+$ or a $\div$ and the number of seconds. Or by an $=$ when the perception time is normal. The same tuning fork is used. The normal perception time of the tuning fork must be added.

a^1M means the perception time of the tuning fork a^1 (435 v. d.) upon the mastoid process (M $=$ mastoideus, bone conduction). The normal perception time is added in parenthesis, the perception time for the right or left ear of the patient above and below, all indicated in seconds. In case only the difference in time is measured this is noted with a $+$ and a $\div$, or in a superficial examination without adding the number of seconds, simply $+$, i. e., lengthened, or $\div$, i. e., shortened, are used. Normal perception by the patient in the latter case is indicated by $=$. The normal perception time of the tuning fork must be added in such cases where only the difference in time is measured. Instead of a^1, another tuning fork, for example, c^2, can be used.

a^1A means the perception time of tuning fork a^1 (435 v. d), held directiy in front of the meatal opening (A $=$ aer, air conduction). Otherwise the symbols are the same as in the bone conduction). c^4A means the perception time of tuning fork c^4 (2048 v. d.), held directly in front of the meatal opening.

R means *Rinne's* test, and measures the difference in time between air conduction and bone conduction, or between bone conduction and air conduction, and the number of seconds are added, accompanied by a $+$ if the air conduction is greater, and by a $\div$ if the bone conduction. If the perception time for air and bone conduction is the same, an $=$ is placed. In superficial examinations, the simple $+$ or $\div$ may be used without addition of the number of seconds. If the fork is heard only by air conduction, this is shown by a $+t$; if it is heard only by bone conduction a $\div$; while the difference is shown by $t \div$, t meaning air conduction and v bone conduction. If in the Rinne's test the difference time is estimated, the normal difference time for the fork must be given in parenthesis. Tuning fork a^1 (435 v. d.) is used.

H means *Horologium*, watch. The normal distance for meters is shown in parenthesis, the hearing for the right and left ear of the patient above and below. In case the watch is heard only in contact with the auricle a. c. $=$ ad concham is written.

P means the *acumeter* of *Politzer*. The hearing distance is written in meters similar to the watch.

V means *Vox* (voice), and indicates the ordinary conversation tone; v means *whisper*. The hearing distance is given in meters and the word used in testing is added in parenthesis. If all the words used in testing are heard in the greatest distance at the physician's command, so that it could be supposed that at least some words might be heard at a greater distance, a > is added. If the voice is understood only very close to the ear, 0.01, i. e., 1 cm., is written. If the test is made with equiintensor and isozonal words, according to Quix, the values for the different groups are joined by brackets, with the value for the deepest group first.

LI, *Limes inferior*, means the lower limit. When possible, it is always estimated by the series of tuning forks of Bezold, and the lowest tone heard is put down with its musical name or the number of vibrations of the corresponding pitch. If the examiner has not such a series, but must use a series of C forks of the different octavos, a < is added to the symbol of the deepest fork still heard, to show that in this case possibly a still deeper tone could be heard. It must be noted what series was used.

LS means *Limes superior*, upper border. If this is estimated with Edelmann-Galton's whistle, the vibrations of the corresponding pitch are given. Otherwise, the pitch and the corresponding source of the pitch, Schulze's monochord, König's rods, etc., must be added in the text accompanying the test. The highest tone heard must always be given as the limiting value.

Under certain circumstances, certain examinations can be omitted, such as the watch and Politzer's acumeter; furthermore, Schwabach and Rinne may be omitted if bone or air conduction alone are tested, as, on the other hand, bone and air conduction may be omitted when Schwabach and Rinne are under investigation. In case any tuning fork is used, except the one designated, it must be described exactly. If other tuning forks are used than those indicated in the formula, the symbols of these, as well as their time of perception, may be used after the chief formula. Gelle's test, etc., must be added with their complete designation. If the quantitative test is made, it, as well as its graphic representation, must be exactly

explained. The pitch of the tuning forks and other sources
of sound are designated in the following way:

The notes are c, d, e, f, g, a, h. The intervening notes are
designated in the manner usually employed in the German
musical notation, by addition of s or es to the symbol of the
note to indicate a lowering of a half tone (e. g., des, es, as),
and the raising of a half tone by addition of is (e. g., fis, gis,
ais). The octave is shown in the following manner: C_2, C_1,
C, c, c^1, c^2, c^3, c^4, c^5, a C indicating 16, 32, 64, 128, etc., vibrations. The vibrations of the tuning fork are always given in
double vibrations (v. d.). As an example a couple of imaginary tests will be given.

$$\frac{AD}{\frac{W}{AS}} = \frac{\div 5}{\underset{=}{a^1 M}(20)} \quad \frac{0}{a^1 A}(60) \quad \frac{\div 20}{c^4 A}(30) \quad \frac{5.0}{V(28)} \quad \frac{0.60}{v(28)} \quad \frac{C}{LI} \quad \frac{15000}{LS}$$
$$\frac{}{\div 20} \qquad \frac{}{\div 10} \quad \frac{}{15.0} \quad \frac{}{3.0} \quad \frac{}{A_1} \quad \frac{}{40000}$$

This reads: Tuning fork on the skull not lateralized. Right
ear: bone conduction shortened, air conduction for a^1 gone,
for c^4 shortened. Aural acuity for conversation and whisper,
test word 28, considerably diminished, lower limit decidedly
raised, upper limit somewhat contracted. Left ear: bone
conduction shortened, aural acuity for conversation and whisper somewhat lessened, lower limit somewhat raised, upper
limit normal. Diagnosis: combined middle ear and labyrinth
on the right side, simple middle ear trouble on the left side.

$$\frac{AD}{\frac{Wo}{AS}} \quad \frac{\div}{a^1 A(20)} \quad \frac{\div}{c^4 A(30)} \quad \frac{+2}{R(35)} \quad \frac{0}{H(30)} \quad \frac{0.1}{P(15.0)}$$
$$\frac{}{\div} \qquad \frac{}{\div} \qquad \frac{}{+20} \quad \frac{}{a.c.} \quad \frac{}{0.5}$$

$$\frac{1.5-1.0-1.0}{V} \qquad \frac{0}{v} \qquad \frac{16}{LI} \quad \frac{15000}{LS}$$
$$\frac{}{2.0-1.5-1.0} \quad \frac{}{0.4-0.1-0.01} \quad \frac{}{16} \quad \frac{}{9000}$$

This reads: Tuning fork on the skull not heard. Air conduction on both sides shortened, Rinne positive, the tuning
fork not heard from the right mastoid process, watch on the
right side not heard at all, on the left side only in contact.
Politzer's acumeter heard on the right side 10 cm. away, left

side 50 cm. away. Conversation tested according to Quix with three groups of words, heard only very close, those of high tone, which normally are heard much further than those of deep tone. Whisper not heard at all on the right side, on the left side only very close, high tones heard only when spoken directly into the ear. Lower limit normal (16 v. d. $= C_2$); upper limit decidedly low. Diagnosis bilateral labyrinth affection.

This resolution of the committee was accepted by the representative of Denmark (Möller), Germany (Panse), Holland (Quix), Italy (Gradenigo), Austria (Politzer), Switzerland (Siebenman). The commission requests that every reader of this exert himself among his colleagues to the end that the above rules be used in every test for hearing.

LXII

A PLASTIC MASTOID OPERATION—A NEW OPERATION FOR ACUTE MASTOIDITIS.*

By Frank T. Hopkins, M. D.,

New York.

Although the technic for the mastoid operation for acute mastoiditis is generally well understood and satisfactorily done, we have, as yet, accomplished little in shortening the length of time required for the after-treatment, which remains still a labor of many weeks' duration. In recent years, however, two methods have been proposed with this end in view: (1) the blood-clot method, [1] [2] [3] and (2) the so-called modified blood-clot method. In the blood-clot method the posterior wound (the skin incision) is closed absolutely, and the bone cavity is supposed to fill up with a blood clot which shall later become organized. In the modified method there is no blood clot at all. The wound is sutured throughout, with the exception of a small opening at its most dependent portion, through which the drainage of the cavity is secured. The granulations are left to take care of themslves, and the drain is removed when the granulations have sufficiently filled the cavity to make the introduction of the drain difficult.

While in some cases both of these methods have given brilliant results, yet in other cases very serious accidents have followed—due to the loose piling up of granulations and the burrowing of pus through easily formed fistulous tracts. The surgeon has no control over the granulating process, and no knowledge of the burrowing of pus, until some abscess, more or less deeply placed, produces unfortunate results.

In this connection we may mention Plummer's[4] method which, with the modified blood clot as a basis, endeavors to fill up the greater part of the bony cavity by bodily pushing back

*Read before the Section on Otology, New York Academy of Medicine, January 8, 1909.

the posterior wall of the membranous canal, having lowered the bony wall to do this, and holding this membranous wall in approximation to the bony surface by firmly packing the canal. The posterior wound is then partially sutured and drained. Here the same objection obtains as in the former method—that of an uncontrolled granulating process in a closed cavity.

In 1877 Wolf[5] suggested making an opening for drainage through the posterior canal wall, after removing the bony wall to do this, and then closing the initial incision throughout except at its lower angle, which was to be left open, thus affording opportunity for thorough irrigation of the bone cavity. I do not know whether the later methods are based on Wolf's suggestion or not, but his method did not, at that time, meet with much favor; and for acute mastoiditis no essential change in after-treatment was made until the blood-clot method was proposed.

The method which I am about to describe, and which I have called a plastic mastoid operation, consists, in a word, of: first, making a meatal opening through the concha and posterior canal wall; secondly, the complete closure of the posterior, or initial, incision; and finally, the cicatrization of the excavated mastoid surface; in other words, the application to acute cases of the plastic methods now used only in radical operations. In the details of the operation my method follows along the lines of the Heath operation for chronic purulent otitis media, which Heath[6] proposed in 1906, and which, with more elaborate technic, was described by Ballenger[7] in 1908, but which has not been used by either of these surgeons for cases of acute mastoiditis. My method is simple and free from danger, and the time required for postoperative treatment is much shorter than by the present method of filling the bone cavity with granulations.

In the method I propose the usual mastoid operation is done, and with the same care and attention to detail. When in all other respects the mastoid operation is complete, the outer portion of the posterior bony wall of the cavity is cut away about the level of the floor of the canal, so that it shall offer no hindrance to free drainage. This removal extends as far inwards as the outer wall of the antrum, but the outer wall of the antrum, unless necrotic, should be left intact. An opening is then made in the concha and posterior fibrocartilaginous

wall of the meatus, exactly as is done in the radical operation;
but in doing this the precaution must be observed that no traction be made on the membranous canal which shall disturb the
position of the membrana tympani.   The style of the incision—
the shape of the meatal flap, is unimportant; either a Ballance
incision, curved and tongue-shaped, or a Panse incision, T-
shaped, and giving two quadrilateral flaps, may be chosen; the
object being to furnish a window of sufficient size to give drainage and make the excavated mastoid surface accessible through
the meatus.   The cartilage included in the flaps must be
dissected out, the flaps turned back to line the mastoid cavity,
—the raw surface against the raw posterior surface of this
canal wall,—and should be secured in this position by cat-gut
sutures.   These sutures must be passed through the periosteum
or through an aponeurosis of muscle, but not through muscle
tissue, or they will be apt to pull out and permit the flap to
sag, which will eventually leave the opening inconveniently
small.   When the flaps have been secured the cavity is packed
with a strip of iodoform gauze, and the end of the gauze
brought out through the meatus.   The posterior wound is
sutured throughout with silk-worm gut, and the usual dressings applied.   At the end of five days the dressings are removed, the stitches of the initial incision are taken out, and this
wound should be found healed throughout by first intention.
The packing is carefully removed through the meatal opening,
and the cavity, after cleansing by irrigation and by swabbing,
is again somewhat lightly packed.   For a day or two longer a
light protective dressing may be applied behind the ear.

The subsequent treatment consists of applications through
the meatus, which should be made daily.   If granulations are
exuberant, the curette or silver bead.   When cicatrization has
begun there should be no packing, and usually swabbing is
better than syringing.   Most important is the careful attention

In considering this mastoid excavation and the healing of it,
we must disabuse our minds of any idea of a cavity to be filled
up with granulations.   This is not the case.   Rather, it is a
surface which, having granulated, is to be covered with cicatricial tissue, and so must be treated as the similar surface of
the radical operation, though it may be a little more extensive
in its area, since it dips downward into the region previously
occupied by the mastoid tip.

to exuberant granulations, especially in the posteroinferior angle, where they often escape notice and become very troublesome. Cicatrization will soon be found spreading up over the antrum and along the vault of the cavity. The whole surface may be expected to be dry in five or six weeks.

To lessen even this short period of the time required for healing we may have recourse to skin grafting. At the end of two weeks a firm and satisfactory granulating surface will give opportunity for a graft to take. This may be applied through the meatus and, if successful, will materially shorten the time of cicatrization; or the posterior wound may be reopened and a Thiersch graft inserted, and the wound sutured again, as in secondary grafting in radical cases.

In case the skin is inflamed at the time of the primary operation the suturing may be postponed a few days, in the mean-. time packing the wound. The same method holds good if it has been necessary to open the sinus.

The advantages which I claim for this method are its simplicity, its ease of handling, its better appearance, its rapid healing with perfect safety and the better hearing which results. Although the operation itself is more troublesome and requires a little longer time than the usual operation, the after-treatment is easier and more quickly done each day and less painful to the patient. Again, it avoids the disfigurement of a wide scar behind the ear, or the equally unpleasant postaural depression occasionally seen. Third, my method gives more rapid healing. It is rare that an ordinary mastoid wound is fully healed under eight weeks, while here we may obtain healing in from five to six weeks. And aside from the great advantage of the more rapid healing of the whole wound, is the great importance of the prompt healing of the postaural incision, for with this method the bandage may be entirely discarded in ten days. In general, also, by this method the hearing is better than by our present method of operation, because the canal is not narrowed, as is now often the case, by a partial prolapse of the posterior wall, but, on the contrary, it is widened, leaving a free canal.

As I have thus far done this operation in only five cases my paper is offered as a preliminary report on a new operative procedure; but as these cases include very severe mastoid conditions, in which my results have been exceedingly satisfactory,

I have felt justified in offering for your consideration this description of the operation, and will give a brief resumé of my cases, and show you three patients:

CASE 1. (H. W.) The first case on which I did this operation was that of a simple mastoid with mixed infection in a man 24 years of age. There was in this case an exostosis of the posterior canal wall, which made it necessary to open the membranous canal. The dressing of this case was difficult on account of a congenital subluxation of the inferior maxilla which distorted the canal. The ear, however, was dry in nine weeks, while the posterior wound was completely healed under the first dressing.

CASE 2.—(M. H.) A man 31 years of age. The discharge had been present three weeks. The smear showed a streptococcus capsulatus infection. In operating it was necessary to expose the sinus over a large area. Under the first dressing the posterior wound healed throughout, with the exception of half an inch at the lower angle, which healed under the second dressing. The rest of the wound was dry in eight weeks.

CASE 3.—(N. L.) A woman 35 years of age with a four days' history of discharge, which showed a streptococcus infection. The operation exposed the sinus over a large area, including the knee. The zygomatic cells were also involved. The posterior wound healed under the first dressing. The wound was dry in a little less than eight weeks.

CASE 4.—(P. D.) A woman 47 years of age. The discharge had been present 19 days and showed a pneumococcus infection. The case was a very severe one. On admission there was a large subperiosteal abscess. The canal was so much narrowed by swelling that the membrana tympani could not be seen. The mastoid destruction was very extensive and involved also the zygomatic cells. There was, besides, a large epidural abscess in the middle fossa, and a perisinus abscess; and both of these exposures were covered with thick, velvety granulations. Here, on account of the superficial inflammation caused by the subperiosteal abscess, the incision behind the ear did not heal by first intention through its lower half, but was closed by a second suturing at the end of a week, and healed promptly. In this case, at the end of two weeks, I inserted a small skin graft through the meatal opening. Part of this graft took, and helped to make the cicatrization more rapid. The cavity healed in five weeks and two days.

CASE 5.—The last case is yet under treatment, and so I cannot give any definite report on it at this time.

All my cases have been operated on at the New York Eye and Ear Infirmary, and all were ward cases.

REFERENCES.

[1]Reik. Jour. A. M. A., March 31, 1906.
[2]Sprague. Laryngoscope, September, 1906.
[3]Bryant. Annals Rhinology and Laryngology, September, 1906.
[4]Plummer. Journal A. M. A., November 24, 1906.
[5]C. Wolf. Berlin. klin. Woch., 1877; xv. p. 205.
[6]Heath. Lancet, August 11, 1906.
[7]Ballenger. Journal A. M. A., September 26, 1908.

LXIII

A CASE OF PRIMARY CARCINOMA OF THE TRACHEA.

By T. P. Berens, M. D.,

New York.

At the meeting of this Association in 1906, Theisen read an exhaustive paper on the subject of Primary Carcinoma of the Trachea. After excluding all doubtful cases, both as regards diagnosis and location, he gathered 27 cases and reported one case from his own practice, making in all 28 cases. In 1908 Nager (*Archiv fuer Laryngologie und Rhinologie*), in a lengthy article quoted 8 cases, including one of his own. Of these 8 cases, one was Theisen's case, one was a case reported by Schroetter, Jr. (*Klinik der Bronchoskopie*, 1907), and the remaining six quoted by him had already been quoted by Theisen. The writer, after a somewhat arduous search through the literature, accepts Theisen's classification as correct, and has found to date but 30 cases of primary tracheal carcinoma,—to which number he would add the following report of a case from his own practice:

The patient, a man 55 years old, was seen in consultation with Dr. J. M. Bleyer, who gave the following history: The patient had always been healthy; there was no specific history, but a brother had recently died from carcinoma of the stomach. The patient had consulted the doctor about nine months before, because of a persistent cough. The cough grew worse, and attacks of dyspnea had become a marked symptom, increasing in severity and frequency. A subglottic tumor had been seen by Dr. Bleyer. The patient was a large man, weighing 175 lbs., with a short, thick neck. Examination revealed both vocal cords reddened and slightly thickened. Beginning at the second ring of the trachea was a grayish-pink velvety appearing mass, which occupied all sides of the trachea, and diminished its lumen to about one-third of its natural size. The mass was higher and thicker on the right side, and apparently faded into what appeared to be thickened mucous membrane on the left side, where the third tracheal ring was visible. Dyspnea was marked; and he was placed in the Manhattan Eye, Ear and Throat Hospital, where, the day following, under general anesthesia, the following operation was performed: After, division of the soft parts and ligation of the isthmus of the thyroid gland, the trachea was incised from the larynx to the sternal notch. A successful effort was made not to wound the mucous membrane of the trachea until the rings had been divided. Adrenalin was then applied, and the mucous membrane incised without bleeding. The larynx was likewise split without hemorrhage. The larynx was found to be free, but beginning at the second ring the walls of the trachea were occupied by an infiltrating 'fungoid appearing growth that extended an inch below the sternal notch. The surface of this growth was velvety and of a grayish rose-pink color. Owing to its extension so deeply down the trachea, exsection of the latter was out of the question; so that an attempt was made to remove the mass by means of a sharp bone curette, and apparently the attempt was largely successful, for the result of the curettage left normal appearing tissue. The growth was not adherent to the rings and did not extend beyond the limits of the trachea. A large and long tracheotomy tube was inserted and the wound stitched. The silver tube was not sufficiently long and a large rubber drainage tube was inserted through it. Although the operation consumed less than an hour and the loss of blood was insignificant, the patient suffered considerably from shock. There was but silght fever, at no time more than 101 degrees; but the patient did badly and died of pulmonary edema and heart failure three weeks after the operation. Postmortem examination was not allowed. Examination by Dr. Jonathan Wright of the tissue removed showed it to be a columnar epithelioma.

ABSTRACTS FROM CURRENT OTOLOGIC, RHINO-LOGIC AND LARYNGOLOGIC LITERATURE.

I.—EAR.

A New Treatment for the Meniere's Symptom Complex.

HERZER (*Münch. med. Wochenschr.*, No. 20, May 18, 1909). In a typical case of Meniere's disease which had proved incurable by other methods of treatment, Herzer used with brilliant success the vibrations massage of the nasal mucous membrane.

Horn.

Three Lectures from the Domain of Ear Diseases.

SCHWARTZE, Halle (*Münch. med. Wochenschr.*, No. 21, May 25, 1909), again warns against the use of Bier's hyperemia in acute otitis. He considers it dangerous, only to be carried out in a hospital and where a suspicion of an intracranial complication is present, absolutely contraindicated. With the prompt alleviation of pain which always follows the use of the elastic bandage, goes hand in hand a destruction of the mastoid process and thrombus of the sinus, until finally we are suddenly confronted with a very dangerous condition.

The use of the pressure sound of Lucae in sclerotic conditions is fully discussed, and Schwartze warns against its use in all atrophic conditions of the drum, and wherever a hyperemia of the promontory can be seen. In·sclerosis he has seen no improvement from the use of phosphorus, after the method of Siebenmann. In early cases one may perhaps be justified in its use, in late cases never. The etiologic basis of otosclerosis is considered. Where a suspicion of hereditary syphilis is present, and the disease not more than six weeks old, an energetic mercury cure may lead to a permanent improvement. The cold water cure, sea-bathing and high altitudes are strictly contraindicated. The use of fibrolysin is yet a debatable question. In a series of 75 cases treated in his clinic, two were unquestionably improved. The use of the leech, in otitis media acuta, has been too much neglected, and he warmly recommends its more general application.

Horn.

The Quantitative Measurement of the Caloric Nystagmus in Acute Inflammation of the Middle Ear.

OSCAR BECK (*Beitrag. z. Anat. Phys., etc., des Ohres, Nasen. u. des Halses,* Bd. 11, 1908, p. 190), after a very careful study of three cases, says that the time of the appearance of a caloric nystgamus after the beginning of the injection of the water, in cases of acute inflammation of the middle ear, depends upon the degree of inflammation. That is, in individuals with normal labyrinths the time of the appearance of the nystagmus depends upon extralabyrinth conditions, such as the quality of the conduction of the heat due to the intensity of the inflammation in the middle ear. This dependency is sufficient to permit one to judge the degree of inflammation in the middle ear by the time of the appearance of the nystagmus. The time of the persistence of the caloric nystagmus, however, is entirely independent of the degree of middle ear inflammation.

Wood.

A Case of Entotic Tinnitus Objectively Perceptible.

H. HALASZ (*Monat. für Ohrenheilkunde sowie für Kehlkopf, Nasen, Rachenkrankheiten,* Vol. XLII. p. 408-411) says that there have been about 40 cases reported of ear noises which have been objectively perceivable. He reports a case of his own in a woman 35 years old, who for one year had had a blowing tinnitus in the left ear, which was so loud as even to disturb her sleep. This was accompanied by a finer, higher tone, which was very transitory. Anyone who was near her left ear could hear these sounds. No pathologic lesion could be found in the nasopharynx, or middle ear. The superficial temporal artery, however, could be easily felt with the finger, and pressure on this artery caused cessation of the tinnitus. The tinnitus could be heard with a stethoscope placed over the artery. Halasz proposed to tie the artery. but the patient refused to have the operation done. *Wood.*

A Case of Cerebellar Abscess.

SACK (*Monatssch. f. Ohrenh.. etc.,* Heft 7. 1908, p. 360) reports a case of cerebellar abscess of otitic origin which was due to an infection of spirillum and Vincent's bacillus. The patient, a girl 5 years old, came into the dispensary with severe general symptoms and a left-sided facial paralysis. She had had otorrhea for two years. Her symptoms were marked drowsiness, pain in the left ear, no headache, temperature normal, pulse 115, no rigidity of the neck muscles, horizontal nystagmus, more marked to the left, uncertain atactic gait and a tendeney to fall toward the left. A radical operation was done and a sequestrum of a part of the labyrinth, including one and a half turns of the cochlea, was removed. The dura was exposed in the middle cerebral fossa, but was found normal. After the operation the pulse fell from 115 to 62, and the nystagmus became more marked towards the right. A second operation was refused, and the patient died on the fourth day after the operation. At the postmortem the cerebrum and dura were found to be normal. The left half of the cerebellum was enlarged, and while normal on the outside contained two abscesses each about the size of a cherry in which were found a spirillum and Vincent's bacillus.   *Wood.*

The Treatment of Otosclerosis With the Faradic Current.

Zitowitsch (*Monatssch. f. Ohrenh., etc.,* Vol. XLII, 1908, p. 597-627) reports 20 cases of otosclerosis which he treated by faradization, with more or less success. With one or two exceptions all the cases showed increase in the hearing and decrease in the tinnitus, though the extent of the improvement varied considerable in the different patients. Zitowitsch says that the lack of resiliency of the drum membrane in these cases is due to the inactivity of the tensor tympani muscle, which is in turn accompanied by a lack of activity of the stapedius muscle. This absence of muscular action within the tympanic cavity causes a decreased movement of the ossicles and gives rise to a lymph stagnation and vascular congestion in the region of the round window and promontory. Politzeration and pneumatic massage are harmful because they tend to increase the congestion and do not bring about active movement of the tensor tympani. In the application of the faradic current one electrode should be introduced into the mouth of the Eustachian tube and pressed against the upper wall, while the second electrode is placed in the interval between the angle of the jaw and the mastoid process. The intensity of the current depends on the individual and should be about as strong as the patient can bear. The treatment should last three or five minutes and not repeated oftener than three times a week.

Wood.

Concerning Venous Evacuation in Otitic Thrombosis of the Lateral Sinus and Pyemia.,

KARL THEIMER (*Monats. für Ohrenh., etc.,* Vol. XLII, 1908, p. 527), who has been working in Alexander's clinic, reports three cases of otitic pyemia, all of which completely recovered, which were treated by the ligation and resection of the internal jugular and the establishment of a jugular fistula after the method of Alexander. He says that the establishment of the fistula affords good drainage to the sinus and the jugular bulb. Ligation of the vein before the operation on the ear prevents the possibility of aspiration of air during the operation on the sinus, and also it makes it impossible for any thrombosis which may possibly be loosened during the operation to enter the general circulation. Just as soon as the diagnosis of otitic pyemia of sinus thrombosis can be made, the ligation of the jugular and its resection should be undertaken.   *Wood.*

A New Method for the Detection of Complete One-Sided Deafness.

PROF. D. O. VOSS (*Beitrage z. Anat. Phys. u. Ther. des Ohres, der Nasen u. des Halses,* Bd. 11, 1908, p. 145-152), after trying several methods found that in cases of one-sided deafness the good ear could be made, for the moment, completely deaf by blowing a continuous stream of air directly into the ear. This was most easily done by a compressed air outfit. While the air was being blown into the ear, the very loudest tones, noises and calling were absolutely imperceptible. The application of the test can best be done by producing a tone, especially selected for testing the degree of deafness, in close proximity to the deaf ear. Air is then blown into the good ear, and if the tone disappears to reappear on cessation of the air stream, it shows that the tone was perceived by the good ear and not the one being tested.   *Wood.*

Concerning Deafness Following Typhoid Fever.

PAUL MANASSE (*Arch. für Ohrenh.,* Vol. 79, 1909, p. 145) had for some time noticed that during epidemics of typhoid fever a number of cases showed clinical evidence of a labyrinthine or nerve deafness. The majority of these patients recovered easily, and only rarely did the condition persist. Recently, in one case in which the typhoid deafness persisted,

Manasse was able to obtain an autopsy and make a careful microscopic examination of the petrous bone. The condition found was a chronic fibrotic change of the internal ear cousequent upon an acute process, and followed by a secondary atrophy of the labyrinth. A similar case had been reported by Sporlader in 1900, in which there was fibrotic degeneration so that both the ganglion cells in the spiral ganglia and the finer nerve fibers in the cochlea were replaced by connective tissue fibers. Manasse, though acknowledging the material at hand is too small to make any positive conclusion, believes that the deafness of typhoid fever outside of otitis media may be due either to an inflammation of the internal ear or of the auditory nerve, and that in the majority of cases this inflammatory process completely heals, though occasionally under certain conditions it may become chronic and permanent deafness result. *Wood.*

Nasal and Nasopharyngeal Conditions as Causative Factors in Middle Ear Diseases.

GEO. A. LELAND (*Boston Medical and Surgical Journal,* September 30, 1909) advocates a more comprehensive inspection and a more thorough treatment of the nose and nasopharynx as a preventive of the pathologic conditions of the ear. With very few exceptions, the nose and nasopharynx are the initial offenders in ear diseases. A normal middle ear depends upon perfect ventilation, normal nasal respiration and a normally functionating Eustachian tube. The aurist should begin as a rhinologist. His treatment should be prophylactic rather than palliative. All nasal and nasopharyngeal obstructions should be corrected, particular attention being directed to the fossae of Rosenmüller and the regions of the Eustachian tubes.

With a perfectly ventilated middle ear, conditions ranging from permanent deafness to isolated symptoms, such as pain, fullness, tinnitus and vertigo, would for the most part have no inception. *Ryder.*

Mastoiditis Complicated by Purulent Leptomeningitis, Epidural Abscess, and Sinus Thrombosis.

ALFRED BRAUN (*Medical Record,* October 16, 1909) reports a case of complicated mastoiditis, unoperated, of considerable interest from the fact that an autopsy revealed a condition not at all in accord with the clinical picture. The classical symptoms of mastoid involvement, tenderness, and inflammatory signs in the membrana tympani, were absent. The drum was merely dull and thickened, possibly a little pinkish. Five weeks previous the patient had a painful, discharging right ear, with some deafness and tinnitus, which had lasted about six weeks. Slightly turbid cerebrospinal fluid following a lumbar puncture pointed to central involvement, but there was no rigidity of the neck, no Kernig's sign or Babinski's, no hyperesthesia, no anesthesia, and no pupillary changes.

The autopsy showed the mastoid process reduced to a mere shell, with pus in the middle ear, antrum, and mastoid cells. There was also a purulent leptomeningitis, with an extension of the purulent process from an epidural abscess to the pia through an apparently normal intact dura. *Ryder.*

Superficial Dermatitis of the External Auditory Canal.

CLARENCE J. BLAKE (*Boston Medical and Surgical Journal,* August 5, 1909). Its peculiar glandular structure, its function, and its relation to an important organ of sense make the skin lining the external auditory canal of more importance than it would otherwise be. Under normal conditions, by a well-defined movement of the epidermis of the drum head and the inner part of the canal wall outward, the effete epidermis is disposed of. An obstruction to this normal disposition results in an accumulation of detritus. In accordance with the differences in structure of the skin lining the canal, there are differing degrees of vulnerability and different symptoms of disturbance, but in all the primary mechanism is a dermal hyperemia with serous transudate and elevation of the thin epidermal layer which, under maceration disintegrates and, mixing with the serum, affords an outflow macroscopically simulative of pus.

Treatment.—Thorough cleansing by syringing with a weak solution of sodium bicarbonate, carefully drying, and repeating until the exfoliated epidermis has been removed. Paint the denuded surface with silver nitrate, 12 to 15 per cent strength, and touch any spot of ulceration or granulomata with stronger solution. *Ryder.*

Diagnosis of Otogenic Meningitis.

HOLGER MYGIND, Copenhagen (*Journal of the A. M. A.,* September 11, 1909). In contrast to the usual impression of middle ear retention in otogenic meningitis, Dr. Mygind has found, as a rule, no otoscopic signs of retention of pus, and in only one-half of the cases has he found any mastoid tenderness or infiltration. The nature of the suppuration, combined with the anatomic relations of the petrous portion of the temporal bone and the mastoid process, play the most important part in the pathogenesis of otogenic meningitis. In most cases of otitis media causing meningitis there is a very marked osteitis of the mastoid process. It may be produced through a suppuration of the labyrinth. Sigmoid sinusitis is not infrequently the medium. It is often combined with suppurative otitis intima and with sinus phlebitis. The diagnosis is difficult, as it is difficult to decide whether the meningitis is due to the otitis media present or the latter is a complication. It must be distinguished from any infectious disease or from pneumonia. It may simulate or be simulated by "meningeal irritation" or "meningismus." The one unfailing sign is turbidity of the cerebrospinal fluid. Two other points of diagnostic value are: the examination of the hearing and the static function of the labyrinth; total deafness speaking in favor of a labyrinthine suppuration with secondary meningitis. If the static part of the labyrinth is destroyed, there is no nystagmus when the ear is syringed with cold water. Destruction of the static portion of the ear points to meningitis produced by suppuration of the inner ear.   *Ryder.*

Adequate Drainage the Essential Step in the Successful Surgery of Brain Abscess.

FRED WHITING (*Medical Record,* January 23, 1909) thinks that the high mortality in brain abscess cases (accurately diagnosed and skillfully evacuated) depends to a great extent upon the failure of proper drainage. The findings at two autopsies, showing discolored and softened areas of brain substance around the cavity and drainage channel, he attributed to trauma, resulting from improper methods of establishing drainage. The introduction of the finger into the abscess cavity he considers a bad surgical procedure and has devised an instrument called an encephaloscope, which allows minute inspection of the abscess cavity and the opening thereto.

Points to be observed in drainage are as follows:

Complete evacuation. Careful and minute inspection of the entire cavity wall, thereby locating any pocket or channel of communication. For the drain itself iodoform gauze is the best. In acute cases, after complete evacuation, there is little danger of the cavity refilling. A single small wick to the bottom of the cavity is sufficient. This is changed at intervals of 48 hours. In chronic cases the treatment is entirely different. The cavity must remain open until the dense, firmly resisting, fibrinoplastic membrane sloughs away or undergoes absorption. Daily dressings, carefully wiping out the entire cavity and its walls, and then introducing enough gauze to balloon the cavity. This procedure is to be continued until the purulent discharge stops. Complete evacuation and thorough drainage, done under inspection and not palpation, are the salient points in the after-treatment.   *Ryder.*

The After-Treatment of the Radical Operation on the Middle Ear.

A. JANSEN (*Monat. für Ohrenheilkunde sowie für Kehlkopf, Nasen, Rachenkrankheiten*, Vol. XLII, p. 400-408). Jansen, on account of the disadvantages of continued packing of the wound after a radical operation, has of recent years done away with the packing after the first eight days, and simply applies a solution of nitrate of silver. He claims that the advantages of the nitrate of silver solution, when used in the proper strength, are that active stimulation produces a sufficient amount of granulation tissue; that the cicatrization is likewise stimulated; that the granulation tissue is protected by the white coagulum, and that the excretion from the wound is kept at a minimum. The use of nitrate of silver should be carried out only in cases of complete exenteration of the middle ear, in which some plastic operation has been done on the canal and the posterior wound closed. Jansen's technic is briefly as follows:—After the completion of the operation, the wound is dusted with iodoform powder, and iodoform gauze is carefully packed into the tympanic cavity and into the antrum. This dressing remains in situ for eight days if no contra-indications develop. The wound is then lightly packed, preferably with xeroform gauze. This second packing remains for two days and then the wound is left free. The whole wound surface is, after the removal of the packing, touched with a 5 per cent solution of nitrate of silver. A quarter of an hour later the wound is dried with cotton and again touched with the silver solution. In half an hour the wound is again dried, and a simple protective dressing applied. Six hours later the wound is again dried and painted, and still again on the next day, but after this last dressing the wound is left free, and the patient is instructed to re-apply the dressing only. if any secretion appears at the end of the canal. In children it is better to leave the dressing on a few days longer. The wound is repainted with the solution every second day four to five times. After this, if there is excessive granulation tissue, this is gently touched with a 10 per cent solution. In the last six cases treated after this manner, in all of which there was complete healing, the length of time averaged four weeks.

Wood.

The Common and Uncommon Localization of Otitic Brain Abscess, as Illustrated by Two Cases, With Recovery.

B. Sachs and A. A. Berg (*New York Medical Record*, January 23, 1909). Abscess following otitic and mastoid diseases is usually situated in the temporosphenoidal lobe or in the cerebellum, being far less common in other parts of the brain. When situated in the temporosphenoidal lobe, in addition to the usual symptoms of headache, somnolence, nausea, vomiting, and optic neuritis, there will be slight hemiparesis and symptoms of speech disturbance, sensory aphasia from left temporosphenoidal involvement, and dysarthria from right. If in the cerebellum, there will be, in addition to the general symptoms, cerebellar ataxia, diminution or increase of the deep reflexes, abducens paresis, or palsy, acoustic nerve symptoms, and possible cerebellar seizures. If in other parts of the brain, symptoms due to involvement of that special part, provided it is not a silent part, will be present in addition to the general symptoms already referred to. When situated in the motor region. doubt may arise as to the site on account of the relatively slight intensity of the localizing symptoms. There may be paresis instead of paralysis, and the deep reflexes may be less exaggerated than we are accustomed to find in neoplasms of the motor area.

Two cases are reported, successfully localized and operated;

one in the temporosphenoidal lobe and the other in the motor area. The point of interest in the second case is limited largely to the question of localization.

In the surgical treatment of brain abscess there are three important considerations: First, wide exposure of the area where the disease is supposed to lie; second, protection of the meninges; third, proper drainage of the abscess cavity.

Diagnosed promptly and localized correctly, otitic brain abscess has proved the most promising of all brain lesions calling for operative interference.   *Ryder.*

The Conservation of Hearing in the Radical Mastoid Operation.

SEYMOUR OPPENHEIMER, New York (*Medical Record,* January 9, 1909). In the radical operation for the cure of chronic suppurative otitis media, it should be the aim, so far as is consistent with the safety of the patient, to restore the auditory organ to as nearly perfect condition as possible, and with due consideration of its function. To this end as much as possible should be saved, provided, of course, that no alterations have taken place in the labyrinth. The continuity of the ossicular chain must be carefully taken into consideration, and if the hearing tests previous to operation show that the ossicles are of some value in the conduction of sound, much will be gained by their retention. Even though superficial necrosis be present in part, it is unnecessary in all cases to remove the tympanic membrane in its entirety, as its retention after drainage has been provided for, will materially aid in retaining the auditory acuity. Probing should be very carefully done, and while all granulation tissue in the antrum, aditus and mastoid cells should be thoroughly removed, that in the tympanum itself should be dealt with very carefully and allowed to remain, unless there is extensive tissue destruction.

The main focus in nearly every case of chronic aural suppuration is the antrum, and this is the primary objective point in all operative procedures. The diseased tissue being removed from this area, the drainage areas lying below these parts will heal when the source of irritation has been removed.

While in some cases it is absolutely necessary to remove all the contents of the tympanum, irrespective of the effect upon the hearing, in many others it will be found that with care sufficient drainage can be obtained, the tympanic contents preserved, and an improvement in hearing acuity follow operation.   *Richards.*

The Treatment of Acute Catarrhal Conditions of the Middle Ear.

WALB (*Deutsche medicinische Wochenschrift,* November 19, 1908) gives the treatment under three headings—acute middle ear catarrh, acute inflammation of the middle ear and acute suppurative middle ear trouble.

Acute Catarrh.—The upper portion of the tympanic membrane is reddened, but there is no swelling. The position of the hammer and the short process can be clearly determined. The patient complains of slight darting pains in the ear, with some deafness. The general condition is not disturbed and, as a rule, there is no fever. Acute catarrhal conditions of the nose and nasopharynx are the most important factors etiologically, the middle ear trouble being the result of a direct extension of the inflammatory process through the Eustachian tube.

This form of middle ear trouble often gets well without treatment of any kind, although this is not always the case. People who are subject to recurring attacks of this kind develop a gradually increasing deafness, with the attending changes in the middle ear. The author believes that inflation of the middle ear by the Politzer method is the best method of treatment for these cases. This has the effect of restoring the ventilation of the middle ear and removing secretions from the Eustachian tube. Wrong methods of treatment are syringing the ear and dropping solutions into the external canal. The application of cold or heat is usually unnecessary. Laxatives and the withdrawal of tobacco and alcoholic stimulants are recommended during the attack.

In considering acute otitis media, the author states that in this form the inflammatory symptoms predominate. It follows an infection, in which the pneumococcus and the streptococcus mucosus are the organisms usually found. The treatment for the first stage should be mainly antiphlogistic. The ice bag and the application of leeches in front of and behind the ear are of the greatest service.

Competent aurists may accomplish the withdraw of blood by superficial incisions in the congested parts of the drum membrane and superior wall of the canal. This antiphlogistic method of treatment should be continued until the active inflammatory process has subsided. During this time inflations of the middle ear are strictly contraindicated, because they favor the development of complications. After the acute inflammatory process has subsided, inflations with the Politzer bag may be carefully used. When a severe desquamative myringitis develops with a throwing off of masses of epithelial scales, irrigations may have to be used, although here, as in the first variety, the author does not favor irrigations. When there is danger of perforation, paracentesis is indicated.

Later on, inflations should be continued until the hearing becomes normal. If improvement has not resulted in eight or ten days and mastoid symptoms develop, a prompt paracentesis should be performed, and in many cases this will clear up the mastoid complication. In this form of middle ear trouble also, inflammatory conditions in the nose and nasopharynx play an important role, and this is particularly the case in children with adenoids and enlarged tonsils. In children who have recurring attacks of acute otitis media, a hyperplasia of the lymphatic ring should always be thought of and proper operative procedures promptly carried out.

In the third form, acute purulent otitis media, a perforation of the tympanic membrane is characteristic. The symptoms in young children, before perforation occurs, are often very alarming (delirium and unconsciousness being sometimes present), and if there is no discharge from the ear, the condition may be mistaken for meningitis. The treatment should be that of an acute infectious process. The patient should be kept in bed and a light diet given. The severe pain in the ear can be controlled only by narcotics, although the ice bag does, some good. The tympanic membrane should be incised just as soon as bulging can be determined. Spontaneous perforations, if not large enough for good drainage, should be enlarged, or if they have not occurred in a favorable place incisions in other parts of the membrane should be made. For securing good drainage from the middle ear the author recommends the use of an antiseptic bandage. The canal should be first carefully washed out to remove all accumulated secretion, a 1 per cent normal salt solution or a boracic acid solution being used for this purpose. A strip of gauze is then inserted in the canal, being carried to the drum membrane, sterile gauze placed against the ear, and a gauze bandage carried around the head. The dressings should be changed as often as necessary, depending upon the amount of discharge.

If this method is effective and the secretions are not retained in the ear, further irrigations are not necessary.

In concluding his consideration of the treatment, the author condemns the use of the Bier treatment in cases of suppurative otitis media. In 20 cases in which this treatment was used unfavorable results were obtained, and a much larger percenatge of the cases had to have the mastoid operation. The cases seemed to improve at first, but then there would be a sudden onset of dangerous symptoms which necessitated a prompt mastoid operation. Attention has previously been called to the fact that the Bier stasis masks one of the most important and serious complications of a suppurative middle ear trouble, a brain abscess. It was found that the Bier treatment relieved the severe and constant localized pain, which is often the only indication of a brain abscess, concealing this important symptom in some cases until it was too late to operate. The Bier method is absolutely contraindicated in cases of suppurative otitis media in which mastoid complications are present.   *Theisen.*

II.—NOSE.

Empyema of the Middle Turbinate.

ANDREGA (*Deutsch. med. Wochenschr.*, No. 8, 1909, p. 372). By removal of the middle turbinate it was found that the bone was entirely destroyed and nothing remained but a pus sack, lined with swollen mucous membrane.   *Horn.*

The Avery Nasal Septatome.

JOHN W. AVERY, New York (*Medical Record*, February 6, 1909). The instrument is intended to take the place of the small knife usually used for the septal incision. It has a blade adjustable to cut a depth varying from 1/32 to 6/32 of an inch. This blade prevents too deep a cut and so lessens the danger of perforation. An indicator on the handle registers the length of the exposed portion of the blade, and hence the depth of the incision.   *Richards.*

On the Treatment of Chronic Suppurative Nasal Conditions by the Use of Lactic Acid Bacteria.

J. L. GOODALE, Boston (*Boston Med. and Surg. Jour.*, July 15, 1909). A series of cases of atrophic rhinitis with ozena and chronic suppuration of the various sinuses were treated with the bacillus bulgariens, as prepared by the Lederle Laboratories, with the result that a distinct effect was produced by the culture in some cases of ozena characterized by generalized crust formation. In localized chronic suppurative sinusitis, attended by hypertrophy and polyp formation, no effect could be detected.   *Richards.*

The Treatment of Nasal Diseases by Means of Negative Pressure.

WALB (*Deutsch. med. Wochenschr.*, No. 1, 1909, p. 22) reviews the uses of negative pressure in the diagnosis and treatment of diseases of accessory cavities and repeats the conclusions already arrived at in the more extensive work of himself and Horn, viz.:

1. Negative pressure enables us to make a better diagnosis than was formerly possible.

2. Negative pressure is a means of treatment, in the acute cases in an absolute sense; in chronic cases, in a relative sense, as we are enabled to at once relieve distressing symptoms, and where the secretory symptoms form the principal complaint, to bring about a cure. When an extensive pathologic alteration of the mucous membrane of the cavities is present a cure is not to be expected.

3. A careful control of the degree of pressure used by means of the quicksilver manometer is of great importance.

4. A constant pressure is only possible with a metal pump. Rubber balls are not to be depended on.

5. The pressure in acute cases should not exceed 8-10 cm. of mercury; in chronic cases, from 12-17 cm.

6. Too much pressure brings about a hemorrhage.

7. In the after-treatment of all operations on these cavities the method has proved of enormous value.   *Horn.*

A Method of Approach to the Upper Respiratory Tract.

LUDWIG LOWE (*Monatschr. f. Ohrenh.*, etc., Vol. XLII, 1908, p. 516) suggests the following procedure for exposing the interior of the nose and sinuses to operative attack. After tamponing of the nasal fossa with packing soaked in 1-4000 adrenalin and injecting the same into the outer surface of the gum, he makes an incision starting at the base of the gum opposite the last molar and carries it forward to the frenum of the lip. The periosteum covering the anterior surface of the maxillary bone is elevated, and the nasal mucous membrane is incised along the edge of the pyriform aperture from the mouth wound. The mucous membrane is now elevated from the lateral wall of the nasal fossa, and then the bony edge of the aperture removed outward to where the thin clear bone of the canine fossa commences, and inward along the outer wall of the nasal fossa until the anterior end of the inferior turbinal is included. The rest of the inner wall of the antrum is now taken away, including the mucous membrane on both the antral and nasal sides, and also the whole of the inferior turbinal. An open path is thus made to the interior of the nose, from which the antral, ethmoidal and sphenoidal sinuses can be easily reached as well as any neoplasm occupying the nasal fossa. *Wood.*

Empyema of the Antrum of Highmore: Its Relation to Other Diseases, and Its Treatment.

WOLFF FREUDENTHAL (*Medical Record*, October 23, 1909). Numerous cases are cited to show how certain conditions may be aggravated by and oftentimes caused by antral sinusitis. Aprosexia nasalis, affections of the stomach and intestines, epilepsy, and eye diseases are often so closely related to antral involvement that great relief and many times permanent cure follows the proper antral treatment. Wertheim's findings, that almost one-third of patients who had died of tuberculosis had empyema of one or more of the accessory sinuses. he thinks is an underestimate.

Treatment.—In certain slight involvements the intranasal method (puncture through the nasal wall) is sufficient. The resection of the anterior part of the inferior turbinate and any considerable amount of the nasoantral wall leaves the sensitive mucosa of the antrum exposed to the varying conditions of temperature, dust. etc., and consequent unpleasant reactions. If after a reasonable time the conditions do not improve; if there is much degeneration of the mucosa; if a bony septum is diagnosed or suspected. a radical operation through the canine fossa is the only satisfactory procedure. *Ryder.*

Acute Inflammation of the Accessory Sinuses, Symptoms, Diagnosis and Treatment.

D. BRADEN KYLE (*Journal of A. M. A.*, September 25, 1909). Acute inflammations of the accessory cavities are usually secondary to acute inflammation of the nasal mucous membranes. Irregularities in the nasal cavities, narrow, poorly developed nostrils, spurs, deviations, and large turbinates, by interfering, first with normal nasal drainage, and then with the drainage and ventilation of the accessory cavities, are predisposing factors.

The symptoms, varied to a certain extent by the location of the sinus, are, for the most part, local, and as follows: Pain of a boring character, swelling, tenderness, bone soreness and a mucopurulent or purulent nasal discharge. Systemic infection is not, as a rule, marked. The sinus is a walled-in-cavity, and consequently there is not much absorption. Of considerable importance in regard to both local and systemic phenomena are the size and shape of the cavity and the variations in the thickness of its walls. Brain abscess may result from perforation of a wall of the frontal sinus. Again, if the superior wall of the antrum is thin, there will be marked eye symptoms, while in another case, with a thick, bony wall, the eye will not be affected.

Diagnosis is made from the clinical history, physical examination, and the X-ray. Transillumination is not reliable. The use of the X-ray cannot be overestimated. It shows the extent of the involvement, the relation to the structures and the formation of the cavity.

The treatment, in a great majority of cases, should be conservative, directed toward the re-establishing of the normal drainage. A careful and persistent shrinking of the tissues at the orifice of the cavity in conjunction with measures directed toward the nasal mucous membrane will usually be sufficient. Such palliative measures will not always be successful, but a great many cases now operated upon would respond to such treatment.   *Ryder.*

Two Cases of Septicemia Following Submucous Resection of the Septum; One Death, One Recovery.

HAROLD HAYS, New York (*American Journal of Surgery*, November, 1909), reports two cases of septicemia following

· submucous resection; one death and one recovery. The histories of the two cases were similar, as were the physical appearances of the patients. Both operations were simple, consuming each less than one-half hour.

Case number one complained of a frontal headache at the time of removal of the packing, two days after the operation. There was moderate bleeding and considerable edema of the mucoperichondrial flaps and a frothy, bloody, serous discharge. A thorough examination between the two layers of septal mucous membrane failed to reveal pus, although the probe went well up to the cribriform plate. Five days after operation the patient was sent to the hospital. Complaints: Violent headache, high fever, and marked exophthalmos, blood count 15,000. One dram of slightly turbid fluid, under pressure, was removed by lumbar puncture. The patient grew gradually worse, dying eight days after operation.

The history of the second case was the same, except that there was no exophthalmos. A careful examination of the nasal chambers under chloroform was made and pus located well up above the middle turbinates. Following its evacuation recovery immediately took place.

Both had symptoms of septicemia, the first probably complicated by cavernous sinus thrombosis and possibly meningitis. Dr. Hays has no doubt that the second case would also have ended fatally had the pus focus not been located. In studying the lymphatic and blood supply of the upper portion of the septum, he finds intercommunicating branches between the arteries and veins of the septum and the arteries and veins communicating with the sinus; hence the possible infection.

Ryder.

The Operative Treatment of Deflection of the Nasal Septum.

CHARLES W. RICHARDSON, Washington (*American Journal of the Medical Sciences*, February, 1909). Gummi of the septum must be ruled out before any operation is done. General anesthesia is preferred, since although cocain answers fairly well for the first half or two-thirds of the operation, if the operation is at all prolonged. the most trying part comes at the end, and many patients suffer quite a little pain and shock, and sometimes become so demoralized as to render the completion of ·the operation extremely difficult. There   is more bleeding under general anesthesia, but, on the whole, the author finds this method more satisfactory than local anesthesia.

He does the submucous resection, protecting the two flaps with the Killian or some type of nasal speculum, which prevents injury to the flaps. He does not think there is ever a reproduction of cartilage or bone in the area from which it is taken. The flaccid septum becomes tense and later gives a certain firmness of sensation. He has not seen any sinking in of the dorsum of the nose. When sufficient bony structure is left above and a fair bridge of cartilage anterior to the seat of the operation, sinking in does not take place.

He has had three per cent of perforations, these often developing from pin-point incisions made into the opposite mucoperichondrium at the point opposite the primary incision. If this occurs, a new incision should be made a millimeter or so farther back, and the perichondrium separated from the septum at that point rather than at the point of primary incision. Perforations are not usually attended by crust formation and give no annoyance to patients, who are not conscious of their existence unless informed of it. The raising of the mucoperichondrium is the crucial point of the operation, requiring great patience and plenty of time. It is best to commence at the upper end of the incision.

The older methods of operating required a shorter time and the wearing of a splint. There was considerable pain and discomfort, with confinement to bed for several days, with the patient uncomfortable and feverish until the splint was removed. In the submucous method there is no postoperative pain, and the patient is practically well at the end of 48 hours. The submucous method offers the greatest advantages in the hands of the operator thoroughly skilled in its technic, but in unskilled and inexperienced hands much more harm can be done by this method than by the methods formerly in use.

Richards.

Concerning an Approach to the Sphenoidal Sinus and the Neighboring Portion of the Basis Cerebri.

LUDWIG LOEWE (*Monats. für Ohrenh. und Laryngo-Rhinologie*, Vol. XLIII, Heft 3, 1909) goes over the whole question of methods of approach to the region of the hy-

pophysis. In 1904 he described the method of operating by
which he divided the nasal bones and turned them outwards,
fracturing through the lamina papyracea. He describes, further, the Chassaignac-Bruns procedure, consisting in reflecting the nose as a whole to one side. Seven cases are reported
as having been treated by the nasal method, one only dying as
a result of the operation. The usual method of gaining access to the nasopharynx for large surgical procedures are so
severe that the patients would generally stand very little more
operative work. His attention was called to the suprahyoid
pharyngotomy by Jeremitsch, who had noticed in the case of
a suicide that the wound gave a very good view of the nasopharynx and surrounding structures. The suprahyoid pharyngotomy is much superior to the subhyoid operation, because
the muscles of the tongue permit an easy closure of the wound
by means of serial sutures, and there is also a great deal less
danger of aspiratory pneumonia. Loewe's method of operating is briefly as follows:—Gauze strips are introduced into
each side of the nose and brought out at the mouth and their
ends firmly tied so as to act as a palate retractor, then with
the head hanging backward over the end of the operating
table, an incision is made about ten meters long just above
the hyoid bone, through the skin platysma and fascia. The
mylohyoid, geniohyoid and medial portion of the hyoglossus
are cut across sufficiently high above the hyoid bone to leave
stumps large enough for later suturing. Under guidance of
the finger in the mouth, the mucous membrane of the valle-
culae is cut by the knife placed through the suprahyoid wound.
The cut edges of the pharyngeal mucous membrane should be
immediately caught and sutures placed in them, as this makes
the subsequent closure of the wound much more easy. Hemorrhage is almost entirely absent and it is almost impossible
to cut the lingual arteries. A broad slip of gauze is now
placed in the wound and brought out of the mouth and both
ends tied firmly over the chin. This brings the tongue forward and opens a good view into the nasopharynx. For operating on the sphenoid from this suprahyoid pharyngotomy
the instruments must be much longer than ordinary, as the
distance from the wound to the roof of the nasopharynx is
about 12 centimeters. The shaft of the instruments ought
to be about 29 centimeters long, and on account of this length

considerably heavier than usual, to keep them from bending. The mucous membrane on the under surface of the sphenoid is split in the middle line down to the bone, and a sagittal incision made across the tops of the choanae. The periosteum is now shoved back on either side and the under surface of the sphenoid bone and the basal surface of the occipital bone laid bare back to the pharyngeal tubercle. The removal of the floor of the sphenoidal sinus should be begun immediately at the tops of the choanae, and after the cavities have once been entered they then can be enlarged backwards. In removing the lateral portions of the floor, great care must be exercised not to wound the upper and outer walls of the sinus because of the important structures in relation to it. Any cavities which may exist in the pterygoid processes are opened up in a posterior direction and the intersphenoidal septum removed. The roof of the sinus is now easy to attack, and the hypophysis and surrounding region of the basis cerebri easily uncovered. In after-treatment, Loewe prefers not to pack the cavity, as he believes that packing interferes with drainage. *Wood.*

The Radical Operation on the Antrum of Highmore From Within.

RETHI (*Wiener medicinische Wochenschrift,* No. 1, 1909) first described the method of opening the antrum of Highmore through the nose seven years ago.

The important point in this operation is to make a large opening into the antrum through the nasoantral wall. The lower turbinate and the lateral wall of the inferior and middle meatus are first thoroughly cocainized and adrenalin applied, and then the anterior two-thirds of the inferior turbinate removed.

An opening is then made with a chisel behind the anterior end of the turbinate and is enlarged with bone forceps up towards the middle meatus as well as in the inferior, so that a wide communication is made between the antrum of Highmore and the nose.

The diseased mucous membrane and any granulations are then scraped out.

The advantages of this method are as follows:—The operation is much simpler than the radical Caldwell-Lue operation through the canine fossa. It can be performed in a few minutes (four or five), after the cocain and adrenalin have been applied.

The author emphasizes the necessity for removing enough of the inferior turbinate; taking off simply the anterior third is not sufficient. He also states that it is important to have the opening into the antrum extend to the middle meatus, and not confine it to the inferior.   •

A small opening closes very rapidly and does not allow sufficient drainage.

Almost all authors give the preference to the Caldwell operation through the canine fossa if conservative methods have not been effective.   '

The operation through the nose is not followed by the severe pain that often goes with the Caldwell operation.

The criticisms that have been frequently made against the operation through the nose are that the antral cavity cannot be thoroughly inspected after the operation, and that it is hard to reach with the curettes, that is, every part of it. This the author states, is not a fact, if a large enough opening has been made. Small mirrors can be carried through the nasal opening into the antrum so that it can be inspected.

The author believes in doing the radical operation in the first place in cases of chronic maxillary sinusitis, rather than to try palliative measures, such as a small opening through the inferior meatus.

The operation through the canine fossa does not cure a larger percentage of the cases than the one through the nasal wall.

Chiari states that in some chronic cases treated in this way he did not obtain a cure in a single case, that is, the discharge did not entirely stop.   .

Out of fifty-eight cases operated on by the writer, by this method, forty-nine were cured. That is, the discharge of pus has entirely stopped. Nine cases were improved, but not cured.   *Theisen.*

III.—PHARYNX.

Dangers Associated with Removal of the Tonsils and Adenoid Growths.

F. C. ARD, Plainfield, N. J. (*Medical Record*, March 6, 1909), has made a careful study of the literature of recent years, and finds that the removal of the tonsils and adenoid growths has been accompanied by many accidents and not a few deaths. The various methods used to combat the accidents are given. The article should be studied in its entirety. In a case of the author's in which secondary hemorrhage of the tonsil had occurred five days after its removal, he used lactate of calcium with satisfaction. *Richards.*

Tonsil Removal, Opsonic Index, and Immunity.

BRYAN D. SHEEDY, New York (*Medical Record*, September 25, 1909). Normal tonsils are most active during the first two or three years of life, and are not absolutely necessary to the well-being of the individual after the period of childhood. They should not therefore be removed in young children unless they are so far diseased as to have their normal functions interfered with, in which case, instead of being a protection against the inroads of bacteria, they become the portals by which the enemies of health gain their admittance.

Richards.

The Significance of Certain Pathologic Conditions in the Fossae of Rosenmüller.

J. W. JERVEY, Greenville, S. C. (*Medical Record*, September 18, 1909), has found that the removal of the web-like bands oftentimes found attached to the posterior lip of the Eustachian tube is followed by improvement of hearing in many cases. These adhesions and granulations should always be sought for in cases of catarrhal deafness, and, when present, removed. "The index finger is passed through the mouth into the postnasal space and the fossae are firmly and completely swept, to their very bottoms, of all obstructing formations, first one side and then the other being attended to without withdrawing the finger. This is followed by the application of a solution of nitrate of silver or argyrol." *Richards.*

Clinical Manifestations of Adenoids in Adults.

OTIS ORENDORFF (*Journal of A. M. A.*, September 23, 1909) calls attention to the fact that the adenoid as a source of trouble is often overlooked in the adult. There is a history of adenoids in childhood, with obstruction. As the child matures, the fauces and nares enlarge and the symptoms of

obstruction disappear, although the adenoids may not atrophy.
The patient then complains of trouble of a different type.   Inspection in these cases shows the usual high arched palate
with the adenoid fringe, an enlargement of the lingual papillae
with nodules on the posterior pharyngeal wall—granular
pharyngitis. No other treatment than complete removal is
satisfactory.   ·   *Ryder.*

Spoon Enucleation of the Tonsil.

A. Morgan MacWhinnie, Seattle (*American Journal of
Surgery*, November, 1909), concludes that hemorrhage following tonsil operations is due, for the most part, to the fact that
some of the tonsil capsule is left, or it may occur if some fibers
of the superior constrictor muscle have been brought away. A
stubborn hemorrhage of the oozing variety occasionally met
with is probably due to the fact that the tonsil capsule is composed of fibrous tissue. He has devised a spoon instrument
with which he is able to remove the tonsil with capsule intact
and with no injury to the pillars or the superior constrictor
muscle.

His technic is as follows: The tonsil is grasped well into
the supratonsillar and intratonsillar fossae, so as to engage the
capsule as well as the tonsil. The spoon is then entered between the posterior pillar and the tonsillar capsule and made
to rapidly separate from below upward to the supratonsillar
fossa. The same process is carried out inferiorly and anteriorly.

The spoon fits so accurately over the tonsil that injury to
the pillars need not be considered, and the extreme traction
brings the tonsils so well forward into the pharynx that very
little separation is necessary. He finds no difficulty in removing tonsils under local anesthesia.   *Ryder.*

The Functional Relation of the Tonsil to the Teeth.

George H. Wright (*Boston Medical and Surgical Journal*)
calls attention to the fact that there are four periods in the
development of an individual, from two to eighteen years of
age, when the tonsil may become enlarged, without infection.
These periods correspond to the time of eruption of the four
groups of molar teeth, from two years, six years, twelve
years, and eighteen years. He claims that under prophylactic
treatment and care the tonsils will return to normal after the

eruption of the teeth. Following out the anatomy and histology of the teeth and their intimate relation to the lymphatic
system, he maintains that the tonsils are simply physiologically
enlarged from excessive functional activity, the equilibrium
of the glandular system being disturbed by the amount of
activity necessitated by the elaboration of the 48 teeth and
the jaws and the taking care of the accompanying waste. This
may be further disturbed by pathogenic organisms derived
from carious teeth, etc. Following the eruption of the teeth
and with the necessary care of the carious ones, the glandular
activity ceases and the tonsils return to normal. He records
150 cases followed out successfully (tonsils not removed) and
cites other cases of glandular enlargement (tonsils previously
removed) clearing up after eruption of the teeth. In the
treatment of the tonsil by the specialist he would include as a
routine the observation of carious teeth and a recognition of
the four periods of eruption coincident with slight enlargement.   *Ryder.*

The Local Treatment of Acute Inflammations of the Throat From the Standpoint of Pathology.

J. L. GOODALE (*Boston Medical and Surgical Journal,* No.
26, 1908). In selecting this subject the author states that he
was influenced by the analogy existing between staphylococcus infections of the throat and those of the skin. In both
conditions we find the same organisms generating toxin at the
point of inoculation, and giving rise to a localized inflammation. We are unable, the author states, to formulate fundamental points of distinction between the local phenomena excited by the staphylococcus, the streptococcus, the pneumococcus, the influenza and the diphtheria bacillus. The clinical differences depend upon the strength of the toxin generated. In his paper the author presents the results of examinations into the effects of local applications upon infectious
processes of the tonsils and pharynx. The investigations were
made with special reference to the effect of antiseptics upon
the course of the clinical phenomena. About 40 cases of acute
tonsillitis were treated by various antiseptic preparations.
Bacteriological examination was made only for the purpose
of excluding diphtheria, and it was therefore not possible in
most of them to specify whether the organism was a staphyl-

ococcus, streptococcus or pneumococcus. It was observed in a number of cases of acute reddening of the pharynx and tonsils that local applications of various remedies were followed by complete subsidence of the local inflammation. In a further series of cases that were seen early, these applications, particularly the silver salts, were followed by disappearance of the local acute inflammatory manifestations, and the patient appeared for a few hours or a day apparently well, after which time inflammation appeared in a neighboring region, and in several cases which were carefully studied it seemed that the total duration of the inflammation was more protracted than would have been the case if a simple acute tonsillitis had been allowed to take its natural course. When the local manifestations were more advanced and accompanied by general symptoms, as fever and prostration, no improvement was noticed from the employment of local antiseptics. In two cases of severe lacunar tonsillitis, the crypts were irrigated several times a day with permanganate of potash and hydrogen peroxide, with the object of sterilizing, if possible, the focus of infection. On each occasion the immediate effect was to produce pain and swelling in the cervical lymph nodes, which lasted for several hours and then subsided. The author summarizes the results as follows:

1. Acute tonsillitis in the early stage before the appearance of white spots or systemic depression, was apparently aborted in some cases by local antiseptics.

2. In some cases acute tonsillitis, when seen early, was apparently checked by local antiseptics, but inflammation appeared in neighboring organs and seemed to be of protracted duration.

3. The introduction of antiseptics into the crypts was followed by an increase of the local inflammatory process and in some cases by increased systemic absorption.

All the pathogenic bacteria present in the tonsils in acute inflammations of these organs cannot be completely destroyed except perhaps in the earliest stage.

Here there is reason for believing that if a given pathogenic microorganism has developed in the mouth and about the orifices of the tonsils, its activity may be checked by suitable antiseptic applications if the process has not gone too far. If, however, the multiplication of the organisms has extended beyond a certain point, so that tissue changes are involved, or the system exhibits evidence of toxic absorption, it is improbable that antiseptic applications could destroy completely the organisms present. *Theisen.*

IV.—LARYNX.

Concerning the Use of Bronchoscopy in Cases of Asthma.

GALEBSKY (*Monatssch. f. Ohrenh., etc.,* Heft 7, 1908, p. 359), by means of the bronchoscope, applied cocain and adrenalin directly to the bronchial mucous membranes in two cases of asthma. In the first place there was a distinct reddening of the mucosa in the left bronchus due to a localized bronchitis. In this patient the asthma was temporarily improved by the first cocain and adrenalin application, but a later application for a recurrence did not seem to have much effect. In the second case the cocain and adrenalin stopped almost immediately a very severe attack. and the patient was free from any interference with her breathing for a month and a half.

Wood.

The Technic of the Treatment of Larynx Tuberculosis with Sunlight.

KRAUS (*Münch. med. Wochenschr.,* No. 13. March 30. 1909) speaks of the favorable results obtained by the use of sunlight in this disease and describes a conveniently mounted mirror, by which the patient can reflect the sun rays into his mouth and against the larynx mirror. In patients without fever he recommends a daily treatment of 20 minutes.

Horn.

The Technic of the Treatment of Larynx Tuberculosis with Sunlight.

LISSAUER (*Münch. med. Wochenschr.,* No. 18. May 4. 1909) uses, instead of an ordinary larynx mirror, one with a concave surface. He can by this method so concentrate the rays that an active hyperemia can be brought about. and the patient experiences a sensation of warmth in the larynx. He considers the method as too dangerous to be put into the hands of the patient. but must be carried out by the physician.

Horn.

The Therapeutics of Larynx Tuberculosis with Special Attention to the Sunlight Treatment.

JANNSEN, Davos (*Deut. med. Wochenschr.*, No. 19, 1909) recommends the treatment and has favorable results. Uses plane mirror and warns against the concave form.   *Horn.*

The Further Report of a Case of Tracheal Scleroma.

EMIL MAYER, New York (*American Journal of the Medical Sciences*, February, 1909). This case has been previously reported. Ten months later there was a recurrence of the growth, with hoarseness and very marked dyspnea. At this time the new growth was grayish-white in appearance, resembling soft mucous polyps, readily breaking down, and extending one and one-half inches below the larynx. · On account of the dyspnea, tracheotomy was required on March 30, 1907. Röntgen-rays in five to six minute exposures were used at intervals of two to three days, from April 1st to May 11th, 1907. On May 17th the patient was discharged well. A year later there is no recurrence and the author considers the case as cured.   *Richards.*

Early Diagnosis of Malignant Disease of the Larynx.

WALTER CHAPPELL (*Medical Record,* October 16, 1909). In the early recognition of malignant diseases of the larynx lies the only hope of approaching anything like permanent relief. The usual doctor and patient treat chronic hoarseness in a most casual manner, and months may pass before there is any suspicion that the hoarseness may mean anything serious. The early symptoms are vague and the clinical picture obscure, but an early recognition is possible.

In intrinsic cancer the age and sex (male over 40) ; location of the growth (the anterior part of the cords more favorable to non-malignancy) ; infiltration: decreased mobility of the cord; and the slowly but constantly increased dyspnea from the diminished mobility of the cord, are the important points. Added to this may be the microscopical findings.

Beginning extrinsic cancer presents a picture somewhat varied by the location. Epiglottic involvement causing cough, slight dysphagia, and occasional "slips" of food into the larynx. When situated in the ventricles of Morgagni the diagnosis is more difficult, as in the early stages the growth is not visible. ˉ Slight disturbances in the mobility of the corresponding cord are suspicious. Implication of the interarytenoid folds causes a very early hoarseness and dyspnea with early glandular involvement. Pain in the first stage is due to pressure and not to ulceration.

No one symptom is diagnostic, nor is the microscope reliable, exclusive of the clinical picture. The diagnosis may be made from the symptomatology, objective and subjective, confirmed, but not disproved, by the microscopical findings.

Ryder.

Stenosis of the Larynx.

RICHARD H. JOHNSTON, Baltimore (*Boston Medical and Surgical Journal*, August 19, 1909), believes that laryngeal stenosis is best treated by the introduction of increasingly larger intubation tubes. By direct laryngoscopy, especially in children, the diagnosis is easily made and the proper treatment thereby instituted. If the stenosis be incomplete, resort at once to intubation as the only logical method of treatment. In complete closures the difficulties are much increased. Several years may be necessary for a cure. We may succeed in making an opening through the direct laryngoscope and then keep it open by intubation.

Rogers, who has had more experience than any one else in this country, is opposed to any form of external operation and believes that any case may be cured by retained intubation tubes. ·He removes the tracheal canula as soon as possible on account of danger of tracheal stenosis from prolonged wearing of the canula.

· Of three cases of laryngeal stenosis coming under the observation of Dr. Johnston, two were successfully treated by the intubation method. The third case left the hospital before treatment was begun. In one case, after a period of four and one-half months, the larynx, from a condition of complete stenosis, had been successfully opened and the intubation tube introduced. The opening was gradually dilated until a three-year-old tube was comfortably worn. One year from the time first seen the patient died from intercurrent pernicious malarial fever. The second case, after three months of gradual dilatation with increasingly larger intubation tubes, was sent home apparently cured and did not return.

The laryngologist should impress the general profession
with the fact that in the early stage, when the difficulty in
breathing appears, it is of paramount importance to have the
larynx examined for the cause of the trouble.   *Ryder.*

Tracheotomy for Foreign Bodies in the Air Passages; Based Upon Fifty-three Successful Cases.

W. F. WESTMORELAND, Atlanta (*American Journal of Surgery,* November, 1909). Weist, from the study of a thousand
cases, concluded that the presence of a foreign body in the air
passages does not make bronchotomy necessary, nor should it
be done unless indicated by dangerous symptoms. .

Westmoreland, on the other hand, says that these cases demand immediate surgical interference and that tracheotomy
should be done.

Remembering that three-fourths of these operations will be
done upon a trachea considerably smaller than a lead pencil
and within the length of an inch, and this crossed by vessels
and also the isthmus of the thyroid, such accidents as cutting
through the trachea or missing it altogether will be easily
avoided.   A general anesthetic should be used, carried only to
the point of quieting.   Tracheotomy tubes are not to be used,
as the trachea will remain sufficiently patent. A silk thread
passed through each edge of the tracheal incision gives perfect
control.   In a majority of cases the foreign body is expelled
immediately upon opening the trachea.   If not, the wound is
left open until the body is expelled.   No instruments should
be introduced into the trachea.

After opening the trachea he divides the cases into three
classes, management depending upon the class.   The first two
classes are those in which the body has been expelled at time
of operation.   In the first of these the trachea is closed at
once.   In the second class the body is expelled promptly, but
drainage is indicated on account of irritation and subsequent
infection with its accompanying accumulation of mucus.   The
wound is left patent with aseptic dressings.   The third class
includes those cases in which the body is not promptly expelled; the wound again being left open until the body escapes
and inflammation subsides.   When drainage is no longer indicated the patient is anesthetized and the wound closed.

The symptoms of foreign bodies he divides into three stages.

Obstructive symptoms immediately following the accident; second, irritation produced by its presence; third, inflammation at a later period.

Westmoreland bases his conclusions upon the successful issue of 53 cases. *Ryder.*

A Case of Myxofibroma of the Temporal Bone Combined with Multiple Paralysis of the Cranial Nerves.

SCHWABACH and BIELSCHOWSKY (*Deut. med. Wochenschr.*, May 18, 1909), describe a case with autopsy findings which was at first diagnosed as a tumor of the acoustic nerve. Full description of the clinical side and the nervous findings.

Horn.

Clinical Experience with Calcium Lactate in Hemorrhages of the Upper Air Tract.

W. K. SIMPSON, New York (*Medical Record*, September 25, 1909) concludes as follows:

1. "Clinical experience shows that calcium lactate has a controlling influence in hastening the coagulation of the blood.

2. Its efficacy is more marked in hemophiliac cases. where the coagulation is delayed, than in cases of normal coagulation time.

3. Before operation, especially on tonsils and adenoids. careful inquiry should be made relative to any hemophilic heredity or tendency.

4. In suspicious cases the coagulation period should be determined before operation.

5. It is questionable, if not positively contraindicated. whether such operations should be undertaken in hemophilic cases, other than under the most extreme urgency.

6. In all cases of operations for the removal of tonsils and adenoids, calcium lactate should be given for a period prior to and after the operation, both for its possible effect in diminishing the immediate hemorrhage and in preventing secondary surface hemorrhage.

7. Of the calcium salts. the lactate is more positive in its results, is more agreeable to administer and is less irritating to the stomach." *Richards.*

The Use of Ethyl Chlorid as a General Anesthetic for Operations in the Throat as Especially Applied to Children.

E. MATHER SILL, New York (*Medical Record,* October 23, 1909). Ethyl chlorid given by means of the Ware inhaler is the easiest of all the anesthetics to give. Two or three thicknesses of gauze should be used over the inhaler and the tube removed at intervals to see that the gauze does not become frosted over, in which case it should be changed. When the inhaler with the rubber bag is used, the ethyl chlorid stream goes directly through the small metal tube into the rubber bag, and this precaution is not necessary. The author considers this preferable. When properly given, the patient is under the anesthetic in from two to five minutes. Profound anesthesia is not necessary. Operation can be begun as soon as there is complete relaxation, the conjunctival reflex being present to a slight degree. Immediately upon the completion of the operation and removal of the mouth gag, consciousness returns. The operation is done with the patient lying flat on the operating table and the head slightly lowered. This anesthetic is especially suited for the operation of removal of adenoids and tonsils in children. Where long operations are necessary, ethyl chlorid anesthesia is first obtained, and deep anesthesia continued with ether by the drop method.

Richards.

Brain Tumor with Unusual Symptoms.

J. E. DALE, Fort Collins, Colo. (*Medical Record,* August 7, 1909), reports a case of brain tumor with unusual symptoms; unusual from the fact that the temperature was subnormal during the whole time of observation, and there was no headache. The patient was a male, sixteen years old. He was under observation from July 7, 1908, to September 28, 1908. When first seen there was occasional vomiting, the abdomen was tender to touch, temperature 97° and pulse 75. After the bowels were cleaned out the vomiting ceased, but temperature remained subnormal. On September 3d, following obstinate constipation, there was an attack similar to the first, only more severe. Temperature was 97.5. Between the two attacks the temperature varied from 96 to 97.5. On September 28th, following two days of complaining bitterly of difficulty in breathing, although respiration was apparently normal, the patient died. Paralytic symptoms appeared one hour before death. The usual headache symptoms were entirely absent. Autopsy showed a small warty growth (endotheliomata) attached to the roof of the fourth ventricle, slightly to the right of the median line, directly over a point in the floor slightly posterior to the center. The late effect on the respiratory center was to be expected from the situation of the tumor. The early and constant effects on the heat centers is hard to explain unless from leucocytic infiltration. *Ryder.*

Recent Advances in the Field of Laryngo-Rhinology.

VON EICKEN (*Deutsch. med. Wochenschr.*, No. 1, 1909, p. 22). The original work done in this field during the last two years is carefully reviewed. In almost every branch something new has been discovered. Especially discussed is: The method of Killian for the treatment of hay fever; the use of hard paraffin in the treatment of ozena; the use of suprarenal extracts as an aid in the diagnosis of nasal conditions; the light therapy of Brunnings in acute accessory sinus disease; the use of negative pressure as an aid in the diagnosis of diseases of the nasal cavities, according to the methods of Walb and Horn; the radical operations of Killian, Denker and Luc-Caldwell in the treatment of this class of cases. Tremendous strides have been made in the use of the Roentgen photography, but the work is not nearly completed. Horseley, Semon, du Bois-Reymond, Onodi, Kuttner and others have contributed important work on the innervation of the larynx, but the question is still unsettled. *Horn.*

Observations on the Relation of Diseases of the Upper Air Passages to Asthma, Cough and Disorders of Digestion.

THOMAS R. FRENCH (*Long Island Medical Journal*, October, 1909). Many of the neuroses of modern civilization are so obscure and shadowy that we do not pretend to understand them. What we do know is from empirical clinical experience. Enthusiasm and hasty judgment of some of the writers have led them too far. Their claims have not been verified and the theory of reflex irritation has been rejected. The direct relationship between nasal abnormalities and reflected phenomena is not always evident, but it is beyond dispute that such relationship does exist. Polypi and hypertrophy of the turbinated structures do in certain cases cause asthma, and the correction of a deflected septum will cure a cough.

French takes up three phases of the subject, viz.: First, the nose in relation to asthma; second, the nose in relation to cough; third, nasopharyngeal catarrh in relation to gastric and intestinal indigestion.

The Nose in Relation to Asthma.—In determining the cause of spasmodic asthma he thinks it wise to eliminate other conditions, thoracic, abdominal and pelvic, and then examine the nose. Hypersensitive nasal mucous membrane may have as an underlying cause some gross fault of elimination, a diatbesis, or some organic disease. Turgescence of the erectile nasal mucous membrane may be and often is caused by transmitted vasomotor irritation from distant parts of the economy. When swollen tissues or sensitive areas in the nose are suspected, carefully test the same. Shrink the swollen tissues and touch with the probe the suspected areas and note results. While the correction of gross nasal lesions holds out the brightest hopes, the relief is often only temporary. Results with the cautery have not been as successful in his hands as in others. but it does occasionally give relief. Great care should be taken in advising operation for relief and still greater care to convey a correct idea of our expectations.

The Nose in Relation to Cough.—While almost any diseased condition of the nose may cause cough, he calls attention especially to that condition caused by contact of the middle turbinate with the septum. If the middle turbinate is flattened to any considerable extent against the septum; if the contact cannot be seen, but the turbinate is prominent and part of it hidden; if there is a high septal deflection against a normal middle turbinate, the introduction of a probe at the suspected point of contact, or the shrinking of the swollen tissues, maintaining the contraction for several days will often settle the diagnosis.

Nasal and Pharyngeal Catarrh in Relation to Gastric and Intestinal Indigestion.—By continuity and reflex action disorders of digestion make their impress upon the mucous membrane of the nose and pharynx. Long experience in viewing these parts will enable one to detect the diseased pharynges due to gastrointestinal irritation. In acute and subacute pharyngitis the deep red congestion of the posterior wall with little or no redness of the pillars of the fauces or palate points to gastrointestinal trouble. A red tip and swollen nose sometimes accompanies an attack of duodenal catarrh. An impairment of the innervation of the larynx resulting in the weakness and loss of voice may occur during an attack of diarrhea. It is difficult to say whether these conditions occur from reflex action or from continuity.

The factor is an ever-changing one, and the same group of symptoms seemingly produced by the nose and throat in one individual may be induced in another by some other organ. While the nose and throat must be looked upon as factors of large importance in the production of reflex phenomena they cannot be regarded as constant. To obtain gratifying results the laryngologist must also become an internist.   *Ryder.*

BOOK REVIEWS.

Verhandlung des Vereins Deutscher Laryngologen, 1909.

A. Stuber's Verlag, Würzburg. Price, 5 marks. The proceedings of the German Laryngological Society, which met in May of this year, are of more than usual interest. To review all of the papers or even to give a list of them would demand too much space. It is not only the articles, but the discussions which are of importance. A requirement for the reading of a paper was originality, and, as I said in my review of the Proceedings for 1908, the matter is not to be found in any other journals. The papers which perhaps created the most interest were: Brunnings, "New Instruments for 1909"; Siebenmann, "Experience with the Galvanocaustic Treatment of Larynx-tuberculosis"; Gutzmann, "The Treatment of Functional Diseases of the Voice"; Meyer, "On Difficult Décanalement"; Schoenemann, "Further Contributions to the Pathology and Treatment of Ozena," etc.

Of the 363 members present, only two were from the United States and one from England. *Horn.*

Die Stirnhöhle (The Frontal Sinus).

By Prof. A. Onodi. Published by Alfred Hölder, Wien. Price, 6.80 marks. The fifth of Prof. Onodi's monographs on the surgical and topographic anatomy of the accessory cavities of the nose, completes a series which has covered many years of most painstaking investigation. His former work on the relation of the optic nerve to the nasal accessory cavities was undoubtedly the basis for the modern conception of orbital pathology. The present monograph will prove a similar stepping stone to a better knowledge of intracranial complications as influenced by diseases of the frontal sinus.

After reviewing the various theories regarding the development of the frontal sinus, he shows by his Röntgen photographs that not until the sixth year is the frontal sinus recognizable as a well-defined cavity.

The comparative value of transillumination as compared to Röntgen photographs is shown by the following figures. In

1200 skulls the frontal sinus was found absent, by transillumination, in 30 per cent on both sides, in 10 per cent on the right side and 10 per cent on the left side. By the radiographic method, on the same skulls, both sides were found wanting in 5 per cent, and right and left, about 1 per cent. The differences in the extent of the sinus, both in a horizontal and vertical direction, varies enormously by the two methods. The various plates simply emphasize the fact that, putting aside for the moment the present questionable position of radiography as a diagnostic agent in pathological conditions, as a preliminary step to a radical operation on the sinus, there is no shadow of a doubt as to its real value.

The text is beautifully illustrated with over 100 life-sized plates. Presswork and paper leave nothing to be desired.

Horn.

Diseases of the Nose, Throat and Ear, Medical and Surgical.

By WILLIAM LINCOLN BALLENGER, M. D. Published by Lea & Febiger, Philadelphia and New York.

The first edition of Ballenger's book received such a hearty reception that a second edition has been necessitated within a year. The author has taken the opportunity thus afforded to review the entire work, to make some important changes and to add some entirely new matter made necessary by the development of the surgery of the accessory sinuses of the nose, the more recent studies on the labyrinth, etc. In our review of the first edition, it was stated that modernity was the keynote. It certainly was a striking feature of the publication, but here we see already in the revision how quickly the changes are developing. We still commend the book for the clearness of its description of operations and the definiteness which characterizes the illustrations.

Tuberculosis of the Nose and Throat.

By LORENZO B. LOCKARD, M. D. Published by C. V. Mosby Book & Publishing Co., St. Louis, Mo., 1909.

The publication of this timely book will be well received by laryngologists, who desire to have a complete treatise upon the subject. The author has divided his theme logically so that the various chapters are rendered acceptable to anyone who desires to study any particular phase. Of special interest are the chapters devoted to the history, etiology, diagnosis and surgical treatment. The illustrations in color, sixty-four in number, are executed with faithful accuracy and bring out the details to be seen in but very few illustrations of this character. ·

The author considers formalin as the drug of greatest value for the treatment of the ulcerative and infiltrative types of laryngeal tuberculosis, summing up the advantages as follows:

(1) It surpasses all other bactericides in solutions of a strength which can be tolerated.

(2) In tuberculous ulcers it is fully the equal of, and probably superior to lactic acid.

(3) Its effect upon vegetations is prompt and pronounced.

(4) In infiltrative cases it is by far the most satisfactory remedy.

(5) It is the only drug of the curative class that can with safety be placed in the hands of the patient, thus making it possible to maintain a continuous, cleansing, germicidal and absorbent action.

(6) Its field of usefulness comprises all the varied types of the disease.

Taking it altogether, the work is a most creditable addition to the literature of tuberculosis and to the publications of American medicine in general.

SOCIETY PROCEEDINGS.

NEW YORK ACADEMY OF MEDICINE.

SECTION OF OTOLOGY.

Regular Meeting, November 13, 1908.

A. B. DUEL, M. D., CHAIRMAN.

Case of Chronic Suppurative Otitis Media During Pregnancy in a Fifteen-Year-Old Patient; Sinus Thrombosis; Operation; Pulmonary Abscess and Other Complications.

DR. M. D. LEDERMAN said he considered himself especially fortunate in being able to present this patient as a picture of health after all that she had passed through. She was sent into the Lebanon Hospital (Medical Service) with a tentative diagnosis of intestinal or blood infection, and was not seen by Dr. Lederman until the ninth day after her admission. The patient was 15 years old, father living and well, mother died of tuberculosis, one younger sister living and well. She had measles when 2 years old, and since then had not been ill up to the present time. Her menstrual history began at the age of 13, and has always been regular. Date of the last menstruation three months prior to admission. Five days before admission patient developed a severe frontal headache, followed by fever, which had continued. The day before admission she had several chills, followed by fever, little sweating, and headache. The next day headache again. No pain in any other part of the body. Admitted to the hospital suffering from chills, fever, headache.

The patient seemed to be in good condition, face flushed and eyes bright. Pupils equal and reacted to light and accommodation.

Physical Examination.—Heart normal; pulse regular, but rapid. Lungs, sonorous rales heard over the chest. Spleen palpable at free border of ribs. Cervix soft, admits one finger;

fundus of uterus felt at umbilicus. Diagnosis of pregnancy about fourth or fifth month.

July 28. Temperature 102.6°.

July 29. Had several chills during day. Vomited yellowish fluid at times, but complained of no pain anywhere. Following a chill at 7:30 p. m. the temperature rose to 107.4° F. Slight tenderness in right iliac region.

On July 30 had chills, which seemed to be at regular intervals. Blood examination showed high polynuclear count, but was otherwise negative.

August 4. Temperature 100.2° F. Patient continues to vomit food. Following an afternoon chill, temperature rose to 104° F.

She had a chill almost every day.

On August 5th the patient was comfortable and the temperature was normal. No pain anywhere.

August 6th. Complete physical examination revealed nothing other than a foul-smelling discharge in the right ear. Antistreptococci serum was given. No pain about the mastoid. Right eye showed signs of approaching choked disk. Pain persisted in the right iliac region. Patient was transferred to surgical division, and came under my observation on the following day.

August 7. Some tenderness over the mastoid tip and along the sternomastoid muscle were present, together with slight rigidity of the neck. Chilly sensations were noted.

Upon the above history and symptoms a diagnosis of infective sinus thrombosis was made, and patient was prepared for operation. On removing the mastoid cortex the sinus was found to be discolored and occupying an abnormal position close to the external auditory canal. The parietal wall of the sinus was black and sloughing. A foul-smelling thrombus was removed from the lumen of the vessel, extending nearly the entire length of the sigmoid division. Free pus was seen in the region of the antrum. The diseased sinus wall was cut away with scissors the entire length of bone wound and its inner wall curetted. A return flow of blood was established both from the torcular and from jugular end; but as the current of blood from the bulb did not seem adequate, the internal jugular vein was ligated by Dr. H. Roth, one of the attending surgeons, who was present during the operation. Two ligatures were placed about the vein, an inch apart, just above the clavicle. No resection was attempted, owing to the patient's condition. The neck wound was closed with sutures.

The same evening the temperature dropped from 106° to 98.2°, and remained there for three readings—12 hours. It then rose to 102°. No chill was observed at any time after the operation. On August 10, three days after operation, the patient aborted a five-month fetus, followed by a slight rise in temperature (to 102.4°). The temperature remained between 103 and 104 for a week. The wound in the neck became infected and had to be reopened. Considerable pus came away.

About this time there were physical signs of pulmonary involvement on right side posteriorly at base of lung. Considerable cough, with a foul-smelling purulent expectoration. These symptoms lasted a little over three weeks. In the meantime, the mastoid and sinus wounds progressed satisfactorily. On account of an increased intracranial pressure an incision one inch in length was made into the visceral wall of the sinus, but only clear fluid, with some disintegrated tissue (resembling brain structure), came away.

On September 8 the patient gave signs of suspected empyema in the right chest posteriorly. She was aspirated and 2 cc. of clear serous fluid was obtained. On the next day the pus expectoration diminished considerably.

On September 16 the temperature was normal.

On September 20 the patient was out of bed, her symptoms having apparently cleared up.

On the 22d she complained of toothache and was found to have quite a large alveolar abscess. This was opened, and in two or three days the swelling in the jaw subsided.

On September 30 the patient was apparently well, temperature normal, and two days later she was discharged from the hospital.

There is no doubt that in this case an earlier operation would have prevented the spread of the infection.

One point of interest is that during the time when the chills and septic temperature were being recorded blood cultures were negative. Repeated examinations showed the polynuclear percentages to be increased in varying degrees, but at no time were bacteria found.

DR. DENCH inquired whether he was right in understanding Dr. Lederman to say that the jugular vein was tied in two places, high up and low down. The case shows clearly the wisdom of taking out the jugular vein, for there is liability of septic infection if it is allowed to remain in. If one examines a specimen, the clot will ordinarily be found running down into the jugular and tapering to a point. The septic material is usually carried into the general circulation through the facial vein, and it is, therefore, Dr. Dench's practice to take out the jugular from a point low down in the neck to a point above the origin of the facial vein.

The case was a most interesting one, and shows the beneficial result of operative treatment in such cases; it also shows how the clinical history may be misleading, and no attention given to the ear unless aural symptoms are particularly inquired into.

Dr. Dench said that he had seen only one case of jugular sinus thrombosis complicated by abscess of the lung, and the patient died 48 hours after the operation from acute gangrene of the lung.

DR. LEDERMAN said that his reason for not removing the vein was that the patient had been on the table so long that further operative procedure was not warranted; the physical aspect of the vessel did not indicate any involvement of its structure.

Thrombosis of the Sigmoid and Lateral Sinus.

DR. W. SOHIER BRYANT demonstrated the case of a boy, 16 years of age, who had had thrombosis of the left sigmoid and lateral sinus, and the adjacent dura mater, and the subjacent cerebrum and cerebellum. A radical operation was performed on the ear, and the jugular vein examined. Later metastatic arthritis and double pyothorax developed.

Final recovery, after two months of sepsis, with the temperature ranging between 97° and 106° F. The temperature reached 105½° on the fifty-fourth day. Efficient nursing in an out-of-door world seemed to be the chief factor contributing to final recovery.

Hernia Cerebri.

DR. W. SOHIER BRYANT demonstrated the case of a girl, 18 years old. When the patient was first seen she had had chronic purulent otitis for a long period. Double radical operation had not controlled the discharge. The last two years she had been incapacitated by extremely severe headaches, chiefly on the left side. The left ear appeared to have the tympanic cavity filled with polypus. A radical operation was performed on the ear. The polypus proved to be a hernia of the dura mater, protruding through the tegmen. In front of this hernia there was a small sinus, leading directly up into the temporal lobe, discharging thin pus.

The opening in the meninges was enlarged and the hernia replaced after extensive exposure of the dura mater. The patient did well for a week, when the symptoms increased with marked signs of cerebral pressure. In a second operation the dura mater was opened wide and explored. About 3½ drams of pus were liberated from the brain. The wound was packed. All went well for five days, when, on account of severe headaches, the nurse cut the bandage, and a hernia cerebri followed, as large as an egg. This was amputated. A second hernia, similar to the first, formed, which was also amputated. A very copious flow of cerebrospinal fluid followed. This flow lasted 25 days. The wound healed solid, but there remained a slight bulging area at the opening in the calvarium. Six months later the patient was seized with a violent headache, became unconscious, and in about three hours was relieved by a spontaneous and very copious flow of cerebrospinal fluid from the fundus of the ear. The fluid came from the opening in the skull. The flow gradually decreased, and in a week the sinus closed, and has since remained closed. The suppuration stopped in both ears.

The eye-grounds remained normal throughout the course of the illness. There were no definite symptoms of aphasia, except at times of the caries.

DR. DENCH said that the difficulty in causing a cessation of the flow of the cerebrospinal fluid, in a case of this kind, was very great. In order to effect a cure it was necessary to secure some method of causing an absorption of the fluid. He believed that the method sometimes employed in cases of hydrocephalus in children might be well suited to a case of this kind. This procedure was suggested by Chene and Sutherland, and had also been employed by Keen. Dr. Dench was indebted for his knowledge of the procedure to its mention in the recent work of Mr. Charles A. Ballance. "Some

Points in the Surgery of the Brain," published about two years·
ago. The procedure consists in draining the lateral ventricle
into the anachroid space by inserting a bent tube into the
cranial cavity, one end of the tube entering the lateral ventricle,
while the other end terminates in the subdural space. In cases
of hydrocephalus the lining of the ventricles seemed to lose
its power of absorbing the cerebrospinal fluid, and this same
condition may well apply to the cases under discussion. Dr.
Dench thought that the procedure was certainly worthy of
trial.

Dr. JOHNSON said that he had a patient with a fracture of
the base of the skull, in which the ventricle had been opened
and a tremendous flow of cerebrospinal fluid had occurred
from the ear—as much as a teaspoonful in a minute. The.
flow continued for ten days, and when it finally ceased the
patient became very much depressed until the reabsorbent
function of the ventricle again came into play. The patient
would become restless or unconscious, the temperature would
mount up, and death would seem imminent. The re-establishment of the ventricular absorption seemed finally to relieve
him, however, and he made a satisfactory recovery.

In another case—a fracture of the occipital bone—there was
an extensive flow from the ventricle, which continued for over
three weeks. In each of these cases, when the cessation of the
flow came, the patient would become very uncomfortable and
restless, and when this period of discomfort subsided, after a
day or two, the patient's condition improved and he had
recovered.

In a case like the one reported, in which operative removal
of a cerebral hernia was followed by so large a flow of ventricular fluid, the condition would seem somewhat analogous
to cases of traumatism such as he had just related.

Dr. LEDERMAN said that Dr. Bryant's remarks recalled a fact
in the case which he himself has just reported—that there was
increased cranial pressure. When he made an incision into
the visceral wall of the sinus a large quantity of clear fluid
came away with what seemed to be a quantity of broken-down
brain tissue, but no pus. A cerebral hernia appeared through
this incision, about the size of a large hickory nut. This was
left alone, and finally it disappeared without further annoyance.

Dr. Kopetzky said that the case presented very interesting features, but, in regard to the brain hernias, he thought that early attempt should be made to replace the protruding part of the brain. When thus attempted at an early stage in the procedures, before retaining adhesions had formed, the protruding part of the brain is gradually pushed back by graduated pressure exerted by pads placed over the hernia. He did not think it wise to cut off the protruding brain substance, although sometimes that was an unavoidable act. In regard ·to the flow of · cerebrospinal fluid, he had observed a case wherein, after incision of the meninges to relieve a serous meningitis, a very free flow of fluid kept up for many days. but the patient recovered, and the flow gradually stopped. It was to be expected that a free flow of fluid would follow opening of the meninges, and was regarded by him as a rather favorable prognostic sign.

Dr. Duel said that not many years ago such a case would have caused much discussion, but they are now seen so frequently that we hear very little about them.

Case of Labyrinthine Disease.

Dr. A. B. Duel presented a man, colored, 47 years old, a Porto Rican, who had lived in New York for many years. His history dates back nearly 17 years ago, when he first had an acute abscess in the middle ear, with a discharge which continned for several weeks, perhaps months.

Later, when he first went to a clinic for treatment, "a large mass of foul-smelling material was removed from the ear." At that time he had most interesting attacks of vertigo. and certain experiences—as when he looked upon "the sudden running up of a curtain" would cause him to faint. Certain sounds also would cause him to fall on account of vertigo. Following removal of the material from the ear the discharge ceased: At intervals of two or three years he has had similar large masses—always ill-smelling—removed from the ear. . When he came under Dr. Duel's observation, he had removed. after considerable effort a cholesteatomatous mass as large in diameter as an index finger. The bony excavation was very large in the attic and hypotympanic region. Part of the drum and ossicles still remain.

An interesting point in this case is the fact that the lower tone limit is very good (90 V. S.), and that his upper tone limit is not much lowered; his hearing distance is as good for both the acumeter and whisper as in most successful radical operations.

Another interesting point is the possibility of his having had a labyrinthine suppuration which affected only the semi-circular canals. He has entirely recovered his equilibrium, and has fairly good hearing remaining on the affected side.

In reply to an inquiry from Dr. Dench, as to whether the patient had had any nystagmus, Dr. Duel replied that he now has a slight horizontal nystagmus on looking away from the affected side; none on looking toward the affected side.

After rapid turning toward the diseased side, a nystagmus —still more marked—was noticeable. Both the spontaneous and the induced nystagmus were in the direction of the sound ear.

Dr. Lederman recalled the case of a colored woman whom he had presented before the section. She had been shot with a 32-caliber revolver, held about six inches from her head. The bullet went through the tragus and carried away the posterior portion of the drum, lodging against the under and posterior portion of the middle ear. The injury had taken place three years before Dr. Lederman examined the patient. She complained of a facial paralysis, and severe vertigo, with attacks of nausea. She was unable to walk alone, and never ventured out without being accompanied by another person. After the injury she was unconscious for over three weeks. At that time some attempt had been made to remove the bullet through the external auditory meatus, but the manipulation caused such dizziness that further treatment was discontinued.

When the patient came under Dr. Lederman's care the facial paralysis, vertigo, and deafness still persisted. On closing the eyes in the erect position the woman fell toward the affected (left) side. There was a purulent discharge from the left ear, and a fibrous growth filled the external auditory canal, being attached to the internal wall of the middle ear. After its removal, the bullet could be seen in position, surrounded by some osseous deposit. It was impossible to move the foreign body through the canal, so a radical operation was performed the following day. The bullet was found imbedded in the inner wall of the middle ear, causing pressure over the horizontal semicircular and facial canals. The lead had to be chiselled away, as a bony framework held the bullet in position. Seventy grains of lead were collected after the operation.

On the fifth day following the surgical treatment the patient was able to sit up in a chair and the dizziness was considerably improved. In two weeks she was able to walk quite well without support, something she had not accomplished in three years. At this time the ordinary speaking voice was plainly heard with the good ear closed. Before the operation only a loud voice could be faintly heard in the affected ear. It was interesting to note that the facial paralysis of three years' duration was slowly improving without additional treatment.

Dr. Richards had nothing to add to the discussion, excepting to call attention to the interesting phenomenon illustrated by the case—that waves of sound affect not only the acoustic but the non-acoustic labyrinth also; and the marked degree to which equilibration may be influenced through this source (when the labyrinth is in a condition of irritability) is well shown.

Dr. Duel said Weber's test showed that the patient lateralized to the affected side, as would be the case where the cochlear portion of the labyrinth was not involved.

Large Mastoid Sequestrum.

Dr. W. C. McFarland presented a large mastoid sequestrum, which was removed last March from a boy 8 years of age, who had had scarlet fever four months previously. At the time of operation he had a large subperiosteal abscess. The whole mastoid cortex was found detached and bathed in pus. It was removed in two pieces. Half an inch down in the mastoid, about the region of the semicircular canals, was a small sequestrum, which on removal left the dura of the middle fossa and of the cerebellum uncovered. The small specimen, taken from the depth of the mastoid, had been decalcified to determine whether any of the labyrinth was involved.

Sequestrum from Mastoid Antrum.

Dr. Myles presented a sequestrum taken from the mastoid antrum, measuring 20 by 15 by 10 mm. He saw the patient, a man, 45 years, for the first time two weeks ago. The case

was a very interesting one. Patient gave a history of a discharge from the left ear since last June. He had had marked
vertigo for some time. He walked with a very peculiar gait—
one foot would go over the other—and he could hardly get
about without assistance. There was a brawny feeling over
the mastoid, and a quantity of pus flowed from the middle
ear and attic. The cortex of the mastoid was removed, together with large masses of granulations, which were sarcomatous in appearance. These granulations appeared rich
in vitality. There was a decided pulsation of the entire mass,
apparently transmitted from the brain beneath. The inner
mastoid plate was absent over an extensive area, and within
the antrum this sequestrum was found. There was carious
bone in the region of the semicircular canals, and, thinking
there might be a specific tubercular or sarcomatous element in
the case, and knowing how nature throws off a gummatous
or tubercular process, the curetting in that region had
been conducted with great conservatism. The cavity meas-
used one and five-eighths inches in depth from the skin, upward and inward. The only way to account for this was
that the pressure from the contents of the cavity had become
so great as to push the cranial contents upward.

The symptoms of dizziness and disturbed locomotion disappeared practically at once after all necrotic tissue had been
removed, and the patient had no untoward symptoms. One or
two necrotic spicules of bone have since been removed, and the
cavity seems to be granulating properly. The patient is
gaining in weight, his pulse is good, and he is improved in
every way. The microscopical examinations were negative. The progress of the case is being watched with a
great deal of interest. It has been deemed advisable to keep
the wound wide open, with a view to possible developments
requiring a second operation. The further developments in
the case will be reported later.

Large Mastoid Sequestrum.

DR. JOHN B. RAE presented a large sequestrum, removed
from the mastoid of a little boy of 7 years, who was admitted
to the New York Eye and Ear Infirmary on June 28th, 1904.
He was suffering from a right-sided chronic purulent otitis
media, and presented, in addition, a very large subperiosteal,

abscess. Over the lower part of the mastoid process could be seen the scar of a small incision, quite healed, and presumably the evidence of a former Wilde operation. On investigation of the abscess cavity a very large cortical perforation was discovered high up over the antrum. The interior of the mastoid was in great part occupied by granulation tissue, and lying within, or loosely connected with this mass of granulation, so that they were easily removed by means of a thumb forceps, were the two sequestra which the doctor presented. The larger included the bony meatus, and the smaller a portion of the bone forming the glenoid fossa. The mastoid having been thoroughly cleaned out, the meatus was enlarged by incision into the concha and removal of cartilage, and the post-auricular wound partially closed by sutures above and below.

Two weeks later the cavity was skin-grafted and the post-auricular incision closed by suture, except at the very lowest corner.

As far as could be determined, the loss of bone caused no inconvenience to the child in eating or in any other way.

On discharge, six weeks after operation, the house surgeon's notes read: "Wound is clean, except for slight serous discharge. Case ran no temperature above 99°."

DR. LEWIS said that a number of years ago a little girl, 8 to 10 years of age, came to the infirmary, with marked discharge from the ear and with a facial paralysis. Upon operation he found the middle ear filled with large masses of granulation, and deep in the granulation a movable mass of bone. After careful manipulation, requiring some little time, this was dislodged and found to be a sequestrum, containing a portion of the cochlea and of the carotid canal.

Paper: Two Tests for the Diagnosis of Ossicular Ankylosis.

By E. P. FOWLER, M. D.

DR. KOPETZKY said that in his opinion the test shown by Dr. Fowler was quite dissimilar to the Gelle test. The latter depended entirely upon bone conduction. The test shown this evening does not depend upon bone conduction, but rather upon the conduction of the vibrations of the fork through a column of air condensed in the cup by the increase of air pressure produced through the action of the hand bulb. According to physical laws, sound will be increased in intensity when the medium through which it is transmitted is increased in density. Therefore it follows that an increase in loudness is to be expected when the air through which the sound is transmitted is made more dense. This constitutes a factor of possible error in the calculation of the results obtained by Dr. Fowler. It will be interesting to note just how far the results obtained from the Fowler test will coincide with those obtained from the Gelle test. Such evidence is as yet not at hand, and until it is given no conclusion can be reached as to the practical value of the Fowler test.

Dr. DENCH said that the manometric observations showed that pressure on the round window was three times as efficacious in increasing labyrinthine pressure as pressure upon the oval window. He thought that this was one reason why Gelle's test could not be depended upon in making a differential diagnosis of ankylosis of the stapes. Of course, if the stapes is immovable, pressure on the round window would cause very little difference in labyrinthine tension, owing to the fact that fluids are practically incompressible.

Dr. DENCH thought the work done by Dr. Fowler was certainly in the right direction, that it was of great value, and the doctor deserved much credit for his painstaking labors. The speaker was extremely skeptical, however, as to the practical value of his experiment as a means of making a diagnosis of stapes ankylosis.

Dr. FOWLER, in closing the discussion, said that in so far as the density of the air in the apparatus is concerned, he understood that the density of the air has no effect unless it is the air in which the sound is generated. In this apparatus the sound is generated partly inside the apparatus, as is proved by the fact that the results obtained with it are similar to those obtained with the apparatus containing an internally mounted fork.

The explanation of the fact that the stronger pressure on the head diminished the sound is that it stops the cup from vibrating so strongly, but these changes, if listened to, are so distinct from the changes brought about by compression that they are easily perceived to be not of the same character.

The tests do not depend upon the pressure of the apparatus against the side of the head. It takes so slight an air pressure to bring out the tests—only a fraction of a millimeter—that this is not enough to cause a great diminution of sound through the variations in intensity due wholly to the altered vibration or other peculiarities of the apparatus. Although the density and elasticity of the air in the cup increase with the pressure, suction has exactly the opposite effect, and yet the sound is diminished as before. The increased density also slightly increases the temperature, and condensation would do the opposite, but changes due to these factors are so slight that they would not affect the accuracy of the experiments.

A Case of Cavernous Sinus Thrombosis Following an Acute Tonsillitis—Death—Report of Autopsy Findings.

DR. ROBERT LEWIS, JR., reported a case of cavernous sinus thrombosis following acute tonsillitis, as follows: On the evening of July 21st I was called to St. Francis Hospital to see a boy, aged 12 years, with the following medical history:

On July 17th the boy complained of sore throat and stiffness of the left side of the neck. That evening he had a chill. On the afternoon of the fourth day following he was admitted to St. Francis Hospital. At that time he complained of pain in the left side of the neck, pain in the left eye and in the right side of his chest. His temperature was 102½° F.

When I saw him at 10 p. m. of that day his temperature was 104° F. Pulse 96. Respiration 30. There was present a chemosis of the conjunctiva of the left eye and eyelid. No strabismus was present, but there was a marked exophthalmus and a paralysis of the left side of the face. A purulent exudate covered the left tonsil. The ears were normal. There was no headache and no vomiting. The pain in the left eye was very severe. The patient talked rationally when spoken to, but was somewhat drowsy. On attempting to walk he staggered and would have fallen had he not been supported. The reflexes were somewhat exaggerated.

The fundus of the eye was examined the next day by Dr. Lynch and found to be normal. Dr. Donavan found a pneumonia at the base of the right lung. On July 22nd, at 8 a. m., his temperature was 105 4/5° F. Pulse 136. Respiration 24. At 6 p. m. of the same day his temperature was 106 2/5° F. Pulse 150. Respiration 28. Patient died at 8:15 p. m.

AUTOPSY BY DR. JOHN LARKIN.

Liver—Pale, anemic, flabby, no abscess. Adhesions between upper border of transverse colon, gall bladder and lower surface of liver.

Right Lung—Upper lobe consolidated, covered with suppurative exudate, adhesions between visceral and lateral pleura, multiple septic infarcts in lung.

Left Lung—Lower lobe confluent lobular pneumonia and hypostatic pneumonia; rest of lung aerated.

Heart—No valvular lesion.

Thymus—Persistent.

Left Tonsil—Moderately enlarged and seat of active suppurative inflammation; no diffuse cellulitis around tonsil.

Right Tonsil—Normal.

Left Internal Jugular Vein—Not dilated, but contained post-mortem thrombus, which was removed without difficulty. Antemortem condition normal.

Muscles of Left Side of Neck and Left Submaxillary Gland—Cellular infiltration.

Meninges—O. K.

Brain—No pathologic changes.

Left Cavernous Sinus—Contained broken-down thrombus and pus.

Right Cavernous Sinus—Filled with pus secondary to infection of left sinus.

Left Inferior Petrosal Sius—Filled with thrombus.

Orbital Veins—Thrombosed. Orbital cellulitis.

Our hands are always tied in the presence of these, always fatal cases. The possibility of developing an operative technic that may be the means of saving these hopeless cases is very questionable, on account of the inaccessibility of the sinus involved. The route which is followed in the removal of the Gasserian ganglion has been attempted on two occasions, once by Dwight and Germain, and again by Hartley and Knapp. Langworthy suggests the following route, which he has done only on the cadaver: "After elongating the usual frontal sinus incision downward along the nasal bone and retracting the eye out of the field, the inner wall of the orbit is removed over a considerable area, together with the nasal 'bone on that side. The entire structures within the nasal fossa, ethmoid labyrinth and turbinates are then curetted out. This at once brings one down on the anterior surface of the body of the sphenoid, with the opening of the sphenoidal sinus in plain view. The anterior wall of the sphenoidal sinus is next to follow and also the external or lateral wall, against which rests the cavernous sinus. From this point one can do considerable on the cadaver with a prick of the knife and a properly curved blunt dissector. If unsuccessful in opening the cavernous sinus, the external wound is easily closed, the eye remains uninjured, and nothing is lost by the attempt."*

I think the fact that, notwithstanding the thrombosis of the orbital veins, as well as of the cavernous sinuses, the fundi of the eyes were found to be normal should be emphasized.

DR. DENCH said that he had approached the cavernous sinus by the Gasserian route in making some experiments on the cadaver, and had been very much impressed with the ease with which the sinus might be exposed. He mentioned the fact that Dr. Hartley some years ago was able to remove a small clot from the circular sinus. This operation is certainly more difficult than the removal of a clot from the cavernous sinus. He had had no experience with the Langworthy operation, either on the cadaver or on the living subject, but thought that this method of approaching the cavernous sinus presented many difficulties.

DR. LEWIS said that his reason for presenting the report was that the path of infection from the tonsil to the cavernous sinus is rather rare.

---

*Laryngoscope, July, 1906.

NEW YORK ACADEMY OF MEDICINE.

SECTION ON OTOLOGY.

Regular Meeting, December 11, 1908.

ARTHUR B. DUEL, M. D., CHAIRMAN.

A Case of Acute Mastoiditis, Complicated by Sinus Thrombosis, Extradural Abscess, Encephalitis and Meningitis.

DR. SEYMOUR OPPENHEIMER first saw the patient, a girl of 12, on March 3, 1908. For two weeks previously she had had a slight cold, but not enough to keep her from school. During this period the mother noticed a slight discharge from the ear. Two days prior to coming under observation she complained of pain in the left ear, which became more pronounced during the day. The following day the temperature varied between 102° and 103°, the pain in the ear was less, and there was some discharge. The patient was in bed and comfortable. During the night she became irritable and complained of much pain. The day of examination she was very irritable and restless, and complained of headache. Discharge from the ear profuse. Temperature 104°. At 10 a. m. she had a pronounced chill, and gradually sank into coma. At 11 she was completely unconscious. At 1 p. m. Dr. Oppenheimer saw her in consultation. Temperature then 106.5°. The patient was comatose and presented all the evideuces of severe acute mastoiditis, and the physical condition indicative of intracranial involvement. No convulsions had been noticed. Slight generalized spasticity of the extremities, and double Kernig and McEwan's signs were present. She was removed to the private pavilion of Mt. Sinai Hospital and immediately operated upon.

The usual curvilinear incision was made through the skin and periosteum over the mastoid process. The entire mastoid process was involved in an acute inflammatory process of severe type. The bone was of a greenish-yellow hue; cells infiltrated with thick greenish fluid. Culture showed streptococci. The entire mastoid process was removed, the extensively necrosed bone being removed en masse. The sigmoid sinus plate was necrotic. and its removal exposed the sinus wall. The vessel was contracted and appeared to be thrombosed. The mastoid emissary vein was exposed and traced to its ending in the sinus; it also was thrombosed. On removing the cells over the mastoid antrum, a fistulous tract was seen through the roof, through which pus escaped. This opening was enlarged, and about two drams of greenish pus under great tension. were liberated. The dura was further exposed anteriorly by removing a large plate of bone from the squamous plate of the temporal bone. The antral and tympanic roof were also removed. The dura was then seen to be markedly congested, bluish black, and bulged pronouncedly. It was freely incised. The brain was much congested, having a friable appearance over a large area, with exudation. The pia arachnoid was greatly congested. Fresh adhesions between the pia arachnoid and dura were bluntly separated, and a gauze drain was inserted into the subdural space. The brain was pulsating, bulging, and markedly softened. The vertical limb of the sigmoid sinus was then compressed above and below and was incised. A fresh reddish brown clot presented, after which there was an escape of blood. Free hemorrhage was established from the distal and proximal ends of the vessel. The blood culture showed four colonies of streptococci to each ccm.; polymorphonuclear count 90%; white blood count 31,000.

On the day after the operation the patient was in a state of wild delirium, and lumbar puncture was resorted to for relief of the cranial pressure. The cerebrospinal fluid escaped under great tension and was cloudy. but bacteriologically negative. Polymorphonuclear count 25%: albumin increased. Prior to the receipt of the laboratory report on the cerebrospinal fluid, antistreptococcic fluid had been injected into the spinal canal. The next day the patient was still delirious and was aroused with difficulty. Lumbar puncture was followed by a flow of clear fluid still under great pressure. Blood culture now sterile. The next day the patient was somewhat rational. From this time the patient gradually improved until the 18th of March, when she again became extremely irritable and sank into a stuporous state. Her temperature rose abruptly to 106°; polynuclear count 84%.. Lumbar puncture resulted in the escape of a large quantity of turbid fluid under great pressure. Smears and culture of fluid negative. Polymorphonuclear count 5%; mononuclears 95%. During the next day the patient's condition showed no improvement, and she was very noisy and unmanageable. On the 20th, the temperature came down to 101°, and she seemed markedly improved. The condition of the last few days was attributed to a local encephalitis rather than to a general cerebral process. From this time her improvement was gradual and uninterrupted, and ended in complete recovery.

Dr. CHAMBERS said that the doctor, as well as the family, should be congratulated on the fortunate outcome in so remarkable a case.

A Case of Sinus Thrombosis.

Dr. E. GRUENING. Boy, aged 10, admitted to Mt. Sinai Hospital March, 1908, with a temperature of 105° and symptoms of sinus thrombosis. A blood culture was taken on the operating table and the streptococcus found in the blood. In the operation the sinus plate was completely removed and the jugular bulb exposed according to Grunert's method. It was not difficult to do this. The transverse process of the first cervical vertebra was not in the way, as in the first case reported by Grunert. The internal jugular vein was ligated and exsected. The clots were removed from the sigmoid and lateral sinuses.

The next day the temperature rose to 107° and within a few hours fell to 95°, a drop of 12°. It remained at 95° four hours and then rose to 106°. A blood culture taken 24 hours after the operation was negative.

A few days later the streptococcus reappeared in the blood. Mastoiditis was found on the right side and a disintegrated clot in the left lateral sinus. The necessary operations performed. Then he had a number of abscesses in different parts of the body, viz.: in the muscles of the thigh, in the muscles of the arms, in the perineum, in the suprapubic region and in the right knee joint. Dr. Howard Lilienthal aspirated and immobilized the knee, and although eight ounces of streptococcic pus were withdrawn from the knee the boy has a perfect joint.

Paper: Sinus Thrombosis and Streptococcemia.[*]

By Emil Gruening, M. D.

DISCUSSION.

Dr. Duel said that Dr. Gruening was to be congratulated upon presenting so remarkable a series of very severe cases, with such a very low mortality. They represented a triumph of modern surgery.

The early recognition of streptococcemia by means of blood culture would undoubtedly lead to earlier operation and, consequently, more gratifying results in many doubtful cases of septic sinus thrombosis.

Dr. Libman: I have but little to add to what I said at the meeting of the section last year. When a patient has recurrent chills and temperatures, and streptococci are found in the blood, even if there is no evidence whatsoever of otitis media, recent or old, it is essential, when no other primary focus can be found, to expose the mastoid and the sinus. The other conditions in which repeated chills with fever occur, and in which streptococci are found in the blood, are infective thromboses of the pelvic veins arising in the male or female genito-urinary tract, infective thromboses of the cerebral sinuses or of the veins of the extremities, and in infective endocarditis. In cases of infective thromboses of the extremities there is local evidence of the disease. In infective thromboses of the pelvic veins there is always a history of a primary focus. The infective thromboses of the cerebral sinuses, excluding the lateral, which is under discussion now, generally have local symptoms and a demonstrable etiologic factor. When the veins of the portal system are involved, although there may be repeated chills and fever, there are generally no bacteria in the blood unless cholangitis is present, and in that case clinical symptoms are present. There are cases with repeated chills and fever in which there is an infection of the veins leading from the throat, but in all such cases the clinical features

[*]This paper, elaborated and more fully discussed, was read at the meeting following.

are distinct. This shows how easy it is in many cases to arrive
by exclusion at the possible source of the infection, and how
important a clew a slight otitis media may give. The cases of
acute infective endocarditis are, as a rule, not difficult to
diagnose. When it is doubtful whether an acute endocarditis
is present or not, it will be found wiser, in the presence of any
evidences of ear trouble, recent or old, to make an exploration
of the sinus.

A point of great interest has been brought out by this work
on sinus thrombosis. The work has shown the rapidity with
which bacteria are gotten rid of by the body fluids. When the
jugular vein is tied off and there have been streptococci in
the blood, the organisms disappear from the blood quite rapidly. In one case we found the blood free eight hours after
operation. These observations have the demonstrative value
of an experiment and show the great difference that exists
between tissue immunity and blood immunity.

Dr. LEDERMAN asked Dr. Libman in a case of sinus
thrombosis which has existed for some time how long he would
expect to find bacteria in the blood, provided no operation was
done? In a cases of sinus thrombosis which has existed some
time, would or would not the blood take care of the bacteria,
even after the clot had become infected? In a case which he
had presented at the last meeting, where symptoms of infected
sinus thrombosis had existed ten days before the speaker had
seen the patient, and operated at once, at no time when the
blood was examined were any bacteria found in the blood.
There were lung complications, breaking down in the neck,
with involvement of the knee joint without suppuration.

Dr. LIBMAN: Dr. Lederman's question is a very pertinent
one, although the answer cannot be made categorically. In
early cases of sinus thrombosis it appears that the blood cultures are practically always positive. This is probably so
because the blood is in part or entirely parietal and bacteria
are washed off by the blood stream. Of course, if there were
an aseptic thrombosis present, there could not be any bacteria
in the blood. There is also a possibility that an infective clot
might have below it a non-infective clot. In the next place, the
blood might acquire such a high bactericidal property in the
course of a short time that the bacteria would be killed off
rapidly.

The main reason, however, why bacteria are at times not present in cases of longer standing is that in these cases pieces of clot are broken off, which are carried to the lungs and are deposited there, the bacteria traveling no further. There may be extensive metastases in the lungs and no bacteria present in the peripheral circulation. We are dealing here with what might be called a partial or incomplete bacteriemia.

DR. HARRIS said that he was not able to contribute anything of value to the discussion, for he had no personal experiences in such blood work as Dr. Gruening had reported, but he wished to express his appreciation of the paper. Through long years of experience he has come to feel that anything which Dr. Gruening may contribute is well worthy of attention. This remarkable series of cases with so low a mortality is a most important showing, and he was particularly impressed with the manner in which the histories were stated, showing how thoroughly they were studied. He had always been impressed with the importance of blood examination, and if this paper has the wide circulation which it deserves it will doubtless have the effect of causing more blood examinations to be made. This ought to be a part of the routine work in all hospitals. Supplemented with what Dr. Libman had said, it has established itself as an important aid in the diagnosis of sinus thrombosis.

DR. SEYMOUR OPPENHEIMER said that he had had the privilege of observing with Dr. Gruening many of the cases of sinus thrombosis with bacteriemia which he had referred to this evening, and wished to express himself as thoroughly in accord with the views contained in the paper. While he did not think that otologists should depend upon the laboratory to establish the diagnosis of sinus thrombosis, yet he had come to regard blood culture examinations as a definite part of the examination. In Dr. Gruening's service at Mt. Sinai Hospital it has been the practice in many cases to have a blood culture taken at the time of the mastoid operation. This has demonstrated almost conclusively that mastoidal disease per se does not produce a bacteriemia. Therefore the value of a positive blood culture is self-evident. In view of the number of atypical cases of thrombosis which have come under observation, in which clinical signs did not allow of the establishment of a definite diagnosis, the value of this work cannot be overestimated. For example, in one of the first cases reported by Dr. Gruening, the patient was admitted to the hospital in a state of coma. The general physical examination was negative, chronic suppurative otitis was noticed, but no mastoidal symptoms; blood culture positive—diagnosis of sinus thrombosis made and proven at operation.

Another point: While he recognizes, after exposing the sigmoid sinus, the usual operatively construed indications for proceeding or not proceeding further and ligating the jugular, yet he feels that in the positive blood culture we have a much more definite and accurate working basis. For example, a mastoid operation having been performed and evidences of sinus thrombosis subsequently develop or are present at the time of the primary operation—the sinus is operated, blood culture found positive and remains positive even in the presence of no evidence of jugular involvement. The logical deduction is that the general systemic invasion is still going on; that the jugular is the main channel through which this invasion can with reasonable certainty be said to be the case, in view of the constant conversion of positive into negative cultures after jugular ligation.

In the last case which he had observed, blood culture eight hours after operation on the jugular gave a negative result, but unfortunately in this case metastases in lungs and joints came several days after the blood was free from bacteria, due to bacteria lodged earlier. Dr. Libman has called attention to the fact that all the foci in which bacteria have been deposited do not show activity at once.

DR. OPPENHEIMER then referred to two cases in a series of his own; the first a young woman upon whom a mastoid operation was performed, followed by operation upon the sigmoid sinus. This was the first case in which he had any experience with the blood culture taken after a sinus operation. It showed a bacteriemia of four or five colonies of bacteria to each cc. Subsequent cultures showed increasing colonies up to sixty. The clinical signs were not sufficient to justify opening the mastoid. The case was atypical and did not suggest the presence of a septic thrombus in the jugular vein. Subsequently the patient developed a chill and high temperature, and thereupon the jugular vein was ligated and a thrombus found.

In another case, a mastoid operation was performed upon a

young man. Three weeks after the operation, although he was running a practically normal temperature, never above 100°, yet he was not looking right. He had frontal headache, and looked septic, although the temperature did not suggest it. A blood culture was taken and showed 230 colonies of the streptococci to each cc. of blood. The jugular vein was ligated and found to be thrombosed. One portion of the thrombus was well organized and the other had broken down.

Both of these patients made excellent recoveries, and in both the diagnosis was made by the blood culture and not by the clinical signs.

DR. CHAMBERS said that Dr. Oppenheimer had spoken of using antistreptococcus serum, and he would like to know how many times it was employed.

Dr. Gruening, in his report, makes no record of its use. From the report he gathered that Dr. Gruening feels that one must be satisfied that there is no clot left in the sinus or in the jugular vein, but one must go down to the clavicle, and to the bulb, and to the lateral sinus, as necessary, until the blood flows freely from both ends of the opening in the vein. So he supposes Dr. Gruening does not use antistreptococcus serum.

DR. OPPENHEIMER, replying to Dr. Chambers, said that one injection of antistreptococcus serum was made in the cerebrospinal canal, and it did not modify the temperature.

In view of the fact that 90 per cent of the cases observed at Mt. Sinai, in which the operation had been performed on the sigmoid sinus, and in which blood culture had been positive, the jugular vein had to be subsequently ligated, he would like to know whether Dr. Gruening would not be inclined to go a step further and say that the presence of a positive blood culture would not be an indication for the primary ligation of the jugular.

DR. LEWIS inquired whether Dr. Gruening had done more than one Grunert operation on the jugular bulb. It seems to be a very difficult operation, and he himself had had no experieuce with it. He would like to know also if other members of the section had had experience with it.

DR. GRUENING said that he generally ties the jugular in thrombosis of the lateral sinus and does so before the removal of the thrombus. He had performed the Grunert operation three times in children, and found no particular difficulty. It may not be so easy in the adult.

Sequestrum of Labyrinth—History.

BY FRANK T. HOPKINS, M. D.

DISCUSSION.

DR. GERHARD H. COCKS asked Dr. Hopkins to which test he referred. when he used the term experimental nystagmus. Did he mean caloric nystagmus (hot and cold water), or did he refer to Barany's compression and aspiration nystagmus?

DR. HOPKINS replied that he referred to caloric nystagmus —produced by hot or cold water.

NEW YORK ACADEMY OF MEDICINE.
SECTION ON OTOLOGY.

Transactions of the Meeting, January 8, 1909.

RORERT LEWIS, M. D., CHAIRMAN.

A New Method for Inflating the Eustachian Tube and Middle Ear.*
By EDMUND PRICE FOWLER, M. D.

NEW YORK.

Necrosis of the Cochlea. Report and Analysis of a Case.†
By ALFRED MICHAELIS, M. D.,

NEW YORK.

DISCUSSION.

DR. FOWLER asked if any of the heat and cold tests produced nystagmus.

DR. MICHAELS replied that he had made no nystagmus tests, nor heat and cold tests. He had not noticed any nystagmus.

DR. KERRISON said that there could be no doubt that the tones which appeared to have been heard in this case by the ear from which the labyrinth had been removed, had in reality been heard by the sound ear—this in spite of the closure of the meatus by the finger. This seems to be the correct conclusion from the tones which the patient did hear. Take, for example, any patient with a moderate grade of tympanic deafness or impairment, and ask him to close both ears with a finger pressed in each meatus. It will be found that the lower tones, i. e., 18 d. v. to 128 d. v., will not be heard, while it may be quite impossible to exclude the upper tones, e. g., 1024 d. v.—2048 d. v. Now, it is just these higher musical tones which the patient is reported to have heard, and it seems clear

---

*See page 852.
†See page 511, September Annais.

that they must have been heard by the sound ear, and not by the ear in which the labyrinth had been destroyed.

DR. LEWIS said that the case was a very interesting one, taking into consideration the conservative treatment which had brought about the desired results.

DR. KENEFICK said that the point mentioned by Dr. Lewis was the one which he wished to emphasize—the conservative or expectant treatment in certain cases of chronic suppuration, with granulation and polypi present. In two cases at the New York Eye and Ear Infirmary—cases of long-continued suppuration, in which it seemed best to try and relieve the situation by conservative treatment—they began treatment, not by removing the polypi in the first place, for the canal was so swollen that nothing could be done that way, but by cleansing the ear, gradually reducing the swelling, and later syringing, removed the malleus and incus. It now appeared probable that the patient would escape the radical operation. In the second case, which is still under care at the Infirmary, the granulation tissue was removed in the clinic, and the patient was kept in the hospital for observation. She had slight attacks of vertigo and nausea, and the day before a small piece of bone was syringed from the ear. The nurse in charge was inexperienced, and the bone was thrown away, but she spoke of it as a very small spicule, evidently an ossicle. We frequently see in the clinic cases in which the canal appears to be occluded and completely epidermatized at the fundus, cases in which no operation has ever been done, and the patient will give a history of very long-continued suppuration. It would seem that in these cases which have had no treatment, such as would be considered proper to-day, nature proceeds along these lines, finally expelling the ossicular sequestrum, and the fundus becoming epidermatized, the case is closed. That is the ideal radical operation which we try to produce artificially, but we see very few ossiculectomies or radicals which close up as beautifully as the cases which were never operated upon.

DR. MICHAELIS said that the discovery of this case was largely accidental, for if he had not found the sequestrum it would have been overlooked. These sequestra frequently elude discovery. He is observing a young man of 17 or 18 years now, in the expectation of getting a sequestrum. The diagnosis of labyrinthine necrosis is absolutely clear. There is facial paralysis, a perforation through Shrapnells', with exuberant granulations protruding, and several severe attacks of vertigo. The granulations were cleared out as well as possible, securing better drainage, with the result that the patient improved. The facial paralysis improved very much, and with the exception of a little twitching of the muscles the patient is apparently all right.

Bezold says that he has noticed that sequestra were often found beneath granulations which were teat-like and partially perforated. This was true of the case he had just spoken of. During the treatment he had noticed a teat-like protrusion on the membrana tympani, a little distance from the perforation. This gradually became perforated, and a drop of pus would come through. Then it would close, and a week or two later it would go through the same cycle. It seems probable that there is a sequestrum beneath it, trying to get out.

The patient is seen once a week and is carefully watched, and all danger symptoms are explained to him, by which he should be guided in case they arise. Much can be done without resorting to the knife, and many of these cases can be saved from the radical operation.

Paper: A Plastic Mastoid Operation—A New Method of Operating in Acute Mastoiditis.*

By Frank T. Hopkins, M. D.

DISCUSSION.

Dr. Kenefick said that he was much interested in some of Dr. Hopkins' cases while under treatment, and while the immediate closure of the posterior wound is a very attractive and most desirable procedure, still there are certain cases where the bone wound is especially extensive and irregular, in which the closure of the posterior flaps would make it very difficult for one unfamiliar with the wound to carry out the subsequent treatment. In other words, if he himself performed this operation, he would wish to carry it through the healing process himself, and not entrust the subsequent care of the case to any one who was not familiar with the wound. From a cosmetic point of view, in cases where that would be of great

*See page 864.

importance, as in actors or actresses, the operation might serve a very excellent purpose. He would like to try it in some cases, but in general could not help feeling that he preferred to see the open wound and watch its granulation from every part.

DR. HOPKINS, replying to an inquiry from Dr. Lewis as to whether there was not quite a sulcus in the anterior wall of the posterior portion of the canal, as in a radical mastoid operation, said that he had such a sulcus in one of the cases reported, but in the others which are still under observation there was not much of a sulcus. This, however, he could determine more definitely later, some time after the operation, when the chances of retraction are greater. One patient now has a good deal of sulcus which he did not have soon after the operation. The other cases have not yet shown this, but they may develop it later.

DR. RAE could not admit Dr. Hopkins had proved his point by the cases he had presented, whatever might be the results of later experience. There was no gain in the time of healing, nor were the posterior scars better than the average treated by older methods. His cases had, in addition, the deformity of the meatus, due to the formation of the flap. Experience with rapid methods of closure, as opposed to the open method, has already shown that the most grave complications may arise and be unsuspected for some time. This criticism can certainly be applied to the method advocated by Dr. Hopkins, and while no method can be entirely free from the risk of complications, the proportion of their occurrence should be less, and their detection earlier, when the old method of treating the post-auricular wound as an open one is followed. The one positive advantage of the method—frequently of great importance where a living for the patient and those dependent upon him must be considered—is the early removal of the unsightly dressing.

DR. LEWIS thought that in these cases one would have somewhat the same conditions arise as in the radical mastoid operation, where there is always a deep sulcus in the excavated mastoid process, where cerumen and broken-down epithelial cells often collect, and which have to be removed with more or less frequency. The same condition is likely to be present here. That would be more of a detriment than to have the wound take a little longer to heal, and when healed be without any such deformity in the meatus. He agreed with what Dr. Rea had said regarding the dangers resulting from such closure of the wound, especially when the sinus or dura was exposed. He could not see that the time of healing had been shortened to any great extent. One case had healed in five weeks, but the others took eight weeks, the ordinary time of healing under the usual method.

Dr. Hopkins, replying to the remarks of the chairman as to the length of time required for the healing, said, that although it had been shortened to five weeks in the last case, and in other cases could be made much shorter, for each succeeding case healed in a shorter time than the previous one. The actual length of time required for the healing of a case, however, was only a part of the benefit which he claimed for the operation. The most important benefit was the closure of the posterior wound, which gave the patient the opportunity to go about his business without the bandage on the head, which is so great a detriment with the ordinary mastoid operation, where it cannot be removed for many weeks. It is certainly a great advantage to a majority of patients to go about as in the natural order of things and not appear so long in the surgeon's hands.

NEW YORK OTOLOGICAL SOCIETY.

DR. J. E. SHEPPARD, PRESIDENT.

Meeting November 28, 1908.

DR. GRUENING reported a case of

Double Lobule of the Ear, One Lateral and One Median.

He also reported a case of

Serous Meningitis Secondary to Mastoiditis.

The patient was admitted to the hospital with a temperature of 105°, in a semi-comatose condition. The leucocyte count was high. A lumbar puncture was made, showing a clear fluid. The next day the patient was decidedly better. A mastoid operation was performed, and there was a prompt recovery.

DISCUSSION.

DR. McKERNON said that he had recently seen a case of serous meningitis, following the mastoid operation, where an attempt had been made to close the wound by the blood clot. The wound itself, when seen by him, looked excellent. The patient, however, complained of intense pain in the head. There was a leucocyte count of 22,000, and a polynuclear percentage of 92 per cent. The wound was reopened and necrotic bone discovered. That night the patient had high temperature and was unconscious. A lumbar puncture was made and 60 cc. of clear fluid drawn off. In eighteen days nine lumbar punctures were made—all showing sterile fluid. Patient made good recovery. Dr. McKernon thinks that the lumbar puncture saved the patient's life.

DR. ROBERT LEWIS, JR., reported a case of

Cavernous Sinus Thrombosis

which he had recently seen. The patient, a boy, when seen by Dr. Lewis had been suffering for four days from an attack of acute tonsillitis. There was an exophthalmus of the left eye, a chemosis of the conjunctiva of the left eye and the left eyelids; the fundus of the eye was normal; a pneumonia of the base of the right lung was present. There was no strabismus; no headache, and no vomiting. The patient was drowsy, but rational when spoken to; when attempting to walk he would have fallen had he not been supported. The temperature was 104° F. The ears were normal. The boy died twenty-four hours later. A postmortem showed, besides pneumonia, a thrombosis of the cavernous sinuses of the left inferior petrosal sinus and of the left orbital veins; the lateral sinus and the jugular vein were normal. The infection evidently spread from the tonsillar structures to the sinuses through the pterygoid plexus of the veins.

DR. GRUENING spoke of a case of thrombosis of almost all the sinuses of the dura mater without optic neuritis. This sems to corroborate the view that optic neuritis is due to an increase of the intracranial pressure and not to the obstruction of the veins alone.

DR. MCKERNON spoke of a case of cavernous sinus thrombosis in a child of six years. An operation for adenoids had been performed by a physician in the country six days before. There was a characteristic swelling of the eyelids. Death took place in four days. In this case there was a thrombosis of both cavernous sinuses.

DR. MCKERNON reported having seen in consultation three cases of

Sinus Thrombosis Following the Simple Mastoid Operation, Where an .Attempt Had Been Made to Induce Healing by the Primary Blood Clot Method.

Two of the cases died. In the third case the vein was ligated. Complications manifested themselves on the 6th, 12th and 14th days, respectively, in the three cases. All three were seen within the past eight months. As a result of these and other cases reported, Dr. McKernon was strongly of the opinion that this method of promoting healing was not sound surgery.

DISCUSSION.

DR. GRUENING repeated the views he had previously expressed in condemnation of the method, stating that his objections had been a priori, while Dr. McKernon's were a posteriori.

DR. DENCH agreed with the views expressed by Dr. McKernon, although he himself had done three cases successfully by this method.

DR. BRYANT stated that he did not believe in completely closing the wound, but in leaving a small opening for the insertion of a drain. In this way he had had no bad results; and in 80 to 90 per cent of his cases the clot had not broken down sufficiently to interfere with the course of healing. He laid stress upon as complete an obliteration of the disease processes as possible, and applying a skin flap into the wound. He regarded complete healing within 14 days as a fairly satisfactory results. Otorrhea does not occur.

DR. RAE emphasized the fact that the method pursued by Dr. Bryant was not in reality a healing by the blood clot, and only differed from the usual method pursued in a more complete closure of the wound.

DR. BERENS said that he had seen a number of these cases, and spoke especially of the case of a child where he had had a most satisfactory result, the patient being well in two weeks. The discharge, however, recurred through the ear, and persisted during the summer, compelling him this fall to do a radical operation. At this time a large pus sac was discovered beneath the natural-looking soft parts, and in spite of the thorough primary operation granulations were found in the attic, and necrosis in the region of the semicircular canals.

DR. DUEL had attempted healing by the blood clot method in a number of cases. At first he had good results superficially. Then one case in this number which had healed promptly developed a sinus thrombosis and died. He believed that the method was not based on sound surgical principles, and in the future should be satisfied with slower healing with the least possible opportunity for disaster. He called attention to the value of the usual method of drainage of the attic by gauze (which in the case of acute mastoiditis is usually full of granulations). Rapid subsidence of the inflammation in the middle ear, which results from good posterior drainage, conserves the hearing functions very materially.

DR. HASKIN spoke of a case in his own practice of prompt healing where this method had been pursued. In nine months, however, pain and discharge compelled a secondary operation, and a sinus was discovered extending to the bottom of the wound, from the region of the former attic. The blood clot had apparently become organized and showed new bone formation.

DR. SHEPPARD had pursued the method in only six or seven cases, in three of which he had primary union, the others having required reopening.

DR. BERENS reported a case of

Mastoiditis Complicated by Diabetes Mellitus.

in a man of 34. The percentage of sugar was not determined. When seen by Dr. Berens, there was a swelling all around the ear. The disease had lasted for six or seven weeks. There was no temperature and no pain. On account of the failure of the mastoiditis to improve, and recognizing the hazard entailed, a mastoid operation was performed by him, and a large sequestrum was removed. Its removal exposed the dura and the knee of the lateral sinus. Death 40 hours later in coma. Ether had been used by the drop method, as the anesthetic— not more than three ounces in all. Death was attributed to diabetic coma from shock rather than from the ether.

DISCUSSION.

DR. GRUENING spoke of a case of mastoiditis complicated by diabetes, with 4 per cent of sugar, acetone, and diacetic acid. Operation was performed under ether, narcosis lasting 20 minutes. Good recovery. He felt that the presence of diabetes should in no way retard operation when necessary.

DR. HASKIN spoke of mastoiditis, complicated by diabetes, where he had operated under local anesthesia—cocain 1 per cent, and adrenalin chlorid 1-1000, equal parts. A good recovery took place.

DR. COWEN referred to a case of mastoiditis complicated by diabetes where he had operated under gas and ether narcosis. The operation lasted only 25 minutes. Death followed from 48 to 72 hours later from internal stomachic hemorrhage.

DR. DENCH reported a case of

Mastoiditis, Epidural Abscess, and Sinus Thrombosis.

Three weeks previously an operation had been performed on the nose, followed by acute inflammation of the ear, for which the drum had been incised. When seen by Dr. Dench there was marked mastoid tenderness and a fusiform swelling, extending from behind the ear into the neck, indicating a Bezold perforation. There was a profuse aural discharge. A complete mastoid operation revealed an epidural abscess and a destruction of the lower part of the lateral sinus. The swelling in the neck was found to be a mass of lymphatic glands, which were excised and the jugular vein ligated and excised. An interesting fact was that there was so little evidence of general sepsis. It was a streptococcus infection.

DISCUSSION.

DR. GRUENING had seen a similar case in a soldier. Here the mastoid cells were found to be filled with serum. There was a thrombosis of the leg. No temperature. The lateral sinus was not opened. Good recovery.

DR. McKERNON inquired into the size of the remaining portion of the sinus. Dr. Dench replied that it was rather small.

DR. HASKIN mentioned a case of

Pulmonary Tuberculosis Complicated by Tubercular Mastoiditis and Swelling of the Neck.

Here the operation showed a large sequestrum involving the superior part of the petrosa. The healing in the mastoid wound had progressed favorably, but it was necessary later to open the swelling in the neck, which was due to enlarged glands. The lateral sinus was not involved.

DR. HASKIN recommended the hypodermic use of adrenalin chlorid underneath the periosteum of the canal after general anesthesia had been induced. In this way he had been able to greatly reduce the amount of bleeding in the radical operation for chronic suppuration.

DR. HARRIS reported a case of

Vertigo.

in a man of 45, which had persisted for over a year, which had been preceded for a short time by a tinnitus in the left ear. The onset of the vertigo followed a severe blow on the temple bone of the left side from a falling plank. This stunned him for a moment, but there was no other apparent damage. Family and personal history negative. He was a mechanic. He had been under the care of a number of good physicians, who had given him pilocarpin, strychnin, and potash, without benefit. He was first seen by Dr. Harris last August. Functional tests showed entire absence of all internal ear disease. There was prolonged Schwabach and raising of the lower tone limit in the Hartmann series of tuning forks. There was no history of previous disease of the ear, and the drum was normal. Under these circumstances, Dr. Harris felt that there was very probably present a binding down of the ossicular chain, and under local anesthesia he removed the malleus and incus. There was satisfactory improvement for a period of three or four weeks, but at the end of that time the vertigo returned and persisted. He 'had never been able until recently to discover any nystagmus, but had noted this condition the day previously. The nystagmus. however, was contradictory; that is, it appeared both away from and toward the affected eye. The caloric test was also· unsatisfactory, in that the left ear gave the same contradictory reaction, and it was impossible with cold water to get nystagmus in the healthy ear. Nothing abnormal has been discovered in the eyeground or in the urine.

Dr. Wilcox, the clinician of the hospital, reported that the man had a distinct arteriosclerosis. There is nothing characteristic about the vertigo. The man does not fall in any one direction. The attacks are for the most part not severe, and there is a vertiginous condition rather than a complaint of isolated attacks. The case is of interest from a diagnostic and therapeutic standpoint. Dr. Harris is inclined to believe that the condition is largely functional, being in all probability dependent on the original trauma.

DISCUSSION.

Dr. Haskin, who has seen the case from time to time, agreed that the disease was probably located in the semicircular canals.

Dr. McKernon, who had also seen the case, felt that from the history of the vertigo developing after the injury, there· was probably a clot in the semicircular canal.

Dr. Duel called attention to the fact that the whole cochlea had to be destroyed in order to produce a loss of bone conduction. In some instances, where only a portion of the cochlea had been destroyed, Weber was referred to that side, and Rinne was negative on that side.

Injury Over the Mastoid, Followed by Immediate Loss of Hearing.

Dr. Kenefick referred to a case of injury of the head in a longshoreman whom he has seen. The injury was received over the mastoid, and was followed by immediate loss of hearing. There was no involvement of the middle ear.

DR. JOHN L. ADAMS, PRESIDENT.

Meeting January 26, 1909.

DR. JAMES F. McKERNON presented a specimen showing a
Sequestrum of the Entire Labyrinth.

This was removed in the course of an operation on the ear
of a child 3½ years of age. There was history of otorrhea
since 3 years of age. When seen by him there was a complete facial paralysis. Three days later the child became unconscious; temperature 104°. There was a spontaneous nystagmus toward the healthy side. He operated the same day.
The mastoid was found extensively diseased. A Schwartze-
Stacke operation was performed, in the course of which a
sequestrum, representing the entire labyrinth, was removed.
The dura was extensively exposed. Following the operation
the temperature fluctuated and the child remained unconscious. Six days later the sinus was opened, and the blood
current found normal. Four days later a lumbar puncture was
made, showing a turbid fluid containing many bacteria. This
was followed by a subarachnoid drainage with chromosized
gut. Two days later another puncture was made, and a large
amount of fluid withdrawn. A similar drainage was introduced at another point. For the first time now there was a
return of consciousness. The posterior wound was closed on
the twenty-ninth day, and the child made a good recovery.

McKernon dwelt upon the importance of puncture and
drainage in cases of meningitis, and stated that in his belief
many cases which we have lost in the past might have been
saved if such a course had been pursued.

DISCUSSION.

DR. WHITING referred to a case in a child of seven suffering from facial paralysis, where he had removed in the course
of an operation a sequestrum of the entire labyrinth. The
sequestrum was so large that he hesitated at first to remove it
en masse, and attempted to take it out piecemeal.

Dr. Bryant reported the autopsy of a man who died recently in one of the hospitals for the insane in this city. The autopsy showed

Streptococcic Infection; Left-Sided Chronic Otorrhea; Thrombosis Extended from the Right Ear Almost to the Left Jugular Bulb; Thrombosis of Longitudinal Sinus, Forward to the Motor Area; and Thrombosis of the Cerebral Veins Between the Thrombosed Sinuses. Cause of Death Was Metastatic Thrombosis in Lungs.

History.—The patient had been seized with a maniacal attack about three weeks previous to his death, and had been admitted as insane. The psychic diagnosis was toxic, depressant insanity. The patient remained inaccessible. No motor symptoms were noted during life. No note of the ear condition was made until 12 days before death, when it was noted that one ear was discharging. No cause for the mental condition was determined previous to the autopsy. There is a rumor that cases come to autopsy from time to time where death is consequent to central complications of ear infection, but where no antemortem suspicion exists that the mental state depends upon an ear lesion.

Sinus Thrombosis Three-fourths of an Inch From the Seat of Inflammation.

Dr. Lewis reported an operation for mastoiditis where, owing to erosion of the inner table of the mastoid process, it was necessary to expose the sinus from a little beyond the knee to within a few mm. of the bulb. The sinus was healthy. During the two weeks following, the process of healing was in every way satisfactory, save a small spot over the knee of the sinus. The patient left the Infirmary, returning to the Clinic for dressing. One evening after a hard defecation he found the bandage soaked with blood. When later the dressing was removed a very severe hemorrhage followed. He was again put to bed; forty-eight hours later a chill occurred, followed by a rise of temperature. An operation for sinus thrombosis was performed the next day, and a clot was found, not at the point of ulceration of the vein, but some distance below in the jugular bulb. The internal jugular vein was tied and excised. The patient is making a good recovery.

The interesting points are: First—The minute area of

sinus apparently involved in the area of ulceration, not more than one mm. in circumference. Second—The fact that the seat of thrombosis was at least three-fourths of an inch beyond the inflammatory area. Third—The hemorrhage occurring spontaneously, a condition which, as far as I am aware of, has not been hitherto mentioned, and of course (fortunately) must be rare, as usually the thrombus forms in the vein around the inflammatory area, and thus prevents any such accident.

Dr. Whiting reported two cases in children of a

Swelling in the Zygomatic Fossa.

Incision revealed that it contained a large quantity of pus. The mastoid antrum was healthy. There was a subdural abscess. The pus had escaped from the tympanum, through the Rivinian fissure. The inner table showed an erosion the size of a twenty-five cent piece. The second case was similar, save that it had burrowed in the region of the suprameatal triangle.

Dr. Quinlan reported a

Fatal Case of Mastoiditis.

in a man 39 years of age. An operation had been performed on the mastoid for acute typical condition, and apparently convalescence was assured. The wound healed and the man was discharged from the hospital five weeks after the operation. The patient returned two weeks later with well-marked redness along the line of incision, and with intense tenderness on the entire process. This was accompanied with a chilly sensation and a temperature of 103°. Ordinary conservative remedies were applied, but the case indicated surgical interference. A second operation was done Christmas Day. The wound was found to be filled with granulations, no pus, but upon close inspection it was noticed that the roof of the tympanum was absent. It had apparently been eroded away, and the dura sagged through the opening. An incision was made into the dura, bringing away only some serum mixed with blood. An inch of gauze was inserted to establish drainage, but the patient, some days later, developed convulsions and remained in a semicomatose condition for five days, when death followed.

DR. DENCH said that he had seen several similar cases. The first was that of a woman suffering from an acute otitis media. Some mastoid tenderness was present when she first presented for treatment, but this disappeared after free incision of the drum membrane. Some weeks later the patient returned to the hospital, suffering from symptoms of mastoid involvement. The mastoid operation was performed, and extensive destruction of the mastoid process found. Convalescence was rapid, and the patient was discharged from the hospital. Four or five weeks after her discharge from the hospital, she again came under observation. The mastoid wound had almost entirely healed, and seemed to be in a thoroughly healthy condition. The patient, however, complained of headache, pain in the back and lower extremities, as well as general malaise. The temperature was 103 degrees. The patient was admitted to the hospital. A differential blood count showed no deviation from the normal standard. The temperature fell to normal on the day after admission to the hospital, and for several days the patient seemed perfectly well. Three or four days after admission, the patient suddenly complained of headache, the temperature rose to 104 degrees, and she rapidly developed symptoms of meningitis. The lateral ventricle on the affected side was drained, but the patient died.

In a second case a fatal meningitis followed an apparently successful mastoid operation. Here Dench drained the fourth ventricle. In his opinion, we have yet much to learn about these meningeal complications. Lumbar puncture is of decided value here, and can be profitably resorted to before any operation on the meninges is performed.

DR. LUTZ reported a fatal case of mastoiditis, occurring in a man who had a history of an otorrhea for six weeks. When first seen by him the man was complaining of severe pain on the side of the affected ear. There was a small quantity of pus in the ear, which seemed to come from an erosion in the posterior wall of the canal. There was no elevation of temperature or pulse. The operation was at first refused. Several days later, when he was called in to operate he found a sinus leading down into the antrum. There was pus in the zygomatic cells. The pus was found to proceed through the dura, beneath which a large abscess cavity was discovered. This was thoroughly drained. The pus was not offensive. Eight days after the operation the temperature began to rise. On the tenth day the patient became unconscious; paralysis of arm and leg of opposite side, and death. No autopsy. The interesting point in the case was the extra large size of the abscess cavity, which occupied almost all of the left half of the cerebrum.

DR. DENCH reported a

Radical Operation for Double Suppurative Otitis Media.

No labyrinthine symptoms were present before operation. At the time of operation the oval window was found open and covered with granulations. No trace of the stapes was discovered. The granulations were carefully removed, but the labyrinth was not drained. The temperature rose to 101° after the operation, and for a few days there was slight nystagmus and staggering gait. Both of these symptoms rapidly disappeared, and the patient made a good recovery.

The reporter wished to know whether, in the opinion of the society, in the absence of labyrinthine symptoms, and the mere fact that the oval window was found open at the time of the operation, these conditions would be a sufficient indication for the institution of free labyrinthine drainage.

DISCUSSION.

DR. McKERNON saw no reason for labyrinthine drainage in this case.

DR. WHITING was of the same opinion as Dr. McKernon. He referred to an operation which he had performed for encapsulated cholesteatoma, where a bud of granulation was found in the oval window. A probe showed it firm, so he let it alone. The patient recovered.

DR. DUEL reported a case which he had recently seen where the

Smear Taken From the Secretion Following an Incision Made in the Drum Membrane Showed the Colon Bacillus.

This was a case of a patient suffering from a slight stuffiness in both ears, associated with sore throat. There was no elevation of temperature and no pain. Examination showed a redness and loss of lustre of the right drum membrane ; congestion in Schrapnell's and along the malleus, without loss of lustre in the left. A solution of adrenalin chlorid was ordered locally. Next day the redness had disappeared from the left drum membrane, but had increased in the right. The day following, this membrane was incised under gas anesthesia, as it was distinctly bulging, dark red in color, and without lustre. There was no pain or rise in temperature. A gush of red fluid followed. The smear showed the colon bacillus. The drum membrane healed and the patient recovered, without complication, in ten days.

NEW YORK OTOLOGICAL SOCIETY.

JOHN L. ADAMS, M. D., PRESIDENT.

Regular Meeting March 23, 1909.

DR. ALDERTON presented the brain of a patient who had died from temporosphenoidal abscess, with the following history:

Case of Brain Abscess of Otitic Origin.

Albert H. Age 44 years; laborer; German. Admitted to the King County Hospital, December 5, 1908. Family and previous history could not be obtained because of the patient's inability to talk; but patient points to the throat and claims to have had trouble for four months.

Patient is a fairly well-nourished male, weighing about 140 pounds. He has ptosis of the left eye, left facial paralysis; the tongue is dry and coated and deviates to the left. There is a large amount of muco-pus in the pharynx, which he is unable to expel; also, paralysis of soft palate, and patient is unable to swallow even small quantities of fluid. There exists a purulent discharge from the right ear; no tenderness, edema or redness over either mastoid; no cording along neck. Heart and lungs are normal.

December 6, 1908. Patient has developed considerable post-cervical rigidity; left pupil contracted and sluggish; considerable photophobia; paresis of left arm and leg, but no absolute hemiplegia; left knee jerk increased; slight left ankle clonus; all left arm jerks increased; is in a semicomatose condition and has large quantities of mucus in pharynx.

December 7, 1908. Patient is brighter this morning; left-sided paresis decreased.

December 8, 1908. Patient sinking into coma at 1 a. m.; lungs filling up; pulse rapid and weak; respiration rapid and labored. 4:30 a. m. patient died.

On December 6th Dr. Tilney was called in consultation and diagnosed an inoperable brain abscess; his report is appended.

The neurological examination made of the patient on December 6th brought out the following facts:

The Reflexes.—All the reflexes on the left side of the body were exaggerated both in force and degree of excursion as compared with those of the right side. Babinski reflex positive on the left side. A slight transitory clonus was observed in the left foot. Negative on the right side.

Voluntary Movements.—Voluntary movements in the left arm and leg apparently abolished. Nurse reports that during this entire day the left extremities have not been observed to move, although the patient is able to respond to all commands which have reference to the right arm and leg.

Sthenic and Tonic Muscular Conditions.—A marked rigidity of the sternocleidotrapezius group on the left side was observed. All the flexor and adductor groups of the left arm and leg, so that the limbs were held in partial flexion and adduction. That this rigidity was of the lower neuron type was evidenced by the fact that the muscular tonicity was not in any degree influenced by the will, although it was apparent that the patient could be made to understand all requests with reference to movements of the limbs.

No change was noted in the volume or consistency of the muscles, nor were any tremors, twitchings or irregular involuntary acts reported or observed. Such coordination as the patient presented in the right extremities was good, but, due to the paresis on the left side, this could not be accurately adjudged.

The patient could neither walk, stand nor maintain the sitting posture.

The semicomatose condition of the patient prevents any exact statements as to the sense qualities, subjectively as well as objectively. Sense perception appared to be normal to such tests as were applicable. A very definite area of sensitiveness was mapped out in the right neck region and about the right mandibular and mastoid processes.

Cranial Nerve Innervations.—Observations as to special senses could not be depended upon. Muscles of both eyeballs were apparently normal in their innervation. A slight left ptosis and paresis of the left orbicularis palpebrarum was noted. The ocular reflexes were all normal.

The entire left side of the face was paralyzed. Mastication was normal, but the act of deglutition was accompanied by considerable regurgitation per nares. Left-sided paresis of

the muscles supplied by the spinal division of the spinal accessory nerve, and also a left hypoglossal paresis.

Mental Status.—Patient was stuporous, but could be aroused
to respond to some requests and answer questions.

The diagnosis of a right-sided brain abscess was based on
the following:

1. The febrile action, which, in conjunction with the characteristic leucocytosis, indicated a purulent process.

2.·Evidence of a purulent otitis media of the right side.

3. Presence of a left hypertonic hemiparesis.

Autopsy.—December 9th, 1908. Dura, after removal of the
calvarium, slightly adherent. The sigmoid sinus contained
blood, coagulated and in the fluid state. The pia mater shows
marked congestion of the veins. The subarachnoidal space
of the convexity of the brain contains no pus. After removal
of the brain, purulent fluid containing shreds and parts of destroyed brain tissue flows off into the middle cerebral fossa
and collects upon the tentorium cerebelli. Dura and pia are
adherent in different places at the base of the temporal lobe,
and in taking the brain out its substance is here torn in a spot
exactly corresponding to a place where an abscess within the
temporal lobe was most superficial. This spot corresponds exactly to a perforation of the dura just above the tegmen tympani and antri of the right temporal bone, through which a
probe passes easily into the antrum of the right ear. The
dura of the median cerebral fossa, above the tegmen tympani
and above the glenoidal fossa, is bulging considerably towards
the cranial cavity; this bulging. is caused by a substance of
dough-like consistency presenting the appearance of cholesteatomatous masses mixed with creamy pus.

The microscopical examination of these masses shows detritus, pus cells, epithelial cells, cholesterin crystals and numerous
diplococci (micrococcus lanceolatus).

The spot where the probe penetrates through the dura and
tegmen tympani into the antrum corresponds exactly to a perforation of the temporal lobe, leading into a stalked multilocular abscess of the temporal lobe, about the size of a walnut.

DISCUSSION.

In reply to a question from Dr. Rae, Dr. Alderton stated
that he did not operate because the neurologist who had seen
the case thought the condition did not permit any operation,

but he was inclined to believe that another time he would have operated in spite of the neurologist's opinion.

DR. ALDERTON presented a case of

Entotic Tinnitus

with the following history:

Case of aural tinnitus; subjectively and objectively perceptible:

A young lady, 31 years of age, was referred to Dr. A——, January 12th, 1909, by Dr. Pendleton of Brooklyn.

She complained of noise in both ears, which had persisted for from five to six weeks; with this there was some blurring of the hearing; also, at times, sharp, shooting pains from throat to the ear. History of discharge from the right ear eight years previously, following the grip.

Examination.—A. D.: Canal normal; membrana tympani irregular in texture, slightly retracted, but of good lustre. Watch heard 2 feet. Lower tone limit c^2; C ac>Bc; C^2ac>Bc. Upper tone limit normal.

• A. S.: Canal normal; membrana tympani same as A. D. Watch heard 1½ feet.

L. t. l., c^2; C ac>Bc; C^2ac>Bc. Upper tone limit normal.

Both Eustachian tubes patent. Nose shows moderate deviation of septum to the right.

On using the otoscope a bruit is heard in both ears, which is synchronous with the pulse; which varies in intensity when present and which disappears entirely from time to time. Pressure on the carotids sometimes will not influence the tinnitus. Changing the position of the head will sometimes cause the tinnitus to disappear when present, but does not seem to cause it to appear when absent. During inflation with the Eustachian catheter the tinnitus will sometimes disappear when present. There is no goitre.

DISCUSSION.

DR. BERENS spoke of the variation in the rate and duration of the pulse during his examination.

DR. DENCH spoke of the possible involvement of the cervical sympathetic.

DR. GRUENING suggested the possibility of pressure in the region of the cavernous sinus.

DR. COWEN referred to a case presented by him to the society many years ago where pressure on the carotid stopped the noise, but the patient could not endure continuous pressure in that region.

Dr. Alderton was inclined to think that the condition was a muscular one and was partially under the patient's control.

Dr. May reported a case of

Atypical Erysipelas Simulating Disease of the Lateral Sinus.

The patient was a child of ten who, two weeks previous to being admitted to the hospital, suffered pain in the left ear, necessitating the opening of the drum. A good recovery followed. On admission to the hospital there was a temperature of 105 with chill. Pain was elicited on pressure over mastoid. There was edema in this region. The left drum was red and a little swollen. The mastoid was opened and found healthy. The sinus was then opened and also found healthy. The blood culture was negative. The temperature fell after the operation. Twenty-four hours later there was another chill with high temperature. The right mastoid became tender. The right drum was red. The mastoid operation was performed on the right side; no disease was found. The right sinus was also exposed and found normal. The following day erysipelas developed, the redness starting at the nose.

DISCUSSION.

Dr. Bacon inquired if there was edema of the scalp.

Dr. May stated that the edema did not extend beyond the mastoid. The gland below the tip was enlarged, suggesting involvement of the lymphatics.

Dr. Gruening did not think that the symptoms as given by Dr. May pointed to mastoiditis.

Dr. Berens stated that he had reported a case of extensive destruction of the mastoid where the drum was normal.

Dr. Lewis referred to a case of mastoiditis under his care some time ago where the only symptom was headache—there was no otorrhea. The operation showed a cortical perforation with epidural and perisinous abscess.

Dr. Toeplitz spoke of the difficulty of diagnosis in children between erysipelas and mastoiditis.

Dr. Cowen thought that the closer we keep to the association between the middle ear and mastoiditis the less chance of error. Primary mastoid disease was very unusual.

Dr. May stated that he operated only because of the serious condition of the child and in spite of the absence of distinct localizing symptoms.

· Dr. Gruening thought that the initial stage of erysipelas may simulate sinus thrombosis.

Severity of Mastoiditis.

Dr. Quinlan inquired if cases of mastoiditis this winter in the practice of members of the society had been severe ones. Those under his care had been very severe. He spoke of the case of a girl whom he had operated upon in St. Vincent's Hospital. Blood examination showed leucocytes of 14,000 and a differential count of 73 to 74 per cent. The operation showed involvement of the deep tip cells.

DISCUSSION.

Dr. Bacon stated that as far as his experience was concerned he had seen about the usual run of cases this winter.

Bacillus Pyocyaneus in the Middle Ear.

Dr. Bacon reported two cases with unusual pathologic findings. One was the case of an adult; the other a case of a child, in both of which a smear made after the opening of the drum showed the bacillus pyocyaneus.

DISCUSSION.

Dr. Dench inquired if a second smear had been made. He had seen a case where the first smear gave the bacillus pyocyaneus, but the second smear showed an error in diagnosis.

Dr. Alderton reported a case of

Mastoiditis Without Localizing Symptoms, but With Profuse, Long Continued Discharge From Ear.

The case was a male who had been treated by a local physician for discharge from the ear, from May until the following November. Repeated incisions had been made into the drum, which showed no material improvement in discharge. When first seen by Dr. Alderton there was a pin-point perforation, with slight bulging and thick pus. Dr. Alderton advised a cross-cut incision, and, if no improvement, a mastoid operation. The general health continued good, but the discharge did not let up, and at the next visit by the patient an operation was advised and was accepted. The operation showed the tip full of pus. An uneventful recovery followed.

DR. ALDERTON reported a second case of a girl, where the operation showed the

Outer Table Involuted So That the Mastosquamosal Suture Was Present.

Only the antrum was diseased. There was a well-defined line of healthy bone between the diseased areas.

DR. DENCH reported a case of a girl, who suffered from a

Swelling in Front of the Zygoma.

The drum membrane was of normal luster and showed only slight bulging and slight sinking of the canal wall. Membrane incised, found normal. Two days later swelling was opened. The usual mastoid operation then was performed, showing well-established evidences of disease.

INDEX OF AUTHORS.

INDEX OF TITLES.